Neuronal Signaling

Neuronal Signaling

Editor: Christian Manning

AMERICAN
MEDICAL PUBLISHERS
www.americanmedicalpublishers.com

AMERICAN
MEDICAL PUBLISHERS
www.americanmedicalpublishers.com

Cataloging-in-Publication Data

Neuronal signaling / edited by Christian Manning.
p. cm.
Includes bibliographical references and index.
ISBN 979-8-88740-314-4
1. Neural transmission. 2. Neurotransmitter receptors. 3. Neurons.
4. Neuroglia. I. Manning, Christian.
QP364.5 .N48 2023
599.018 8--dc23

American Medical Publishers,
41 Flatbush Avenue,
1st Floor, New York,
NY 11217, USA

ISBN 979-8-88740-314-4 (Hardback)

Contents

Preface

The cells within the brain and the nervous system, which are responsible for receiving sensory information from the outside world and sending motor commands to the muscles, are known as neurons. They comprise of a cell body, an axon and dendrites. The process of signaling between the neurons is both electrical and chemical in nature. Neurons are electrically excitable and can communicate with other cells through connections known as synapses. There are also voltage gradients across their membranes. These allow them to generate an electrochemical pulse if the voltage changes significantly over a short interval. These electrochemical pulses are known as action potential. They are broadly categorized into sodium-based action potentials and calcium-based action potentials. This book contains some path-breaking studies in the field of neurology and neuroscience. It is a valuable compilation of topics, ranging from the basic to the most complex researches on neuronal signaling. This book will serve as a reference to a broad spectrum of readers.

This book is a comprehensive compilation of works of different researchers from varied parts of the world. It includes valuable experiences of the researchers with the sole objective of providing the readers (learners) with a proper knowledge of the concerned field. This book will be beneficial in evoking inspiration and enhancing the knowledge of the interested readers.

In the end, I would like to extend my heartiest thanks to the authors who worked with great determination on their chapters. I also appreciate the publisher's support in the course of the book. I would also like to deeply acknowledge my family who stood by me as a source of inspiration during the project.

Editor

1

Function of P2X4 Receptors is Directly Modulated by a 1:1 Stoichiometric Interaction With 5-HT$_3$A Receptors

*Paola Soto, Pablo S. Gaete, Christian Fuentes, Benjamin Lozano, Pamela A. Naulin, Xavier F. Figueroa and Nelson Patricio Barrera**

Department of Physiology, Faculty of Biological Sciences, Pontificia Universidad Católica de Chile, Santiago, Chile

Correspondence:
Nelson P. Barrera
nbarrera@bio.puc.cl

Interacting receptors at the neuronal plasma membrane represent an additional regulatory mode for intracellular transduction pathways. P2X4 receptor triggers fast neurotransmission responses *via* a transient increase in intracellular Ca^{2+} levels. It has been proposed that the P2X4 receptor interacts with the 5-HT$_3$A receptor in hippocampal neurons, but their binding stoichiometry and the role of P2X4 receptor activation by ATP on this crosstalking system remains unknown. *Via* pull-down assays, total internal reflection fluorescence (TIRF) microscopy measurements of the receptors colocalization and expression at the plasma membrane, and atomic force microscopy (AFM) imaging, we have demonstrated that P2X4/5-HT$_3$A receptor complexes can interact with each other in a 1:1 stoichiometric manner that is preserved after ATP binding. Also, macromolecular docking followed by 100 ns molecular dynamics (MD) simulations suggested that the interaction energy of the P2X4 receptor with 5-HT$_3$A receptor is similar at the *holo* and the *apo* state of the P2X4 receptor, and the interacting 5-HT$_3$A receptor decreased the ATP binding energy of P2X4 receptor. Finally, the P2X4 receptor-dependent Ca^{2+} mobilization is inhibited by the 5-HT$_3$A interacting receptor. Altogether, these findings provide novel molecular insights into the allosteric regulation of P2X4/5-HT$_3$A receptor complex in lipid bilayers of living cells *via* stoichiometric association, rather than accumulation or unspecific clustering of complexes.

Keywords: receptor-receptor interaction, atomic force microscopy, stoichiometry, P2X4 receptor, 5-HT$_3$A receptor, intracellular Ca^{2+}, ATP

INTRODUCTION

Receptor-receptor interaction has been an extensive research area with enormous implications in neuronal crosstalking transduction mechanisms, which usually provide new molecular ways to tune and regulate the receptor function (Barrera et al., 2005b; Ferre et al., 2007). Ionotropic receptors located at the central nervous system, such as those belonging to the cys loop family, have been found to form macromolecular complexes composed by two or more different receptors (Ferre et al., 2007). In particular, P2X2 and 5-HT_3A receptors are co-expressed at the plasma membrane and physically interact with each other in myenteric neurons and heterologous systems. This interaction depends on the second intracellular loop of the 5-HT3A subunit and an unknown region of the P2X2 receptor that was initially thought to be the C-term tail (Boué-Grabot et al., 2003). As a functional consequence, the inhibition of the additive responses attained with serotonin and ATP was observed. Similar receptor-receptor interactions and inhibitory crosstalking have been observed between P2X and nicotinic acetylcholine (nACh) receptors (Barajas-López et al., 1998) and between P2X and GABA receptors (Jo et al., 2011). Recently, Emerit et al. (2016) showed that the 5-HT_3A receptor can colocalize with the P2X4 receptor at the plasma membrane of hippocampal neurons. Nevertheless, it remains unknown the stoichiometry of these interacting receptors, whether the interaction is controlled by the agonist binding and the functional role of this regulatory mechanism.

P2X4 receptor is also regulated by direct interactions with phospholipids. In this context, phosphoinositides PI(4,5)P2 (PIP_2) and PI(3,4,5)P3 (PIP_3) can modulate P2X4 activity, apparently, by direct interactions with the proximal C-terminal domain of the receptor (C360–V375), which was shown to be required for the development of full receptor function, since depletion of PIP_2 and PIP_3 dramatically inhibits the P2X4-mediated Ca^{2+} signal activated by ATP (Bernier et al., 2008). Therefore, as it has been proposed that 5-HT_3A receptor may interact with the C-term tail of P2X receptors (e.g., P2X2 receptor), the potential interaction between this receptor and P2X4 receptor may also represent a relevant control mechanism of the phospholipids-mediated P2X4 regulation.

A variety of methods have been continuously developed to tackle the molecular architecture of interacting membrane proteins, from high resolution, such as x-ray crystallography, to complementary biophysical approaches, including cryo-electron microscopy, mass spectrometry and atomic force microscopy (AFM). Based on the surface scanning of the sample, AFM has already been used to characterize the molecular architecture of individual P2X and 5-HT3 receptors (Barrera et al., 2005a,c, 2007; Antonio et al., 2011), among others.

Herein, *via* pull-down assay of interacting receptors, AFM imaging, macromolecular docking, molecular dynamics (MD) simulations, and total internal reflection fluorescence (TIRF) microscopy analysis, we propose that P2X4 receptor physically interacts in a 1:1 stoichiometric manner with 5-HT_3A receptor, which is maintained after ATP binding. By measurements of intracellular Ca^{2+} levels, we further confirmed that the interacting 5-HT_3A receptor inhibits the response to ATP of the P2X4 receptor. Altogether, these findings provide insights into the inhibitory responses triggered *via* stoichiometric binding of interacting receptors, which consequently support the notion that interacting receptors in specific numbers rather than receptor aggregation are involved in crosstalking neuronal responses.

MATERIALS AND METHODS

Expression of P2X4/5-HT_3A Receptor Complexes on tsA201 Cells

tsA201 cells (Sigma–Aldrich, St. Louis, MO, USA. Cat. # 96121229-1VL) were grown in DMEM medium (Gibco, Grand Island, NY, USA), supplemented with 10% fetal bovine serum (FBS, Gibco, Grand Island, NY, USA), 100 unit/ml penicillin (Sigma–Aldrich, St. Louis, MO, USA) and 100 μg/ml streptomycin (Sigma–Aldrich, St. Louis, MO, USA). Cells were maintained at 37°C in a humidified 5% CO_2–95% air atmosphere incubator. To induce the expression of P2X4 and 5-HT_3A receptors, tsA201 cells with a confluence of 40–60% were transfected with the pDNAs of P2X4 and 5-HT_3A receptors using polyethyleneimine (PEI, Sigma–Aldrich, St. Louis, MO, USA) as transfection reagent. Briefly, 10 ml of DMEM without serum were mixed with 275 μl of 1 mg/ml PEI alone (mock transfection) or plus pDNAs for P2X4 and/or 5-HT_3A (25 μg each) and left for 15 min at room temperature. Then, cells were incubated with this mixture for 24 h at 37°C. For transfection, the following constructs were used; rat P2X4 (*Rattus norvegicus*, GenBank: U47031.1) with a C-terminal hemagglutinin (HA) tag and human 5-HT_3A (*Homo sapiens*, GenBank: AK304630.1) with a C-terminal MYC/His-6 epitope tag, subcloned into the vector pcDNA3.1 (Invitrogen). Immunofluorescence analysis and Ca^{2+} measurements were performed using cells seeded onto sterile glass coverslips.

Measurements of Intracellular Ca^{2+} Levels

Ca^{2+} measurements were performed using the fluorescent Ca^{2+} indicator, Fluo 4, as described recently by Lillo et al. (2018). To upload Fluo 4, cells were incubated with 5 μM Fluo 4-AM for 45 min in a MOPS-buffered solution (composition in mM: 118 NaCl; 5.4 KCl; 2.5 $CaCl_2$; 1.2 KH_2PO_4; 1.2 $MgSO_4$; 11.1 glucose and 5 MOPS) adjusted to pH 7.4. The fluorescent indicator was washed out and the experiments started after 15 min of equilibration. Cells were visualized using an Olympus BX50 WI microscope and the fluorescent signal was recorded using an intensified CCD camera (Retiga Fast 1394, QImaging) and IPLab software. Images were acquired every 2 s at basal conditions and during 2 min of stimulation. Changes in intracellular Ca^{2+} levels were expressed as the variations of the fluorescence intensity along the time (F/F_0), where F is the fluorescence detected during the recording and F_0 is the basal fluorescence, or the maximum net fluorescence observed after stimulation ($\Delta F/F_0$). Three concentrations of ATP (1, 10 and 100 μM) were tested and, to confirm the activation of P2X4 receptors, 30 μM PPADS was preincubated during 15 min before the ATP application. Both reagents were poured over the cultured cells.

Confocal and Epifluorescence Microscopy

Cells were fixed with 1% formaldehyde and then washed with PBS solution (composition in mM: 136.9 NaCl; 2.68 KCl;

10.44 NaH_2PO_4; 1.76 KH_2PO_4) adjusted to pH 7.4. Nonspecific protein binding sites were blocked with PBS containing 0.1% FBS. Cells were incubated overnight with an anti-MYC monoclonal antibody to detect 5-HT_3A receptor (1:250, Thermo Fisher Scientific, Cat. # PA1-981, Rockford, IL, USA) and an anti-HA monoclonal antibody to label P2X4 receptor (1:250 Thermo Fisher Scientific, Cat. # 26183, Rockford, IL, USA). Cells were washed three times for 10 min with PBS and then incubated for 1 h with a secondary antibody conjugated to Alexa Fluor® 555 for anti-MYC (1:500, Cat. #A-21424, Molecular Probes, Eugene, OR, USA) or Alexa Fluor® 488 for anti-HA (1:500, Cat. # A-11029, Molecular Probes, Eugene, OR, USA). Then, cells were washed and mounted with Fluoromount-G (Electron Microscopy Sciences, Cat. # 17984-25, Hatfield, PA, USA). The fluorescent signal was examined using either an Olympus IX81 confocal inverted microscope coupled with an ORCA R2 Hamamatsu CCD camera or an Olympus BX41 WI microscope coupled with a Jenoptik ProgRes C5 CCD camera. As a negative control, primary antibodies were omitted.

TIRF Microscopy

TIRF microscopy imaging was performed using a NIKON Eclipse Ti2-E microscope with the module NIKON H-TIRF with a 100X magnification and up to 100 nm sample depth. Sample preparation was similar to the confocal experiments except for using PBS as mounting protocol and secondary antibodies conjugated to Alexa Fluor® 555 and Alexa Fluor® 488 to identify anti-HA and anti-MYC primary antibodies, respectively.

Quantification of P2X4 Receptor Expression and Colocalization of P2X4/5-HT_3A Receptor Complexes

Fluorescence intensity of P2X4 receptor expression attained by TIRF and epi microscopies were quantified using the ImageJ software (Schneider et al., 2012). Window and level parameters were optimized to select the Regions of Interest (ROIs) and exclude background noise. Fluorescence intensity was measured as the mean intensity of each ROI in raw images ± SE. For the colocalization analysis of P2X4/5-HT_3A receptor complexes, coloc2 plug-in implemented in ImageJ allowed to evaluate the correlation between the pixel's intensity on each channel *via* Pearson's R coefficient. Note that protein colocalization and expression experiments were performed using the same instrumental acquisition parameters such as light intensity and exposure time for all the images.

Purification of P2X4/5-HT_3A Receptor Complexes

Cells (five flasks of 150 cm^2 for each condition) were washed with HBS solution (composition in mM: 50 HEPES; 100 NaCl; 2 EDTA) adjusted to pH 7.6, and then, removed by shaking. Cells were collected in falcon tubes and centrifuged at 6,500 g at 4°C for 5 min. The pellet was resuspended in a solubilization solution (9 ml, composition in mM: 10 Tris-HCl; 100 NaCl; 5 EDTA, adjusted to pH 7.6), 1% Triton X-100 (Sigma–Aldrich, Cat. # 9002-93-1), a protease inhibitor mixture (complete, EDTA-Free, Roche) and 10 μl PMSF. The sample was incubated on a rotating wheel for 1 h at 4°C. The supernatant was placed in a Beckman centrifuge tube and subjected to ultracentrifugation at 50,000 *g* at 4°C for 1 h. The supernatant, corresponding to the positive control for the plasma membrane protein and named MEMBRANE fraction in Western blot analysis, was mixed with pre-washed anti-HA agarose beads (Thermo Fisher Scientific) and incubated for 3 h at 4°C. Beads were washed with 10 ml washing buffer (solubilization buffer containing 1% w/v Triton X-100) and centrifuged at 6,500 *g* three times. One last washing step was performed including a solution of 0.1% CHAPS (3-[(3-Cholamidopropyl)dimethylammonio]-1-propanesulfonate; Cat. # 220201, Calbiochem). Finally, proteins were eluted from beads by incubating them with 200 μl of 0.1% CHAPS plus 6 μl HA peptide (Thermo Fisher Scientific). An identical purification protocol was followed when tsA201 cells were expressing only P2X4 receptors. The ELUTION fraction (200 μl), representing the purified receptor or complex, was stored to perform Western blot analysis and AFM imaging. Five independent purification series were performed for the complex. Note that 100 μM ATP was applied in the eluted sample in solution during 30 min at room temperature, before protein adsorption (50 μl) onto mica.

When P2X4/5-HT_3A receptor complexes were pulled down *via* His6 tag, the purification procedure was similar to that used with the HA tag, except that in this case HisPur Ni-NTA agarose beads were used (Thermo Fisher Scientific) to carry out the extraction of His6 tagged proteins. Later, beads bound to the 5-HT_3A-MYC/His6 receptors were deposited in purification columns (Cat. # 450015, Invitrogen), and 200 mM imidazole was used for elution. An identical protocol was followed in tsA201 cells expressing only 5-HT_3A receptors. Five independent purification series were performed for each receptor.

Western Blot Analysis

Purified proteins were separated by 10% SDS-PAGE and transferred onto a nitrocellulose membrane (BioRad, CA, USA). Primary antibodies: anti-MYC (1:500, Thermo Fisher Scientific, Cat. # PA1-981, Rockford, IL, USA), or anti-HA (1:500 Thermo Fisher Scientific, Cat. # 26183, Rockford, IL, USA) were incubated overnight in a PBS solution containing 4% milk at 4°C. HRP-labeled secondary antibodies (1:1,000, Cat. # 621040, Molecular Probes, Eugene, OR, USA) were incubated at room temperature for 1 h in a PBS solution containing 4% milk. The SuperSignal® West Femto chemiluminescent substrate (Thermo Fisher Scientific) was used to detect protein bands. Molecular mass was estimated with prestained markers (Bio-Rad Laboratories, Hercules, CA, USA). The MyECL™ Imager (Thermo Fisher Scientific) was used to reveal the membrane.

AFM Imaging

Purified protein samples (50 μl from eluted samples) were placed on muscovite micas (Electron Microscopy Sciences, Cat. # 71855-01, Hatfield, PA, USA) to be adsorbed. After incubation for 15 min at room temperature, the mica was washed with Milli-Q water and dried with nitrogen gas. Images of dry samples were acquired in an AFM (MFP-3D-SA Asylum Research, CA, USA) using the intermittent contact mode. Cantilever was used with a drive frequency of ~300 kHz and a spring constant of 40 N/m.

The force applied to obtain the images was kept as low as possible. The target amplitude was ~0.5 V and amplitude setpoint ~0.4 V. Each image (4 μm^2) was obtained in 15 min and 50 images were analyzed. The molecular volumes of the adsorbed receptor and complex particles were determined from the height and radius of the particle obtained by AFM (Barrera et al., 2008). The molecular volume was calculated from the equation:

$$Vm = (\pi h/6)(3r^2 + h^2) \quad (1)$$

where h is the height of the particle and r is the radius at half the height. The equation considers the protein molecule as a sphere. Histograms of molecular volumes were fit by Gaussian distribution.

To calculate the individual receptor or complex concentration for the analyzed samples, the following equation was used:

$$M = \frac{\text{total mica area } (\mu m^2) \times \text{particle number per scanning area } (\frac{particle}{\mu m^2}) \times 10^6 (\frac{\mu l}{L})}{\text{elution volume in mica } (\mu l) \times \text{Avogadro Number } (\frac{particle}{mol})} \quad (2)$$

where M represents the molarity of the purified particle sample obtained from AFM imaging. For P2X4 receptors, 5-HT$_3$A receptors and P2X4/5-HT$_3$A receptor complexes, molecular volume cut-offs corresponding to their peaks were 403 and 431 (Antonio et al., 2011), 726 and 788 (Barrera et al., 2005a), and 991 and 1209 (**Figure 3**), respectively. Calculated values are derived from five independent purification processes for each sample, where all the samples were adsorbed in the same mica type surface during 15 min.

Molecular Docking and Molecular Dynamics Simulations of the P2X4/5-HT$_3$A Receptor Complex

The amino acid sequence of rat P2X4 subunit was obtained from UNIPROT (entry P51577) and aligned against the sequence of the zebrafish crystallized structures of P2X4 receptor (Hattori and Gouaux, 2012; PDB codes 4DW0 for the *apo* structure and 4DW1 for the *holo*-structure) by using MultAlin (Corpet, 1988). One hundred homology models for the *apo* and *holo*-structures were generated by using Modeller 9.18 (Webb and Sali, 2017) and the one having lowest DOPE score for each case was selected and verified by using the web servers MolProbity (Chen et al., 2010) and ProSA (Wiederstein and Sippl, 2007) to evaluate both stereochemical and energetics of each model. From the two final models, N and C-term tails were cut from MET 1 to VAL 28 and from LEU 358 to GLU 388, respectively.

The amino acid sequence of the human 5-HT3A subunit was obtained from UNIPROT (entry P46098) and aligned against the sequence of mouse 5-HT$_3$A receptor structure (Basak et al., 2018; PDB code 6BE1). One hundred homology models for the *apo* structures were generated by using Modeller 9.18 (Webb and Sali, 2017) and the one having the lowest DOPE were selected and verified by using the web servers MolProbity and ProSA to evaluate both stereochemical and energetics. From the final model, the N-term tail was cut from MET 1 to THR 30 and the intracellular loop consisting from CYS 356 to ALA 411 was cut as well.

Docking of ATP into the P2X4 receptor was performed in AutoDock (Morris et al., 2008). Binding pockets had volumes of 22.5 × 22.5 × 22.5 Å^3 and the center of each box was placed as the ligand is seen in the crystal structure. The 100 best conformations were saved and grouped in clusters of root mean square displacement (RMSD) less than 2 Å. Selected dockings for each binding pocket had a negative binding energy and a similar spatial orientation as the crystallized bound ATP.

Due to pentameric and trimeric symmetry of both 5-HT$_3$A and P2X4 receptors, respectively (Hattori and Gouaux, 2012; Basak et al., 2018), there are several possible combinations depending upon their interaction surface. However, we used two experimental evidence to take an appropriate orientation for the receptor complex: (1) choosing the minimal distance between both receptors at the second intracellular loop of the 5-HT$_3$A receptor, which has been postulated as a domain involved in the physical P2X2/5-HT$_3$A receptor interaction (Emerit et al., 2016); and (2) rotating, in the perpendicular plane of the bilayer, all possible conformations of the complex until the largest interaction surface was found since it has been shown that bigger interaction surfaces are more energetically favorable between macromolecular complexes (Casuso et al., 2012). To have a similar comparison between the two dockings, the P2X4 receptor *apo* structure was aligned to the first resulting docking of the P2X4 *holo*/5-HT$_3$A receptor complex.

The homology model of the P2X4 receptor in its *holo* state was combined with three ATP molecules in their binding pocket. Later both *apo* and *holo*-structures in the designed position were merged with the structure of the 5-HT$_3$A receptor and were protonated accordingly to the physiological pH. Both complexes were inserted in a pre-equilibrated POPC bilayer (of size 204 × 124 Å^2) created using the Visual Molecular Dynamics suite (VMD; Humphrey et al., 1996). To do this, both the bilayer and the receptor complex were aligned and all overlapped lipids (nearer than 0.8 Å) and water molecules (nearer than 3 Å) were deleted. The complex of receptor-bilayer was solvated by using the TIP3 water model and NaCl was added to both neutralize and provide a physiological concentration of salt. Simulations were performed using NAMD 2.12 with the temperature at 310 K and pressure at 1 atm with periodic boundary conditions (PBC). The first step was to minimize the energy by simulating 10,000 steps in the NVT ensemble, and then, the NPT ensemble was simulated. One hundred ns MD simulations for both P2X4 *apo*/5-HT$_3$A and P2X4 *holo*/5-HT$_3$A receptor complexes were carried out, which correspond to a similar simulation time already applied in our group to study allosteric regulation of P2X4 receptor by ivermectin (Latapiat et al., 2017). To maintain temperature and pressure constant, Langevin dynamics and Nosé–Hoover Langevin piston methods were used for temperature and pressure coupling. To calculate electrostatic interactions, Ewald sums were used with a grid density of 1 Å. Ligand parameterization (ATP) was done using the SwissParam webserver (Zoete et al., 2011) and the CHARMM27 forcefield was used for lipids and protein. Electrostatic and van der Waals interactions between both receptors (or between P2X4 receptor and ATP molecules) within 12 Å cut off, corresponding to the total interaction energy, were measured by using VMD plugin "NAMDEnergy" every 40 ps during the simulation.

Reagents

MOPS, ATP and all chemicals of analytical grade were obtained from Sigma–Aldrich (St. Louis, MO, USA). Fluo 4-AM was purchased in Life Technologies (Eugene, OR, USA) and pyridoxalphosphate-6-azophenol-2′,4′ disulfonic acid (PPADS) in Tocris Bioscience (Ellisville, MO, USA). ATP and PPADS were dissolved in water. Fluo 4-AM was dissolved in DMSO.

Statistical Analysis

Values are represented as means ± SE. Comparisons between groups were made using unpaired student's *t*-test or 1-way ANOVA plus Newman–Keuls *post hoc* test, as appropriate. A value of $p < 0.05$ was considered significant.

RESULTS

First, the P2X4 receptor function in transfected tsA201 cells was evaluated by measuring the changes in free intracellular Ca^{2+} concentration observed in response to ATP application. Stimulation with 100 μM ATP evoked a Ca^{2+} signal that showed two components: a first fast-transient component that peaked at ~12 s and decreased thereafter, and a second slow component that starts after ~60 s (**Figures 1A,B**). In tsA201 cells co-transfected with P2X4 and 5-HT$_3$A receptors, the transient increase in intracellular Ca^{2+} was blunted (**Figure 1B**) whereas the time course of the second component was similar to that observed in P2X4 transfected cells. Although the Ca^{2+} response was evaluated at a range of ATP concentrations (1–100 μM), the most striking difference in the initial Ca^{2+} signaling (first 60 s) between cells transfected with P2X4 receptor alone or co-transfected with P2X4 and 5-HT$_3$A receptors was attained with 100 μM ATP (**Figure 1C**). As expected, the intracellular Ca^{2+} concentration was not affected by ATP in non-transfected cells (mock, **Figures 1B,C**). Consistent with the activation of P2X4 receptors, the response induced by ATP was almost completely blocked (~85%) by 15 min pre-incubation with the preferential P2X receptor antagonist PPADS (**Figure 1D**; Lê et al., 1998). Interestingly, the response of co-transfected cells was inhibited by PPADS in the same proportion to that observed in cells transfected with P2X4 alone. As PPADS blocks access to the orthosteric ATP-binding pocket (Huo et al., 2018), these results suggest that the Ca^{2+} influx *via* transfected P2X4 receptors is inhibited by the presence of 5-HT$_3$A receptors without interfering with the ATP binding site through direct steric interaction or *via* a downstream effect.

To test whether or not both P2X4 and 5-HT$_3$A receptors interact with each other, tsA201 cells co-expressing P2X4 and 5-HT$_3$A receptors were identified by confocal, TIRF and epifluorescence analysis using anti-HA and anti-MYC antibodies. As shown in **Figures 2A–C**, confocal imaging revealed that both receptors colocalize in the same cell at the plasma and intracellular membranes. Then, the colocalization of P2X4 and 5-HT$_3$A receptor complexes at the plasma membrane was quantified using TIRF microscopy (**Figures 2D–F**) analysis, which showed a significant colocalization Pearson R index of 0.88 ± 0.09 (**Figure 2G**).

To evaluate a potential direct interaction, P2X4 or 5-HT$_3$A receptors were purified with HA or Ni^{2+} bound agarose beads from tsA201 cells expressing only one type of receptor. The success and specificity of the purification process was confirmed by Western blot analysis against HA or MYC tag epitopes for P2X4 or 5-HT$_3$A receptors, respectively (**Figures 2J,L**). Electrophoretic migration for each subunit (55 kDa for 5-HT$_3$A and 70 kDa for P2X4) reached a similar molecular weight of that previously published (Barrera et al., 2005a) for 5-HT$_3$A (55kDa) and slightly larger of that reported (Antonio et al., 2011) for P2X4 (65kDa). The difference observed in the electrophoretic migration of P2X4 subunit could correspond to a bigger glycosylation state, which is a posttranslational modification commonly observed for P2X receptors (Barrera et al., 2005c; Ormond et al., 2006; Antonio et al., 2011), since, according to its primary sequence, P2X4 subunit should have a molecular weight of 43.5 kDa. Once both P2X4 and 5-HT$_3$A receptors were co-expressed in tsA201 cells, the purification process was based on pull-down experiments targeting the HA tag epitope in the P2X4 receptor. As a negative control, 5-HT$_3$A receptors expressed alone were not detected in pull-down experiments using the HA-based purification protocol (data not shown). Western blot analysis demonstrated the presence of the P2X4 receptor in the eluted samples, but also a band corresponding to the 5-HT3A subunit was detected by anti-MYC antibody binding, demonstrating that both P2X4 and 5-HT$_3$A receptors interact each other in cells co-expressing both receptors (**Figure 2K**). A similar finding was observed after pulling down the complex by targeting the His6 tag epitope in the 5-HT$_3$A receptor, where a band corresponding to the P2X4 subunit was detected by anti-HA antibody binding (**Figure 2M**). To analyze the stoichiometry of the interaction, complexes formed by interacting P2X4/5-HT$_3$A receptors were recorded by AFM imaging (**Figures 3A–D**). The molecular volumes of the purified samples showed 2 peaks at 489 ± 24 nm^3 and 1100 ± 109 nm^3, which are consistent with the detection of P2X4 alone (417 nm^3; Antonio et al., 2011) and a P2X4/5-HT$_3$A receptor complex with a stoichiometry 1:1; this is 417 nm^3 and 757 nm^3 (Barrera et al., 2005a; **Figure 3B**). After stimulation of the purified sample with 100 μM ATP in solution before adsorption onto mica for AFM imaging, the proportion of the complex marginally increased from 42% to 51% (area under the double Gaussian curve fit, cut off 800 nm^3) with no change on the peak values (505 ± 15 nm^3 and 1236 ± 62 nm^3; $p > 0.05$; **Figure 3D**). All the peaks at histograms were derived from non-linear Gaussian distributions and were elected those that presented the best fits, R^2 values corresponding to 0.9307 and 0.9126 for the P2X4/5-HT$_3$A receptor complexes in the absence and presence of ATP, respectively.

To determine the protein concentration of the purified samples obtained from cells transfected with P2X4 or P2X4/5-HT$_3$A receptor complexes, we used the number of protein particles adsorbed into mica, as an indicator of the concentration

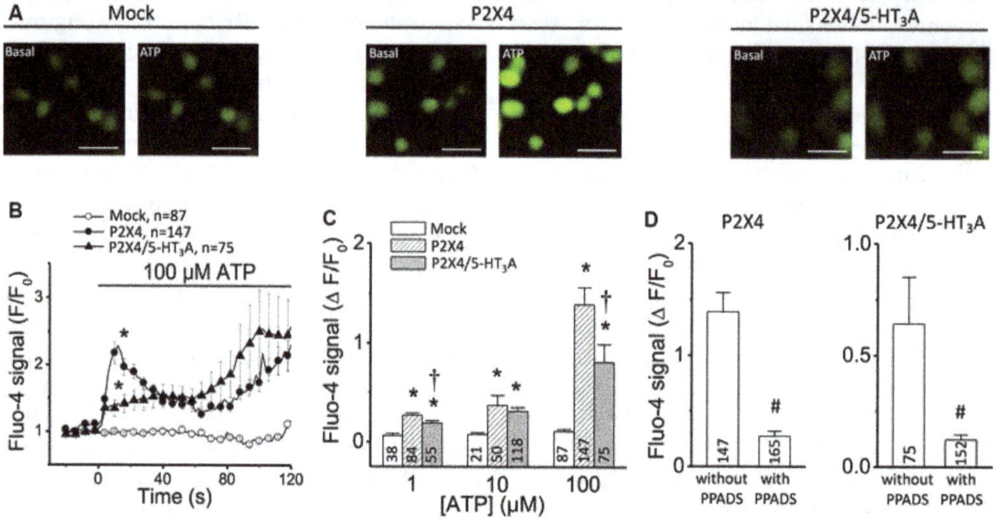

FIGURE 1 | Ca^{2+} measurements in tsA201 cells expressing P2X4 receptor alone or P2X4/5-HT_3A receptor complexes. **(A)** Representative images of Ca^{2+} measurements in mock-transfected cells, cells transfected with P2X4 receptor alone and cells co-transfected with P2X4 plus 5-HT_3A receptors. Changes in intracellular Ca^{2+} concentration were detected using the Ca^{2+} indicator Fluo-4. Images were captured before (Basal) and 20 s after the addition of 100 μM ATP. Scale bars represent 30 μm. **(B)** Time course of Fluo-4 fluorescence signal in cells stimulated with 100 μM ATP. The horizontal bar indicates the stimulation period. **(C)** Analysis of the maximum increase in intracellular Ca^{2+} levels observed after stimulation with 1–100 μM ATP. **(D)** Analysis of the maximum increase in intracellular Ca^{2+} levels observed in cells transfected with P2X4 receptor alone (left) or co-transfected with P2X4 and 5-HT_3A receptors (right) after application of 100 μM ATP in the absence or presence of 30 μM PPADS, an inhibitor of P2X receptors. Three independent Ca^{2+} measurements were carried out for each condition from different batches of cells. Numbers inside bars indicate the number of cells analyzed. Values are the mean ± SE. $^{*}p < 0.05$ vs. Mock by 1-way ANOVA plus Newman–Keuls *post hoc* test; $^{\dagger}p < 0.05$ vs. P2X4 by 1-way ANOVA plus Newman–Keuls *post hoc* test; $^{\#}p < 0.05$ vs. without PPADS by unpaired student's *t*-test.

determined by the Avogadro Number relationship (equation 2). This analysis showed that P2X4 receptors from single transfected cells and P2X4/5-HT_3A receptor complexes from cotransfected cells had a similar concentration of 3.3 ± 0.6 pM and 3.7 ± 1.3 pM ($p > 0.05$), respectively. However, AFM imaging of purified samples from cotransfected cells also presented an abundant peak at approximately the volume of individual P2X4 receptors, which suggests that pulling down the HA-tagged protein (P2X4 receptor) from the plasma membrane purified the complexes as well as P2X4 receptors alone and, therefore, increased the overall P2X4 expression at the plasma membrane. This correlates well with the TIRF microscopy analysis, where the P2X4 receptor expression in the cotransfected tsA201 cells was approximately two-fold higher than that observed on single transfected cells (**Figure 2H**). Interestingly, according to the analysis of epifluorescence imaging, the total cellular P2X4 receptor expression in tsA201 cells was similar in single and cotransfection experiments (**Figure 2I**), indicating a cellular redistribution of P2X4 receptors depending upon the presence of 5-HT_3A receptors.

To calculate interaction energy between P2X4 and 5-HT_3A receptors, macromolecular dockings for the interacting receptors were followed by 100 ns MD simulations, considering domains involved in the physical crosstalking between P2X and 5-HT_3 receptors (Boué-Grabot et al., 2003; Emerit et al., 2016), and the larger interaction energy between membrane protein complexes observed through larger subunit interfaces (Casuso et al., 2012; **Figures 3E,F**). Total interaction energy (van der Waals and electrostatic energies) of P2X4 receptor at the *apo* state with 5-HT_3A receptor was −301 ± 9 kcal/mol (mean ± SE; **Figure 3E**), which was not statistically different ($p > 0.05$) from that observed with P2X4 receptor at *holo* state (−278 ± 12 kcal/mol; **Figure 3F**). Also, the binding interaction energy of 3 ATP molecules to P2X4 receptor *holo* (−310 ± 12 kcal/mol) was significantly larger than that observed in the presence of interacting 5-HT_3A receptor (−168 ± 3 kcal/mol, $p < 0.05$), suggesting that the inhibitory effect of 5-HT_3A receptor could be allosteric, reducing the ATP affinity of the P2X4 receptor.

DISCUSSION

The P2X4 receptor activation by ATP binding triggered an initial transient increase in intracellular Ca^{2+} level that was followed by a slow component, where only the transient increase was strongly inhibited by the 5-HT_3A receptor, which could correlate well with a reduced Ca^{2+} influx through P2X receptors. Our data brings a novel outcome for the P2X4/5-HT_3A receptor complex interaction. A functional cross-inhibition has been demonstrated between P2X2 and 5-HT_3A receptors (Boué-Grabot et al., 2003), but that study was based on simultaneous activation of the receptors by parallel stimulation with ATP and 5-HT. This current report demonstrates that the mere presence of the 5-HT_3A interacting receptor in the complex, independent of its agonist, is sufficient to inhibit the P2X4 receptor. A similar inhibitory response has been observed for the mGlu5a

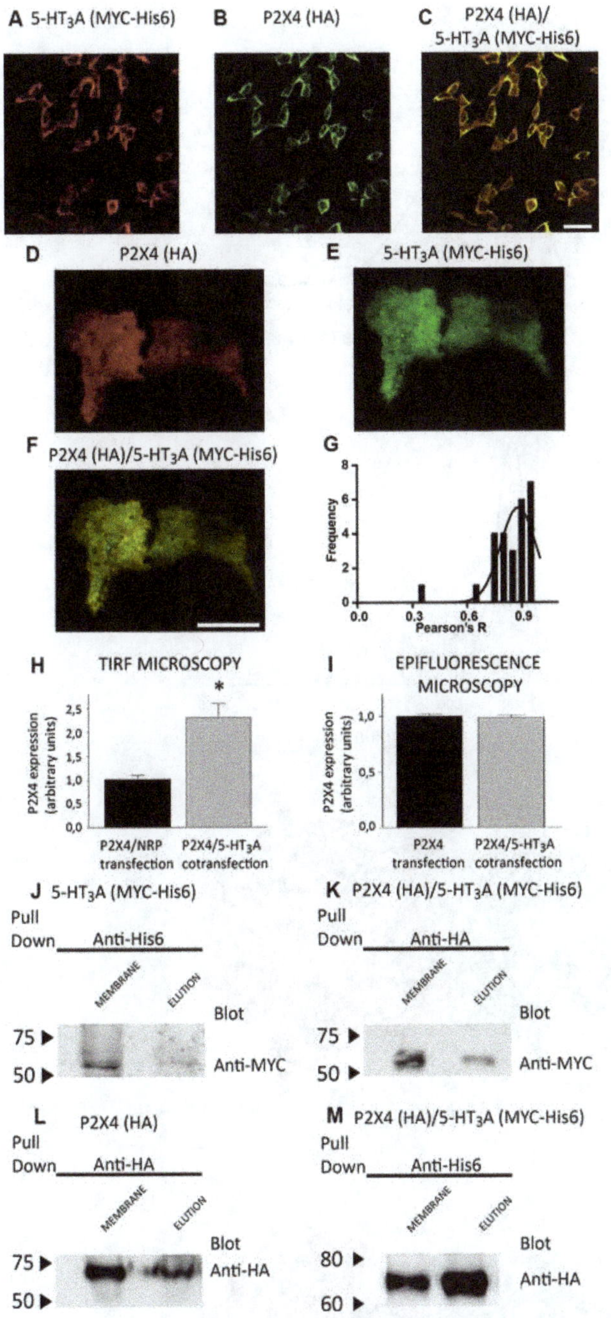

FIGURE 2 | Expression and purification of P2X4/5-HT_3A receptor complexes. **(A,B)** Detection of co-expressed 5-HT_3A **(A)** and P2X4 **(B)** receptors by confocal immunofluorescence in tsA201 cells *via* anti-MYC (1:250) and anti-HA (1:250) antibodies, followed by their corresponding secondary antibodies conjugated to Alexa Fluor® 555 and Alexa Fluor® 488, respectively. The merge of panels **(A,B)** is shown in **(C)**, where scale bar represents 30 μm. **(D,E)** Analysis by total internal reflection fluorescence (TIRF) microscopy of co-expressed P2X4 **(D)** and 5-HT_3A **(E)** receptors individually and merge images **(F)** in tsA201 cells *via* anti-HA (1:250) and anti-MYC (1:250) antibodies, followed by their corresponding secondary antibodies conjugated to Alexa Fluor® 555 and Alexa Fluor® 488, respectively. Scale bar in **(F)** represents 3 μm. **(G)** Colocalization analysis of the P2X4/5-HT_3A receptor complexes in tsA201 cells (n = 26 from two

(Continued)

FIGURE 2 | Continued

independent experiments). **(H,I)** P2X4 receptor expression analysis in tsA201 cells through TIRF (**H**, n = 26 for P2X4/NRP and P2X4/5-HT_3A transfections from two independent experiments) and epifluorescence (**I**, n = 273 for P2X4 and 254 for P2X4/5-HT_3A transfections from two independent experiments) measurements. Non-related plasmid (NRP) corresponds to pDNA IRES-GFP (0.5 μg each well) used in the same amount as the other receptor plasmids. Data are shown as mean ± SE. $^*p < 0.05$ vs. P2X4/NRP expression by unpaired t-test. **(J,L)** Western blot analysis of the purified samples from tsA201 cells expressing only 5-HT_3A **(J)** or P2X4 **(L)** receptors identified by anti-MYC or anti-HA antibodies, respectively. Specific bands in plasma membrane enriched fraction (MEMBRANE) and purified (ELUTION) samples were observed at 55 kDa **(J)** for 5-HT3A and 70 kDa **(L)** for P2X4 subunits. **(K,M)** Western blot analysis of purified samples from tsA201 cells co-expressing 5-HT_3A and P2X4 receptors after pulling down the complexes with either the HA-tag purification **(K)** or His6-tag purification **(M)** method. Bands corresponding to 5-HT3A (anti-MYC antibody; **K**) and P2X4 subunits (anti-HA antibody; **M**) were detected at similar molecular weights compared to those present after single transfection. Arrowheads indicate molecular mass markers in kDa.

receptor agonist-independent effect on the NMDA receptor (Perroy et al., 2008). Nevertheless, it remains to be determined whether the activation of the 5-HT_3A receptor can further inhibit the P2X4 receptor-dependent ATP response or the P2X4 receptor *apo* could be able to inhibit the activated 5-HT_3A receptor, which would enlighten the whole mechanistic scenario of these ionotropic receptors' interaction.

Our data are consistent with the notion that P2X4/5-HT_3A receptor interaction results in an allosteric inhibition of ATP-induced P2X4 activation. To further support this proposal, we performed additional experiments to reach the saturation of the concentration-response curve elicited by ATP in cells transfected with P2X4 receptor alone or co-transfected with P2X4 and 5-HT_3A receptors. However, stimulation with 1 mM ATP induced an increase in intracellular Ca^{2+} concentration in non-transfected cells (mock cells), which precluded the direct comparison of the response observed at different ATP concentrations (data not shown), and then, the analysis of the Emax and EC50 observed in response to ATP, as required to confirm the presence of an allosteric interaction of 5-HT_3A receptors with P2X4 receptors.

An alternative explanation to the inhibitory action of 5-HT_3A receptors on the P2X4 receptor-triggered Ca^{2+} increase would be a reduction of the expression of P2X4 receptors at the plasma membrane in cotransfected cells. Conversely, we found a similar total expression of the P2X4 receptor between transfected tsA201 cells containing P2X4 and P2X4/5-HT3A subunits. Furthermore, the expression of P2X4 receptors specifically at the plasma membrane, revealed by TIRF microscopy analysis, indicated a two-fold increase of the purinergic receptor in cotransfected cells. Interestingly, a redistribution of P2X4 receptor from intracellular locations to the cell surface without changing total cellular expression has been demonstrated after activation of the C-C chemokine receptor type 2 in microglial cells, which is mediated by delivery of lysosomal P2X4 receptor to the plasma membrane (Toyomitsu et al., 2012). Besides, the P2X4 receptor has been shown to colocalize with the 5-HT_3A receptor at the cell surface of

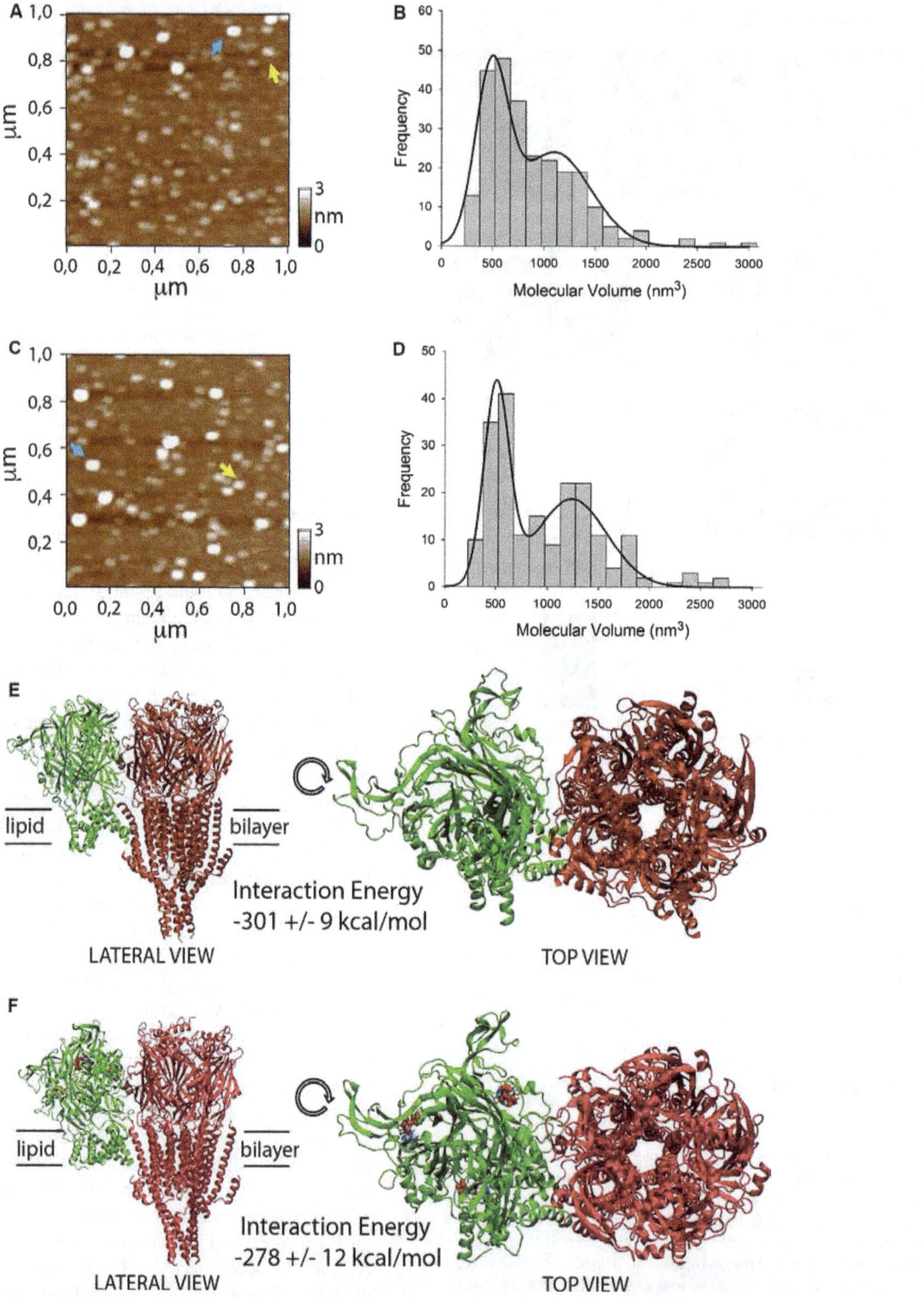

FIGURE 3 | Stoichiometry and interaction energy on P2X4/5-HT_3A receptor complexes. **(A–D)** Atomic force microscopy (AFM) imaging of purified P2X4/5-HT_3A receptor complexes in the absence **(A,B)** and presence **(C,D)** of 100 μM ATP. Yellow and blue arrows indicate molecular volumes of 493 nm^3 and 1,194 nm^3 **(A)** and 486 nm^3 and 1,125 nm^3 **(C)**. Histogram of molecular volumes of particles fitted by double Gaussian peaks in the absence **(B)** and presence **(D)** of 100 μM ATP. **(E)** Molecular docking of the complex formed between P2X4 receptor *apo* (green) and 5-HT_3A receptor (red). **(F)** Molecular docking of the complex formed between P2X4 receptor *holo* (green) and 5-HT_3A receptor (red). ATP molecules are depicted as colored blobs. Interaction energy values for both complexes are indicated as mean ± SE after 100 ns molecular dynamics (MD) simulations.

hippocampal neurons when its internalization motif is replaced by a FLAG epitope (Emerit et al., 2016). Our results have shown that this mutation is not needed for a significant plasma membrane expression of both receptors; however, it has yet to be determined whether the physical interaction between P2X4 and 5-HT$_3$A receptors is enough to trigger the protein trafficking or requires intracellular signaling pathway. Remarkably, the expression pattern of purified P2X4/5-HT$_3$A receptor complexes vs. the P2X4 receptor alone, revealed by AFM imaging, resembles relatively well to that observed on the plasma membrane in living cells. Almost half of the particles of the purified samples from tsA201 cells coexpressing P2X4 and 5-HT$_3$A receptors correspond to the assembled complex and present an identical concentration to that from cells expressing only P2X4 receptors. If we consider the other half of particles that match the molecular volume of free P2X4 receptors, then the total purinergic receptor should increase almost twice, reinforcing our notion that the purification process is highly enriched in the plasma membrane fraction.

Our AFM results demonstrate for the first time that the P2X4/5-HT$_3$A receptor complex is formed with a stoichiometry 1:1, which is maintained by the presence of the P2X4 receptor agonist. To propose a molecular way for the allosteric inhibition of 5-HT$_3$A receptor on P2X4 receptor function, we embarked on testing a docking between both receptors, considering the postulated domains for physical crosstalking (Boué-Grabot et al., 2003; Emerit et al., 2016), and interfaces with larger surfaces that maintain a trimeric/pentameric symmetry, which has been already postulated as variables energetically favorable for interacting macromolecules (Casuso et al., 2012). After 100 ns MD simulations, no differences in interaction energy between the P2X4 receptor *apo* or P2X4 receptor *holo* complexed with 5-HT$_3$A receptors were found. Also, the presence of the interacting 5-HT$_3$A receptor decreased the ATP binding interaction energy of ATP molecules to the P2X4 receptor, which is consistent with a negative allosteric effect of 5-HT$_3$A receptors that preserves the 1:1 stoichiometric interaction between both receptors. Nevertheless, further bioinformatic analysis should be performed to corroborate these findings, in particular, to explore extensively other receptor-receptor surface dockings *via*, for example, coarse-grained approaches, which would result in the same or additional conformations of the receptor complex.

Crosstalking mechanisms lead to more complex neuronal signaling by providing additional regulatory roles of agonists and receptors. Taken together, we have shown here that the P2X4 receptor is inhibited by a physical interaction with the 5-HT$_3$A receptor in a 1:1 stoichiometry and ATP maintains this complex. As 5-HT$_3$A receptor can interact with other P2X receptors subtypes such as P2X2 and P2X3 (Emerit et al., 2016), it remains to be solved if the same stoichiometry and steric mechanism participate in the functional regulation of these receptors. Furthermore, as P2X4 receptors can be modulated by membrane phosphoinositides (Bernier et al., 2008), it could be further explored whether or not the 5-HT$_3$A receptor and phospholipids can coexist to control the P2X4 receptor function *via* modifications of the stoichiometric binding.

AUTHOR CONTRIBUTIONS

PS performed AFM experiments and data analysis, immunofluorescence and western blot experiments. PG performed Ca^{2+} measurements and helped writing the article. CF performed homology modeling, molecular docking, and data analysis. BL performed western blot and TIRF experiments, followed by a quantitative analysis of immunofluorescence images. PN performed western blot and TIRF experiments. XF supervised Ca^{2+} measurements and helped writing the article. NB designed and supervised the investigation, analyzed the data and wrote the article.

FUNDING

Millennium Scientific Initiative ICM P10-035F, Newton Picarte PCI-DPI Conicyt grant 20140080 and FONDECYT grant 1181326 funded NB. FONDECYT grants 1150530 and 3160348 funded XF and PG, respectively. PS holds a PhD scholarship from Pontificia Universidad Católica de Chile. CF holds an MSc scholarship from CONICYT. This work was supported in part by the Advanced Microscopy Facility UMA-UC.

ACKNOWLEDGMENTS

To Prof. Michael Edwardson (University of Cambridge, UK) for providing the P2X4 and 5-HT$_3$A receptor constructs and scientific feedback on the experimental design, analysis, and procedure.

REFERENCES

Antonio, L. S., Stewart, A. P., Xu, X. J., Varanda, W. A., Murrell-Lagnado, R. D., and Edwardson, J. M. (2011). P2X4 receptors interact with both P2X2 and P2X7 receptors in the form of homotrimers. *Br. J. Pharmacol.* 163, 1069–1077. doi: 10.1111/j.1476-5381.2011.01303.x

Barrera, N. P., Ge, H., Henderson, R. M., Fitzgerald, W. J., and Edwardson, J. M. (2008). Automated analysis of the architecture of receptors, imaged by atomic force microscopy. *Micron* 39, 101–110. doi: 10.1016/j.micron.2006.12.006

Barrera, N. P., Henderson, R. M., Murrell-Lagnado, R. D., and Edwardson, J. M. (2007). The stoichiometry of $P2X_{2/6}$ receptor heteromers depends on relative subunit expression levels. *Biophys. J.* 93, 505–512. doi: 10.1529/biophysj.106.101048

Barrera, N. P., Herbert, P., Henderson, R. M., Martin, I. L., and Edwardson, J. M. (2005a). Atomic force microscopy reveals the stoichiometry and subunit arrangement of 5-HT3 receptors. *Proc. Natl. Acad. Sci. U S A* 102, 12595–12600. doi: 10.1073/pnas.0503253102

Barrera, N. P., Morales, B., Torres, S., and Villalon, M. (2005b). Principles: mechanisms and modeling of synergism in cellular responses. *Trends Pharmacol. Sci.* 26, 526–532. doi: 10.1016/j.tips.2005.08.003

Barrera, N. P., Ormond, S. J., Henderson, R. M., Murrell-Lagnado, R. D., and Edwardson, J. M. (2005c). Atomic force microscopy imaging demonstrates that

$P2X_2$ receptors are trimers but that $P2X_6$ receptor subunits do not oligomerize. *J. Biol. Chem.* 280, 10759–10765. doi: 10.1074/jbc.m412265200

Basak, S., Gicheru, Y., Samanta, A., Molugu, S. K., Huang, W., Fuente, M., et al. (2018). Cryo-EM structure of 5-HT3A receptor in its resting conformation. *Nat. Commun.* 9:514. doi: 10.1038/s41467-018-02997-4

Bernier, L. P., Ase, A. R., Chevallier, S., Blais, D., Zhao, Q., Boué-Grabot, E., et al. (2008). Phosphoinositides regulate P2X4 ATP-gated channels through direct interactions. *J. Neurosci.* 28, 12938–12945. doi: 10.1523/JNEUROSCI.3038-08.2008

Barajas-López, C., Espinosa-Luna, R., and Zhu, Y. (1998). Functional interactions between nicotinic and P2X channels in short-term cultures of guinea-pig submucosal neurons. *J. Physiol.* 513, 671–683. doi: 10.1111/j.1469-7793.1998.671ba.x

Boué-Grabot, E., Barajas-López, C., Chakfe, Y., Blais, D., Bélanger, D., Emerit, M. B., et al. (2003). Intracellular cross talk and physical interaction between two classes of neurotransmitter-gated channels. *J. Neurosci.* 23, 1246–1253. doi: 10.1523/JNEUROSCI.23-04-01246.2003

Casuso, I., Khao, J., Chami, M., Paul-Gilloteaux, P., Husain, M., Duneau, J. P., et al. (2012). Characterization of the motion of membrane proteins using high-speed atomic force microscopy. *Nat. Nanotechnol.* 7, 525–529. doi: 10.1038/nnano.2012.109

Chen, V. B., Arendall, W. B. III., Headd, J. J., Keedy, D. A., Immormino, R. M., Kapral, G. J., et al. (2010). MolProbity: all-atom structure validation for macromolecular crystallography. *Acta Crystallogr. D Biol. Crystallogr.* 66, 12–21. doi: 10.1107/S0907444909042073

Corpet, F. (1988). Multiple sequence alignment with hierarchical clustering. *Nucleic Acids Res.* 16, 10881–10890. doi: 10.1093/nar/16.22.10881

Emerit, M. B., Baranowski, C., Diaz, J., Martinez, A., Areias, J., Alterio, J., et al. (2016). A new mechanism of receptor targeting by interaction between two classes of ligand-gated ion channels. *J. Neurosci.* 36, 1456–1470. doi: 10.1523/JNEUROSCI.2390-15.2016

Ferre, S., Ciruela, F., Woods, A. S., Lluis, C., and Franco, R. (2007). Functional relevance of neurotransmitter receptor heteromers in the central nervous system. *Trends Neurosci.* 30, 440–446. doi: 10.1016/j.tins.2007.07.001

Hattori, M., and Gouaux, E. (2012). Molecular mechanism of ATP binding and ion channel activation in P2X receptors. *Nature* 485, 207–212. doi: 10.1038/nature11010

Humphrey, W., Dalke, A., and Schulten, K. (1996). VMD: visual molecular dynamics. *J. Mol. Graph.* 14, 33–38, 27–38. doi: 10.1016/0263-7855(96)00018-5

Huo, H., Fryatt, A. G., Farmer, L. K., Schmid, R., and Evans, R. J. (2018). Mapping the binding site of the P2X receptor antagonist PPADS reveals the importance of orthosteric site charge and the cysteine-rich head region. *J. Biol. Chem.* 293, 12820–12831. doi: 10.1074/jbc.ra118.003737

Jo, Y. H., Donier, E., Martinez, A., Garret, M., Toulme, E., and Boue-Grabot, E. (2011). Cross-talk between P2X4 and γ-aminobutyric acid, type A receptors determines synaptic efficacy at a central synapse. *J. Biol. Chem.* 286, 19993–20004. doi: 10.1074/jbc.m111.231324

Latapiat, V., Rodríguez, F. E., Godoy, F., Montenegro, F. A., Barrera, N. P., and Huidobro-Toro, J. P. (2017). P2X4 receptor *in silico* and electrophysiological approaches reveal insights of ivermectin and zinc allosteric modulation. *Front. Pharmacol.* 8:918. doi: 10.3389/fphar.2017.00918

Lê, K. T., Babinski, K., and Séguéla, P. (1998). Central P2X4 and P2X6 channel subunits coassemble into a novel heteromeric ATP receptor. *J. Neurosci.* 18, 7152–7159. doi: 10.1523/JNEUROSCI.18-18-07152.1998

Lillo, M. A., Gaete, P. S., Puebla, M., Ardiles, N. M., Poblete, I., Becerra, A., et al. (2018). Critical contribution of Na^{+}-Ca^{2+} exchanger to the Ca^{2+}-mediated vasodilation activated in endothelial cells of resistance arteries. *FASEB J.* 32, 2137–2147. doi: 10.1096/fj.201700365rr

Morris, G. M., Huey, R., and Olson, A. J. (2008). Using AutoDock for ligand-receptor docking. *Curr. Protoc. Bioinformatics* 24, 8:8.14.1–8.14.40. doi: 10.1002/0471250953.bi0814s24

Ormond, S. J., Barrera, N. P., Qureshi, O. S., Henderson, R. M., Edwardson, J. M., and Murrell-Lagnado, R. D. (2006). An uncharged region within the N terminus of the $P2X_6$ receptor inhibits its assembly and exit from the endoplasmic reticulum. *Mol. Pharmacol.* 69, 1692–1700. doi: 10.1124/mol.105.020404

Perroy, J., Raynaud, F., Homburger, V., Rousset, M. C., Telley, L., Bockaert, J., et al. (2008). Direct interaction enables cross-talk between ionotropic and group I metabotropic glutamate receptors. *J. Biol. Chem.* 283, 6799–6805. doi: 10.1074/jbc.M705661200

Schneider, C. A., Rasband, W. S., and Eliceiri, K. W. (2012). NIH Image to ImageJ: 25 years of image analysis. *Nat. Methods* 9, 671–675. doi: 10.1038/nmeth.2089

Toyomitsu, E., Tsuda, M., Yamashita, T., Tozaki-Saitoh, H., Tanaka, Y., and Inoue, K. (2012). CCL2 promotes P2X4 receptor trafficking to the cell surface of microglia. *Purinergic Signal.* 8, 301–310. doi: 10.1007/s11302-011-9288-x

Webb, B., and Sali, A. (2017). Protein structure modeling with MODELLER. *Methods Mol. Biol.* 1654, 39–54. doi: 10.1007/978-1-4939-7231-9_4

Wiederstein, M., and Sippl, M. J. (2007). ProSA-web: interactive web service for the recognition of errors in three-dimensional structures of proteins. *Nucleic Acids Res.* 35, W407–W410. doi: 10.1093/nar/gkm290

Zoete, V., Cuendet, M. A., Grosdidier, A., and Michielin, O. (2011). SwissParam: a fast force field generation tool for small organic molecules. *J. Comput. Chem.* 32, 2359–2368. doi: 10.1002/jcc.21816

2

Estradiol-Mediated Axogenesis of Hypothalamic Neurons Requires ERK1/2 and Ryanodine Receptors-Dependent Intracellular Ca^{2+} Rise in Male Rats

*Lucas E. Cabrera Zapata[1], Mariana Bollo[1] and María Julia Cambiasso[1,2]**

[1]Instituto de Investigación Médica Mercedes y Martín Ferreyra, INIMEC-CONICET, Universidad Nacional de Córdoba, Córdoba, Argentina, [2]Cátedra de Biología Celular, Facultad de Odontología, Universidad Nacional de Córdoba, Córdoba, Argentina

***Correspondence:**
María Julia Cambiasso
jcambiasso@immf.uncor.edu

17β-estradiol (E2) induces axonal growth through extracellular signal-regulated kinase 1 and 2 (ERK1/2)-MAPK cascade in hypothalamic neurons of male rat embryos *in vitro*, but the mechanism that initiates these events is poorly understood. This study reports the intracellular Ca^{2+} increase that participates in the activation of ERK1/2 and axogenesis induced by E2. Hypothalamic neuron cultures were established from 16-day-old male rat embryos and fed with astroglia-conditioned media for 48 h. E2-induced ERK phosphorylation was completely abolished by a ryanodine receptor (RyR) inhibitor (ryanodine) and partially attenuated by an L-type voltage-gated Ca^{2+} channel (L-VGCC) blocker (nifedipine), an inositol-1,4,5-trisphosphate receptor (IP_3R) inhibitor (2-APB), and a phospholipase C (PLC) inhibitor (U-73122). We also conducted Ca^{2+} imaging recording using primary cultured neurons. The results show that E2 rapidly induces an increase in cytosolic Ca^{2+}, which often occurs in repetitive Ca^{2+} oscillations. This response was not observed in the absence of extracellular Ca^{2+} or with inhibitory ryanodine and was markedly reduced by nifedipine. E2-induced axonal growth was completely inhibited by ryanodine. In summary, the results suggest that Ca^{2+} mobilization from extracellular space as well as from the endoplasmic reticulum is necessary for E2-induced ERK1/2 activation and axogenesis. Understanding the mechanisms of brain estrogenic actions might contribute to develop novel estrogen-based therapies for neurodegenerative diseases.

Keywords: hypothalamic neurons, axogenesis, estradiol, ERK1/2, Ca^{2+} signaling, ryanodine receptors

INTRODUCTION

For many years, estrogens have been recognized as one of the main orchestrators of the sexual differentiation of the brain, acting during critical periods of development to organize neural circuits in a way that determines the modulatory/activational effects of gonadal hormones in adulthood. Testosterone secreted by male rodent testes during development is aromatized in neurons to 17β-estradiol (E2), which displays multiple cellular processes that finally set the masculine phenotype (McCarthy, 2008; Wright et al., 2010). More recently, accumulating evidence indicates that E2 is not only a reproductive hormone but also a brain-derived neuroprotective factor, coordinating multiple signaling mechanisms that protect the brain from neurodegenerative diseases, affective disorders and cognitive decline (Arevalo et al., 2015). These beneficial actions in the brain have positioned estrogens as promising therapeutic compounds against different brain pathologies such as Parkinson and Alzheimer diseases, schizophrenia, multiple sclerosis, stroke, neuroinflammation, among others (Dye et al., 2012; Villa et al., 2016; McGregor et al., 2017; Giatti et al., 2018).

Classical estrogenic actions are mediated *via* intracellular estrogen receptors (ERs) that function as ligand-activated transcription factors to regulate the expression of estrogen-responsive genes. Additionally, estrogens generate a wide diversity of rapid "non-classical" effects, which occur in a range from some seconds to a few minutes *via* membrane-initiated mechanisms (Arevalo et al., 2012), including the triggering of Ca^{2+} signals (Beyer and Raab, 1998; Picotto et al., 1999; Wong et al., 2012), and the activation of several signaling pathways, such as phospholipase C (PLC)/inositol 1,4,5-trisphosphate (IP_3) and diacylglycerol (Le Mellay et al., 1997; Chaban et al., 2004), nitric oxide synthase/nitric oxide (Kelly and Levin, 2001), adenylate cyclase/AMPc/protein kinase A (PKA; Beyer and Karolczak, 2000), phosphoinositide-3 kinase (PI3K; Garcia-Segura et al., 2010), PKC, and extracellular signal-regulated kinase 1 and 2 (ERK1/2) cascades (Wu et al., 2005).

Currently, it is known that E2 prevents cell death, promotes neuronal survival, and enhances neuritogenesis and synaptic plasticity in the brain (Carroll and Pike, 2008; Spence et al., 2013; Acaz-Fonseca et al., 2014; Khan et al., 2015; Lai et al., 2017; Céspedes Rubio et al., 2018). The induction of neurite outgrowth by E2 was first demonstrated by Toran-Allerand (1976, 1980) and Toran-Allerand et al. (1983) working with organotypic explant cultures of the preoptic area, hypothalamus, and cerebral cortex. This neuritogenic effect of the hormone was then observed in other brain regions, both directly related and unrelated with reproduction (Nishizuka and Arai, 1981; Reisert et al., 1987; Cambiasso et al., 1995; Murphy and Segal, 1996). Hypothalamic neurons *in vitro* undergo several intermediate stages of development from unpolarized to fully polarized cells (Díaz et al., 1992). Most of the neuritogenic effects of E2 were demonstrated in polarized neurons (stage III of development), which are characterized by the presence of axon (Díaz et al., 1992; Cambiasso et al., 1995). Previous studies from our laboratory have shown that E2 induces axonal growth through ERK1/2 activation in hypothalamic neurons of male embryos *in vitro*. Both axogenesis (Cambiasso and Carrer, 2001) and ERK1/2 activation (Gorosito and Cambiasso, 2008) mediated by the hormone are dependent on a membrane-initiated mechanism since E2-bovine serum albumin (BSA; a membrane-impermeable conjugate of E2) was as effective as free E2. Interestingly, decreasing intracellular Ca^{2+} by the Ca^{2+}-chelator BAPTA-AM or blocking Ca^{2+}-dependent PKC isoforms by Ro 32-0432 significantly decreased these E2 effects (Gorosito and Cambiasso, 2008). These findings strongly suggested an important role for Ca^{2+} in E2-induced ERK1/2 pathway activation and axonal growth; however, the results did not provide the mechanism of E2-induced Ca^{2+} signaling in hypothalamic neurons.

In this study, we found that E2 evoked activation of Ca^{2+} entry *via* L-type voltage-gated Ca^{2+} channels (L-VGCCs) and promoted Ca^{2+} release through ryanodine receptors (RyRs). This early Ca^{2+} response underlies E2-induced ERK1/2 activation and axogenesis in hypothalamic neurons. Altogether, these results bring new insights about the mechanism of brain estrogenic actions and might contribute to developing novel estrogen-based therapies for neurodegenerative diseases.

MATERIALS AND METHODS

Animals and Cell Cultures

Embryos were obtained from pregnant Wistar rats at embryonic day 16 (E16). The day of vaginal plug was set as E0. Experimental procedures for handling and sacrificing animals were approved by the Animal Care and Use Committee at our institution (CICUAL-IMMF, INIMEC-CONICET-UNC; Córdoba, Argentina) and followed the NIH guidelines for care and use of laboratory animals. The minimum number of animals required was used for these experiments and suffering was minimized. Primary neuronal and astroglial cultures were prepared as previously described in Cambiasso et al. (2000). Pregnant rats were sacrificed by cervical dislocation under CO_2 anesthesia, and the fetuses were dissected from the uterus. The male fetuses used for cultures were identified by visualization of the spermatic artery on the developing testes. Ventromedial hypothalamic and mesencephalic regions were dissected out and stripped off the meninges for primary neuronal and glial cultures, respectively. At E16, the axogenic effect of E2 is contingent on the presence of astroglia (Cambiasso et al., 1995) or astroglia-conditioned media from a target region (Cambiasso et al., 2000; Cambiasso and Carrer, 2001; Brito et al., 2004). The basal medium (BM) was (1:1) DMEM:Ham's F12 Nutrient Mixture, supplemented with 0.043% l-alanyl-l-glutamine (GlutaMAX I), 0.15% glucose, 100 U/ml penicillin and 100 μg/ml streptomycin. All cultures were raised under phenol red-free conditions to avoid "estrogen-like effects" (Berthois et al., 1986). For neuronal cultures, the dissociated cell suspension was seeded on different supports pre-coated with 1 mg/ml poly-D-lysine depending on the experiment: 60 mm × 15 mm dishes (Corning Life Science, Tewksbury, MA, USA) for protein assays, 25 mm coverslips (Assistent, Germany) for Ca^{2+} imaging, and 12 mm coverslips (Assistent, Germany) for morphological studies.

Western Blot

Hypothalamic neurons derived from male fetuses plated 1–2 h before were fed with astroglia-conditioned media for 2 days *in vitro* (DIV). After a 2 h washout period using BM, neuronal cultures were treated for 1 h with nifedipine (2 μM; Sigma-Aldrich, St. Louis, MO, USA), inhibitory ryanodine (50 μM; Santa Cruz Biotechnology, Santa Cruz, CA, USA), 2-APB (100 μM; Santa Cruz Biotechnology, Santa Cruz, CA, USA) or U-73122 (10 μM; Sigma-Aldrich, St. Louis, MO, USA), and then pulsed with 100 nM E2 (Sigma-Aldrich, St. Louis, MO, USA) for 15 min. Hormone concentration used was determined by dose dependence (1–100 nM) experiments previously performed by our group (Gorosito and Cambiasso, 2008; Gorosito et al., 2008). ERK phosphorylation was maximally increased after the application of 100 nM E2. This dose was then used for all further acute stimulation studies. We have used compounds at final concentrations that did not alter cell viability or morphology in control conditions.

After treatment, hypothalamic neurons were washed and harvested at 4°C in RIPA buffer [150 mM NaCl, 0.1% NP40, 0.5% sodium deoxycholate, 0.1% sodium dodecyl sulfate (SDS), 50 mM Tris, pH 7.5] with protease and phosphatase inhibitors (1 μg/ml aprotinin, 1 μg/ml leupeptin, 1 μg/ml pepstatin A, 5 μg/ml chymostatin, 5 μg/ml antipain, 100 μg/ml PMSF, 50 μM NaF, 10 μM $Na_4P_2O_7$, and 1 mM $NaVO_4$). Protein samples (20 μg/lane) were separated by 10% SDS-PAGE and transferred onto polyvinylidene fluoride membrane (Bio-Rad, Hercules, CA, USA). ERK1/2 phosphorylation was detected by using a rabbit monoclonal anti-phospho-p44/42 MAPK (Cell Signaling Technology, Danvers, MA, USA), which specifically detects both Thr202 and Tyr204 ERK phosphorylation forms of ERK [molecular masses (kDa) for ERK1 and ERK2 are 44 and 42, respectively]. Total ERK1/2 was detected by using a mouse anti-p44/42 MAPK (Cell Signaling Technology, Danvers, MA, USA). Secondary antibodies conjugated to horseradish peroxidase (Jackson, West Grove, PA, USA) were used for the detection by enhanced chemiluminescence on X-ray film. After incubation with the antibody against phospho-ERK1/2, blots were stripped and then re-probed with anti-total ERK1/2 to ensure equal protein loading. The resulting film samples were scanned and analyzed with an image analysis program (ImageJ; NIH, Bethesda, MD, USA). Data are presented as a ratio of phospho-ERK1/2/total-ERK1/2 of 3–4 different experiments (independent cultures) performed in duplicate.

Ca^{2+} Imaging

After 2 DIV, hypothalamic neurons were treated (or not) with 50 μM ryanodine or 2 μM nifedipine for 1 h and incubated with 3 μM acetoxymethyl (AM) ester form of the organic Ca^{2+}-dye Cal-520 (AAT Bioquest, Sunnyvale, CA, USA) for 30 min at 37°C in a Ca^{2+}-containing HEPES buffered salt solution (Ca^{2+}-HBSS) composed of (mM): 135 NaCl, 5.4 KCl, 2 $CaCl_2$, 1 $MgCl_2$, 10 HEPES, and 10 glucose; pH = 7.4 set with NaOH at RT. Following loading, neurons were washed twice with warm Ca^{2+}-HBSS and were imaged in the same buffer. To analyze the participation of extracellular Ca^{2+}, the cells were resuspended in an EGTA-containing buffer composed of (mM): 135 NaCl, 5 KCl, 0.5 $CaCl_2$, 1.2 $MgCl_2$, 5 HEPES, 14 $NaHCO_3$, and 1 EGTA; pH = 7.4 set with NaOH at RT.

Imaging of cytosolic Ca^{2+} signals was performed using a 60× oil immersion objective of an Olympus IX81 inverted microscope [equipped with a Disk Spinning Unit (DSU), epifluorescence illumination (150 W Xenon Lamp), and a microprocessor], an ORCA AG (Hamamatsu) CCD camera and OSIS software. Frames were collected at a continuous rate of 2.5 per second during 5 min (790 frames). Cal-520 was excited at a wavelength of 492 nm, and emitted fluorescence was collected at 514 nm. E2 (100 nM) was added 30 s after starting the recording. 10 μM thapsigargin (tg) was added at 3 min of recording as a positive control of normal endoplasmic reticulum Ca^{2+} content. The fluorescence intensity of the Ca^{2+} indicator was analyzed using ImageJ (NIH, Bethesda, MD, USA) software and plotted as the change in fluorescence (ΔF) of 2 × 2 pixels divided by mean resting fluorescence [(Fo; ΔF/Fo)] over time. We measured both the peak fluorescence value and the integrated area under the ΔF/Fo curve with OriginPro 8 SR0 software (OriginLab Corporation, Northampton, MA, USA). The integrated area roughly corresponds to the total amount of Ca^{2+} released over the recording period.

Immunocytochemical Staining

To analyze the effect of ryanodine in E2-stimulated axon growth without affecting the normal polarization of neurons, we performed the experiment after 1 DIV (stage III of development). After 2 h in absence of E2, the cultures were treated for 1 h with 50 μM ryanodine before the addition of 10 nM E2 for an additional 24 h. The hormone concentration used to study the neuritogenic effect of E2 was chosen based on previous studies of our laboratory (Gorosito et al., 2008; Scerbo et al., 2014).

After 2 DIV, neuronal cultures were fixed for 20 min with warm 4% paraformaldehyde in PBS containing 0.12 M sucrose and rinsed in PBS. Neurons were immunocytochemically stained with antibodies against β-tubulin class III (SDL.3D10). The details of the immunocytochemical procedure were as specified by Díaz et al. (1992). Briefly, the fixed cells were permeabilized in 0.2% Triton X-100 for 5 min at RT, preincubated with 5% BSA, incubated in mouse anti-β-tubulin class III (Sigma-Aldrich, St. Louis, MO, USA), rinsed in PBS, and finally incubated with appropriate biotinylated secondary antibody. Incubation with secondary antibody was followed by washing in PBS, incubation for 2 h in VECTASTAIN ABC immunoperoxidase reagent (Vector Laboratories, Burlingame, CA, USA), and a final reaction with 1.4 mM 3,3'-diaminobenzidine in phosphate buffer with H_2O_2. Coverslips were then dehydrated with ethanol, cleared with xylene, and mounted on glass slides for morphometric analysis. No immunostaining was detected when primary antibodies were replaced by 5% BSA.

Morphometric Analysis

The morphometric analysis of stained neuronal cultures was performed on digitized video images using JAVA as an image processor (Jandel Inc., Richmond, CA, USA) controlled by a host computer. Images were acquired through an optic microscope (Carl Zeiss, Germany). Microscope slides were coded, and the person conducting the analysis was blind to the experimental group. All labeled cells that could be identified as one individual neuron were measured in random fields at 40× magnification. Neural processes were classified as minor processes or axons according to accepted morphological criteria (Dotti et al., 1988; Blanco et al., 1990; Díaz et al., 1992). Minor processes are two or three short neurites that emerge from the cell body; axons are much longer, unique, thin, and relatively uniform in diameter. Neurons were considered to have developed an axon

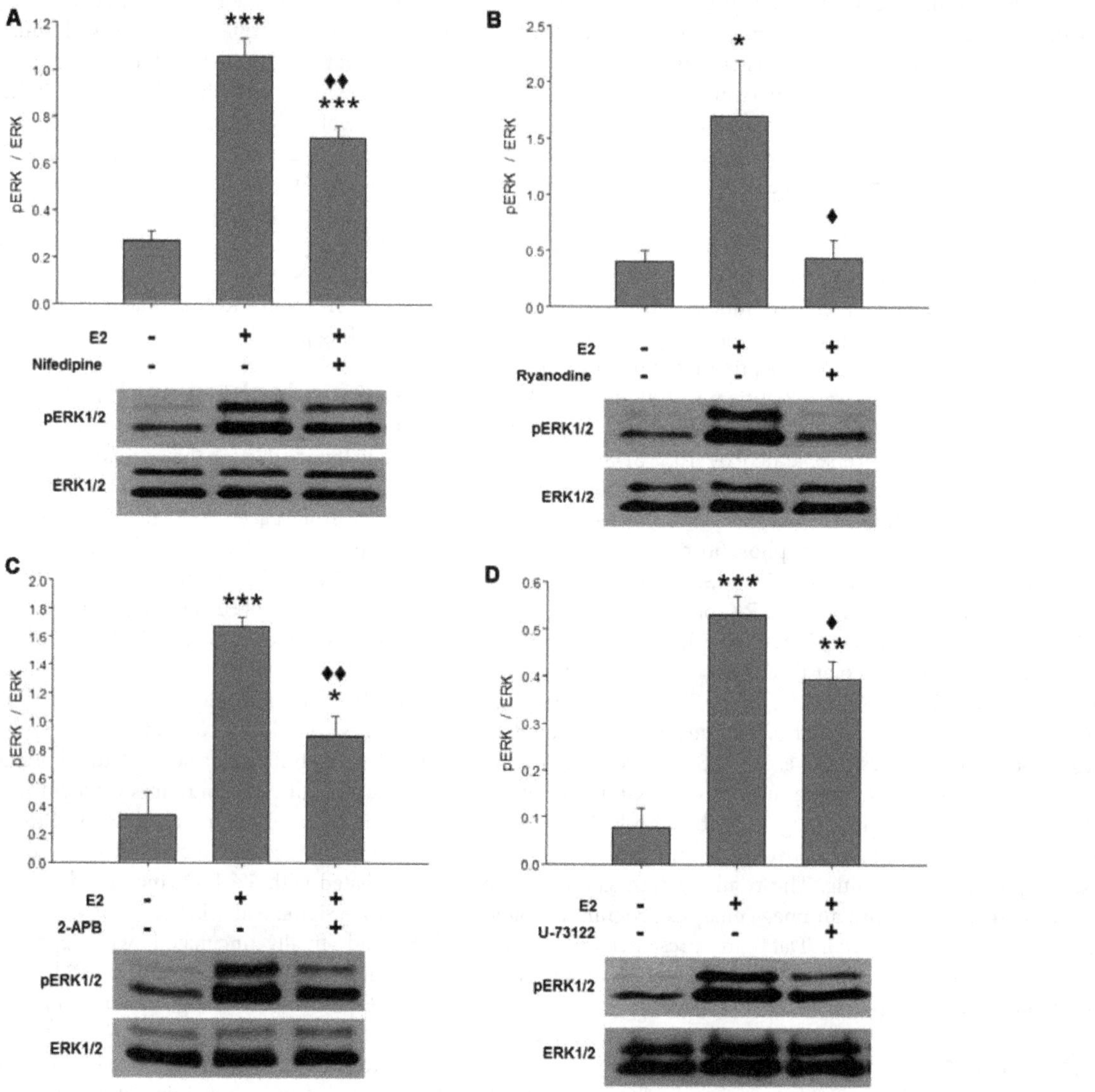

FIGURE 1 | E2-induced extracellular signal-regulated kinase 1 and 2 (ERK1/2) activation depends on cytosolic Ca^{2+} increase mainly mediated by ryanodine receptors (RyRs). Effects of **(A)** 2 μM nifedipine, **(B)** 50 μM ryanodine, **(C)** 100 μM 2-APB or **(D)** 10 μM U-73122 on E2-induced ERK phosphorylation. After washing for 2 h, the cultures were treated with the inhibitors for 1 h and were then pulsed for 15 min with 17β-estradiol (E2) and harvested for Western blotting. Top: ratio of readings for pERK/ERK bands in arbitrary densitometric units. Bottom: examples of immunoblots showing a decrease of hormone-induced ERK phosphorylation in cultures pretreated with the inhibitors. Molecular masses (kDa) for ERK1 and ERK2 are 44 and 42, respectively. Blots shown are representative of the mean ± SEM of 3–4 different cultures. **(A)** Nifedipine: ANOVA $F_{(2,10)} = 52.78$; $p \leq 0.001$. Least significant differences (LSDs) test indicated ***$p < 0.001$ vs. control and ♦♦$p < 0.01$ vs. E2. **(B)** Ryanodine: ANOVA $F_{(2,6)} = 5.856$; $p = 0.04$. LSDs test indicated *$p = 0.05$ vs. control and ♦$p = 0.05$ vs. E2. **(C)** 2-APB: ANOVA $F_{(2,6)} = 27.203$; $p \leq 0.001$. LSDs test indicated ***$p < 0.001$ and *$p = 0.05$ vs. control and ♦♦$p = 0.01$ vs. E2. **(D)** U-73122: ANOVA $F_{(2,6)} = 34.891$; $p \leq 0.001$. LSDs test indicated ***$p < 0.001$ and **$p = 0.01$ vs. control and ♦$p \leq 0.05$ vs. E2.

if they showed one neurite three to five times longer than the rest (stage III of development). Soma area, length of minor processes, total axonal length, and the number of neurites per cell were recorded. At least 60 neurons were measured for every experimental condition in each culture; at least three separate cultures were made for every condition.

Statistical Analysis

Data were statistically evaluated by one-way ANOVA, followed by Fisher's Least Significant Difference (LSD) *post hoc* test (Statistica; StatSoft Inc., Tulsa, OK, USA) where $p < 0.05$ was considered statistically significant.

RESULTS

E2-Induced ERK1/2 Activation Is Mainly Mediated by RyRs

Our previous results suggested that E2-induced ERK1/2 phosphorylation is Ca^{2+}-dependent. Here, we further

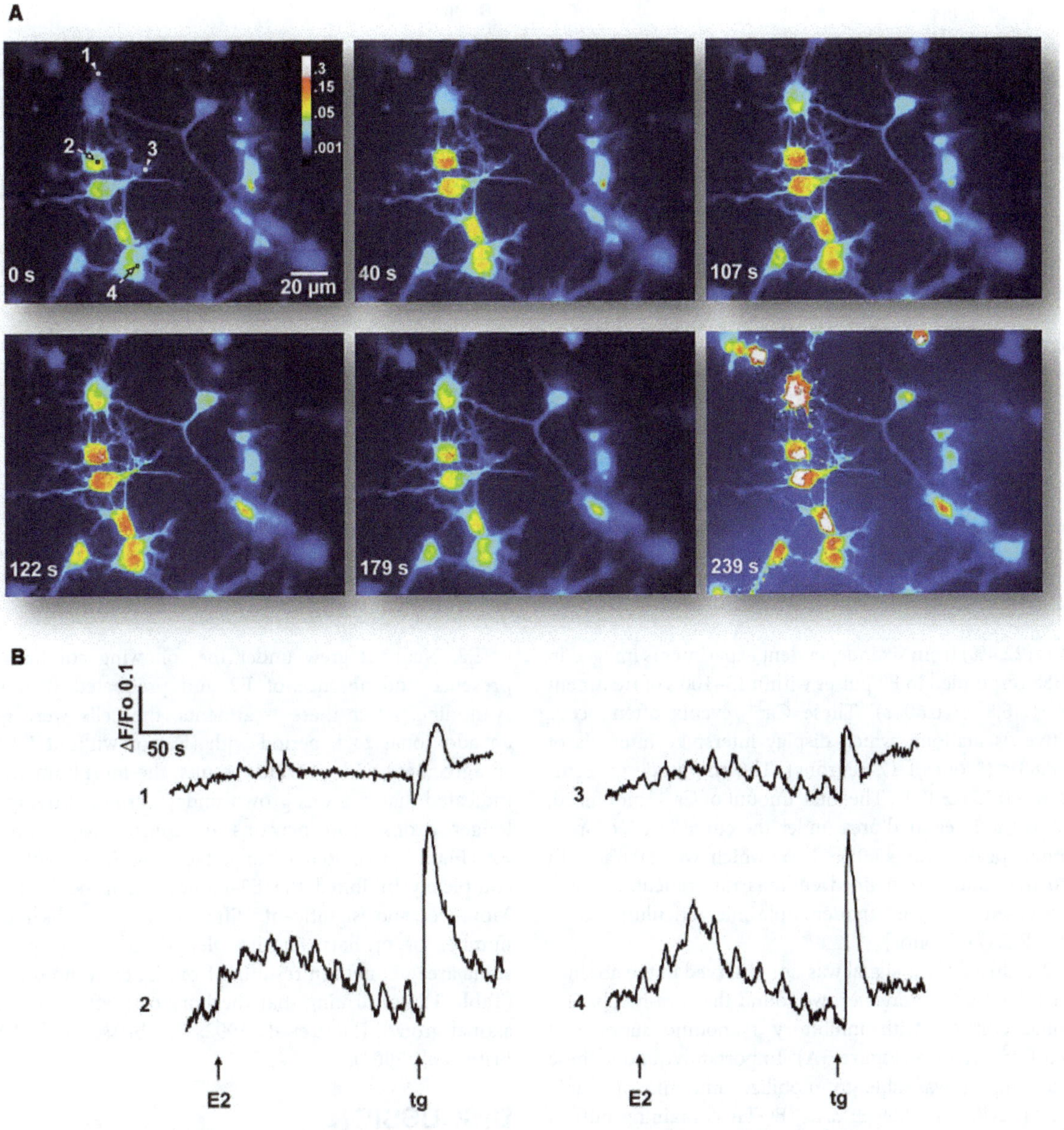

FIGURE 2 | 17β-estradiol (E2) induces Ca^{2+} oscillations. **(A)** Hypothalamic neurons were loaded with Cal-520 AM for 30 min at 37°C, maintained in a Ca^{2+}-containing buffer (Ca^{2+}-HBSS) and changes in cytosolic Ca^{2+} concentration were measured using confocal microscopy [Olympus IX81 inverted microscope equipped with a Disk Spinning Unit (DSU)]. Time series of Cal-520 pseudocolor images is shown, before and after the addition of E2 and thapsigargin (tg). Pseudocolor scale bar: 0.3–0.001 arbitrary units. Length scale bar: 20 μm. **(B)** Representative Ca^{2+} traces [regions of interest labeled 1–4 in **(A)**] plotted as changes over time in fluorescence intensity of the indicator (ΔF) respect to resting values (Fo). Arrows indicate the addition time of E2 (30 s) and tg (3 min). Data are from one representative experiment out of six independent experiments.

investigated the Ca^{2+} response involved in ERK activation mediated by E2. Hypothalamic cultures grown with E2 for 48 h were washed in BM for 2 h and pre-treated with specific compounds for 1 h before a pulse of E2 for 15 min. In agreement with previous reports, E2 induced a strong phosphorylation of ERK at 15 min (**Figure 1**). This effect was completely abolished by inhibitory ryanodine (**Figure 1B**) and partially attenuated by nifedipine (**Figure 1A**), IP_3R inhibitor 2-APB (**Figure 1C**), and a PLC inhibitor U-73122 (**Figure 1D**).

E2 Induces Rapid Ca^{2+} Increase Depending on Ca^{2+} Influx and RyRs

As E2-activation of the ERK1/2 signaling cascade depends on extracellular as well as intracellular Ca^{2+} stores, we decided to characterize the Ca^{2+} signal generated by the hormone. The addition of agonist to cell cultures, loaded with the indicator Cal-520 AM and imaged in a Ca^{2+}-containing buffer, induced fluorescence changes that were observed in neuronal soma as well as in minor processes (**Figure 2**). Seventeen out of

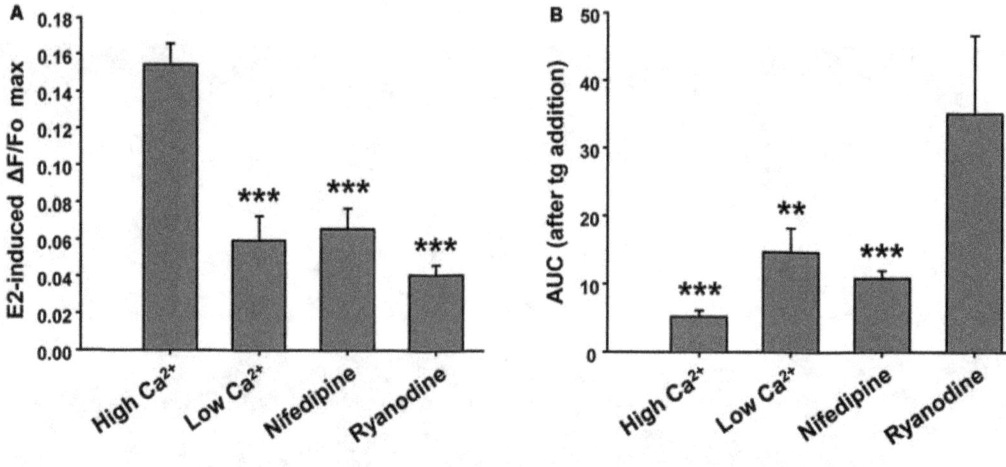

FIGURE 3 | Ryanodine, external Ca^{2+} and nifedipine modulate E2-induced Ca^{2+} increase. **(A)** Mean values of maximal ΔF/Fo for Ca^{2+} mobilized by 17β-estradiol (E2) in hypothalamic neurons recorded either in the presence or absence of extracellular Ca^{2+} (Ca^{2+}-HBSS/EGTA-containing buffer, named High Ca^{2+}/Low Ca^{2+}), or after a pre-incubation period (1 h) with ryanodine or nifedipine. ANOVA $F_{(3,41)} = 22.94$; $p \leq 0.001$. LSDs test indicated $^{***}p < 0.001$ vs. Ca^{2+}-HBSS. **(B)** Mean values of integrated area under ΔF/Fo curve (AUC) after thapsigargin (tg) addition during Ca^{2+} imaging [same conditions as **(A)**]. ANOVA $F_{(3,26)} = 9.18$; $p \leq 0.001$. LSDs test indicated $^{***}p < 0.001$ and $^{**}p = 0.01$ vs. ryanodine. Bars represent mean ± SEM; n = 4–6 different cultures.

76 neurons (22.4%) from six independent experiments imaged in Ca^{2+}-HBSS responded to E2 pulses within 15–100 s of treatment (average = 46.8 ± 6.60 s). These Ca^{2+} events often occur in repetitive oscillations, which display interspike intervals of 21.58 ± 8.83 s (9 out of 17 neurons). The amplitude in terms of ΔF/Fo was 0.154 ± 0.01. The total amount of Ca^{2+} mobilized, measured as the integrated area under the curve (AUC) for all E2-generated peaks, was 4.69 ± 1.03, which was 90.6% with respect to the control [remained endoplasmic reticulum Ca^{2+} content released by tg, a sarco/endoplasmic reticulum Ca^{2+}-ATPase (SERCA) inhibitor].

This E2-induced Ca^{2+} signal was not observed in the absence of extracellular Ca^{2+}. Moreover, we found that pre-incubation of neuronal cultures with inhibitory ryanodine suppressed E2-evoked Ca^{2+} release (**Figure 3A**). Importantly, under these conditions, the tg was able to mobilize amounts of Ca^{2+}, measured as AUC, of 14.69 ± 3.45 (EGTA-containing buffer) and 35.05 ± 11.54 (ryanodine pre-incubation), five and nine times greater, respectively, than the amounts of Ca^{2+} mobilized by tg in E2-induced control neurons (**Figure 3B**). Moreover, nifedipine reduced the E2-induced Ca^{2+} increase more than 50% (ΔF/Fo = 0.065 ± 0.011; and AUC = 10.779 ± 1.159, n = 4), which strongly suggests the participation of L-VGCCs in this signal (**Figures 3A,B**). Representative Ca^{2+} traces plotted as ΔF/Fo vs. time for EGTA, ryanodine, and nifedipine conditions are provided in **Supplementary Figure S1**.

Taken together, these results indicate that both Ca^{2+} influx and mobilization from intracellular stores contribute to the response.

E2-Induced Axonal Growth Depends on Ca^{2+} Signal Generated by RyRs

Finally, we tested whether the RyR-induced Ca^{2+} response is part of the signaling cascade that mediates the axogenic effect of E2. Neurons grew under the following conditions: in the presence and absence of E2 and pretreated with inhibitory ryanodine. After these treatments, the cells were grown for an additional 24 h period with (E2) or without E2 (control). In agreement with previous results, the morphometric analysis indicated that neurons grown under hormonal treatment show longer axons than neurons in control conditions without E2 (**Figure 4A**). Remarkably, blocking RyRs with ryanodine completely inhibited the E2-induced axogenesis (**Figure 4B**). Moreover, no significant differences were observed in the number of primary neurites, length of minor processes, or soma area per neuron resulting from E2 or ryanodine treatment (**Table 1**), confirming that the hormonal effect is restricted to axonal growth (Díaz et al., 1992; Cambiasso et al., 1995, 2000; Brito et al., 2004).

DISCUSSION

In the present study, results from ERK1/2 phosphorylation, Ca^{2+} imaging and neuronal growth consistently pointed to RyRs as the Ca^{2+} channels necessary to mediate activation of the MAPK/ERK pathway and the final axogenic effect induced by E2. Inhibitory ryanodine completely blocked E2-mediated Ca^{2+} transients, ERK1/2 phosphorylation and axonal outgrowth, which provides valuable evidence to propose that E2 mobilizes endoplasmic reticulum stores of Ca^{2+} through RyRs to activate the signaling cascades that finally affect the axonal elongation of hypothalamic neurons.

In regard to the impact of functional RyRs on cellular response, Dr Hidalgo's group showed that BDNF-induced neural plasticity requires functional RyRs activated by the Ca^{2+}-induced Ca^{2+} release (CICR) mechanism to evoke the larger Ca^{2+} signaling needed to maintain changes during long-term memory storage (Adasme et al., 2011). CICR is a positive

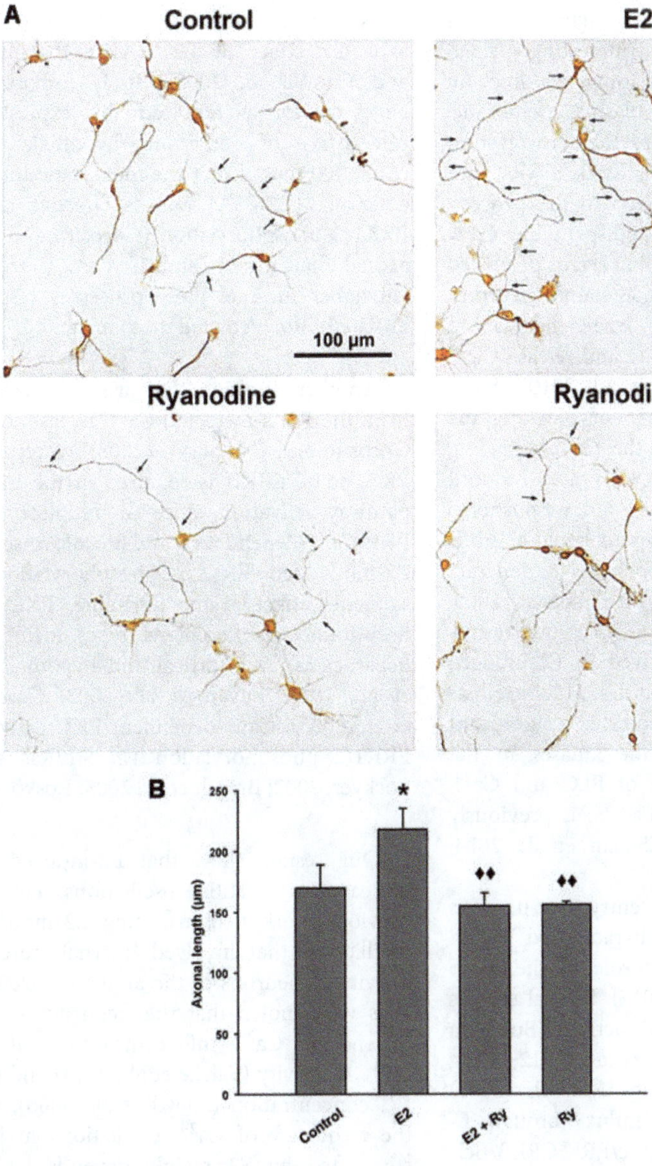

FIGURE 4 | RyR activity is required to the E2-induced axogenesis. (A) Representative images of male hypothalamic neurons cultured for 48 h with (E2) or without (control) 10 nM 17β-estradiol in combination or not with 50 μM ryanodine (Ry) for the last 24 h of incubation (arrows indicate the axons of some neurons). **(B)** Mean of axonal length for each condition in **(A)**. ANOVA $F_{(3,12)} = 4.51$; $p = 0.02$. LSDs test indicated *$p = 0.05$ vs. control and ♦♦$p = 0.01$ vs. E2. Data represent the mean ± SEM; $n = 4$ independent cultures. Scale bar: 100 μm.

TABLE 1 | Number of primary neurites, soma area, and length of minor processes of male hypothalamic neurons grown with or without 17β-estradiol (E2) in 3 combination or not with ryanodine.

Variable	Treatment			
	Control	E2	E2 + Ryanodine	Ryanodine
N° of neurites	4.2 ± 0.2	4.4 ± 0.2	4.3 ± 0.4	4.2 ± 0.2
Soma area (μm^2)	118.9 ± 13.2	116.6 ± 4.5	119.5 ± 10.0	126.2 ± 9.0
Minor processes length (μm)	107.2 ± 7.7	115.6 ± 8.9	94.0 ± 11.5	92.6 ± 5.8

Data represent the mean ± SEM; n = 4 independent cultures.

feedback mechanism by which cytoplasmic Ca^{2+} stimulates Ca^{2+} release from the endoplasmic reticulum through RyRs or IP_3Rs (Bezprozvanny et al., 1991; Berridge et al., 2003; Seo et al., 2015). Moreover, several studies have indicated a regulatory role for estrogens on RyRs activity, for instance, in the human eccrine sweat gland cell line NCL-SG3 (Muchekehu and Harvey, 2008), ventricular myocytes (Yan et al., 2011), detrusor smooth muscle cells (Hristov et al., 2017), and dorsal root ganglion neurons (Ferrari et al., 2016; Khomula et al., 2017). Interestingly, Zhao X. et al. (2005) proposed, in a neuroblastoma cell line, an E2-mediated mechanism starting at the plasma membrane, by which rapid Ca^{2+} signaling potentiates the transcription of genes normally regulated by estrogens; RyRs, IP_3Rs, and N-VGCCs, but not L-VGCCs, were involved in the process. Our results clearly show that RyRs are indispensable Ca^{2+} channels involved in the non-classical signaling events produced by E2 to generate axonal growth in hypothalamic neurons. However, RyRs also require a previous small increase in cytosolic Ca^{2+} from resting levels to activate and release Ca^{2+} by CICR (Hidalgo et al., 2005; Lanner et al., 2010). Since we found that removing extracellular Ca^{2+} or blocking the membrane channels L-VGCCs prevented the Ca^{2+} signaling induced by E2 and that inhibiting L-VGCCs also reduced ERK1/2 phosphorylation modulated by the steroid, we postulate that E2 initially induces a Ca^{2+} influx in hypothalamic neurons *via* L-VGCCs that then enables RyRs opening to generate the final and complete Ca^{2+} signaling event (Hidalgo, 2005; Calin-Jageman and Lee, 2008). Besides L-VGCCs, our results show that the PLC/IP_3Rs system is involved in E2-induced ERK1/2 activation, since both 2-APB and U-73122 used as blockers of IP_3Rs and PLC, respectively, produced a significant reduction in phosphorylation levels of the kinases in the presence of the hormone. The activation of PLC and Ca^{2+} release *via* IP_3Rs induced by estrogens has been previously reported in different cellular systems (Chaban et al., 2004; Fricke et al., 2007).

L-VGCCs are the major route of Ca^{2+} entry into neurons and the most profusely studied and best characterized VGCC type by far, as they play a predominant role in the brain (Striessnig et al., 2014; Vega-Vela et al., 2017). Several studies report that E2 is able to modulate L-VGCCs activity (Bulayeva et al., 2005; Sarkar et al., 2008; Farkas et al., 2012; Feng et al., 2013). Wu et al. (2005) and Zhao L. et al. (2005) indicated that E2 induced rapid Ca^{2+} influx through L-VGCCs, which was required to activate the Src/ERK/CREB/Bcl-2 signaling pathway and finally mediated neuroprotective and neurotrophic responses in rat hippocampal and cortical neurons. The generation of this intracellular Ca^{2+} increase and the downstream activation of ERK depend on the presence of ERs in the membrane of rat hippocampal neurons (Wu et al., 2011). These membrane ER-expressing neurons represented 29% of the cultured cells and all of them co-expressed L-VGCCs. Consistently, our data from Ca^{2+} imaging experiments indicated that approximately 22% of hypothalamic neurons responded to E2.

Although previously it has been reported that E2 induces L-VGCCs-mediated Ca^{2+} influx, the question about how the hormone activates L-VGCCs remains open. Sarkar et al. (2008) reported that E2 potentiated the activity of L-VGCCs by directly binding to specific sites in the channel, independently of ERs. On the other hand, PI3K signaling cascade has been proposed as a candidate to link membrane ER activation with L-VGCCs aperture (Simoncini et al., 2000; Quignard et al., 2001; Wu et al., 2005), although our preceding work blocking PI3K with LY-294,002 did not prevent the axogenic effect of E2 in hypothalamic neurons (Gorosito and Cambiasso, 2008). It is important to note that we have previously reported the expression of ERα on the cell-surface of embryonic hypothalamic neurons (Gorosito et al., 2008), and that the membrane-impermeable E2-albumin construct (E2-BSA) was as effective as free E2 to generate ERK1/2 phosphorylation (Gorosito and Cambiasso, 2008) and axonal elongation (Cambiasso and Carrer, 2001), evidence that altogether indicate these processes respond to a membrane-initiated ERα-mediated mechanism.

Another question that arises is what other elements lead from the RyRs-mediated Ca^{2+} release to ERK1/2 activation. In Gorosito and Cambiasso (2008) we reported that PKC but not PKA nor CaMKII is required in the E2-induced MAPK-ERK pathway activation, since an inhibitor with specificity for the PKC Ca^{2+}-dependent α and βI isoforms, Ro 32-0432, attenuated E2-modulated ERK1/2 phosphorylation and prevented the axogenic effect of the hormone. PKC activation by E2 has been found in different cell types, including breast cancer cells, hepatocytes, and cortical and hypothalamic neurons (Marino et al., 1998; Boyan et al., 2003; Cordey et al., 2003; Qiu et al., 2003). Ca^{2+}-dependent PKC activation can then induce ERK1/2 phosphorylation *via* Src/Ras signaling (Cullen and Lockyer, 2002; Brandt et al., 2003; Roskoski, 2005).

Our results show that E2-induced cytosolic Ca^{2+} often increases as repetitive oscillations. This is in agreement with previous work demonstrating E2-induced intracellular Ca^{2+} oscillations that involved internal stores and PKA and PLC activity in neurons of the arcuate nucleus (Fricke et al., 2007). It is well known that the frequency of Ca^{2+} oscillation may depend on Ca^{2+} influx into the cell (Sneyd et al., 2004), SERCA activity (Falcke et al., 2003) and oscillating cytoplasmic IP_3 concentration (Sneyd et al., 2006). Our data suggest that the frequency of Ca^{2+} oscillations in hypothalamic neurons stimulated by E2 mainly depends on Ca^{2+} entry. Leaving aside its modulation, our results allow us to speculate that the characteristic frequency encodes information to regulate the cellular response (axonal growth) mediated by the hormone Dolmetsch et al., 1998).

In conclusion, we have provided new insights into the non-classical mechanisms triggered by estrogens and its axogenic effect in male rat hypothalamic neurons. The hormone induces ERK1/2 activation in a Ca^{2+}-dependent manner. RyRs inhibition abolished this activation as well as axonal growth. The oscillatory Ca^{2+} signal generated by E2 required functional RyRs and L-VGCCs. This early Ca^{2+} response that underlies E2-induced RyRs and MAPK/ERK activation may transmit a finely tuned message into a neuronal development program, reflecting the need for tight control of a critical event during sexual differentiation of the male brain. The conjunction of XY genotype with adequate estrogen exposure levels at the time of hypothalamic neuronal differentiation may induce the growth of axons towards their appropriate targets. A complete and detailed understanding of the intracellular signaling mechanisms and neuronal processes mediated by estrogens will allow to improve current estrogen-based therapies, such as hormone replacement therapy in postmenopausal women, as well as to develop novel treatments to prevent and/or alleviate neurological pathologies based on its widely proven neuritogenic and neuroprotective effects.

AUTHOR CONTRIBUTIONS

LCZ, MB and MC made the conception and design of research, interpreted results of experiments, wrote the manuscript. LCZ performed all experiments and analyzed the data. LCZ and MB prepared the figures. MB and MC edited and revised the manuscript. MC drafted the manuscript.

FUNDING

This study was supported by grants from Consejo Nacional de Investigaciones Científicas y Técnicas (CONICET; PIP 2013-2015), Agencia Nacional de Promoción Científica y Tecnológica (ANPCyT; PICT 2015 N° 1333) and Secretaria de Ciencia y Tecnología (SECyT)-Universidad Nacional de Córdoba (2016-2017), Argentina to MC and from CONICET (PIP 2014-2016) to MB.

ACKNOWLEDGMENTS

We thank for the technical support from INIMEC animal facility and Dr Quassollo for his invaluable help with imaging. Calcium imaging was generated at National Center of Microscopy, Universidad Nacional de Córdoba, Córdoba, Argentina.

REFERENCES

Acaz-Fonseca, E., Sanchez-Gonzalez, R., Azcoitia, I., Arevalo, M. A., and Garcia-Segura, L. M. (2014). Role of astrocytes in the neuroprotective actions of 17β-estradiol and selective estrogen receptor modulators. *Mol. Cell. Endocrinol.* 389, 48–57. doi: 10.1016/j.mce.2014.01.009

Adasme, T., Haeger, P., Paula-Lima, A. C., Espinoza, I., Casas-Alarcon, M. M., Carrasco, M. A., et al. (2011). Involvement of ryanodine receptors in neurotrophin-induced hippocampal synaptic plasticity and spatial memory formation. *Proc. Natl. Acad. Sci. U S A* 108, 3029–3034. doi: 10.1073/pnas.1013580108

Arevalo, M. A., Azcoitia, I., and Garcia-Segura, L. M. (2015). The neuroprotective actions of oestradiol and oestrogen receptors. *Nat. Rev. Neurosci.* 16, 17–29. doi: 10.1038/nrn3856

Arevalo, M. A., Ruiz-Palmero, I., Scerbo, M. J., Acaz-Fonseca, E., Cambiasso, M. J., and Garcia-Segura, L. M. (2012). Molecular mechanisms involved in the regulation of neuritogenesis by estradiol: recent advances. *J. Steroid Biochem. Mol. Biol.* 131, 52–56. doi: 10.1016/j.jsbmb.2011.09.004

Berridge, M. J., Bootman, M. D., and Roderick, H. L. (2003). Calcium signalling: dynamics, homeostasis and remodelling. *Nat. Rev. Mol. Cell Biol.* 4, 517–529. doi: 10.1038/nrm1155

Berthois, Y., Katzenellenbogen, J. A., and Katzenellenbogen, B. S. (1986). Phenol red in tissue culture media is a weak estrogen: implications concerning the study of estrogen-responsive cells in culture. *Proc. Natl. Acad. Sci. U S A* 83, 2496–2500. doi: 10.1073/pnas.83.8.2496

Beyer, C., and Karolczak, M. (2000). Estrogenic stimulation of neurite growth in midbrain dopaminergic neurons depends on cAMP/protein kinase A signalling. *J. Neurosci. Res.* 59, 107–116. doi: 10.1002/(sici)1097-4547(20000101)59:1<107::aid-jnr13>3.0.co;2-w

Beyer, C., and Raab, H. (1998). Nongenomic effects of oestrogen: embryonic mouse midbrain neurones respond with a rapid release of calcium from intracellular stores. *Eur. J. Neurosci.* 10, 255–262. doi: 10.1046/j.1460-9568.1998.00045.x

Bezprozvanny, I., Watras, J., and Ehrlich, B. E. (1991). Bell-shaped calcium-response curves of Ins(1,4,5)P3- and calcium-gated channels from endoplasmic reticulum of cerebellum. *Nature* 351, 751–754. doi: 10.1038/351751a0

Blanco, G., Diaz, H., Carrer, H. F., and Beaugé, L. (1990). Differentiation of rat hippocampal neurons induced by estrogen *in vitro*: effects on neuritogenesis and Na, K-ATPase activity. *J. Neurosci. Res.* 27, 47–54. doi: 10.1002/jnr.490270108

Boyan, B. D., Sylvia, V. L., Frambach, T., Lohmann, C. H., Dietl, J., Dean, D. D., et al. (2003). Estrogen-dependent rapid activation of protein kinase C in estrogen receptor-positive MCF-7 breast cancer cells and estrogen receptor-negative HCC38 cells is membrane-mediated and inhibited by tamoxifen. *Endocrinology* 144, 1812–1824. doi: 10.1210/en.2002-221018

Brandt, D. T., Goerke, A., Heuer, M., Gimona, M., Leitges, M., Kremmer, E., et al. (2003). Protein kinase C delta induces Src kinase activity via activation of the protein tyrosine phosphatase PTP α. *J. Biol. Chem.* 278, 34073–34078. doi: 10.1074/jbc.m211650200

Brito, V. I., Carrer, H. F., and Cambiasso, M. J. (2004). Inhibition of tyrosine kinase receptor type B synthesis blocks axogenic effect of estradiol on rat hypothalamic neurones *in vitro*. *Eur. J. Neurosci.* 20, 331–337. doi: 10.1111/j.1460-9568.2004.03485.x

Bulayeva, N. N., Wozniak, A. L., Lash, L. L., and Watson, C. S. (2005). Mechanisms of membrane estrogen receptor-α-mediated rapid stimulation of Ca^{2+} levels and prolactin release in a pituitary cell line. *Am. J. Physiol. Endocrinol. Metab.* 288, E388–E397. doi: 10.1152/ajpendo.00349.2004

Calin-Jageman, I., and Lee, A. (2008). Ca_v1 L-type Ca^{2+} channel signaling complexes in neurons. *J. Neurochem.* 105, 573–583. doi: 10.1111/j.1471-4159.2008.05286.x

Cambiasso, M. J., and Carrer, H. F. (2001). Nongenomic mechanism mediates estradiol stimulation of axon growth in male rat hypothalamic neurons *in vitro*. *J. Neurosci. Res.* 66, 475–481. doi: 10.1002/jnr.1238

Cambiasso, M. J., Colombo, J. A., and Carrer, H. F. (2000). Differential effect of oestradiol and astroglia-conditioned media on the growth of hypothalamic neurons from male and female rat brains. *Eur. J. Neurosci.* 12, 2291–2298. doi: 10.1046/j.1460-9568.2000.00120.x

Cambiasso, M. J., Diaz, H., Cáceres, A., and Carrer, H. F. (1995). Neuritogenic effect of estradiol on rat ventromedial hypothalamic neurons co-cultured with homotopic or heterotopic glia. *J. Neurosci. Res.* 42, 700–709. doi: 10.1002/jnr.490420513

Carroll, J. C., and Pike, C. J. (2008). Selective estrogen receptor modulators differentially regulate Alzheimer-like changes in female 3xTg-AD mice. *Endocrinology* 149, 2607–2611. doi: 10.1210/en.2007-1346

Céspedes Rubio, Á. E., Pérez-Alvarez, M. J., Lapuente Chala, C., and Wandosell, F. (2018). Sex steroid hormones as neuroprotective elements in ischemia models. *J. Endocrinol.* 237, R65–R81. doi: 10.1530/joe-18-0129

Chaban, V. V., Lakhter, A. J., and Micevych, P. (2004). A membrane estrogen receptor mediates intracellular calcium release in astrocytes. *Endocrinology* 145, 3788–3795. doi: 10.1210/en.2004-0149

Cordey, M., Gundimeda, U., Gopalakrishna, R., and Pike, C. J. (2003). Estrogen activates protein kinase C in neurons: role in neuroprotection. *J. Neurochem.* 84, 1340–1348. doi: 10.1046/j.1471-4159.2003.01631.x

Cullen, P. J., and Lockyer, P. J. (2002). Integration of calcium and Ras signalling. *Nat. Rev. Mol. Cell Biol.* 3, 339–348. doi: 10.1038/nrm808

Díaz, H., Lorenzo, A., Carrer, H. F., and Cáceres, A. (1992). Time lapse study of neurite growth in hypothalamic dissociated neurons in culture: sex differences and estrogen effects. *J. Neurosci. Res.* 33, 266–281. doi: 10.1002/jnr.490330210

Dolmetsch, R. E., Xu, K., and Lewis, R. S. (1998). Calcium oscillations increase the efficiency and specificity of gene expression. *Nature* 392, 933–936. doi: 10.1038/31960

Dotti, C. G., Sullivan, C. A., and Banker, G. A. (1988). The establishment of polarity by hippocampal neurons in culture. *J. Neurosci.* 8, 1454–1468. doi: 10.1523/JNEUROSCI.08-04-01454.1988

Dye, R. V., Miller, K. J., Singer, E. J., and Levine, A. J. (2012). Hormone replacement therapy and risk for neurodegenerative diseases. *Int. J. Alzheimers Dis.* 2012:258454. doi: 10.1155/2012/258454

Falcke, M., Li, Y., Lechleiter, J. D., and Camacho, P. (2003). Modeling the dependence of the period of intracellular Ca^{2+} waves on SERCA expression. *Biophys. J.* 85, 1474–1481. doi: 10.1016/s0006-3495(03)74580-9

Farkas, I., Sárvári, M., Aller, M., Okada, N., Okada, H., Likó, I., et al. (2012). Estrogen receptor α and β differentially mediate C5aR agonist evoked Ca^{2+}-influx in neurons through L-type voltage-gated Ca^{2+} channels. *Neurochem. Int.* 60, 631–639. doi: 10.1016/j.neuint.2012.02.024

Feng, Y., Wang, B., Du, F., Li, H., Wang, S., Hu, C., et al. (2013). The involvement of PI3K-mediated and L-VGCC-gated transient Ca^{2+} influx in 17β-estradiol-mediated protection of retinal cells from H_2O_2-induced apoptosis with Ca^{2+} overload. *PLoS One* 8:e77218. doi: 10.1371/journal.pone.0077218

Ferrari, L. F., Khomula, E. V., Araldi, D., and Levine, J. D. (2016). Marked sexual dimorphism in the role of the ryanodine receptor in a model of pain chronification in the rat. *Sci. Rep.* 6:31221. doi: 10.1038/srep31221

Fricke, O., Kow, L. M., Bogun, M., and Pfaff, D. W. (2007). Estrogen evokes a rapid effect on intracellular calcium in neurons characterized by calcium oscillations in the arcuate nucleus. *Endocrine* 31, 279–288. doi: 10.1007/s12020-007-0034-7

Garcia-Segura, L. M., Arévalo, M. A., and Azcoitia, I. (2010). Interactions of estradiol and insulin-like growth factor-I signalling in the nervous system: new advances. *Prog. Brain Res.* 181, 251–272. doi: 10.1016/s0079-6123(08)81014-x

Giatti, S., Garcia-Segura, L. M., Barreto, G. E., and Melcangi, R. C. (2018). Neuroactive steroids, neurosteroidogenesis and sex. *Prog. Neurobiol.* doi: 10.1016/j.pneurobio.2018.06.007 [Epub ahead of print].

Gorosito, S. V., and Cambiasso, M. J. (2008). Axogenic effect of estrogen in male rat hypothalamic neurons involves Ca^{2+}, protein kinase C, and extracellular signal-regulated kinase signaling. *J. Neurosci. Res.* 86, 145–157. doi: 10.1002/jnr.21466

Gorosito, S. V., Lorenzo, A. G., and Cambiasso, M. J. (2008). Estrogen receptor α is expressed on the cell-surface of embryonic hypothalamic neurons. *Neuroscience* 154, 1173–1177. doi: 10.1016/j.neuroscience.2008.05.001

Hidalgo, C. (2005). Cross talk between Ca^{2+} and redox signalling cascades in muscle and neurons through the combined activation of ryanodine receptors/Ca^{2+} release channels. *Philos. Trans. R. Soc. Lond. B Biol. Sci.* 360, 2237–2246. doi: 10.1098/rstb.2005.1759

Hidalgo, C., Donoso, P., and Carrasco, M. A. (2005). The ryanodine receptors Ca^{2+} release channels: cellular redox sensors? *IUBMB Life* 57, 315–322. doi: 10.1080/15216540500092328

Hristov, K. L., Parajuli, S. P., Provence, A., Rovner, E. S., and Petkov, G. V. (2017). Nongenomic modulation of the large conductance voltage- and Ca^{2+}-activated K^+ channels by estrogen: a novel regulatory mechanism in human detrusor smooth muscle. *Physiol. Rep.* 5:e13351. doi: 10.14814/phy2.13351

Kelly, M. J., and Levin, E. R. (2001). Rapid actions of plasma membrane estrogen receptors. *Trends Endocrinol. Metab.* 12, 152–156. doi: 10.1016/s1043-2760(01)00377-0

Khan, M. M., Wakade, C., de Sevilla, L., and Brann, D. W. (2015). Selective estrogen receptor modulators (SERMs) enhance neurogenesis and spine density following focal cerebral ischemia. *J. Steroid Biochem. Mol. Biol.* 146, 38–47. doi: 10.1016/j.jsbmb.2014.05.001

Khomula, E. V., Ferrari, L. F., Araldi, D., and Levine, J. D. (2017). Sexual dimorphism in a reciprocal interaction of ryanodine and IP3 receptors in the induction of hyperalgesic priming. *J. Neurosci.* 37, 2032–2044. doi: 10.1523/JNEUROSCI.2911-16.2017

Lai, Y. J., Yu, D., Zhang, J. H., and Chen, G. J. (2017). Cooperation of genomic and rapid nongenomic actions of estrogens in synaptic plasticity. *Mol. Neurobiol.* 54, 4113–4126. doi: 10.1007/s12035-016-9979-y

Lanner, J. T., Georgiou, D. K., Joshi, A. D., and Hamilton, S. L. (2010). Ryanodine receptors: structure, expression, molecular details, and function in calcium release. *Cold Spring Harb. Perspect. Biol.* 2:a003996. doi: 10.1101/cshperspect.a003996

Le Mellay, V., Grosse, B., and Lieberherr, M. (1997). Phospholipase C β and membrane action of calcitriol and estradiol. *J. Biol. Chem.* 272, 11902–11907. doi: 10.1074/jbc.272.18.11902

Marino, M., Pallottini, V., and Trentalance, A. (1998). Estrogens cause rapid activation of IP3-PKC-α signal transduction pathway in HEPG2 cells. *Biochem. Biophys. Res. Commun.* 245, 254–258. doi: 10.1006/bbrc.1998.8413

McCarthy, M. M. (2008). Estradiol and the developing brain. *Physiol. Rev.* 88, 91–124. doi: 10.1152/physrev.00010.2007

McGregor, C., Riordan, A., and Thornton, J. (2017). Estrogens and the cognitive symptoms of schizophrenia: possible neuroprotective mechanisms. *Front. Neuroendocrinol.* 47, 19–33. doi: 10.1016/j.yfrne.2017.06.003

Muchekehu, R. W., and Harvey, B. J. (2008). 17β-estradiol rapidly mobilizes intracellular calcium from ryanodine-receptor-gated stores via a PKC-PKA-Erk-dependent pathway in the human eccrine sweat gland cell line NCL-SG3. *Cell Calcium* 44, 276–288. doi: 10.1016/j.ceca.2007.12.001

Murphy, D. D., and Segal, M. (1996). Regulation of dendritic spine density in cultured rat hippocampal neurons by steroid hormones. *J. Neurosci.* 16, 4059–4068. doi: 10.1523/JNEUROSCI.16-13-04059.1996

Nishizuka, M., and Arai, Y. (1981). Organizational action of estrogen on synaptic pattern in the amygdala: implications for sexual differentiation of the brain. *Brain Res.* 213, 422–426. doi: 10.1016/0006-8993(81)90247-x

Picotto, G., Vazquez, G., and Boland, R. (1999). 17β-oestradiol increases intracellular Ca^{2+} concentration in rat enterocytes. Potential role of phospholipase C-dependent store-operated Ca^{2+} influx. *Biochem. J.* 339, 71–77. doi: 10.1042/bj3390071

Qiu, J., Bosch, M. A., Tobias, S. C., Grandy, D. K., Scanlan, T. S., Ronnekleiv, O. K., et al. (2003). Rapid signaling of estrogen in hypothalamic neurons involves a novel G-protein-coupled estrogen receptor that activates protein kinase C. *J. Neurosci.* 23, 9529–9540. doi: 10.1523/JNEUROSCI.23-29-09529.2003

Quignard, J. F., Mironneau, J., Carricaburu, V., Fournier, B., Babich, A., Nurnberg, B., et al. (2001). Phosphoinositide 3-kinase γ mediates angiotensin II-induced stimulation of L-type calcium channels in vascular myocytes. *J. Biol. Chem.* 276, 32545–32551. doi: 10.1074/jbc.m102582200

Reisert, I., Han, V., Lieth, E., Toran-Allerand, D., Pilgrim, C., and Lauder, J. (1987). Sex steroids promote neurite growth in mesencephalic tyrosine hydroxylase immunoreactive neurons *in vitro*. *Int. J. Dev. Neurosci.* 5, 91–98. doi: 10.1016/0736-5748(87)90054-2

Roskoski, R. Jr. (2005). Src kinase regulation by phosphorylation and dephosphorylation. *Biochem. Biophys. Res. Commun.* 331, 1–14. doi: 10.1016/j.bbrc.2005.03.012

Sarkar, S. N., Huang, R. Q., Logan, S. M., Yi, K. D., Dillon, G. H., and Simpkins, J. W. (2008). Estrogens directly potentiate neuronal L-type Ca^{2+} channels. *Proc. Natl. Acad. Sci. U S A* 105, 15148–15153. doi: 10.1073/pnas.0802379105

Scerbo, M. J., Freire-Regatillo, A., Cisternas, C. D., Brunotto, M., Arevalo, M. A., Garcia-Segura, L. M., et al. (2014). Neurogenin 3 mediates sex chromosome effects on the generation of sex differences in hypothalamic neuronal development. *Front. Cell. Neurosci.* 8:188. doi: 10.3389/fncel.2014.00188

Seo, M. D., Enomoto, M., Ishiyama, N., Stathopulos, P. B., and Ikura, M. (2015). Structural insights into endoplasmic reticulum stored calcium regulation by inositol 1,4,5-trisphosphate and ryanodine receptors. *Biochim. Biophys. Acta* 1853, 1980–1991. doi: 10.1016/j.bbamcr.2014.11.023

Simoncini, T., Hafezi-Moghadam, A., Brazil, D. P., Ley, K., Chin, W. W., and Liao, J. K. (2000). Interaction of oestrogen receptor with the regulatory subunit of phosphatidylinositol-3-OH kinase. *Nature* 407, 538–541. doi: 10.1038/35035131

Sneyd, J., Tsaneva-Atanasova, K., Reznikov, V., Bai, Y., Sanderson, M. J., and Yule, D. I. (2006). A method for determining the dependence of calcium oscillations on inositol trisphosphate oscillations. *Proc. Natl. Acad. Sci. U S A* 103, 1675–1680. doi: 10.1073/pnas.0506135103

Sneyd, J., Tsaneva-Atanasova, K., Yule, D. I., Thompson, J. L., and Shuttleworth, T. J. (2004). Control of calcium oscillations by membrane fluxes. *Proc. Natl. Acad. Sci. U S A* 101, 1392–1396. doi: 10.1073/pnas.0303472101

Spence, R. D., Wisdom, A. J., Cao, Y., Hill, H. M., Mongerson, C. R., Stapornkul, B., et al. (2013). Estrogen mediates neuroprotection and anti-inflammatory effects during EAE through ERα signaling on astrocytes but not through ERβ signaling on astrocytes or neurons. *Brain Behav. Evol.* 33, 10924–10933. doi: 10.1523/jneurosci.0886-13.2013

Striessnig, J., Pinggera, A., Kaur, G., Bock, G., and Tuluc, P. (2014). L-type Ca^{2+} channels in heart and brain. *Wiley Interdiscip. Rev. Membr. Transp. Signal.* 3, 15–38. doi: 10.1002/wmts.102

Toran-Allerand, C. D. (1976). Sex steroids and the development of the newborn mouse hypothalamus and preoptic area *in vitro*: implications for sexual differentiation. *Brain Res.* 106, 407–412. doi: 10.1016/0006-8993(76)91038-6

Toran-Allerand, C. D. (1980). Sex steroids and the development of the newborn mouse hypothalamus and preoptic area *in vitro*. II. Morphological correlates and hormonal specificity. *Brain Res.* 189, 413–427. doi: 10.1016/0006-8993(80)90101-8

Toran-Allerand, C. D., Hashimoto, K., Greenough, W. T., and Saltarelli, M. (1983). Sex steroids and the development of the newborn mouse hypothalamus and preoptic area *in vitro*: III. Effects of estrogen on dendritic differentiation. *Brain Res.* 283, 97–101. doi: 10.1016/0165-3806(83)90085-8

Vega-Vela, N. E., Osorio, D., Avila-Rodriguez, M., Gonzalez, J., Garcia-Segura, L. M., Echeverria, V., et al. (2017). L-type calcium channels modulation by estradiol. *Mol. Neurobiol.* 54, 4996–5007. doi: 10.1007/s12035-016-0045-6

Villa, A., Vegeto, E., Poletti, A., and Maggi, A. (2016). Estrogens, neuroinflammation, and neurodegeneration. *Endocr. Rev.* 37, 372–402. doi: 10.1210/er.2016-1007

Wong, C. K., So, W. Y., Law, S. K., Leung, F. P., Yau, K. L., Yao, X., et al. (2012). Estrogen controls embryonic stem cell proliferation via store-operated calcium entry and the nuclear factor of activated T-cells (NFAT). *J. Cell. Physiol.* 227, 2519–2530. doi: 10.1002/jcp.22990

Wright, C. L., Schwarz, J. S., Dean, S. L., and McCarthy, M. M. (2010). Cellular mechanisms of estradiol-mediated sexual differentiation of the brain. *Trends Endocrinol. Metab.* 21, 553–561. doi: 10.1016/j.tem.2010.05.004

Wu, T. W., Chen, S., and Brinton, R. D. (2011). Membrane estrogen receptors mediate calcium signaling and MAP kinase activation in individual hippocampal neurons. *Brain Res.* 1379, 34–43. doi: 10.1016/j.brainres.2011.01.034

Wu, T. W., Wang, J. M., Chen, S., and Brinton, R. D. (2005). 17β-estradiol induced Ca^{2+} influx via L-type calcium channels activates the Src/ERK/cyclic-AMP response element binding protein signal pathway and BCL-2 expression in rat hippocampal neurons: a potential initiation mechanism for estrogen-induced neuroprotection. *Neuroscience* 135, 59–72. doi: 10.1016/j.neuroscience.2004.12.027

Yan, S., Chen, Y., Dong, M., Song, W., Belcher, S. M., and Wang, H. S. (2011). Bisphenol A and 17β-estradiol promote arrhythmia in the female heart via alteration of calcium handling. *PLoS One* 6:e25455. doi: 10.1371/journal.pone.0025455

Zhao, L., Chen, S., Ming Wang, J., and Brinton, R. D. (2005). 17β-estradiol induces Ca^{2+} influx, dendritic and nuclear Ca^{2+} rise and subsequent cyclic AMP response element-binding protein activation in hippocampal neurons: a potential initiation mechanism for estrogen neurotrophism. *Neuroscience* 132, 299–311. doi: 10.1016/j.neuroscience.2004.11.054

Zhao, X., MacBride, M. M., Peterson, B. R., Pfaff, D. W., and Vasudevan, N. (2005). Calcium flux in neuroblastoma cells is a coupling mechanism between non-genomic and genomic modes of estrogens. *Neuroendocrinology* 81, 174–182. doi: 10.1159/000087000

3

Extracellular Vesicles Secreted by Astroglial Cells Transport Apolipoprotein D to Neurons and Mediate Neuronal Survival Upon Oxidative Stress

Raquel Pascua-Maestro[1], *Esperanza González*[2], *Concepción Lillo*[3], *Maria D. Ganfornina*[1]*, *Juan Manuel Falcón-Pérez*[2,4†] *and Diego Sanchez*[1†]

[1]*Instituto de Biología y Genética Molecular-Departamento de Bioquímica y Biología Molecular y Fisiología, Universidad de Valladolid-CSIC, Valladolid, Spain,* [2]*Exosomes Group, Metabolomics Unit and Platform, CIC bioGUNE, CIBERehd, Technology Park of Bizkaia, Derio, Spain,* [3]*Instituto de Neurociencias de Castilla y León, IBSAL, Universidad de Salamanca, Salamanca, Spain,* [4]*IKERBASQUE, Basque Foundation for Science, Bilbao, Spain*

***Correspondence:**
Maria D. Ganfornina
opabinia@ibgm.uva.es

†These authors have contributed equally to this work and are senior authors

Extracellular vesicle (EV)-mediated glia-to-neuron communication has been recognized in a growing number of physiological and pathological situations. They transport complex sets of molecules that can be beneficial or detrimental for the receiving cell. As in other areas of biology, their analysis is revolutionizing the field of neuroscience, since fundamental signaling processes are being re-evaluated, and applications for neurodegenerative disease therapies have emerged. Using human astrocytic and differentiated neuronal cell lines, we demonstrate that a classical neuroprotective protein, Apolipoprotein D (ApoD), expressed by glial cells and known to promote functional integrity and survival of neurons, is exclusively transported by EVs from astrocytes to neurons, where it gets internalized. Indeed, we demonstrate that conditioned media derived from ApoD-knock-out (KO) astrocytes exert only a partial autocrine protection from oxidative stress (OS) challenges, and that EVs are required for ApoD-positive astrocytic cell line derived medium to exert full neuroprotection. When subfractionation of EVs is performed, ApoD is revealed as a very specific marker of the exosome-containing fractions. These discoveries help us reframe our understanding of the neuroprotective role of this lipid binding protein and open up new research avenues to explore the use of systemically administered ApoD-loaded exosomes that can cross the blood-brain barrier to treat neurodegenerative diseases.

Keywords: ApoD, exosomes, extracellular vesicles, astrocytes, neurons, oxidative stress, neuroprotection, glia-to-neuron communication

INTRODUCTION

Nervous system function relies on a complex set of cell types interacting and communicating among them. Cell contact-dependent interactions underlie cell adhesion processes important for neural circuit construction and plasticity. However, communication can also take place by secretion of signaling molecules and neurotransmitters. In this line, the discovery of extracellular vesicles (EVs) have brought a new format of interactions to an already multifaceted communication network.

EVs produced by most cells, including all nervous system cell types (Frühbeis et al., 2013a; Lopez-Verrilli et al., 2013; Basso and Bonetto, 2016; Guitart et al., 2016; Croese and Furlan, 2018), open up a new mechanism of signal transmission (Valadi et al., 2007; Hervera et al., 2018) that is changing our understanding of how glia and neurons communicate (Frühbeis et al., 2013b; Basso and Bonetto, 2016; Krämer-Albers, 2017).

As the lipid, carbohydrate, protein and nucleic acid composition of EVs (Kalra et al., 2012; Keerthikumar et al., 2015; Kim et al., 2015) is cell type and physiological state-specific (György et al., 2011; Müller, 2012), such feature makes them candidate biomarker tools in many human diseases, including neuronal disorders (Müller, 2012; Cheow et al., 2016). Furthermore, the potential therapeutic use of EVs is particularly important in brain illnesses, given that they can cross the blood-brain barrier (Alvarez-Erviti et al., 2011; Ridder et al., 2014; Krämer-Albers, 2017). In this regard, EVs purposely loaded with neuroprotective molecules are a promising therapy for neurodegenerative disorders (Pandya et al., 2013; Spencer et al., 2014; Rufino-Ramos et al., 2017).

The Lipocalin Apolipoprotein D (ApoD) is mostly expressed in the nervous system and upregulated in response to oxidative stress (OS; Ganfornina et al., 2008; Bhatia et al., 2012, 2013), a challenge that accompanies physiological aging and disease (Ganfornina et al., 2008; Perdomo and Henry Dong, 2009; Bhatia et al., 2012, 2013). Not surprisingly, ApoD is one of the few genes consistently over-expressed in the aging brain of all vertebrate species tested so far (Loerch et al., 2008). Moreover, ApoD expression is boosted in an amazingly wide array of neurodegenerative and psychiatric diseases of diverse etiology (Suresh et al., 1998; Reindl et al., 2001; reviewed by Dassati et al., 2014). ApoD is actively secreted by astrocytes and myelinating glia, and is uptaken by neurons during neural development and differentiation (Sánchez et al., 2002; Ganfornina et al., 2008, 2010; García-Mateo et al., 2014; Pascua-Maestro et al., 2017). At the cellular level, ApoD is found in the endosome-lysosome-autophagosomal compartment (Pascua-Maestro et al., 2017). Such subcellular location is finely regulated, both in glia, that express ApoD, and in neurons that uptake ApoD in a paracrine fashion (Pascua-Maestro et al., 2017). Within the lysosome, ApoD is able to prevent and revert OS-triggered membrane permeabilization (Bhatia et al., 2013; Pascua-Maestro et al., 2017). ApoD has been demonstrated to reduce free radical-generating lipid hydroperoxides to inert lipid hydroxides (Bhatia et al., 2012), a biochemical property that enables the protection and repair of OS-damaged membranes, finally resulting in cell survival. Previous work demonstrate that ApoD pro-survival mechanism is mediated specifically by the control of lipid peroxidation levels both in cultured cells and *in vivo* animal models (Ganfornina et al., 2008; Navarro et al., 2010; Bajo-Grañeras et al., 2011).

ApoD is considered to be secreted through a canonical secretion pathway, and is found associated to serum LDL/HDL (Perdomo and Henry Dong, 2009; Dassati et al., 2014). However, proteomic analyses have identified this Lipocalin in EVs from serum and cerebrospinal fluid (Cheow et al., 2016; Przybycien-Szymanska et al., 2016). Thus, we set up to test whether ApoD is present in glial-derived EVs and contributes, in this cell-cell communication format, to improve neuronal viability and function.

MATERIALS AND METHODS

Animals

ApoD-knock-out (KO) mice were generated by homologous recombination (Ganfornina et al., 2008), and maintained in positive pressure-ventilated racks at 25 ± 1°C with 12 h light/dark cycle, fed *ad libitum* with standard rodent pellet diet (Global Diet 2014; Harlan Inc., Indianapolis, IN, USA), and allowed free access to filtered and UV-irradiated water. To avoid potential maternal effects of ApoD, and to generate wild-type (WT) and ApoD-KO mice of homogeneous genetic background, the experimental cohorts used in this study are the F1 generation of homozygous crosses of ApoD$^{-/-}$ and ApoD$^{+/+}$ littermates born from heterozygous crosses of an ApoD-KO line backcrossed for over 20 generations into the C57BL/6J background.

Mice experimental procedures were approved by the University of Valladolid Animal Care and Use Committee, following the regulations of the Care and the Use of Mammals in Research (European Commission Directive 86/609/CEE, Spanish Royal Decree 1201/2005). No human subject was involved in this study.

Cell Culture and Treatments

The human astrocytoma 1321N1 and neuroblastoma SH-SY5Y cell lines were obtained from ECACC (86030402) and ATCC (CRL-2266) respectively. Cells were grown at 37°C in a humidity-saturated atmosphere containing 5% CO_2. Culture medium was replaced twice a week and cells were subcultured at 90% confluence. Cells were counted with Countess Automated Cell Counter (Invitrogen).

1321N1 cells were cultured in Dulbecco-modified Eagle's medium (DMEM; Lonza) supplemented with heat-inactivated 5% fetal bovine serum (FBS), 1% L-glutamine, and 1% penicillin/streptomycin/amphotericin B (PSA).

SH-SY5Y cells were cultured in DMEM supplemented with 4.5 g/l glucose, heat-inactivated 10% FBS, 1% L-glutamine, 1% PS and 1% nonessential amino acids (Lonza). To subculture, we used 0.25% Trypsin-EDTA (Gibco Life Technologies). SH-SY5Y differentiation was achieved by culturing cells on collagen-treated plates with 3% FBS and 10 μM retinoic acid (Sigma-Aldrich) for 72 h.

Primary astrocytes from WT and ApoD-KO neonatal (0–1 days old) mice were cultured as described (Bajo-Grañeras et al., 2011). Cerebral cortices were quickly dissected, their meninges removed by rolling on filter paper, and pieces of cortex placed in Earle's Balanced Salt Solution (EBSS) with 2.4 mg/ml DNAse I and 0.2 mg/ml bovine serum albumin (BSA). The tissue was minced with a surgical blade, centrifuged (200 *g*, 2 min), incubated with 10 mg/ml trypsin for 15 min at 37°C (incubation terminated by 10% FBS addition), mechanically dissociated with a Pasteur pipette, and centrifuged (200 *g*, 5 min). The resulting cells were resuspended in DMEM with 10% FBS, 1% L-glutamine, 1% PSA, plated onto cultured flasks, and incubated at 37°C in 5% CO_2 with 90%–95% humidity. Culture medium was replaced after 24 h and weekly thereafter. Cells were used for experiments after two subculture steps, when >99% of cells are astrocytes (Bajo-Grañeras et al., 2011).

Exogenous addition of ApoD: human ApoD purified from breast cystic fluid (Ruiz et al., 2013) was added (10 nM) to the cell cultures for 2 h.

Paraquat (PQ) treatment: cells were cultured in phenol red-free DMEM supplemented with 1% L-glutamine, 1% PS, and 0.2% charcoal stripped FBS. This medium without additives was used as our low-serum (LS) control condition. Cells were treated for 1–24 h with PQ (500 μM) prepared in LS medium.

To label and track the whole population of EVs produced by a cell (including exosomes and shedding vesicles) the membranous organelles were labeled with Vybrant-DiI (V22888). To label organelles of the phagocytic-endocytic pathway [endosomes, lysosomes and multivesicular bodies (MVB)] we used Dextran-Alexa 488 (D22910), following the manufacturer's specifications (Molecular Probes). Cells were incubated with the dye solution for 48 h. After removing the culture medium and performing three 5 min washes with phosphate-buffered saline (PBS), cells were incubated overnight and then subcultured alone or in different co-culture formats (see below).

Cells remained in co-culture during 48 h before performing flow cytometry or fluorescence microscopy analyses to test for transfer of vesicles between astrocytes and neurons. Two types of co-cultures were used: cells were subcultured to experimental plates in a 50:50 proportion (mixed cultures), or separated by a 0.4 μm pore membrane (Transwell plates, Corning Inc.) to avoid direct cell-cell contact.

Conditioned Media Harvesting for EV Preparations

A standard FBS is used for the culture medium used in the maintenance and amplification of each cell type, and for experiments not directed to EV collection. The experiments described below are performed in EV-free media, where FBS was EV-depleted by ultracentrifugation and added (5%) to phenol red-free DMEM with 25 mM HEPES, 4.5 g/l glucose, 1% L-glutamine and 1% PS.

Conditioned media collection: Cells were cultured in EV-free medium and incubated at 37°C in 5% CO_2 with 90%–95% humidity for 72 h before the culture medium was collected. A total of 24 culture dishes (20×10^6 cells/dish) per condition were necessary for EV preparations from 1321N1 cells, and 66 culture flasks (8×10^6 cells/flask) per conditions of primary astrocytes. After centrifugation at 1,500× *g* for 30 min at 4°C, the culture supernatant was filtered through a 0.22 μm membrane to obtain a debris-free conditioned medium (CM). The filtered culture medium was immediately frozen at −80°C. Two independent pools of media from 1321N1 cells and two from primary astrocytes per genotype were prepared for further vesicle isolation by differential ultracentrifugation (see below).

Isolation, Fractionation and Analysis of Astrocyte-Derived EVs

To isolate EVs, the stored debris-free CM samples were centrifuged at 10,000× *g* for 30 min and the supernatant was centrifuged at 100,000× *g* for 75 min. The supernatant of this centrifugation was collected for some experiments as EV-depleted CM. The resulting pellet was washed with an excess of PBS, and centrifuged again at 100,000× *g* for 60 min. The pellet was resuspended in cold PBS and stored at −80°C.

EVs size distribution and concentration were analyzed using a NanoSight LM10 system equipped with a fast video capture and particle-tracking software. Vesicles are visualized by light scattering using a light microscope with a Nanoparticles tracking analysis (NTA) software that tracks Brownian motion of individual vesicles. NTA post-acquisition settings were kept constant for all samples, and each video was analyzed to calculate the median vesicle size and concentration estimates (Dragovic et al., 2011). The starting EV-free culture medium was subject to NTA as control for comparison. We also characterized EVs by Western Blot and Transmission Electron Microscopy (TEM).

Glia-derived EVs (either from the 1321N1 human astrocytic cell line or from mouse primary astrocytes) were fractionated in a continuous 0.25–2 M sucrose density gradient (Taylor, 2015). The EV sample was placed on top of the gradient and centrifuged for 16 h at 210,000× *g*, 4°C, in a SW40 Ti rotor. Fractions (1 ml) were collected from top to bottom by using an autodensity-flow gradient fractionator (Labconco). After mixing by vortex, 20 μl of each fraction were separated for density measures. Subsequently, the rest of the volume was diluted in 20 mM HEPES (pH 7.4), and centrifuged 1 h at 110,000× *g*, 4°C, in a TLA-110 rotor. The pellets were resuspended in PBS and stored at −80°C for subsequent immunoblot analysis. Using the volume set aside, the refractive index of each fraction was measured with a high-resolution refractometer (Abbe 2WAJ, PCE Americans, Inc.). Values are translated into density values by use of equivalence tables.

Immunoblot Analysis

Cell lysates, cultured media (either directly or concentrated 20× by filter centrifugation with 10 KDa cut-off Centricon YM-10; Millipore), isolated EVs, or EV fractions were analyzed by immunoblot. Denaturing and reducing conditions (0.5% SDS, 25 mM DTT) were used to solubilize proteins prior to electrophoresis in order to detect ApoD. Proteins were transferred to PVDF membranes using standard procedures, and exposed to rabbit serum anti-human ApoD (custom made by Abyntek Biopharma against purified ApoD; Ruiz et al., 2013), goat serum anti-mouse ApoD (Santa Cruz Biotechnology), rabbit serum anti-CD81 (GeneTex), mouse anti-flotillin 1 (Becton Dickinson), or rabbit serum anti-BiP (Sigma), and followed by HRP-conjugated secondary antibodies (Santa Cruz Biotechnology). Membranes were developed with ECL reagents (Millipore) and the signal visualized with a digital camera (VersaDoc; BioRad). The integrated optical density of the immunoreactive protein bands was measured in images taken within the linear range of the camera, avoiding signal saturation.

Electron Microscopy Methods

Primary astrocytes, destined for pre-embedding immunogold labeling of ApoD, were fixed in 4% formaldehyde and 0.3% glutaraldehyde in 0.1 M PB, pH 7.4, for 30 min at 4°C. Following washes in 0.1 M PB, the cells were blocked with 0.1% cold water fish skin gelatin and permeabilized with Tween-20 (0.5%) in Tris-buffered saline (TBS; 20 mM Tris-HCl, 150 mM NaCl). Samples were incubated with rabbit serum anti-human ApoD antibody diluted in blocking solution. After several washes they were incubated with ultra-small gold-conjugated goat anti-rabbit secondary antibodies Electron Microscopy Sciences (EMS) in PBS. After several washes with PBS, samples were post-fixed in 2% glutaraldehyde in PBS for 20 min, washed, and the ultra-small gold particles were silver-enhanced for 20 min at room temperature with AURION R-Gent SE-EM (Silver Enhancement for Electron Microscopy) following the manufacturer indications. Later, samples were post-fixed with 0.5% OsO_4 in PBS for 20 min at 4°C, washed with PBS, dehydrated through a graded series of ethanol and embedded in Epoxy EMbed-812 resin EMS. Ultrathin sections were obtained with an Ultracut E ultramicrotome (Reichert/Leica), contrasted with uranyl acetate and lead citrate, and analyzed using a JEOL JEM-1011 HR electron microscope with a CCD Gatan ES1000W camera with iTEM software.

EV preparations destined to cryo-electron microscopy were directly adsorbed onto glow-discharged holey carbon grids (QUANTIFOIL, Germany). Grids were blotted at 95% humidity and rapidly plunged into liquid ethane with the aid of VITROBOT (Maastricht Instruments BV, Netherlands). Vitrified samples were imaged at liquid nitrogen temperature using a JEM-2200FS/CR transmission electron microscope (JEOL, Japan) equipped with a field emission gun and operated at an acceleration voltage of 200 kV.

Immunocytochemistry

Cells attached to poly-L-lysine (Sigma-Aldrich) treated coverslips were fixed with 4% formaldehyde. Following washes in PBS, cells were blocked and permeabilized with Tween-20 (0.1%) and 1% non-immune (goat or donkey) serum. Cells were incubated with primary antibodies: mouse anti-CD81 (monoclonal JS81), Mouse anti-CD63 (H5C6) or rabbit serum anti-human ApoD. All antibodies were prepared in blocking solution. Cy5, Cy3 (Abcam), Alexa Fluor® 594/488 (Jackson Labs) or DyLight® 405 (Thermo Scientific) conjugated IgGs were used as secondary antibodies. After washes in PBS, cells were mounted in EverBrite™ Mounting Medium with DAPI, and sealed with CoverGrip™ Coverslip Sealant (Biotium).

Image Acquisition and Analysis

Confocal images were obtained with a 63× oil immersion objective (HCX PL Apo CS NA = 1.4; Leica) attached to a confocal DMI 6000B microscope with a TCS SP5 confocal system (Leica) equipped with AOBS and AOTF systems. Fluorophores were excited with WLL laser (Leica) and a 405 line (Leica) controlled by LAS AF software (Leica). Emissions were collected with the AOBS system and three spectral detectors. Laser power and detection gains were set by scanning control samples labeled with secondary antibody alone. We ensured to obtain similar dynamic ranges in our images, and adjusted gain and offset using LUTs. In this manner, bleed through can be neglected. Negative control images showed very weak and homogeneous background. We obtained confocal sections under constant conditions to minimize image acquisition variation. Images were stored as 1,024 × 1,024 pixels and 8-bit TIFF files.

Z-series (xyz scan) were performed in all cases, covering the whole cell *z*-axis dimension. The number of z-stacks was determined by observing the limits of the cell membrane. The focus plane was set to be 3 μm beneath the section surface. The optimal value of the step size was calculated for the wavelength used to fulfill the Nyquist theorem. The optical section thickness was 0.772 μm. Besides, images were taken with a 4× zoom, reducing field size. Pixel size corresponded to 0.06*0.06*0.3777 μm^3. Scanning was performed with a 1.0 Airy unit pinhole size.

Images were processed with a Gaussian Blur filter [Sigma (Radius): 1.00], to facilitate object detection, and analyzed with a Colocalization Indices plug-in (Nakamura et al., 2007) and the 3D Object Counter tool of the FIJI software. To analyze triple-colocalization experiments we used the Image Calculator and 3D Object Counter tools of FIJI. We analyzed 20 cells per condition. Colocalization was quantitated using the intensity correlation quotient (ICQ), as described (Li et al., 2004). A 2 × ICQ was adopted so that colocalization values range from −1 (total exclusion) to +1 (total colocalization), with 0.1 representing the threshold for random association of signals (Pascua-Maestro et al., 2017). The index was referenced either to ApoD signal or to DiI signal.

Flow Cytometry

Cells cultured for 48 h after labeling with Vybrant-DiI or Dextran-Alexa 488 were lifted with 500 μl of Triple (Tryple™ Select, Gibco Life Technologies) after removal of the culture medium and washes with PBS. Suspended cells were analyzed in a FACS Canto II flow cytometer (Beckton Dickinson). DiI signal was collected with the "PE" detector (BP585/42) and Alexa 488 was detected with the "FITC" channel (BP530/30) after excitation with 488 nm laser. Data was processed with Kaluza Analysis software v.1.3 (Beckman Coulter).

MTT-Viability Assay

Cell viability was measured with the 3-(4,5-dimethylthiazol-2-yl)-2,5-diphenyltetrazolium bromide (MTT) colorimetric assay as previously described (Bajo-Grañeras et al., 2011; Pascua-Maestro et al., 2018). After MTT exposure for 3 h, cells were incubated in isopropanol with 10% Triton X-100, and the solubilized formazan was measured by spectrophotometry using the SOFTmax Pro microplate reader (Molecular Devices).

Absorbance was measured at λ = 570 nm after subtracting the λ = 690 nm background.

RT-PCR

RNAs from 1321N1 cells or differentiated SH-SY5Y cells after exposure to 1321N1-derived EVs were extracted with TRIzol (Qiagen). Total RNA (1 μg) was treated with DNaseI and reverse-transcribed with Prime-Script (Takara). The cDNA obtained was used as template for RT-PCR amplifications. To amplify human ApoD and the housekeeping control gene RPL18 we used the following primers: Human ApoD-Forward: 5'-CCACCCCAGTTAACCTCACA; Human ApoD-Reverse: 5'-CCACTGTTTCTGGAGGGAGA; Human RPL18-Forward: 5'-CCATCATGGGAGTGGACAT-3'; Human RPL18-Reverse: 5'-CACGGCCGTCTTGTTTTC.

Statistical Analysis

Statistical analyses were performed with SPSS v.19 (IBM) and SigmaPlot v.11.0 (Systat) software. A p value < 0.05 was used as a threshold for significant changes. The tests used for each experiment are stated in figure legends.

RESULTS

Glia-Neuron Communication *in vitro*

Although extensive data support the role of EVs as mediators of neuron-glia communication *in vivo* (Frühbeis et al., 2013b; Basso and Bonetto, 2016), we tested whether this relationship exists between human astroglial 1321N1 and neuronal SH-SY5Y cells, that have been previously used as a model to unravel the mechanism of action of ApoD (Bajo-Grañeras et al., 2011; Pascua-Maestro et al., 2017). We first studied the possibility of vesicular exchange between these cells by labeling the membranous compartment of 1321N1 astrocytes with the lipophilic compound DiI, and the endo-lysosomal compartment of SH-SY5Y neurons with Dextran-Alexa 488 (see "Material and Methods" section). Co-culturing of labeled cells in EV-free media for 48 h showed colocalization of DiI and Dextran-Alexa 488 in both astrocytes and neurons (**Figures 1C,D**), suggesting an exchange of membranous material among them. In addition, flow cytometry analysis (**Figures 1E–H**) confirms the presence of double-labeled cells (DiI-Dextran co-labeling; **Figure 1H**) and suggests that such transfer of material might be occurring mainly in the astrocyte-to-neuron direction (arrow in **Figure 1H**). However, the pattern of labeled cells observed might also be due to differences in efficiency of the labeling methods.

Analyzing DiI and Dextran-Alexa 488 distribution in 1321N1 and SH-SY5Y respectively by confocal microscopy we found that in both cells some of the labeled organelles colocalize with CD81, a marker of late endocytic compartments (Escola et al., 1998; **Figures 1A,B**). These results suggest that the membranous transfer between cells could be mediated by EVs. Nevertheless, they also could be explained by: (i) a cell-cell direct contact-dependent exchange of material; (ii) endocytosis of cellular debris such as apoptotic bodies generated in the co-cultures; or (iii) endocytosis of EVs produced by either cell type. Thus, to discern between these scenarios we used a Transwell assay, focusing on the transcellular traffic from astrocytes to neurons. Using EV-free media, we cultured DiI-labeled 1321N1 astrocytes as donor cells, on the Transwell insert, and SH-SY5Y neurons as target cells, on the lower compartment. After 48 h of incubation, a DiI positive population of SH-SY5Y recipient cells is detected by flow cytometry (**Figures 2A–C**). These experiments suggest that SH-SY5Y neurons receive and internalize DiI-labeled EVs secreted by 1321N1 astrocytes.

Neurons Uptake Glial-Derived EVs Containing ApoD

As ApoD is secreted by astrocytes and uptaken by neurons (Pascua-Maestro et al., 2017), we wanted to test if EVs play a role in such intracellular communication. In contrast to ApoD-expressing glioma and astrocytic cell lines like 1321N1 cells (Bajo-Grañeras et al., 2011; Pascua-Maestro et al., 2017), no ApoD expression has been detected in SH-SY5Y neuroblastoma cells either by genome-wide transcriptome analyses (e.g., 0.0 FPKM for ApoD in http://systemsbiology.uni.lu/shsy5y/) or by immunodetection of ApoD protein (Pascua-Maestro et al., 2017). We therefore tested whether 1321N1-derived vesicles uptaken by SH-SY5Y neurons contain astrocyte-derived ApoD using the Transwell co-culture system.

When co-cultured with 1321N1 cells in the Transwell insert, we are able to detect ApoD signal in intracellular vesicles of SH-SY5Y (**Figures 2D–F**), with a significant colocalization with the EV markers CD63 (**Figures 2D,G**) and CD81 (**Figures 2E,G**), as well as with the astrocyte-originated DiI signal (**Figures 2F,G**). Although, in general, the detected CD63 and CD81 can be either endogenous (produced by neurons) or transferred in astrocyte-derived EVs, the particular subset of CD63 or CD81-positive organelles that are also ApoD-positive are strong candidates to have an astrocytic origin. Indeed, the high colocalization index ($2 \times ICQ > 0.6$) of CD81 relative to the DiI signal detected in neurons, strongly supports a significant uptake of CD81-DiI-labeled EVs, a fraction of which ($2 \times ICQ > 0.2$), bring ApoD with them (**Figure 2G**). The significant colocalization indexes agree with the high incidence of triple colocalization of ApoD-CD81-DiI (**Figure 2F**).

However, ApoD could be provided externally to neurons as protein or mRNA, or alternatively its expression be induced after treatment with astroglial EVs, since the later have been shown to trigger diverse signaling cascades in cells (e.g., Hervera et al., 2018). To distinguish among these three possibilities we cultured SH-SY5Y neurons with: (1) EV-free standard media (SM); (2) 1321N1-conditioned media (CM); (3) the EV fraction (EVs) obtained by differential centrifugation of CM; and (4) the EV-depleted supernatant (Sup) of CM. We then used immunocytochemistry to detect ApoD protein in neurons, and RT-PCR to monitor *APOD* mRNA expression in the donor and recipient cells involved.

Immunofluorescence analysis of cultured SH-SY5Y showed the absence of ApoD in SM-cultured neurons (**Figure 3A**), thus confirming the absence of endogenous ApoD in control

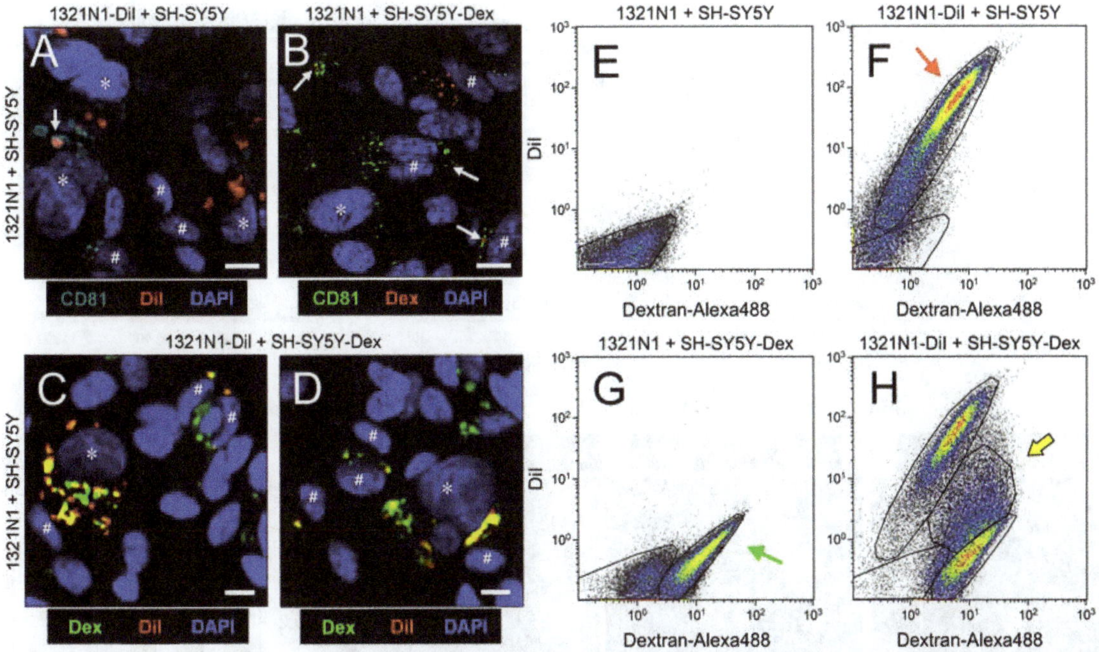

FIGURE 1 | Astrocytes and neurons exchange CD81-positive material. **(A–D)** Single plane confocal microscopy images extracted from Z-stacks obtained from co-cultures of: 1321N1 astrocytes labeled with DiI and unlabeled SHSY5Y neurons **(A)**; unlabeled 1321N1 and SH-SY5Y labeled with Dextran-Alexa 488 **(B)**; 1321N1 labeled with DiI and SH-SY5Y labeled with Dextran-Alexa 488. **(C,D)** Immunocytochemistry with the extracellular vesicle (EV) marker CD81 is shown in **(A,B)**. Arrows point to colocalizing signals. Asterisks and pound signs mark identified nuclei from astrocytes and neurons respectively. N = 20 confocal stacks/condition. Calibration bars: 10 μm. **(E–H)** Flow cytometry analyses plotting the DiI and Dextran-Alexa 488 signals in the different co-culture conditions. The red arrow in **(F)** indicates the DiI-1321N1 population, and the green arrow in **(G)** points to the Dextran-Alexa 488-SHSY5Y population. A double labeled cell population appears when both astrocytic and neuronal cells are labeled (**H**, marked with a yellow arrow).

conditions. ApoD protein is observed in CM-cultured neurons (**Figure 3B**), in agreement with our previous reports showing internalization of exogenously added ApoD in neurons (Pascua-Maestro et al., 2017) and with the results obtained in the Transwell experiments (**Figure 2**). Surprisingly, when CM is separated into EVs and EV-depleted supernatant, ApoD is only observed in neurons after addition of the fraction containing EVs (**Figure 3C**) and no ApoD is obtained after exposure to the EV-depleted supernatant (**Figure 3D**).

Additionally, RT-PCR was performed in order to detect *APOD* mRNA expression in 1321N1 donor astrocytes and SH-SY5Y recipient neurons after 48 h exposure to 1321N1 EVs. While the housekeeping ribosomal gene *RPL18* is present in all samples, *APOD* mRNA was only detected in the donor cells (**Figure 3E**), thus discarding a potential induction of endogenous *APOD* expression in SH-SY5Y neurons upon exposure to 1321N1-derived EVs followed by *de novo* synthesis of ApoD protein.

Characterization of ApoD in Glial EVs: ApoD as a Very Specific Marker of Human Astroglial Exosomes

So far, our results show that 1321N1 astroglia express the EV marker CD81 (**Figure 1A**), that colocalizes with DiI-labeled membranous organelles and can be transferred to neurons (**Figures 2, 3**). Also, MVB can be detected in the cytoplasm of 1321N1 astrocytes by EM (**Figure 4A**). Our previous analysis of intracellular traffic of ApoD (Pascua-Maestro et al., 2017) revealed its presence in the extracellular side of the plasma membrane, and its traffic through the endo-lysosomal and autophagosome compartments. Here, we show by means of immunofluorescence and immunoelectron microscopy that ApoD can also be found both in Lamp2-positive MVBs (**Figure 4B**), and in putative EVs (arrowhead in **Figure 4C**), whose size is in the range of exosomes.

Given the locations of ApoD, would the protein be carried in membrane budding microvesicles (MVs) or in MVB-derived exosomes? When the EV-free medium used to culture cells and the 1321N1-CM collected after 72 h are subjected to NTA (**Figure 4D**), we found that 1321N1 cells secrete several EV populations, absent in the starting culture media, with a group showing a particle size compatible with exosomes (arrow in **Figure 4D**, around 100 nm). Following sucrose gradient fractionation of two independent 1321N1 EV preparations and immunoblot analysis, we uncover that ApoD exclusively partitions in the fractions that contain the known density range for exosomes (1.13–1.20 g/ml; (Salomon et al., 2013; Kharaziha et al., 2015). In the preparation shown (**Figure 4E**), fractions with densities of 1.176 g/ml and 1.232 g/ml are both positive for ApoD and for the exosome marker CD81 (**Figure 4E**). All fractions are negative for other sub-cellular

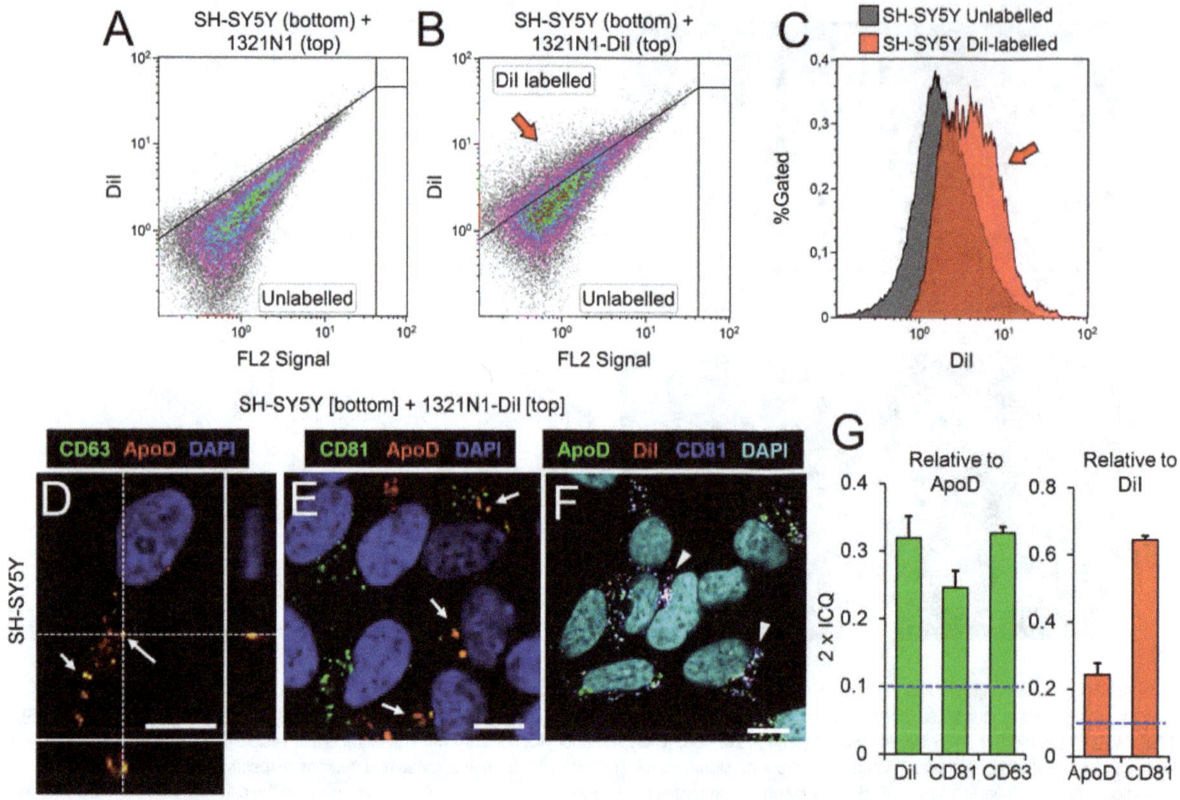

FIGURE 2 | Astrocyte-to-neuron communication is mediated by EVs that carry Apolipoprotein D (ApoD) into neurons. **(A–C)** Flow cytometry analyses of SH-SY5Y cells cultured with 1321N1 cells seeded in a Transwell inset. Astrocytic 1321N1 cells were either unlabeled **(A)** or labeled with DiI. **(B,C)** Dot plots show the existence of a population of DiI-positive SH-SY5Y neurons (arrow in **B**, representing 25.1%) when cultured with labeled 1321N1 astrocytes. The histogram in **(C)** displays the fluorescence increase in DiI-positive neurons (arrow), with median fluorescence increasing from 1.9 to 4.0 (a.u.). **(D–F)** Single plane confocal microscopy images extracted from Z-stacks obtained from unlabeled SH-SY5Y target cells cultured on the lower compartment of a Transwell assay while DiI-labeled 1321N1 donor cells were cultured on the insert. Immunofluorescence with ApoD, CD81 and CD63, and DiI signal are shown with different LUTs to properly display the colocalization of EV markers with ApoD (arrows in **D,E**) or with DiI (arrowheads in F point to triple colocalization DiI-CD81-ApoD). Orthogonal views are shown in **(D)** to visualize the location of vesicular labeling within the cell. *N* = 20 confocal stacks/condition. Calibration bars: 5 μm. **(G)** Average colocalization index (2 × ICQ) referenced either to ApoD signal (green bars) or to DiI signal (red bars) in SH-SY5Y neurons co-cultured in Transwell with DiI-labeled 1321N1 astrocytes. The dotted lines represents the colocalization threshold. Error bars represent SEM (*n* = 20 cells/marker from four independent experiments).

compartment markers (endoplasmic reticulum chaperone BiP; **Figure 4E**). Curiously, the ApoD-containing vesicular fractions present both monomeric and dimeric forms of ApoD (see "Discussion" section). Our results demonstrate that ApoD is specifically enriched in the exosome-containing fractions of 1321N1 astroglial EVs.

ApoD-Containing Exosomes Underlie a Protective Reaction of Glial Cells Against Oxidative Stress and Mediate ApoD-Dependent Neuroprotection

In order to assess whether the presence of ApoD in astrocytic EVs has functional consequences, we tested EV-associated ApoD effect on neuronal viability upon an oxidative insult triggered by the reactive oxygen species (ROS) generator PQ. To address this question we cultured again SH-SY5Y neurons with: (1) EV-free standard media (SM); (2) 1321N1-conditioned media (CM); (3) the EV fraction (EVs) obtained by differential centrifugation of CM; and (4) the EV-depleted supernatant (Sup) of CM.

In the absence of PQ, the exposure of SH-SY5Y neurons to 1321N1 CM or its EVs does not affect their viability (white bars in **Figure 5A**). On the other hand, upon exposure to 2 mM PQ for 2 h (black bars in **Figure 5A**), the decrease observed in SH-SY5Y viability after the OS stimulus is significantly ameliorated after treatment with complete CM or its EV fraction, compared to exposure to PQ in standard medium (SM). Such protection against OS is only partial when the EV-depleted media is used (Sup, black bar, in **Figure 5A**). Since we have demonstrated that ApoD is uptaken by neurons only in EV format (**Figure 3**), these results indicate that a full neuroprotection effect by the 1321N1 secretome can only be achieved when EVs are present in the media. The beneficial effect of EV-associated ApoD is comparable to that obtained with native ApoD purified from human cystic fluid (**Figure 5B**), an effect whose specificity is proven by its reduction when blocking ApoD with a specific antibody.

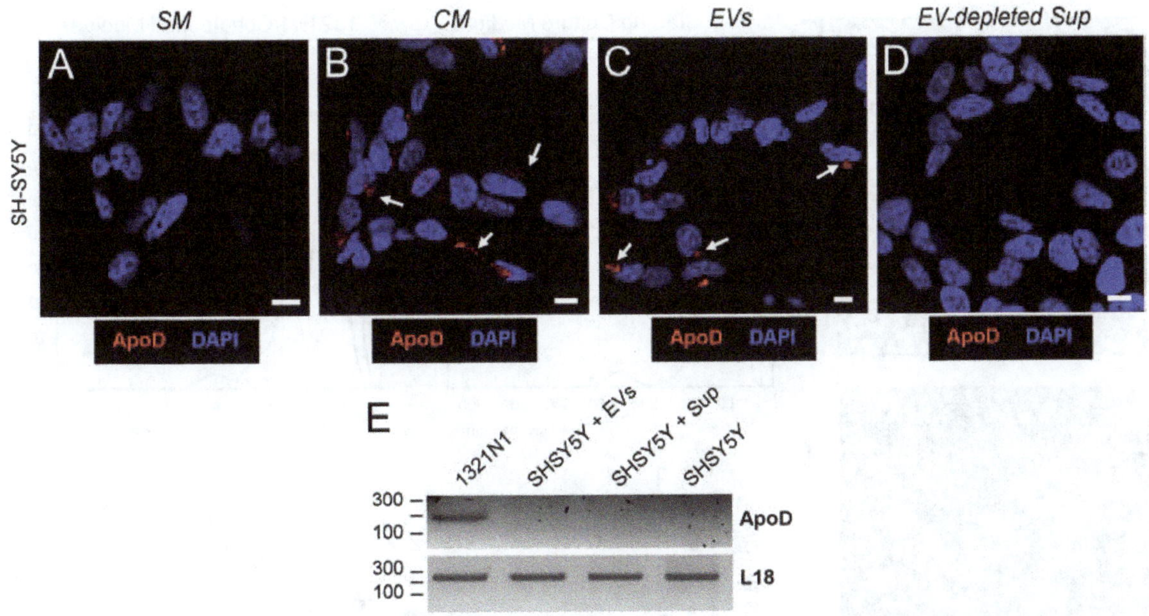

FIGURE 3 | Astrocyte-to-neuron ApoD traffic is exclusively mediated by EVs. **(A–D)** Single plane confocal microscopy images extracted from Z-stacks obtained from SH-SY5Y cells cultured with standard medium (SM; **A**), astrocyte-conditioned medium (CM; **B**), purified astrocyte EVs **(C)**, or EV-depleted astrocyte-derived supernatant, Sup **(D)**. Arrows point to the ApoD vesicular labeling within SH-SY5Y neurons. No signal is detected when SM or EV-depleted Sup is used. Calibration bars: 10 μm. **(E)** RT-PCR analysis of ApoD mRNA expression in the1321N1 donor cells, and in SH-SY5Y differentiated neurons after 48 h exposure to 1321N1-generated EVs. The housekeeping ribosomal gene RPL18 is amplified as control.

In summary, our data demonstrate that a fraction of the ApoD produced by 1321N1 astrocytes is targeted to EVs, and particularly to the fraction displaying exosomal properties. We also show that, surprisingly, it is in this form of cell-cell communication, and not in free soluble form, that ApoD gets internalized by SH-SY5Y neurons, where it is able to protect them from PQ-triggered OS.

A fair amount of data account for the neuroprotective effects of ApoD also on astrocytes themselves (Bajo-Grañeras et al., 2011; Pascua-Maestro et al., 2017). To further contrast this hypothesis and expand the finding to non-immortalized native cells, we used the WT and ApoD-KO mice as experimental model.

First, we performed two additional EV purifications from the culture medium of primary murine cortical astrocytes. Immunoblot analysis (**Figure 6**) demonstrates the presence of ApoD in both the cell homogenate and the EV-enriched fraction from WT primary astrocytes (**Figure 6B**), but not in the ApoD-KO EV preparations (**Figure 6C**), after confirming by EM the presence of EVs in the preparations from both genotypes. As expected, EVs show the markers CD81 and flotillin-1 (also in the whole cell extract) while other subcellular compartment marker (the endoplasmic reticulum chaperon BiP) is absent. Taking into account the starting material for the cell homogenate and the EV-enriched preparations from WT astrocytes (**Figure 6A**), and the relative abundance of ApoD compared with flotillin-1 (**Figure 6B**), we estimate that a significant proportion (around 0.6%) of the ApoD expressed by an astroglial cell is targeted to EVs.

After demonstrating the secretion of ApoD-loaded EVs by primary WT astrocytes, we tested the effect of astrocyte-derived conditioned media on primary astrocytes of WT and ApoD-KO mice exposed to PQ (500 μM, 2 h).

As expected, ApoD-KO astrocytes showed significantly lower viability than WT astrocytes upon exposure to PQ (**Figure 7A**). In both cases, the viability significantly improves after culture with astrocyte-derived conditioned media (collected over a 72 h period), regardless of genotype of the cell originating the conditioned media (**Figure 7B**, gray and black bars). For WT astrocytes, a similar protection effect is attained with media conditioned by either WT or by ApoD-KO cells, which can be explained by the accumulation of various protective factors over time. However, the more vulnerable ApoD-KO astrocytes are significantly better protected when exposed to WT conditioned media (black bar) than when media was conditioned by ApoD-KO astrocytes (gray bar). These results suggest that ApoD, produced by WT astrocytes and present in the extracellular medium, is significantly contributing to protect astrocytes from OS in an autocrine manner.

Together, our results demonstrate that ApoD is present in EVs purified from conditioned media produced by both a human astrocytic cell line and primary murine astrocytes (**Figures 4**, **6**), that ApoD is detected specifically in the exosome-containing fractions of these EVs (**Figure 4**), and that these ApoD-positive EVs become internalized by SH-SY5Y neurons (**Figures 2**, **3**). Moreover, an unexpected result is the absence of detectable ApoD endocytosis into neurons when we use the EV-depleted CM that strongly

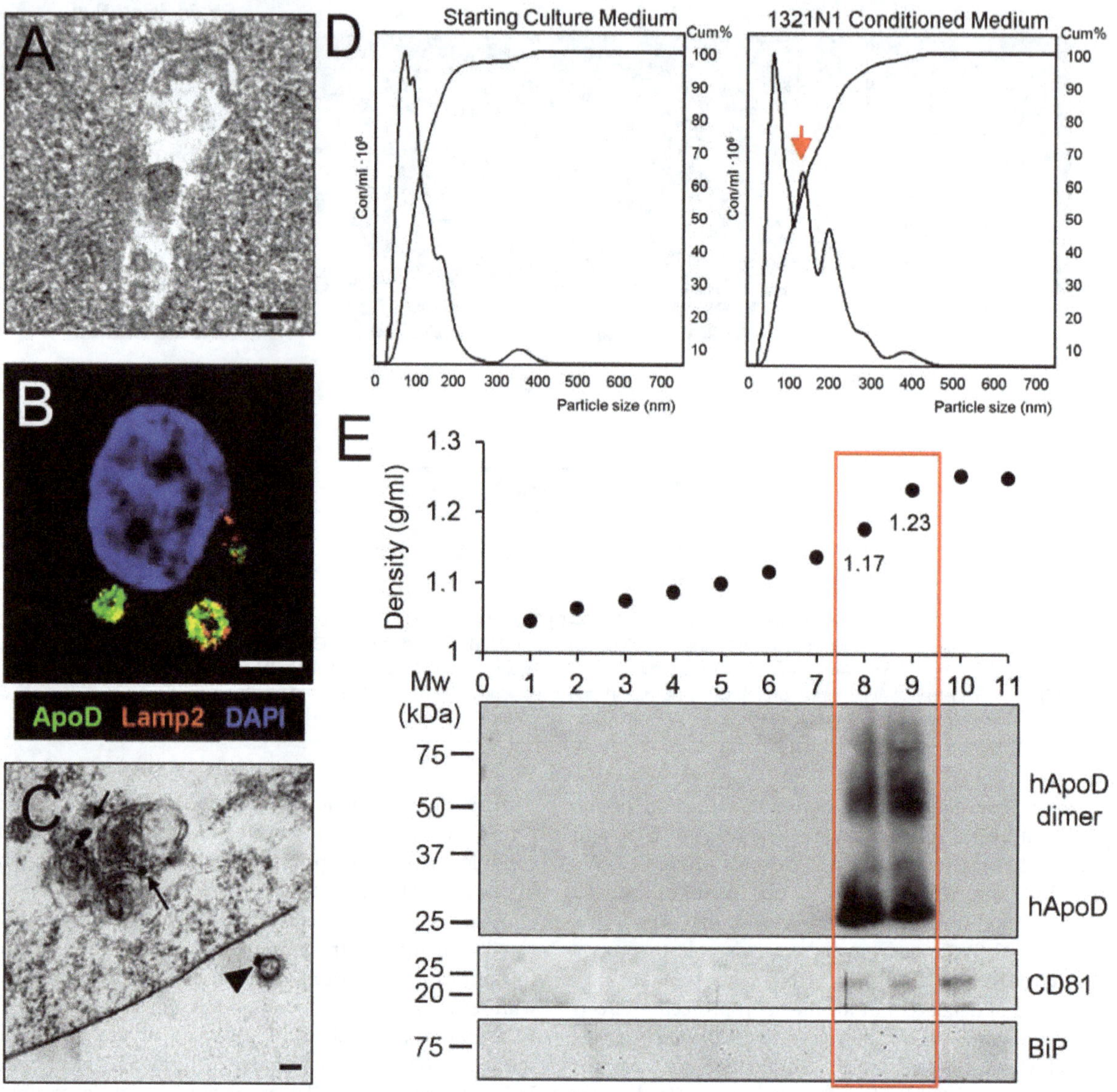

FIGURE 4 | ApoD is specifically found in EV fractions containing astrocyte-derived exosomes. **(A)** Electron microscopy image of a multivesicular body (MVB) in the cytoplasm of a 1321N1 astrocyte. **(B)** Single plane confocal microscopy image extracted from a Z-stack of a 1321N1 astrocyte showing the colocalization of ApoD and Lamp2 in putative MVBs. **(C)** Immunoelectron microscopy image showing ApoD in mature lysosomes of a 1321N1 cell (arrows), and on the external surface of a putative exosome (arrowhead). Calibration bars: **(A,C)**: 100 nm; **(B)**: 5 μm. **(D)** Nanoparticle tracking analysis (NTA) of the starting culture medium or 1321N1-CM shows that 1321N1 astrocytes secrete several EV populations with a group showing particle size compatible with exosomes (red arrow). EV preparations were obtained from two pools of two independent cell culture sets (480 × 10^6 cells/preparation). Particle size: 92 and 97 nm, respectively. Particle concentration: 218 × 10^9 and 222 × 10^9 particles/ml respectively. **(E)** Fractionation of EV preparation from 1321N1 astrocytes by sucrose gradient. The plot shows the fraction density along with the immunoblot analysis of each fraction with ApoD, CD8 and BiP antibodies. Only fractions 8 and 9 are positive for ApoD, while the exosome marker CD81 appears in fractions 8–10.

indicates that the majority of extracellular ApoD produced by 1321N1 astrocytes is associated to EVs and not in a free soluble form, as previously thought. EV-associated ApoD protects both neurons and astrocytes from PQ-induced OS. These results set the stage to study whether we find *in vivo* such an important contribution of exosomes to the ApoD astrocyte-to-neuron traffic both in physiological and pathological situations.

DISCUSSION

Besides a role in cell-cell communication during cellular homeostasis, EVs are shed by cells in response to pathological states (reviewed by Croese and Furlan, 2018; Holm et al., 2018). In the nervous system, glial EVs have been involved both in regulation of neuroinflammation (Dickens et al., 2017; Kumar et al., 2017; Li et al., 2018), and in mechanisms

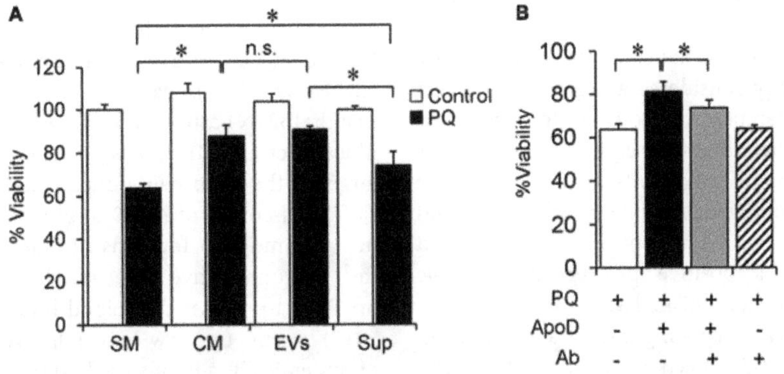

FIGURE 5 | Astroglial EVs promote neuronal survival. **(A)** SH-SY5Y neurons viability in control and oxidative stress (OS) conditions [2 mM paraquat (PQ) for 2 h], measured by the 3-(4,5-dimethylthiazol-2-yl)-2, 5-diphenyltetrazolium bromide (MTT) assay after culture in SM, astrocyte-CM, purified astrocyte EVs, or EV-depleted astrocyte-derived supernatant, Sup. **(B)** Cell viability of PQ-challenged SH-SY5Y neurons (2 mM PQ for 2 h) in the absence or presence of purified native ApoD and/or an equimolar amount of anti-ApoD antibody. Error bars represent SEM ($n = 3$ independent experiments with three technical replicas each). Asterisks represent significant differences ($p < 0.01$) assessed by ANOVA with Holm-Sidak *post hoc* method. (n.s.: non-significant differences) Only the most relevant comparisons are pointed.

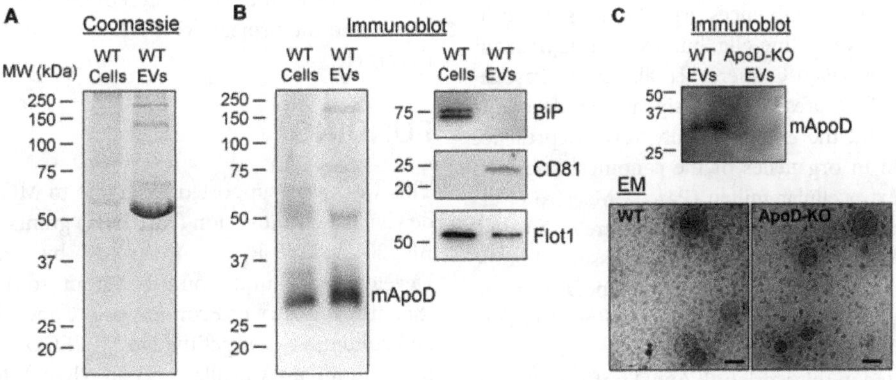

FIGURE 6 | Primary murine astrocytes produce ApoD-positive EVs. **(A)** Coomassie blue staining of whole cell extracts and EV preparation (240 times concentrated, relative to the starting cell culture) from wild-type (WT) primary astrocytes. **(B)** Immunoblot analysis of ApoD, the endoplasmic reticulum marker BiP, and the EV markers CD81 and flotillin-1 in cell lysates and EV preparations from WT primary astrocytes. No signal of BiP is detected in the EV preparation. Intracellular CD81 is not detectable in the cell extract. **(C)** Immunoblot analysis of ApoD in WT and ApoD-knock-out (KO) primary astrocyte EV preparations, confirming the presence of ApoD in WT EVs. Immunoelectron microscopy images of WT and ApoD-KO EVs. Calibration bars: 100 nm.

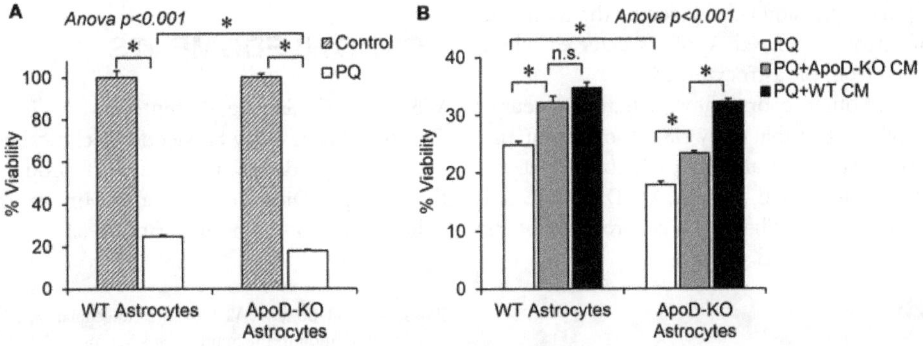

FIGURE 7 | Extracellular ApoD mediates autocrine protection of primary murine astrocytes. **(A)** Percent viability estimated by the MTT assay of WT and ApoD-KO primary astrocytes cultured in SM, in either control or upon an OS challenge with PQ (500 μM, 2 h). ApoD-KO astrocytes are significantly more vulnerable to PQ than WT astrocytes. **(B)** PQ challenge was performed either on SM (white bars), or in astrocyte-CM, either derived from ApoD-KO astrocytes (gray bars) or from WT astrocytes (black bars). Effect of CM on ApoD-KO astrocyte viability is dependent on the genotype of CM origin. Error bars represent SEM ($n = 3$ independent experiments with three technical replicas each). Asterisks point to significant differences ($p < 0.01$) assessed by ANOVA with Holm-Sidak *post hoc* method (n.s.: non-significant differences). Only the most relevant comparisons are pointed.

triggering neuroprotection (Lopez-Verrilli et al., 2013; Guitart et al., 2016).

The production of ROS and a concomitant inflammatory response have been classically considered a negative side-effect of tissue damage that hampers nervous system recovery upon aging and neurodegeneration. Consequently, great efforts have been made to identify antioxidants that can mediate neuroprotection through improvement of neuronal survival and axonal regeneration. However, a recent report has demonstrated that ROS can also play a positive pro-regenerative role upon neural damage by a mechanism based on glia-neuron EV-mediated Nox2-PI3K–pAkt signaling (Hervera et al., 2018). How can a cell control the side effects of ROS, and the levels that can be managed without tilting the equilibrium towards cell-death?

The Lipocalin ApoD has been demonstrated to be a neuroprotectant by controlling the levels of lipid peroxides generated by ROS accumulation with aging or pathological conditions (Ganfornina et al., 2008; Li et al., 2015; Sanchez et al., 2015; Pascua-Maestro et al., 2017). The neuroprotection exerted by ApoD not only influences ApoD-expressing cells such as astrocytes and myelinating glia, but also affects neurons in a paracrine manner (Bajo-Grañeras et al., 2011; Pascua-Maestro et al., 2017). The presence of a signal peptide in the unprocessed protein and the experimentally verified presence of the mature protein in organelles of the canonical secretion pathway and in the extracellular milieu (Pascua-Maestro et al., 2017), result in the annotation of ApoD as a secreted protein (UniProtKB-P51910/P05090). This property was assumed in the interpretation of our previous studies reporting ApoD traffic in astrocytes and neurons under control or OS conditions (Pascua-Maestro et al., 2017).

The results presented in this work link ApoD traffic to the EV compartment of astrocytes, where it appears very specifically in the exosomal subtype of EVs, as determined by the co-expression of classical markers such as CD81 (Tkach et al., 2018). More importantly, the neuroprotective effect that ApoD exerts upon OS-challenged neurons or astrocytes must be entirely based on the protein present in the EVs supplied by reactive astrocytes, since no neuronal ApoD expression is triggered by the EVs, and no incorporation of astrocyte-derived ApoD is detected when EVs have been removed from the astrocyte-CM.

This result agrees with other reports showing that non-neural cells exposed to ROS release EVs that carry OS response proteins and antioxidants (Saeed-Zidane et al., 2017; Chettimada et al., 2018). The fact that EV-associated human ApoD is detected both as monomers and dimers (**Figure 4**), is a readout of its antioxidant activity, since it is known that a consequence of its lipid reducing activity is the formation of stable dimers (Bhatia et al., 2012) that accumulate in advanced stages of Alzheimer's disease patients (Bhatia et al., 2013). Since we know that the1321N1 astrocytic cell line has a basal level of OS (Pascua-Maestro et al., 2017), it is not surprising that they are already targeting the redox pair reduced/oxidized-ApoD to exosomes.

The discovery of ApoD in glia-derived EVs, and particularly in exosome-like fractions, reframes our understanding of the neuroprotective role of this Lipocalin. The capability of EVs to cross the blood-brain barrier (Krämer-Albers, 2017) opens up new research avenues to explore the use of systemically administered ApoD-positive exosomes to treat neurodegenerative diseases.

AUTHOR CONTRIBUTIONS

RP-M, MG, JF-P and DS conceived and designed the project. RP-M, EG, CL and MG designed and performed the experiments. RP, EG, JF-P and DS analyzed the data. DS, MG and JF-P supervised the project. RP-M, EG, CL, JF-P, MG and DS wrote the article.

FUNDING

This work was supported by grants to MG and DS [Ministerio de Ciencia e Innovación (MICINN) grants BFU2011-23978 and BFU2015-68149-R, co-financed by European Regional Development Fund], and by grant to JF-P SAF2015-66312 (Spanish Ministry of Economy and Competitiveness, Ministerio de Economía y Competitividad MINECO). RP-M was supported by a Junta de Castilla y León (JCyL) fellowship to young researchers (call#EDU/1883/2013), financed by the European Social Fund, Operational Programme for Castilla y León and managed by Consejería de Educación (JCyL) and by 1st GEIVEX mobility fellowship. The funders had no role in study design, data collection and analysis, decision to publish, or preparation of the manuscript.

ACKNOWLEDGMENTS

We thank C. Sánchez-Vicente and Y. Noriega at the IBGM Confocal Microscopy Service for technical assistance. C. Pérez-Segurado provided technical support throughout the project. We thank Sergio Diez-Hermano and Miriam Corraliza-Gómez for helpful discussions and inspiring ideas.

REFERENCES

Alvarez-Erviti, L., Seow, Y., Yin, H., Betts, C., Lakhal, S., and Wood, M. J. (2011). Delivery of siRNA to the mouse brain by systemic injection of targeted exosomes. *Nat. Biotechnol.* 29, 341–345. doi: 10.1038/nbt.1807

Bajo-Grañeras, R., Ganfornina, M. D., Martín-Tejedor, E., and Sanchez, D. (2011). Apolipoprotein D mediates autocrine protection of astrocytes and controls their reactivity level, contributing to the functional maintenance of paraquat-challenged dopaminergic systems. *Glia* 59, 1551–1566. doi: 10.1002/glia.21200

Basso, M., and Bonetto, V. (2016). Extracellular vesicles and a novel form of communication in the brain. *Front. Neurosci.* 10:127. doi: 10.3389/fnins.2016.00127

Bhatia, S., Jenner, A. M., Li, H., Ruberu, K., Spiro, A. S., Shepherd, C. E., et al. (2013). Increased apolipoprotein D dimer formation in Alzheimer's disease hippocampus is associated with lipid conjugated diene levels. *J. Alzheimers Dis.* 35, 475–486. doi: 10.3233/JAD-122278

Bhatia, S., Knoch, B., Wong, J., Kim, W. S., Else, P. L., Oakley, A. J., et al. (2012). Selective reduction of hydroperoxyeicosatetraenoic acids to their hydroxy derivatives by apolipoprotein D: implications for lipid antioxidant activity and Alzheimer's disease. *Biochem. J.* 442, 713–721. doi: 10.1042/BJ20111166

Cheow, E. S., Cheng, W. C., Lee, C. N., de Kleijn, D., Sorokin, V., and Sze, S. K. (2016). Plasma-derived extracellular vesicles contain predictive biomarkers and potential therapeutic targets for myocardial ischemic (MI) injury. *Mol. Cell. Proteomics* 15, 2628–2640. doi: 10.1074/mcp.M115.055731

Chettimada, S., Lorenz, D. R., Misra, V., Dillon, S. T., Reeves, R. K., Manickam, C., et al. (2018). Exosome markers associated with immune activation and oxidative stress in HIV patients on antiretroviral therapy. *Sci. Rep.* 8:7227. doi: 10.1038/s41598-018-25515-4

Croese, T., and Furlan, R. (2018). Extracellular vesicles in neurodegenerative diseases. *Mol. Aspects Med.* 60, 52–61. doi: 10.1016/j.mam.2017.11.006

Dassati, S., Waldner, A., and Schweigreiter, R. (2014). Apolipoprotein D takes center stage in the stress response of the aging and degenerative brain. *Neurobiol. Aging* 35, 1632–1642. doi: 10.1016/j.neurobiolaging.2014.01.148

Dickens, A. M., Tovar-Y-Romo, L. B., Yoo, S. W., Trout, A. L., Bae, M., Kanmogne, M., et al. (2017). Astrocyte-shed extracellular vesicles regulate the peripheral leukocyte response to inflammatory brain lesions. *Sci. Signal.* 10:eaai7696. doi: 10.1126/scisignal.aai7696

Dragovic, R. A., Gardiner, C., Brooks, A. S., Tannetta, D. S., Ferguson, D. J., Hole, P., et al. (2011). Sizing and phenotyping of cellular vesicles using Nanoparticle Tracking Analysis. *Nanomedicine* 7, 780–788. doi: 10.1016/j.nano.2011.04.003

Escola, J. M., Kleijmeer, M. J., Stoorvogel, W., Griffith, J. M., Yoshie, O., and Geuze, H. J. (1998). Selective enrichment of tetraspan proteins on the internal vesicles of multivesicular endosomes and on exosomes secreted by human B-lymphocytes. *J. Biol. Chem.* 273, 20121–20127. doi: 10.1074/jbc.273.32.20121

Frühbeis, C., Fröhlich, D., Kuo, W. P., Amphornrat, J., Thilemann, S., Saab, A. S., et al. (2013a). Neurotransmitter-triggered transfer of exosomes mediates oligodendrocyte-neuron communication. *PLoS Biol.* 11:e1001604. doi: 10.1371/journal.pbio.1001604

Frühbeis, C., Fröhlich, D., Kuo, W. P., and Krämer-Albers, E. M. (2013b). Extracellular vesicles as mediators of neuron-glia communication. *Front. Cell. Neurosci.* 7:182. doi: 10.3389/fncel.2013.00182

Ganfornina, M. D., Do Carmo, S., Lora, J. M., Torres-Schumann, S., Vogel, M., Allhorn, M., et al. (2008). Apolipoprotein D is involved in the mechanisms regulating protection from oxidative stress. *Aging Cell* 7, 506–515. doi: 10.1111/j.1474-9726.2008.00395.x

Ganfornina, M. D., Do Carmo, S., Martinez, E., Tolivia, J., Navarro, A., Rassart, E., et al. (2010). ApoD, a glia-derived apolipoprotein, is required for peripheral nerve functional integrity and a timely response to injury. *Glia* 58, 1320–1334. doi: 10.1002/glia.21010

García-Mateo, N., Ganfornina, M. D., Montero, O., Gijón, M. A., Murphy, R. C., and Sanchez, D. (2014). Schwann cell-derived Apolipoprotein D controls the dynamics of post-injury myelin recognition and degradation. *Front. Cell. Neurosci.* 8:374. doi: 10.3389/fncel.2014.00374

Guitart, K., Loers, G., Buck, F., Bork, U., Schachner, M., and Kleene, R. (2016). Improvement of neuronal cell survival by astrocyte-derived exosomes under hypoxic and ischemic conditions depends on prion protein. *Glia* 64, 896–910. doi: 10.1002/glia.22963

György, B., Szabó, T. G., Pásztói, M., Pál, Z., Misják, P., Aradi, B., et al. (2011). Membrane vesicles, current state-of-the-art: emerging role of extracellular vesicles. *Cell. Mol. Life Sci.* 68, 2667–2688. doi: 10.1007/s00018-011-0689-3

Hervera, A., De Virgiliis, F., Palmisano, I., Zhou, L., Tantardini, E., Kong, G., et al. (2018). Reactive oxygen species regulate axonal regeneration through the release of exosomal NADPH oxidase 2 complexes into injured axons. *Nat. Cell Biol.* 20, 307–319. doi: 10.1038/s41556-018-0039-x

Holm, M. M., Kaiser, J., and Schwab, M. E. (2018). Extracellular vesicles: multimodal envoys in neural maintenance and repair. *Trends Neurosci.* 41, 360–372. doi: 10.1016/j.tins.2018.03.006

Kalra, H., Simpson, R. J., Ji, H., Aikawa, E., Altevogt, P., Askenase, P., et al. (2012). Vesiclepedia: a compendium for extracellular vesicles with continuous community annotation. *PLoS Biol.* 10:e1001450. doi: 10.1371/journal.pbio.1001450

Keerthikumar, S., Chisanga, D., Ariyaratne, D., Al Saffar, H., Anand, S., Zhao, K., et al. (2015). ExoCarta: a web-based compendium of exosomal cargo. *J. Mol. Biol.* 428, 688–692. doi: 10.1016/j.jmb.2015.09.019

Kharaziha, P., Chioureas, D., Rutishauser, D., Baltatzis, G., Lennartsson, L., Fonseca, P., et al. (2015). Molecular profiling of prostate cancer derived exosomes may reveal a predictive signature for response to docetaxel. *Oncotarget* 6, 21740–21754. doi: 10.18632/oncotarget.3226

Kim, D. K., Lee, J., Kim, S. R., Choi, D. S., Yoon, Y. J., Kim, J. H., et al. (2015). EVpedia: a community web portal for extracellular vesicles research. *Bioinformatics* 31, 933–939. doi: 10.1093/bioinformatics/btu741

Krämer-Albers, E. M. (2017). Ticket to ride: targeting proteins to exosomes for brain delivery. *Mol. Ther.* 25, 1264–1266. doi: 10.1016/j.ymthe.2017.05.001

Kumar, A., Stoica, B. A., Loane, D. J., Yang, M., Abulwerdi, G., Khan, N., et al. (2017). Microglial-derived microparticles mediate neuroinflammation after traumatic brain injury. *J. Neuroinflammation* 14:47. doi: 10.1186/s12974-017-0819-4

Li, Q., Lau, A., Morris, T. J., Guo, L., Fordyce, C. B., and Stanley, E. F. (2004). A syntaxin 1, Gα_o, and N-type calcium channel complex at a presynaptic nerve terminal: analysis by quantitative immunocolocalization. *J. Neurosci.* 24, 4070–4081. doi: 10.1523/JNEUROSCI.0346-04.2004

Li, H., Ruberu, K., Muñoz, S. S., Jenner, A. M., Spiro, A., Zhao, H., et al. (2015). Apolipoprotein D modulates amyloid pathology in APP/PS1 Alzheimer's disease mice. *Neurobiol. Aging* 36, 1820–1833. doi: 10.1016/j.neurobiolaging.2015.02.010

Li, J. J., Wang, B., Kodali, M. C., Chen, C., Kim, E., Patters, B. J., et al. (2018). *In vivo* evidence for the contribution of peripheral circulating inflammatory exosomes to neuroinflammation. *J. Neuroinflammation* 15:8. doi: 10.1186/s12974-017-1038-8

Loerch, P. M., Lu, T., Dakin, K. A., Vann, J. M., Isaacs, A., Geula, C., et al. (2008). Evolution of the aging brain transcriptome and synaptic regulation. *PLoS One* 3:e3329. doi: 10.1371/journal.pone.0003329

Lopez-Verrilli, M. A., Picou, F., and Court, F. A. (2013). Schwann cell-derived exosomes enhance axonal regeneration in the peripheral nervous system. *Glia* 61, 1795–1806. doi: 10.1002/glia.22558

Müller, G. (2012). Microvesicles/exosomes as potential novel biomarkers of metabolic diseases. *Diabetes Metab. Syndr. Obes.* 5, 247–282. doi: 10.2147/DMSO.S32923

Nakamura, K., Watakabe, A., Hioki, H., Fujiyama, F., Tanaka, Y., Yamamori, T., et al. (2007). Transiently increased colocalization of vesicular glutamate transporters 1 and 2 at single axon terminals during postnatal development of mouse neocortex: a quantitative analysis with correlation coefficient. *Eur. J. Neurosci.* 26, 3054–3067. doi: 10.1111/j.1460-9568.2007.05868.x

Navarro, J. A., Ohmann, E., Sanchez, D., Botella, J. A., Liebisch, G., Moltó, M. D., et al. (2010). Altered lipid metabolism in a *Drosophila* model of Friedreich's ataxia. *Hum. Mol. Genet.* 19, 2828–2840. doi: 10.1093/hmg/ddq183

Pandya, R. S., Zhu, H., Li, W., Bowser, R., Friedlander, R. M., and Wang, X. (2013). Therapeutic neuroprotective agents for amyotrophic lateral sclerosis. *Cell. Mol. Life Sci.* 70, 4729–4745. doi: 10.1007/s00018-013-1415-0

Pascua-Maestro, R., Corraliza-Gomez, M., Diez-Hermano, S., Perez-Segurado, C., Ganfornina, M. D., and Sanchez, D. (2018). The MTT-formazan assay: complementary technical approaches and *in vivo* validation in *Drosophila* larvae. *Acta Histochem.* 120, 179–186. doi: 10.1016/j.acthis.2018.01.006

Pascua-Maestro, R., Diez-Hermano, S., Lillo, C., Ganfornina, M. D., and Sanchez, D. (2017). Protecting cells by protecting their vulnerable lysosomes: identification of a new mechanism for preserving lysosomal functional integrity upon oxidative stress. *PLoS Genet.* 13:e1006603. doi: 10.1371/journal.pgen.1006603

Perdomo, G., and Henry Dong, H. (2009). Apolipoprotein D in lipid metabolism and its functional implication in atherosclerosis and aging. *Aging* 1, 17–27. doi: 10.18632/aging.100004

Przybycien-Szymanska, M. M., Yang, Y., and Ashley, W. W. (2016). Microparticle derived proteins as potential biomarkers for cerebral vasospasm post subarachnoid hemorrhage. A preliminary study. *Clin. Neurol. Neurosurg.* 141, 48–55. doi: 10.1016/j.clineuro.2015.12.012

Reindl, M., Knipping, G., Wicher, I., Dilitz, E., Egg, R., Deisenhammer, F., et al. (2001). Increased intrathecal production of apolipoprotein D in multiple sclerosis. *J. Neuroimmunol.* 119, 327–332. doi: 10.1016/s0165-5728(01)00378-2

Ridder, K., Keller, S., Dams, M., Rupp, A.-K., Schlaudraff, J., Del Turco, D., et al. (2014). Extracellular vesicle-mediated transfer of genetic information between the hematopoietic system and the brain in response to inflammation. *PLoS Biol.* 12:e1001874. doi: 10.1371/journal.pbio.1001874

Rufino-Ramos, D., Albuquerque, P. R., Carmona, V., Perfeito, R., Nobre, R. J., and Pereira de Almeida, L. (2017). Extracellular vesicles: novel promising delivery systems for therapy of brain diseases. *J. Control. Release* 262, 247–258. doi: 10.1016/j.jconrel.2017.07.001

Ruiz, M., Ganfornina, M. D., Correnti, C., Strong, R. K., and Sanchez, D. (2013). Ligand binding-dependent functions of the lipocalin NLaz: an *in vivo* study in *Drosophila*. *FASEB J.* 28, 1555–1567. doi: 10.1096/fj.13-240556

Saeed-Zidane, M., Linden, L., Salilew-Wondim, D., Held, E., Neuhoff, C., Tholen, E., et al. (2017). Cellular and exosome mediated molecular defense mechanism in bovine granulosa cells exposed to oxidative stress. *PLoS One* 12:e0187569. doi: 10.1371/journal.pone.0187569

Salomon, C., Kobayashi, M., Ashman, K., Sobrevia, L., Mitchell, M. D., and Rice, G. E. (2013). Hypoxia-induced changes in the bioactivity of cytotrophoblast-derived exosomes. *PLoS One* 8:e79636. doi: 10.1371/journal.pone.0079636

Sanchez, D., Bajo-Grañeras, R., Del Caño-Espinel, M., Garcia-Centeno, R., Garcia-Mateo, N., Pascua-Maestro, R., et al. (2015). Aging without Apolipoprotein D: molecular and cellular modifications in the hippocampus and cortex. *Exp. Gerontol.* 67, 19–47. doi: 10.1016/j.exger.2015.04.003

Sánchez, D., Ganfornina, M. D., and Martínez, S. (2002). Expression pattern of the lipocalin apolipoprotein D during mouse embryogenesis. *Mech. Dev.* 110, 225–229. doi: 10.1016/s0925-4773(01)00578-0

Spencer, B., Verma, I., Desplats, P., Morvinski, D., Rockenstein, E., Adame, A., et al. (2014). A neuroprotective brain-penetrating endopeptidase fusion protein ameliorates Alzheimer disease pathology and restores neurogenesis. *J. Biol. Chem.* 289, 17917–17931. doi: 10.1074/jbc.M114.557439

Suresh, S., Yan, Z., Patel, R. C., Patel, Y. C., and Patel, S. C. (1998). Cellular cholesterol storage in the Niemann-Pick disease type C mouse is associated with increased expression and defective processing of apolipoprotein D. *J. Neurochem.* 70, 242–251. doi: 10.1046/j.1471-4159.1998.70010242.x

Taylor, D. D. (2015). Isolation and molecular characterization of extracellular vesicles. *Methods* 87, 1–2. doi: 10.1016/j.ymeth.2015.08.006

Tkach, M., Kowal, J., and Théry, C. (2018). Why the need and how to approach the functional diversity of extracellular vesicles. *Philos. Trans. R. Soc. Lond. B Biol. Sci.* 373:20160479. doi: 10.1098/rstb.2016.0479

Valadi, H., Ekstrom, K., Bossios, A., Sjostrand, M., Lee, J. J., and Lötvall, J. O. (2007). Exosome-mediated transfer of mRNAs and microRNAs is a novel mechanism of genetic exchange between cells. *Nat. Cell Biol.* 9, 654–659. doi: 10.1038/ncb1596

4

Sphingolipids as Emerging Mediators in Retina Degeneration

*M. Victoria Simón, Facundo H. Prado Spalm, Marcela S. Vera and Nora P. Rotstein**

Instituto de Investigaciones Bioquímicas de Bahía Blanca (INIBIBB), Departamento De Biología, Bioquímica y Farmacia, Universidad Nacional del Sur (UNS), Argentine National Research Council (CONICET), Bahía Blanca, Argentina

Correspondence:
Nora P. Rotstein
inrotste@criba.edu.ar

The sphingolipids ceramide (Cer), sphingosine-1-phosphate (S1P), sphingosine (Sph), and ceramide-1-phosphate (C1P) are key signaling molecules that regulate major cellular functions. Their roles in the retina have gained increasing attention during the last decade since they emerge as mediators of proliferation, survival, migration, neovascularization, inflammation and death in retina cells. As exacerbation of these processes is central to retina degenerative diseases, they appear as crucial players in their progression. This review analyzes the functions of these sphingolipids in retina cell types and their possible pathological roles. Cer appears as a key arbitrator in diverse retinal pathologies; it promotes inflammation in endothelial and retina pigment epithelium (RPE) cells and its increase is a common feature in photoreceptor death *in vitro* and in animal models of retina degeneration; noteworthy, inhibiting Cer synthesis preserves photoreceptor viability and functionality. In turn, S1P acts as a double edge sword in the retina. It is essential for retina development, promoting the survival of photoreceptors and ganglion cells and regulating proliferation and differentiation of photoreceptor progenitors. However, S1P has also deleterious effects, stimulating migration of Müller glial cells, angiogenesis and fibrosis, contributing to the inflammatory scenario of proliferative retinopathies and age related macular degeneration (AMD). C1P, as S1P, promotes photoreceptor survival and differentiation. Collectively, the expanding role for these sphingolipids in the regulation of critical processes in retina cell types and in their dysregulation in retina degenerations makes them attractive targets for treating these diseases.

Keywords: ceramide, sphingosine-1-phosphate, sphingosine, ceramide-1-phosphate, photoreceptor, glia, pigmented epithelium

---

Abbreviations: AMD, age related macular degeneration; C1P, ceramide-1-phosphate; Cer, ceramide; CerK, ceramide kinase; CerKL, Cer kinase-like; CerS, Cer synthase; CERT, Cer transport protein; DAMP, damage associated molecular pattern; DHA, docosahexaenoic acid; DHCer, dihydroceramide; ER, endoplasmic reticulum; GDNF, glial derived neurotrophic factor; GlucoCer, glucosylceramide; OS, outer segments; PARP1, poly ADP-ribose-polymerase 1; PUFA, polyunsaturated fatty acids; ROS, reactive oxygen species; RPE, retinal pigment epithelium; S1P, sphingosine-1-phosphate; S1PR, S1P receptor; SM, sphingomyelin; SMase, sphingomyelinase; Sph, sphingosine; SphK, sphingosine kinase; SPP, S1P phosphatases; SPT, serine palmitoyltransferase; TNF, tumor necrosis factor; VLCPUFA, very long chain polyunsaturated fatty acids.

INTRODUCTION

Sphingolipids entered the group of Bioactive Lipids about three decades ago; however, they are still regarded by many as newcomers, less familiar than the phosphatidylinositol phosphates, prostaglandins or leukotrienes. Yet, the overwhelming amount of literature accumulated evidences that simple sphingolipids such as Cer, Sph, and their phosphorylated derivatives, S1P and C1P (**Figure 1**) have taken centre stage in controlling normal and pathological cellular processes throughout the organism.

First identified in the brain by Thudichum in the late 19th century, for virtually another century their functions remained as enigmatic as the Sphinx their name honors. Being lipid molecules, they were considered as ubiquitous membrane components both in animal and plant cells for several decades. Even just as such, they have multiple and relevant roles. They are crucial constituents of lipid rafts and regulate their formation and expansion, essential for building signaling platforms (Grassme et al., 2001); they are also critical for receptor function, membrane conductance and cell–cell interactions, and play key roles in pathogen internalization (Huwiler et al., 2000; Gulbins and Kolesnick, 2003; Hannun and Luberto, 2004). The pioneer work from both Hannun and Kolesnick laboratories three decades ago added an additional dimension to their biological relevance; the groundbreaking findings that Sph inhibits protein kinase C and Cer is a "potential second messenger" in the signaling cascade activated by TNF-α provided the first data as to their role as bioactive lipids (Hannun et al., 1986; Kolesnick, 1987; Dressler et al., 1992; Obeid et al., 1993). Sph and Cer were then established to inhibit cell growth and promote cell death upon different cell stressors. The family of bioactive sphingolipids gained in complexity when their phosphorylated counterparts, S1P and C1P were shown to control the opposing processes, proliferation and cell survival. The sphingolipid family also includes GlucoCer, lactosylceramide, several gangliosides and DHCer.

These bioactive lipids respond to a diversity of cell stimuli by modifying their intracellular levels, thus regulating multiple signaling pathways that finally induce major changes in cell fate. Their roles have strikingly extended to include virtually every aspect of cell biology, from cell cycle, differentiation, endosome and exosome formation, adhesion and migration to angiogenesis, immune response, inflammation and cell death, including autophagy and apoptosis. Recent advances have revealed that sphingolipid mediators play important roles in human disease.

This Review focuses on the functions played by simple sphingolipids in the retina during development and particularly in the onset of retina pathologies. Lipids have long been known to be essential for maintaining both the structure and functionality of the visual system. Docosahexaenoic acid (DHA) has been shown to promote photoreceptor survival and differentiation, and docosanoids, such as Neuroprotectin D1, and elovanoids have relevant neuroprotective roles in the retina (Rotstein et al., 1996, 1997; Jun et al., 2017; Bazan, 2018). Conversely, mutations of lipid metabolizing proteins and chronic misregulation of retinal lipid metabolism have been linked to retinal degeneration (Fliesler and Bretillon, 2010; Friedman et al., 2010; Yu et al., 2011). During the last decade, understanding on the relevance of lipids in the retina has expanded to reveal the involvement of sphingolipids in numerous ocular diseases. Here, we briefly present the structural characteristics and metabolism of sphingolipids and a concise description of the physiological and pathophysiological roles of simple sphingolipids as Cer, Sph, S1P, C1P, and DHCer. We then focus on the information that points to both their deleterious and protective functions in the retina and in retina pathologies, supporting the emerging roles of sphingolipids as novel mediators in retina degenerative diseases.

Structure and Metabolism of Sphingolipids

The sphingolipid family encompasses a huge diversity of molecular species that place them among the major lipid classes in eukaryotic cells. Sph, a straight, long chain (18–20 carbon atoms) aminoalcohol, is the common backbone shared by all these species (**Figure 1**). Attachment of a fatty acid to Sph through an amide bond gives rise to Cer, the central molecule in sphingolipid metabolism (Fahy et al., 2005). Further attachment of hundreds of diverse headgroups at the C-1 position of Cer originates the more complex sphingolipids (**Figure 1**). Taking into account than in addition to these huge number of headgroups, sphingolipids are formed by at least sixty different long-chain bases and dozens of fatty acids varying from twelve to over thirty carbons in length, the number of sphingolipid molecular species is likely in the tens of thousands (Merrill et al., 1993). If we add this up to their complex metabolism, and their ability to interconvert upon different and even opposing cell stimuli, we can start to grasp their extraordinary flexibility for modulating an ample range of cell responses.

A key to the multiplicity and diversity of the signaling roles of sphingolipids is in their intricate and highly interconnected metabolism, their constant cross-conversions that modify their levels upon changes in the environment (**Figure 2**). Cer is the central hub among these metabolic pathways and can be synthesized by different pathways, *de novo* synthesis, degradation of sphingomyelin (*sphingomyelinase pathway*) and recycling of Sph and complex sphingolipids (*salvage pathway*). *De novo* synthesis begins in the ER (Mandon et al., 1992) with the condensation of L-serine and palmitoyl CoA, catalyzed by SPT; the resulting 3-ketosphinganine is reduced to sphinganine, which is amino-acylated with a chain of 14 to 32 carbons to form diverse DHCer species; finally, the insertion of a *trans* double bond at the C4 position of the sphingoid base backbone by DHCer desaturase gives rise to Cer. SPT, a heteromeric complex, is responsible for opening the entrance to the sphingolipid network. Interestingly, recent evidence has uncovered that subunit mutations causing hereditary sensory and autonomic neuropathy type 1 (HSAN1) shift SPT preference to use alanine and glycine instead of serine (Penno et al., 2010; Bode et al., 2016). This gives rise to a class of atypical 1-deoxysphingolipids, such as deoxy(dihydro)ceramides and 1-deoxysphingosine, shown to induce cell death in various cell types. When elevated, as in HSAN1, they are neurotoxic and contribute to sensory and autonomic neuropathies affecting both cytoskeletal stability, NMDA receptor signaling and membrane

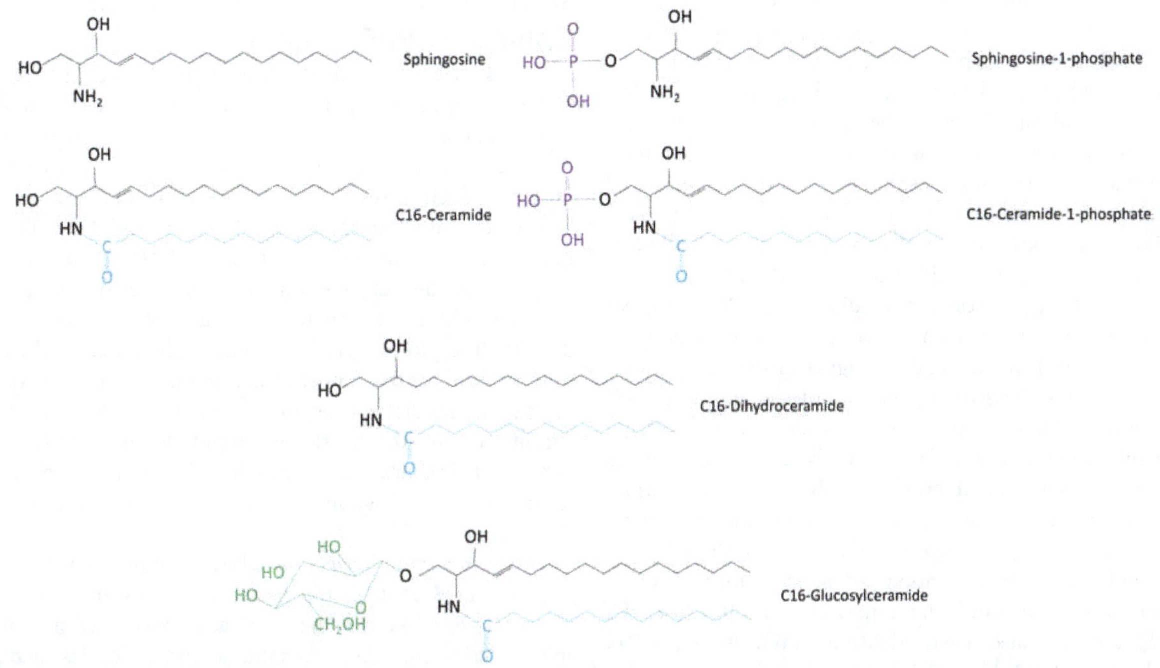

FIGURE 1 | Chemical structures of sphingolipid molecules. The structures of different sphingolipid types are shown. All sphingolipids share a sphingosine backbone (black). This sphingoid backbone is amide-linked to a fatty acid moiety (blue).

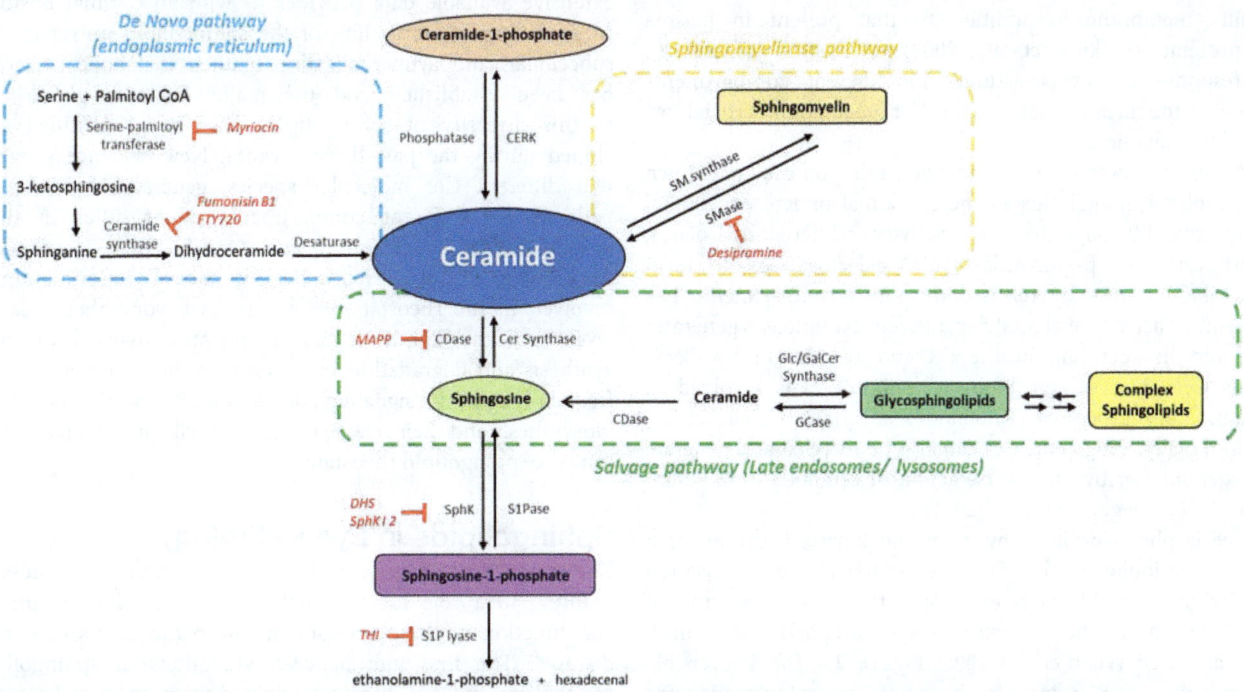

FIGURE 2 | The sphingolipid network: metabolic interconnection between bioactive sphingolipids. Ceramide, the central hub of sphingolipid metabolism, is synthesized by the *de novo* pathway (light blue), from serine and palmitoyl CoA, by the sphingomyelinase pathway, i.e., through hydrolysis of sphingomyelin mediated by sphingomyelinases (SMase) (orange) or by the salvage pathway (green). Ceramide can then be phosphorylated to generate Ceramide-1-phosphate and/or deacylated to form sphingosine, which is then phosphorylated to generate sphingosine-1-phosphate (S1P). The catabolism of S1P mediated by S1P lyase provides the only exit route from the sphingolipid network. CDase, ceramidase; CERK, ceramide kinase; GCase, glucosylceramidase; SMase, sphingomyelinase; SM synthase, sphingomyelin synthase; SphK, sphingosine kinase; SPPase, sphingosine phosphate phosphatase. The inhibitors mentioned in this Review are indicated in red.

properties (Jiménez-Rojo et al., 2014; Güntert et al., 2016). SPT can also change its selectivity for palmitate, using myristate or stearate as substrates (Hornemann et al., 2009; Harmon et al., 2013), further increasing the diversity of sphingolipid molecules.

The newly synthesized Cer can be glycosylated by GlucoCer synthase on the cytoplasmic surface of the Golgi, to render GlucoCer, the precursor of glycosphingolipids, or galactosylated by galactosyl Ceramide synthase in the ER (**Figure 2**; Raas-Rothschild et al., 2004). It can also receive a phosphocholine head group from phosphatidylcholine and thus generate sphingomyelin (SM), a reaction mediated by SM synthases (Tafesse et al., 2006). In turn, these complex sphingolipids can generate Cer through basal or signal-mediated catabolic pathways. The hydrolysis of the phosphodiester bonds in SM, catalyzed by at least five different SMases, renders Cer through the so-called *sphingomyelinase pathway* (**Figure 2**). These enzymes present several isoforms differing in subcellular localization, optimal pH range and cation dependence. A prominent example is neutral SMase; a Mg^{2+} -dependent form is localized in the plasma membrane whereas a cation-independent form is found in cytosol (Marchesini and Hannun, 2004); a mitochondrial neutral SMase has also been identified (Wu et al., 2010; Rajagopalan et al., 2015). The acid SMase gene can also generate, through differential trafficking, a cation-independent acid SMase, found in the endosomal-lysosomal compartment and an acid SMase that is secreted extracellularly and is responsible for hydrolyzing SM in the outer leaflet of the plasma membrane in addition to that present in plasma lipoproteins (Jenkins et al., 2009). Activation of SMases in response to diverse stimuli in different compartments provides the means for a rapid Cer generation, crucial for signal transduction.

A third pathway for Cer generation relies on the breakdown of complex sphingolipids in the lysosomal or late endosomal compartment through the reverse activity of different hydrolases, such as specific β-glucosidases and galactosidases, to form Cer, which cannot be released from this compartment. The subsequent activity of at least five different ceramidases generates Sph and its recycling in the ER and reacylation by CerSs yields Cer; this "salvage pathway" (**Figure 2**) is involved in inflammatory processes (Kitatani et al., 2008; Canals et al., 2018). Finally, exogenous Cer can also be recycled and generate endogenous Cer by the reverse action of ceramidases (Kitatani et al., 2008; Novgorodov et al., 2011).

Cer is phosphorylated by a specific kinase, CerK to form C1P (Wijesinghe et al., 2005). As stated above, deacylation of Cer by ceramidases renders Sph, the phosphorylation of which by one of the two existing SphKs, SphK1 and SphK2, generates S1P (Hait et al., 2006; **Figure 2**). The irreversible degradation of S1P by S1P lyase, at the cytoplasmic side of the ER, yields ethanolamine-1-phosphate and hexadecenal, providing the only release gate from the complex sphingolipid metabolic cycle (Bandhuvula and Saba, 2007). Comprehensive and detailed accounts of sphingolipid molecular diversity and metabolism can be found in excellent previous reviews (Lahiri and Futerman, 2007; Kitatani et al., 2008; Hannun and Obeid, 2011; Canals et al., 2018).

To Be or Not to Be. . ., a Decision for the Sphingolipid Rheostat

By 1995, several seminal findings evidenced that Cer and S1P had opposing cellular roles; whereas growth and survival factors increase S1P levels to stimulate proliferation and survival, different cell stressors promote an intracellular accumulation of Cer, which arrests the cell cycle or induces cell death. The ready interconversion of S1P, Sph, and Cer (**Figure 2**), prompted by numerous cues that stimulate or inhibit the activities of the enzymes involved, provides a significant tool for determining the patterns of intracellular signaling and deciding the physiological outcome. This understanding led to the proposal that the opposite functions of S1P and Cer transform their signal-mediated interconversion in a sensor of intracellular conditions, and the consequent rapid alteration of the balance between their levels in a key switch in the control of cell fate, later termed as the "sphingolipid rheostat" (Gómez-Muñoz et al., 1995; Cuvillier et al., 1996).

Since then, the collective effort of numerous laboratories has shed new light on the molecular actors and the signaling pathways involved in the intricate cross-reactions of these sphingolipids, included new sphingolipid molecules such as C1P and DHCer, and shown that this rheostat is involved in the induction of multiple pathologies, including neurodegeneration (Taha et al., 2006; Hannun and Obeid, 2008; Young et al., 2013; Newton et al., 2015; Wang and Bieberich, 2018). The extensive available data provides us with an optimal position to complete the unraveling of the sphingolipid universe. The subcellular compartmentalization of their metabolic pathways has been established and the major enzymes giving rise to this diversity of sphingolipids have been identified and cloned during the past three decades. New evidence suggests that different Cer molecular species, generated by different pathways in different compartments might differ in their intracellular roles (Hannun and Obeid, 2011; Hernández-Corbacho et al., 2015). Hence, the relevance of the sphingolipids involved in the rheostat model extends beyond their relative levels and the tightly regulated enzymes involved in their synthesis and degradation to encompass the innumerable and frequently opposite signaling pathways they control, their site of biosynthesis and their release to the extracellular milieu, to finely tune the sphingolipid rheostat.

Sphingolipids in Eye Pathology

The last 15 years have seen the buildup of a body of evidence pointing to a role for sphingolipids in normal development and function of the retina and in the pathogenesis of ocular diseases. The first link between alterations in sphingolipid metabolism and eye disease originated from lysosomal storage diseases, collectively denominated sphingolipidoses, which arise in mutations in the enzymes or cofactors involved in sphingolipid degradation. These diseases share an early neurodegeneration and visual impairment, with ocular manifestations including retinal vascular abnormalities, degeneration of ganglion cells, and even blindness (Harcourt and Ashton, 1973; Brownstein et al., 1978; Brownstein et al., 1980; Chen et al., 2014).

In Farbert's disease, Cer accumulation in the retina brings on visual dysfunction, with ganglion cells being the most affected (Zarbin et al., 1988). Brain accumulation of Cer occurs in the juvenile form of Batten disease, in which retina neurodegeneration and blindness are early events (Puranam et al., 1997). These early reports underscored the relevance of sphingolipid metabolism in eye pathogenesis; however, few clues existed on how this accumulation led to ocular manifestations. Thrillingly, work from many laboratories over the last decade has implicated sphingolipids such as Cer, S1P, Sph, and C1P in the progression of ocular diseases, including diabetic retinopathy, retinitis pigmentosa, AMD and other neuronal degenerative diseases. We will first summarize the sphingolipid species present in the eye and then review their roles in retinal cells and in the pathogenesis of these diseases.

Sphingolipid Presence in the Eye

Due to their high complexity, detailed composition analysis of retina sphingolipids is quite recent. Sphingolipids amount to about 11–13 (mole) % of both rat and bovine retinal lipids (Brush et al., 2010). SM is the most abundant species, amounting to 2.4–2.5% of total retinal lipids, whereas Cer and GlucoCer amount to less than 1%. Retinal sphingolipids have abundant (nearly 90%) of saturated, and particularly very long chain saturated fatty acids, with 18:0 and 16:0 being the most abundant fatty acid species. They contain about 2-3% of DHA, 22:6 n-3, the most abundant PUFA, but no VLCPUFA longer than 24 carbons are present (Brush et al., 2010); this is intriguing since the retina is characterized for the abundance of PUFA and VLCPUFA, which are enriched in sphingolipids in other tissues (Aveldaño and Sprecher, 1987; Oresti et al., 2011). In mice retina, almost 80% of Cer contains 16:0 and 18:0, with 21% having 20:0 or longer chain fatty acids (Fox et al., 2006). Bovine rod OS have lower levels of sphingolipids than the whole retina, varying from 3.4 to 6.4 mole % (Brush et al., 2010). SM and Cer from detergent resistant membranes obtained from rod OS are enriched in saturated fatty acids (Martin et al., 2005).

Diverse studies confirm the earlier observations that the sphingolipid profile is modified in retinal pathologies. Cer mass content decreases in retinas from diabetic mice compared to normal retinas, without modifying its fatty acid composition, with a concomitant increase in GlucoCer, and no changes in Sph and SM (Fox et al., 2006). The relevance of particular Cer molecular species in preserving retinal functions has been emphasized by recent findings from the Busik laboratory, demonstrating that overexpression of elongation of very long-chain fatty acids protein 4 (ELOVL4), whose presence is significantly reduced in the diabetic retina, preserves tight junctions and prevents retinal vascular permeability; this effect is parallel to an increase in the levels of Cer having 16 and 24 carbons, and very long chain fatty acids, which localize in and might stabilize tight junctions (Kady et al., 2018). In a retinitis pigmentosa model, the 23H-1 rat, photoreceptor degeneration starts at the beginning of light responsiveness; Cer, S1P and SM increase in the retina early during degeneration, with a reduction in shorter-chain species and an increase in longer-chain species (Stiles et al., 2016).

The fact that sphingolipids are affected during the course of degeneration intuitively makes them likely candidates to have a role in retinal diseases. A combination of studies *in vivo* and *in vitro* has contributed to our understanding of these roles. *In vivo* studies with animal models have provided comprehension on the biological functions of sphingolipids and allowed to test the physiological effects of modulating its levels. Research *in vitro* has allowed dissecting their specific effects on particular cell types and the biochemical pathways involved in these effects. We will now highlight the findings that support that significance of sphingolipids during normal development and in pathologies affecting the retina.

CERAMIDE, A CRUCIAL EXECUTIONER IN RETINAL DEGENERATION

Cer Metabolism

Cer has a central role in the sphingolipid family, both structural and metabolic. Consisting in a Sph molecule bound to a fatty acid of 16 to 24 carbons length (Fahy et al., 2005), these long acyl chains confer Cer its high hydrophobic properties; unable to exist in a free-solution form in the cytoplasm, it is the most hydrophobic lipid in biological membranes (Castro et al., 2014). This apparently static, membrane-confined location of Cer does not preclude it from having key intracellular actions, as the regulation of cell cycle and cell death.

As Cer is synthesized in the ER, its hydrophobic nature demands a transport mechanism to reach its diverse cellular destinations. Cer transport to the *trans* Golgi region, to generate SM, involves a CERT, which carries it in a non-vesicular manner (Hanada et al., 2009). Cer has very different patterns of tissue distribution and functions (Bartke and Hannun, 2009; Kurz et al., 2018). Interestingly, six specific types of CerSs (CerS 1-6) have been identified, each of them attaching acylCoAs differing in their chain length to the sphingoid backbone, thus generating different molecular species of Cer, with distinct cellular effects (Levy and Futerman, 2010; Park and Pewzner-Jung, 2013; Wegner et al., 2016). The distribution of these CerSs differs between organs and even between cell types in the same organ, contributing to a characteristic Cer composition (Laviad et al., 2008; Kremser et al., 2013).

Ceramide Biological Functions

Numerous cellular stressors, such as oxidative stress, absence of trophic factors, chemotherapy, and UV radiation, activate the synthesis of Cer; the consequent increase in Cer levels mediates many cell-stress responses, including the regulation of cell growth, differentiation (Okazaki et al., 1989), senescence (Trayssac et al., 2018), proliferation, necrosis, apoptosis and autophagy (Obeid et al., 1993; Hannun and Obeid, 2008; Scarlatti et al., 2004). These multiple roles of Cer result from its ability to act both at membrane level and as an intracellular messenger. Cer is a key modulator of membrane dynamics; as a cone-shaped lipid, it readily forms non-lamellar phases with increased negative spontaneous curvature, thus promoting membrane invagination, budding and fusion

(Holopainen et al., 2000; Stancevic and Kolesnick, 2010). Cer initiates multiple signaling pathways through the rapid formation or expansion of Cer-enriched microdomains in the plasma or outer mitochondrial membrane. These microdomains allow for the interaction and/or oligomerization of different proteins, such as death receptors in the former or Bax in the later that then signal the activation of diverse death programs (Grassmé et al., 2001; Ganesan et al., 2010).

In addition, Cer triggers many of its effects by acting as a lipid second messenger, through the activation of several intracellular targets. Cer activates protein phosphatase PP1A and PP2A (Chalfant et al., 1999) and regulates protein kinase C zeta (PKCζ) and Akt activity (Wang et al., 2005; Canals et al., 2018; Hannun and Obeid, 2018) as well as raf-1 and the kinase-suppressor of Ras, significantly changing the level of phosphorylation of various key substrates (Ruvolo, 2003).

Among the multifaceted roles of Cer, autophagy and cell death have been those that have drawn more attention. Cer controls both autophagy-mediated cell survival and cell death by regulating nutrient transport, ER stress and mitophagy (Dany and Ogretmen, 2015). Still, Cer has been more frequently identified as a key cell death player (Galadari et al., 2015), activating both the intrinsic and extrinsic pathways of apoptosis. Although its actual contribution to the apoptotic response in living cells has been unclear, multiple *in vitro* studies suggest that Cer might initiate cell death by acting directly on mitochondria. In an interesting recent work, a diverting CERT-mediated Cer transport to mitochondria has been shown to trigger Bax-dependent apoptosis (Jain et al., 2017).

Knowledge on the role of Cer in different pathological processes is vast and constantly expanding, and there are excellent reviews covering its functions (Canals et al., 2018; Hannun and Obeid, 2018; Kurz et al., 2018). We will here focus on Cer functions in retinal physiology and pathologies.

Ceramide in the Retina

Cer and Retina Degeneration

Acharya's group provided the first direct link between Cer and the death of retinal neurons in a *Drosophila* model of retinal degeneration. Using photo-transduction mutants, they demonstrated Cer has a crucial role in photoreceptor fate; keeping Cer levels low by preventing its *de novo* synthesis or by targeting neutral ceramidase suppresses photoreceptor death in the *Drosophila* mutants (Acharya et al., 2003). In functional null mutants of *Drosophila* ceramidase, photoreceptors degenerate in a light-dependent manner, do not respond to light stimulus and have no effective turnover of rhodopsin; in turn, overexpression of ceramidase, even in tissues distant from photoreceptors, suppresses their degeneration in arrestin mutants and facilitates membrane turnover in a rhodopsin null mutant (Acharya et al., 2008). Furthermore, a *Drosophila* mutant in the CerK shows increased Cer levels leading to the loss of phospholipase C activity and inhibition of phototransduction, ultimately accompanied by photoreceptor degeneration (Dasgupta et al., 2009).

Along the last decade, increasing evidence points to a key involvement of Cer in the onset of retina degeneration in mammals (**Table 1**). The gradual loss of photoreceptors observed in a rabbit model of retinal detachment correlates with the

TABLE 1 | Ceramide and sphingosine functions in the retina.

Sphingolipid	Retinal Process
Ceramide (Cer)	**Photoreceptor death**
	↓ Cer levels rescues photoreceptors from death in *Drosophila* RP models (Acharya et al., 2003)
	↑ Cer levels induces photoreceptor loss of function and death in *Drosophila* (Dasgupta et al., 2009)
	Photoreceptor death induced by retinal detachment correlated with ↑ Cer levels in rabbits (Ranty et al., 2009)
	↓ Cer levels by Myoricin treatment (*de novo* Cer synthesis inhibitor) rescue photoreceptors in a *rd10* mouse model (Strettoi et al., 2010)
	↓ Cer levels by inhibiting *de novo* synthesis with FTY720 delays retinal degeneration in P23H-1 rats (Stiles et al., 2016)
	↓expression of acid SMase protects the retina and preserves its function after ischemic injury in an acidic SMase +/− mice model (Fan et al., 2016)
	Intra-vitreal C2Cer injection causes vision loss in rats (Lou et al., 2017)
	C2Cer treatment induces photoreceptor and amacrine cell death in rat retinal neuronal cultures (German et al., 2006)
	Oxidative stress ↑ Cer levels and leads to cone cell death in 661W cell line (Sanvicens and Cotter, 2006)
	Brief C2Cer treatment induces photoreceptor death by activating parthanatos in rat retinal cultures (Prado Spalm et al., 2018)
	Retinal Pigment Epithelium (RPE) dystrophy
	C2Cer induces caspase-dependent death in rat RPE cells (Tomita et al., 2000)
	Oxidative stress ↑ Cer levels and activates cell death in ARPE-19 cells (Sugano et al., 2018)
	C2Cer treatment induces apoptosis in non-polarized, but not in polarized RPE cells (Zhu et al., 2010)
Sphingosine (Sph)	**Photoreceptor death**
	Oxidative stress ↑ Sph synthesis, preceding the onset of photoreceptor death *in vitro* (Abrahan et al., 2010)
	Addition of exogenous Sph induces mitochondrial-dependent photoreceptor death (Abrahan et al., 2010)
	RPE alterations
	Increased levels of Sph in SMase knockout mice match with age-dependent retina degeneration and RPE alterations, and an impaired autophagic flux (Wu et al., 2015)
	Overexpression of acid ceramidase in ARPE19 cells ↑ Sph levels and protects these cells from oxidative stress (Sugano et al., 2018).

production of Cer (Ranty et al., 2009). Intra-vitreal C2-Cer injection causes vision loss in rats, increasing apoptosis and expression of glial fibrillary acidic protein, a marker of gliosis (Lou et al., 2017). A recent work in a mouse model of Farber disease, with a deficiency in acid ceramidase activity, provides direct evidence of accumulation of Cer in the retina, associated to inflammation and severe visual loss (Yu et al., 2018). Ischemia increases the expression of acid SMase, increasing Cer levels and leading to retinal degeneration in wild type mice; reduction of this expression in an acid SMase +/− mouse model decreases Cer levels, protects retina structure and preserves its function after ischemic injury (Fan et al., 2016). However, the maintenance of a basal acid SMase activity is necessary for preserving normal retina structure and function; a total deficiency in acid SMase, as occurs in acid SMase knockout mice, leads to the disruption in lysosomal function and prominent photoreceptor degeneration (Wu et al., 2015). Mandalt's group showed alterations in the sphingolipid profile in P23H-1 rat retinas during degeneration, with an increase in neutral SMase activity leading to higher Cer levels at PN22. Treatment with FTY720, an established CerS inhibitor, partly decreases neutral SMase activity and delays the alterations in retina structure and functionality, granting partial neuronal protection. However, this treatment also leads to a stimulation of acid SMase activity and the consequent increase in Cer levels, which might explain why FTY720 does not fully prevent degeneration (Stiles et al., 2016). This underscores the relevance of establishing not only the pathways leading to Cer increase in each retinopathy but also whether inhibition of a major pathway promotes the activation of further biosynthetic paths, to identify the targets to effectively promote photoreceptor survival.

Diabetic retinopathy is the major cause of blindness among working age adults; increased Cer levels have been associated to reduction of insulin action (Chaurasia and Summers, 2015) and recent research establishes Cer as a relevant player in the progression of this retinopathy. Acid SMase is highly activated in the diabetic retina, particularly in retinal endothelium, elevating Cer levels and contributing to the pro-inflammatory changes in this tissue; noteworthy, DHA, which is decreased in the diabetic retina (Tikhonenko et al., 2010), downregulates the expression of acid SMase in human retinal endothelial cells (Opreanu et al., 2010; Busik et al., 2012; Hammer and Busik, 2017). Acid SMase vascular isoform specifically increases in the retinas of diabetic animal models at the vasodegenerative stage, whereas its absence or downregulation with DHA prevents capillary formation and cytokine production (Opreanu et al., 2010, 2011; Busik et al., 2012; Chakravarthy et al., 2016). Activation of acid SMase and the consequent Cer increase appear as relevant contributors to the pathogenesis of diverse retina degenerations, and reestablishing an adequate balance in sphingolipid levels emerges as essential to maintain retina functionality.

Ceramide and Photoreceptor Death

The work of several groups, including ours, has provided direct links between Cer increase and the onset of photoreceptor death. This death is the hallmark of most retinal degenerative diseases with very diverse etiologies (Chang et al., 1993; Portera-Cailliau et al., 1994; Sancho-Pelluz et al., 2008); hence, uncovering common molecular mechanisms and mediators is essential to identify new therapeutic targets. *In vitro* studies have been fundamental to establish Cer as a mediator of photoreceptor death. Our group demonstrated that oxidative stress increases the *de novo* synthesis of Cer preceding photoreceptor death in rat retina cultured neurons, whereas inhibiting this synthesis with fumonisin B1, a CerS inhibitor, prevents this death (German et al., 2006). These neurons present low levels of DHA, which has been shown to be neuroprotective for photoreceptors (Rotstein et al., 1996, 1997). DHA supplementation protects photoreceptors from C2-Cer and oxidative stress-induced death, promoting the synthesis of GlucoCer (German et al., 2006). Cotter's group extended Cer role in oxidative stress-induced death of photoreceptors; they showed that treatment of 661W cells, a cone cell line, with a nitric oxide donor increases Cer levels by activating acid SMase; inhibition of Cer synthesis by an acid SMase inhibitor (Desipramine) prevents cone cell death (Sanvicens and Cotter, 2006). Interestingly, induction of oxidative stress with H_2O_2 also raises Cer levels and promotes cell death in 661W cells, whereas inhibiting *de novo* synthesis of Cer with Myriocin, a serine palmitoyl transferase inhibitor, prevents Cer increase preserving cell viability (Fabiani et al., 2017). The buildup of Cer, arising from the activation of different biosynthetic pathways in rod and cone photoreceptors, emerges as a death arbitrator in photoreceptors, suggesting that pharmacological prevention of this increase might have therapeutic potential (**Figures 3, 4**).

In vivo studies have supported this hypothesis. Cer levels increase during the peak of photoreceptor degeneration in the *rd10* mouse, a mouse model of Retinitis Pigmentosa, and treatment with Myriocin noticeably prevents photoreceptor loss and preserves both photoreceptor morphology and retina functionality (Strettoi et al., 2010). Although the genetic mutations in Retinitis pigmentosa and in animal models of this disease affect mostly rods, their death is eventually followed by the death of cones; noteworthy, Myriocin was also effective as a strategy to promote cone survival in the same *rd10* model, even after rod death (Piano et al., 2013).

Increasing evidence suggests that Cer activates death pathways alternative to those of canonical apoptosis to induce photoreceptor demise. Cer increase triggers several pathways in 661W cells subjected to oxidative stress; it not only induces the mitochondrial pathway and subsequent activation of caspases, but also promotes Ca^{2+} increases in both mitochondria and cytosol that precede the activation of calpain-mediated death and activates cathepsin D pathway as well (Sanvicens and Cotter, 2006).

We have recently established that Cer activates PARP-1 to induce photoreceptor death. Cer induces photoreceptor death in cultured rat retina neurons in a caspase-independent process, involving generation of ROS, increase in mitochondrial permeability, activation of PARP-1 and calpain, accumulation of poly ADP-ribose polymers and nuclear translocation of AIF (Prado Spalm et al., 2018), which are features of a recently unveiled death process named Parthanatos (David et al., 2009). Notably, inhibition of both PARP-1 and calpain

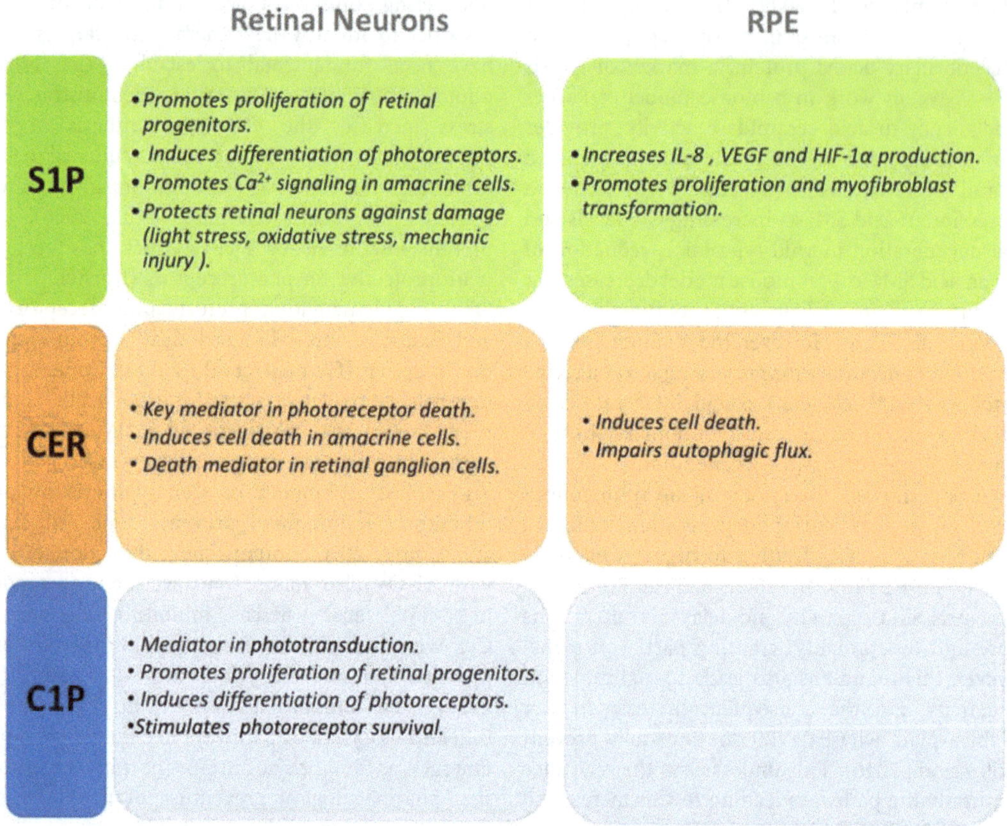

FIGURE 3 | Actions of S1P, Cer, and C1P on retinal neurons and RPE cells. This figure summarizes the effects shown for S1P, Cer, and C1P on different retinal neurons and RPE cells.

activity rescues photoreceptors from Cer-induced death (Prado Spalm et al., 2018). Paquet-Durandt's group established PARP-1 activation as a common non-apoptotic mechanism involved in retinal neurodegeneration in animal models encompassing the major groups of inherited human blindness (Arango-Gonzalez et al., 2014). PARP-1 activity is crucial in the induction of photoreceptor death in the *rd1* and *rd2* mouse models (Sahaboglu et al., 2017). Activation of PARP-1 has only been associated with Cer-induced death in neuroblastoma cells (Czubowicz and Strosznajder, 2014); hence, these findings not only link for the first time Parthanatos with Cer-induced photoreceptor death but support Parthanatos as a novel cell death routine triggered by Cer. Although different retinal neurodegenerative diseases may have particular cell death mechanisms, taking together these studies Parthanatos appears as a central, shared photoreceptor death-process with Cer as a crucial mediator in these degenerations. Targeting Cer overproduction or Parthanatos key molecular actors might provide enticing strategies for novel, disease-independent treatments for retina neurodegenerations.

Cer as a Death Mediator in Other Neuronal Types in the Retina

Cer role as a mediator in the induction of cell damage is not confined to photoreceptors. A 24 h treatment with C2-Cer induces death of amacrine neurons in retina neuronal cultures (German et al., 2006). Optic nerve crush, which triggers the injury to retinal ganglion cells in the rat retina, increases the expression of enzymes involved in Cer biosynthesis (Agudo-Barriuso et al., 2013). Gene expression profiling in injured retinal ganglion cells following overexpression of the *Sox11 transcription factor* revealed that genes associated with Cer biosynthetic and metabolic processes are upregulated, suggesting the activation of a Cer-induced cell death pathway (Norsworthy et al., 2017).

Cer and RPE Degeneration

Cer also plays a pivotal role in diseases affecting RPE function, such as AMD and Stargardt disease. Atrophy of RPE cells followed or accompanied by photoreceptor cell death is usually the final outcome of all forms of retinitis pigmentosa, despite their different etiologies. RPE atrophy, i.e., RPE cell death, in the macular region is the primary event in dry AMD and a common event in early stage wet AMD (Al-Zamil and Yassin, 2017). C2-Cer induces death of human and rat RPE cultured cells, which involves caspase activation and is partially prevented by antioxidants and growth factors (Tomita et al., 2000; Kannan et al., 2004; Sreekumar et al., 2009). Oxidative stress increases Cer levels and induces apoptosis in human RPE cells and this was replicated by using C2- and C6-Cer (Barak et al., 2001). Oxidative stress increases both Cer and hexosyl-Cer

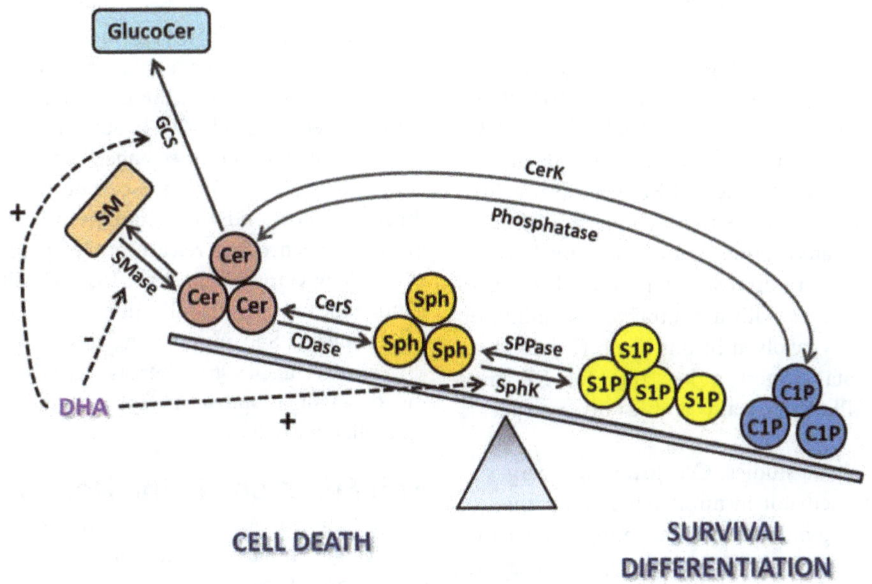

FIGURE 4 | The relevance of the sphingolipid rheostat in retina photoreceptors. Increases in Cer levels through the activation of its *de novo* synthesis or the SMase pathway trigger photoreceptor death; this death is also induced after Cer hydrolysis to increase Sph levels, mediated by ceramidase (CDase). In turn, S1P and C1P promote photoreceptor survival and differentiation. Docosahexaenoic acid (DHA) promotes survival by regulating the sphingolipid rheostat, inhibiting SMase or stimulating the synthesis of glucosylceramide (GlucoCer) to decrease Cer levels or enhancing the synthesis of S1P. Exogenous addition of C1P also promotes photoreceptor survival and differentiation.

levels in ARPE-19 cells, a human RPE cell line, promoting cell death; this death is prevented by over-expression of acid ceramidase, which increases Sph levels but not those of S1P (Sugano et al., 2018). Interestingly, increased serum levels of hexosyl-Cer have been reported in patients with late stage AMD (Pujol-Lereis et al., 2018). Noteworthy, oxidative stress leads to increased S1P levels in control RPE cells, which might reflect an attempt to counteract Cer action toward cell death (Sugano et al., 2018). Laser exposure, a frequent treatment for retina neovascularization, induces human RPE cell death concomitant with Cer overproduction (Barak et al., 2005).

Cer significance as a mediator of RPE cell death is also evidenced by the induction of cell death in ARPE19 cells overexpressing neutral SMase3. Intracellular Cer increase and cell death are proportional to the amount of the transfected enzyme and SMase3 overexpression also inhibits proliferation in ARPE19 cells (Zhu et al., 2010). Intriguingly, C2-Cer treatment induces apoptosis in non-polarized RPE cells but does not affect differentiated and polarized RPE cells (Zhu et al., 2010). This differential susceptibility suggests that while healthy, polarized cells forming the RPE monolayer *in vivo* may be resistant to injures leading to an eventual Cer increase, non-polarized, activated RPE cells, frequent in late AMD lesions and in proliferative vitreoretinopathies, might be more susceptible to increased Cer levels resulting from chronic retina injuries (**Figure 3**).

Cer increase is common to several diseases affecting RPE cells. Excessive acid SMase activation and the subsequent Cer accumulation have been related to the pathogenic changes of RPE cells in diabetic retinopathy. High glucose enhances acid SMase expression, increasing Cer levels in ARPE19 cells. Interestingly, microRNAs (miR) appear as novel players in the modulation of sphingolipid metabolic enzymes. Work from the Busik laboratory showed miR-15a participates in the regulation of Cer levels; its expression is decreased by high glucose whereas its overexpression downregulates acid SMase expression in human RPE cells, restoring normal Cer levels (Wang et al., 2016). This adds an additional complexity to the intricate regulation of sphingolipid metabolism and underscores the usefulness of its modulation in disease treatment.

Acid SMase activation has been shown in aged RPE and in a Stargardt disease mouse model, and the consequent Cer increase impairs autophagic flux, which is crucial for preserving functional RPE and photoreceptor cells (Toops et al., 2015). Efficient endolysosome function in RPE is essential for its phagocytic role and autophagic clearance of cellular debris, and endolysosomal dysfunction is characteristic of neurodegenerative diseases. Recent findings show acid SMase-derived Cer increase and subsequent endolysosomal dysfunction contribute to internalization of the complement protein C3, abnormal levels of which have been implicated in AMD; inhibiting Cer synthesis with desipramine decreases this dysfunction and C3 internalization (Kaur et al., 2018). Significantly, epidemiological studies indicate that the use of tricyclic antidepressants, like desipramine, is associated with a statistically significant protective effect against developing early AMD (Klein et al., 2001), emphasizing the significance of Cer increase in RPE cell dysfunction and AMD progression (**Figure 3**).

Several signaling pathways participate in Cer-induced RPE cell death. C2-Cer induces the over-production of ROS, activating the intrinsic apoptotic pathway, with a subsequent increase in mitochondrial membrane permeability and caspase-3 activation (Kannan et al., 2004). Both H_2O_2 and UV radiation induce ER and stress-activated protein kinase (AMPK) axis, which promote RPE cell death (Yao et al., 2013). Tunicamycin treatment of cultured RPE cells induces NF-κB nuclear translocation, increases in nitric oxide synthase 2 expression and nitrotyrosine formation leading to cell death, which is prevented with a neutral SMase inhibitor, implying Cer generation is involved in this death (Kucuksayan et al., 2014). These data suggest a key role for ER-stress induced by Cer in RPE cell death and a disease-specific activation of SMases.

Taking together the above studies, Cer distinctly emerges as a common pathological mediator in numerous retinopathies of diverse etiologies, activating multiple downstream pathways that induce both the degeneration of rod and cone photoreceptors and RPE dysfunction and death. Pharmacological interventions to prevent Cer increase might provide useful tools for treating multiple retinopathies, in a disease-independent mode. The preservation of retina morphology and functionality by the inhibition of Cer synthesis (Strettoi et al., 2010; Stiles et al., 2016) sustains this proposal. In addition, DHA provides an exciting "proof of concept," emerging as a modulator of several enzymes of sphingolipid metabolism in order to prevent Cer accumulation, thus tilting the sphingolipid rheostat toward cell survival (**Figure 4**).

SPHINGOSINE, A DEADLY MESSENGER IN THE RETINA?

Sph Biological Functions

The finding that Sph inhibits protein kinase C was one of the first supporting a role for sphingolipids in cell signaling (Hannun and Bell, 1989; Merrill et al., 1989). Later work demonstrated that in addition to this modulatory function, Sph, as its precursor Cer, is a crucial signal for cell death. Sph levels increase during the early stages of cell death, and its addition can trigger this death (Cuvillier, 2002). Oxidative stress, radiation and chemotherapy enhance Cer and Sph generation promoting senescence, cell cycle arrest or cell death (Ogretmen and Hannun, 2004; Hannun and Obeid, 2018). Although Sph increase might result from a decreased SphK activity, as occurs in radiation-resistant prostate cancer cells (Nava et al., 2000), the rapid deacylation of Cer is the main source of Sph increase. The increase in Cer usually precedes that of Sph, suggesting that Cer hydrolysis by ceramidases gives rise to this increase (Ohta et al., 1995; Cuvillier et al., 2000). Precisely, the fact that Cer can be hydrolyzed to Sph, and Sph reacylated to generate Cer made it difficult initially to discern their effects. However, exogenous Sph induces apoptosis in cell lines such as Jurkat cells and rhabdomyosarcoma cell lines even when its conversion to Cer is inhibited (Cuvillier et al., 2000; Phillips et al., 2007) and Sph has been shown to act independently from Cer and at an earlier step in the apoptotic pathway in human leukemic cells (Sweeney et al., 1996). Conversely, inhibiting the synthesis of Sph reduces the induction of apoptosis by different stimuli (Lépine et al., 2004; Suzuki et al., 2004). Sph is now an established second messenger, rapidly generated by different apoptotic stimuli to induce cell death. Sph signals this death through mitochondrial membrane permeabilization, formation of ROS, cytochrome c release, and caspase-3 activation (Sweeney et al., 1996; García-Ruiz et al., 1997; Cuvillier et al., 2000, 2001). Mitochondrial permeabilization is crucial for Sph induction of cell death; Sph induces the downregulation of Bcl-2 levels (Sweeney et al., 1996) whereas Bcl-xl overexpression prevents the onset of apoptosis in spite of the increase in Sph levels (Cuvillier et al., 2001).

Sph Functions in the Retina

Scarce information exists regarding Sph roles in the eye (**Table 1**). Initial data in *Drosophila* mutants showed that expression of ceramidase suppresses retinal degeneration in arrestin mutant flies, in parallel to a decrease in Cer levels; however, these mutants show enhanced degeneration of photoreceptors when they are raised with a Sph-enriched diet, suggesting that Sph is not involved in preventing degeneration (Acharya et al., 2003).

Sph functions in mammalian retina are still ill-defined. Sph induces cell death in amacrine and photoreceptor neurons in culture (Abrahan et al., 2010); oxidative stress rapidly enhances Sph synthesis, preceding the onset of photoreceptor death *in vitro*. In turn, inhibition of Sph synthesis by blocking Cer breakdown with an alkaline ceramidase inhibitor, MAPP, markedly decreases oxidative stress-induced photoreceptor death. Moreover, exogenous Sph promotes photoreceptor death, even when Cer synthesis is inhibited, implying that Sph is responsible for this death. As reported in different cell types, Sph promotes apoptotic death by inducing mitochondrial permeabilization in photoreceptors, increasing ROS formation and cytochrome c release, whereas inhibiting Sph synthesis prevents mitochondrial permeabilization (Abrahan et al., 2010).

As occurs with Cer (German et al., 2006), DHA prevents Sph-induced apoptosis, enhancing the expression of SphK1 and its translocation to the plasma membrane (Miranda et al., 2009; Abrahan et al., 2010). Noteworthy, inhibition of SphK1 activity with DHS blocks DHA protection, implying that the decrease in the levels of Sph and/or the generation of S1P are required for DHA protective effect (Abrahan et al., 2010). As a whole, these findings suggest that oxidative stress increases the generation of Cer and Sph in retina photoreceptors, which act as second messengers, inducing mitochondrial dysfunction and increased generation of ROS (Rotstein et al., 2010), to activate cell death. Lowering Sph levels, by preventing its synthesis or promoting its phosphorylation to S1P effectively prevents photoreceptor death, accentuating the relevance of manipulating sphingolipid metabolism in photoreceptor survival.

Whether Sph acts as a deadly messenger promoting degenerative changes in other retinal cell types is still unclear.

In acid SMase knockout mice, increased levels of Sph and normal levels of Cer are found in the retina (Wu et al., 2015), probably due to compensatory changes in the activities of other sphingolipid enzymes, aimed at maintaining Cer levels constant. These mice show age-dependent retina degeneration and RPE alterations, with an impaired autophagic flux (Wu et al., 2015); it still remains to be defined whether Sph increase leads to these changes. Puzzlingly, overexpression of acid ceramidase in ARPE19 cells increases their Sph levels, and protects these cells from oxidative stress, with no concomitant increase in S1P levels (Sugano et al., 2018). Hence, much remains to be investigated regarding Sph actions in the retina in order to design new therapies through the adequately modulation of sphingolipid levels.

SPHINGOSINE-1-PHOSPHATE, A FORMIDABLE DOUBLE-EDGED SWORD IN THE RETINA

S1P Synthesis

Sphingosine-1-phosphate is a crucial lipid intermediate in the complex sphingolipid metabolism. It has a polar head group (phosphate), and a long-chain sphingoid base backbone (Sph) (Saba and Hla, 2004; **Figure 1**). Sph is phosphorylated to generate S1P by two different SphKs, SphK1 and SphK2 (Maceyka et al., 2005; **Figure 2**). SphK1 is found mainly in the cytosol, close to the cell membrane, in nearly every cell type. When activated, it translocates to the plasma membrane, where Sph is localized. Its structure, functions and roles in disease are widely identified. Much less is known on SphK2; predominantly localized in nuclei and mitochondria, its expression is tissue and time of development dependent (Hait et al., 2009; Strub et al., 2011). Its structure, functions and the processes in which it is involved are poorly understood. Its most recognized function is its ability to phosphorylate FTY720/Fingolimod, a Sph analog and the first oral pro-drug to be approved for the treatment of multiple sclerosis by the FDA.

S1P as an Intracellular and an Extracellular Messenger

Notably, in spite of being chemically identical, S1P molecules from nuclei or cytoplasm perform different functions. While nuclear S1P works as a histone deacetylase (HDAC) inhibitor to epigenetically regulate gene transcription (Hait et al., 2009), cytoplasmic S1P acts as a second messenger or as an extracellular ligand. To function as an extracellular ligand, the S1P produced inside the cell is exported by specific transporters, such as Spinster 2 (Spns2) (Osborne et al., 2008; Kawahara et al., 2009; Spiegel et al., 2019) or ABCA1 (Sato et al., 2007), ABCC1 (Mitra et al., 2006), and ABCG2 (Takabe et al., 2010). Once outside the cell, S1P acts in a paracrine or autocrine fashion, a process known as "inside-out signaling" (Takabe et al., 2008). As an extracellular ligand, S1P interacts with five S1P G protein-coupled membrane receptors (S1PRs), termed $S1P_{1-5}$. Most cells express one or more subtypes of S1PRs, and depending on the G-protein they are coupled with, S1PRs exhibit unique properties and regulate different cellular processes. Downstream effectors of S1PRs include adenylate cyclase, PI3-kinase, phospholipase C, protein kinase C and intracellular calcium (Hla et al., 2001; Spiegel and Milstien, 2002). In addition, S1P has been proposed to signal through S1PRs, in a paracrine fashion, upregulating the transcription of SphK1 and thus activating the S1P/SphK1 axis; this "outside-in" signaling pathway has been shown to contribute to the progression of diabetic retinopathy (Huang et al., 2014).

Sphingosine-1-phosphate is a pleiotropic bioactive lipid mediator; its cellular concentration responds to different stimuli and is tightly regulated. Concentrations of S1P in blood and lymph are actually higher than in tissues (Cyster and Schwab, 2012; Olivera et al., 2013; Nagahashi et al., 2016). The final concentration of S1P in any tissue depends on the balance between its synthesis and its degradation, with S1P degrading enzymes playing an important role in maintaining the low tissue levels of S1P. The main enzymes that degrade S1P are S1P lyases and SPP. SPP has two isoforms, SPP1 and SPP2, which catalyze the reversible dephosphorylation of S1P, generating Sph that it is then converted to Cer by CerS (Mandala, 2001; Pyne et al., 2009). S1P lyases are responsible for irreversibly degrading S1P to hexadecenal and ethanolamine-1-phosphate, removing S1P from the sphingolipid metabolic routes and providing the only escape path from this complex metabolism (Bandhuvula and Saba, 2007).

Sphingosine-1-phosphate induces a wide spectrum of cellular effects, including proliferation, differentiation, survival, migration, angiogenesis and immune responses (Tabasinezhad et al., 2013). These pleiotropic effects grant S1P a key role in several diseases, including cancer, inflammation, autoimmunity, atherosclerosis and fibrotic disorders (Knapp, 2011; Maceyka et al., 2012; Takuwa et al., 2013). The highly conserved relevance of S1P and its regulation of important biological functions in organisms ranging from yeast and plants to flies and vertebrates highlight its significance in cell signaling.

The role of S1P in immune functions is well demonstrated, being involved in infections, allergy and chronic inflammation (Aoki et al., 2016). Its key role in neuroinflammation is evident in the successful use of FTY720 in the treatment of multiple sclerosis. S1P acts as an "extracellular siren song," its high plasma concentrations stimulating pathogenic lymphocyte migration and promoting their egress from lymph nodes to blood vessels (Bandhuvula and Saba, 2007). FTY720, and more precisely its phosphorylated form, is a functional antagonist of almost all S1PRs, excepting S1P2, and prevents S1P activation of S1P1 by binding and promoting its internalization and further degradation, thus decreasing S1P1 membrane levels and retaining lymphocytes in the lymph nodes (Paugh et al., 2003; Brinkmann et al., 2010; Chun and Hartung, 2010). In addition, FTY720 has been shown to inhibit *de novo* synthesis of Cer (Berdyshev et al., 2009) and histone deacetylases (Hait et al., 2014). Its efficacy in the treatment of multiple sclerosis has led to an accelerated research on its therapeutic effects in other inflammatory diseases.

Glial cells are key players in neuroinflammation and S1P induces this inflammation in the different glial types (microglia, astrocytes, and oligodendrocytes). S1P has been linked to microglial activation; S1P addition to cultured microglial cell lines increases the release of pro- inflammatory cytokines whereas microglial activation *in vivo* increases SphK1 activity (Nayak et al., 2010; Lv et al., 2016). Astrocytes, which are involved in many central nervous system pathologies, respond to and release inflammatory mediators, and an active crosstalk exists between S1P and these mediators; S1P induces astrogliosis, whereas IL-1 induces SphK1 expression (Sorensen et al., 2003; Paugh et al., 2009). S1P1 expression in astrocytes is critical in the development of animal models of multiple sclerosis, as shown by the protective effect of FTY720 (Choi et al., 2011).

Inflammation, angiogenesis, proliferation and migration are common features in most retinopathies; hence, S1P signaling of these processes makes it an ideal candidate to regulate the onset and progression of these diseases. We will here discuss current knowledge regarding the role of S1P in eye and retina development and during retina pathological disorders, particularly the opposing functions of S1P in both neuronal survival and inflammation and fibrosis in the retina.

S1P, Dr. Jekill or Mr. Hyde in the Retina?

Numerous findings during the last decade have shed new light on S1P functions in the retina (**Table 2**). SphK1 is expressed in photoreceptors whereas SphK1 and SphK2 are expressed both in ARPE19 and in human fetal RPE cells, implying these cells have the molecular machinery required for S1P synthesis (Abrahan et al., 2010; Zhu et al., 2010). A recent work has dissected the distribution of SphKs and S1PRs in mouse retina (Porter et al., 2018). *SphK1* is low in most mouse ocular tissues and highest in the retina and optic nerve, whereas higher levels of *SphK2* are observed in all mouse eye tissues. Interestingly, both SphK2 and SphK1 increase in the retina during early development, peaking at adulthood. *S1p1* and *S1p3* are expressed in the retina, while expression of *S1p2* and *S1p5* is minimal; S1P3 expression remains high and constant during retina development, whereas S1P1 increases gradually. Photoreceptors express both S1P1 and S1P3; S1P1 is highly expressed in RPE cells while S1P3 is localized in ganglion cells (Porter et al., 2018). Müller glial cells also show expression of SphK1 and S1P3 (Simón et al., 2015). Hence, the enzymes and receptors that take part in S1P signaling pathway are present in most retina cell types.

S1P in Eye Development and Neuronal Survival

Sphingosine-1-phosphate has essential functions during normal eye development. Mutations in *Spns2* cause the abnormal fusion of eyelids during rat embryogenesis, which can be reversed by treatment with S1P (Bian et al., 2018). Functional SPNS2 is crucial for retinal morphogenesis, since dysfunctional SPNS2 causes delayed cell-cycle exit of retinal progenitors and retinal laminar disorganization (Fang et al., 2018). A role for S1P signaling in axon guidance has also been reported; S1P promotes repulsive turning and collapse of growth cones from ganglion cell axons in the Xenopus retina, through activation of the S1P5 and RhoA whereas loss of S1P function results in target recognition errors (Strochlic et al., 2008). S1P is also involved in signaling in inner retina cells; S1P increases cytosolic Ca^{2+} levels in cultured amacrine cells, through the activation of S1P1 and S1P3 (Crousillac et al., 2009).

Sphingosine-1-phosphate displays a vital function in preventing neuronal death during retinal injuries. S1P1 contributes to survival and axonal sprout of injured retinal ganglion cells after damage to the optic nerve (Joly and Pernet, 2016) and FTY720 has neuroprotective effects in experimental glaucoma in rats (You et al., 2014). Moreover, the expression of SphK1, S1P2, and S1P3 immediately increases in light-stressed retinas, with S1PRs localizing to the pyknotic nuclei, suggesting the up-regulation of a cytoprotective S1P signaling to counteract the onset of apoptosis (Porter et al., 2018).

S1P as a Mediator in Photoreceptor Survival and Differentiation

Sphingosine-1-phosphate emerges as a pleiotropic mediator for development and survival of photoreceptors. Our group established that 1 μM S1P promotes the proliferation of retinal progenitors and their later differentiation into photoreceptors; S1P increases the expression of specific photoreceptor proteins, and advances the development of rudimentary OS (Miranda et al., 2009). We also evidenced that S1P is a key mediator in photoreceptor survival, preventing photoreceptor death during development *in vitro* and when exposed to oxidative stress (Miranda et al., 2009; Rotstein et al., 2010).

An increase in S1P intracellular levels protects 661W cells from oxidative stress; exogenous addition of S1P or inhibiting S1P lyase with THI preserves viability in these cells when treated with H_2O_2, by decreasing Cer levels, activating the Nrf-regulated antioxidant pathway and increasing the Bcl-2/Bax ratio (Fabiani et al., 2017). Further evidence supports the proposal that S1P is an intracellular second messenger, the synthesis of which is promoted by photoreceptor trophic factors to exert its actions. GDNF promotes the proliferation of photoreceptor progenitors (Politi et al., 2001; Insua et al., 2003), as S1P does, and inhibiting SphK1 with DHS blocks GDNF mitogenic effect (Miranda et al., 2009). Inhibition of SphK1 abolishes DHA neuroprotection of photoreceptors during oxidative stress-induced apoptosis and DHA enhancement of photoreceptor differentiation (Miranda et al., 2009; Abrahan et al., 2010). Cytokines and growth factors, such as Transforming growth factor β and Nerve growth factor (NGF), enhance the expression of SphK1 and promote its rapid translocation and activation to increase the synthesis of S1P, which then acts as a second messenger to exert their effects (Toman et al., 2004; Yamanaka et al., 2004; Wattenberg et al., 2006). Noteworthy, both GDNF and DHA upregulate the expression of SphK1 and promote its translocation to the plasma membrane (Abrahan et al., 2010). Thus, GDNF and DHA might elicit their biological effects on photoreceptors by promoting SphK1 activity and increasing the synthesis of S1P, which then acts as a second messenger, essential for proper development and survival of photoreceptors. As described above, DHA prevents photoreceptor death by promoting Cer glucosylation (German et al., 2006). As a whole, these findings highlight the importance of the "sphingolipid rheostat" and of manipulating sphingolipid metabolism to promote photoreceptor survival in retinal degenerations (**Figure 4**).

TABLE 2 | Functions of Sphingosine-1-phosphate and Ceramide-1-phosphate in the retina.

Sphingolipid	Retinal Process
Sphingosine-1- phosphate (S1P)	**Normal Eye development and function**
	↓ in *Spns2* expression causes abnormal eyelid fusion (Bian et al., 2018), alterations in retinal progenitors cell cycle and laminar disorganization (Fang et al., 2018)
	↑S1P promotes proliferation of retinal progenitors and their later differentiation into photoreceptors (Miranda et al., 2009)
	↑ S1P promotes Ca^{2+} signaling in amacrine cells in the inner retina via S1P1 and S1P3 (Crousillac et al., 2009)
	Protection against Retinal injuries
	↑ S1P through S1P1 promotes neuronal survival and axonal sprouting after optic nerve damage (Joly and Pernet, 2016)
	FTY720 has neuroprotective effects in rat models of glaucoma (You et al., 2014)
	↓ S1P abolishes DHA–mediated protection of cultured photoreceptors from oxidative stress (Abrahan et al., 2010)
	Light- stressed retinas ↑ expression of SphK1, S1P2 and S1P3 (Porter et al., 2018)
	Eye inflammation
	↑ S1P promotes retinal angiogenesis and neovascularization (Eresch et al., 2018)
	↑ S1P increases IL-8 secretion in RPE (Qiao et al., 2012)
	TNF-α promotes ↑ S1P and IL-8 and IL-6 production (Qiao et al., 2012)
	↑ S1P promotes VEGF and HIF-1α production in RPE (Terao et al., 2017)
	↑ levels of S1P1 and S1P lyase in vitreous of patients with proliferative diabetic retinopathy (Abu El-Asrar et al., 2014)
	Retinal fibrosis
	S1P promotes proliferation, myofibroblast transformation and formation of pro- fibrotic proteins in RPE cells (Swaney et al., 2008)
	S1P promotes glial migration (Simón et al., 2015)
	Blockade of S1P with monoclonal antibodies reduces angiogenesis and sub-retinal fibrosis (Caballero et al., 2009) and prevents excessive scarring in animal models of glaucoma (Lukowski et al., 2013)
Cer-1- phosphate (C1P)	**Signaling in photoreceptors**
	C1P regulates lipid metabolism in photoreceptor outer segments (Pasquaré and Giusto, 2008; Pasquaré et al., 2008)
	C1P increases the proliferation of photoreceptor progenitors in retina neuronal cultures (Miranda et al., 2011)
	C1P promotes differentiation and prevents apoptosis in cultured rat retina photoreceptors (Miranda et al., 2011)
	↑ C1P levels in uveitis (Wang et al., 2018)
	Phototransduction
	CerK regulation of Cer levels required for phospholipase C activity and PIP2 production during phototransduction (Dasgupta et al., 2009)

S1P Signaling in Retina Inflammation and Neovascularization

Sphingosine-1-phosphate is a potent mediator in the modulation of inflammatory responses and angiogenesis. It is crucial in the regulation of lymphocyte traffic, an essential step in the pathology of inflammation (Aarthi et al., 2011; Aoki et al., 2016). Several cytokines and chemokines, including TNF-α and interleukin 1-beta (IL1-β), activate SphK1 to produce S1P, which later induces cyclo-oxygenase 2 activity (Snider et al., 2010).

Collective evidence supports the relevance of S1P in retina inflammatory and vascular diseases. Abnormal retina blood vessel growth and macular edema are major complications leading to vision loss in diabetes retinopathy and S1P emerges as a key signal in the induction of neovascularization and in the preservation of retina endothelial barrier integrity (Allende and Proia, 2002; McGuire et al., 2011). In transgenic mice that overexpress SphK2, higher retinal S1P concentration accelerates retinal angiogenesis and increases neovascularization (Eresch et al., 2018). In turn, downregulation of S1P signaling with anti-S1P monoclonal antibodies and in S1P2 null mice in an ischemia-driven retinopathy markedly reduces pathologic neovascularization (Skoura et al., 2007; Caballero et al., 2009). RPE cells express the five S1PRs, and exogenous S1P induces the secretion of Interleukin-8 (IL-8); interestingly, supplementation with TNF-α enhances S1P3 expression, with a subsequent increase in S1P-induced IL-8 and IL-6 production (Zhu et al., 2010; Qiao et al., 2012). S1P also promotes the expression of vascular endothelial growth factor (VEGF) and hypoxia inducible factor-1α in RPE cells, which are crucial angiogenic factors (Terao et al., 2017). A significant increase in the expression of S1P1 and S1P lyase is detected in the vitreous of patients with proliferative diabetic retinopathy (Abu El-Asrar et al., 2014) whereas S1P signaling through S1P1/S1P3 promotes angiogenesis *in vitro*, participating in the changes affecting pericytes and endothelial cells (Durham et al., 2015). Hence, S1P signaling through S1PRs is a driving force in the onset and progression of inflammatory and angiogenic responses in retina inflammatory diseases (**Figure 3**).

S1P and Retinal Fibrosis

Fibrosis is a pathological process characterized by the deregulation of production and deposition of extracellular matrix components, leading to the destruction of normal tissue function and architecture (Wynn, 2007). Initiated by an acute injury or a vascular damage that leads to the recruitment of inflammatory cells, subsequent secretion of pro-inflammatory cytokines, as tumor growth factor (TGF)-β, platelet derived growth factor (PDGF), connective tissue growth factor, IL-3 and also S1P conducts to the excessive production and deposition of extracellular matrix components (Kisseleva and Brenner, 2008). Although the initial damage promotes a physiological fibrotic response to accomplish tissue repair, the chronic exposure to irritation and/ or inflammation leads to the formation of a fibrotic scar that impairs functionality. Many reports establish the role of S1P in fibrotic disorders in lung (Kono et al., 2007; Milara et al., 2012), kidney (Geoffroy et al., 2005; Awad et al., 2011), liver (Davaille et al., 2002; Li et al., 2011; Liu et al., 2011) and heart (Gellings Lowe et al., 2009; Pchejetski et al., 2012). However, S1P involvement in retinal fibrosis is poorly understood.

Many retinal diseases, including AMD, diabetic retinopathy and proliferative vitreoretinopathy, have a common underlying etiology of pathological scar tissue production and the role of TGF-β and PDGF in the development of eye fibrosis is well-known (Connor et al., 1989; Gamulescu et al., 2006; Saika, 2006; Lei et al., 2007). Recent data indicate a crosstalk between S1P and TGF-β in human corneas and orbital connective tissues and suggest that S1P anti- or pro-fibrotic functions in the eye are tissue-specific (Ko et al., 2017; Nicholas et al., 2017).

The available evidence suggests that S1P is involved in retina fibrotic disorders. A monoclonal anti-S1P strategy reduces sub-retinal fibrosis in a mouse model of choroidal neovascularization and prevents the formation of excessive scarring after surgery in animal models of glaucoma (Caballero et al., 2009; Lukowski et al., 2013). Müller glial cells and RPE cells, the two main cell types that support normal retinal function, have protagonic roles in the development of retinal fibrosis (Saika et al., 2008; Bringmann and Wiedemann, 2009). S1P promotes proliferation, myofibroblast transformation, collagen production and pro-fibrotic protein expression in human RPE cells (Swaney et al., 2008). We have shown that S1P has a key role in the regulation of Müller glial cell motility; 5 μM S1P promotes the migration of cultured rat Müller glial cells through activation of S1P3 while inhibiting S1P synthesis using SphK inhibitor 2 (SphKI 2) completely blocks this migration (Simón et al., 2015). We have proposed that Müller glial cells release S1P, which signals through S1P3 and activates the PI3K and the ERK/MAPK pathway to enhance migration (Simón et al., 2015). Taking into account that the deregulation of glial migration is involved in proliferative retinopathies, the S1P/SphK1/S1P3 axis emerges as a key target for controlling these diseases.

The above findings position S1P as a real Jekill and Hyde in the retina. S1P is indispensable for establishing retina structure, regulating proliferation of retinal progenitors and their later laminar distribution in the retina (Miranda et al., 2009; Fang et al., 2018). It is also a pro-survival factor for neurons, promoting their differentiation, preserving normal functioning and granting neuroprotection (Crousillac et al., 2009; Miranda et al., 2009; Abrahan et al., 2010; Joly and Pernet, 2016; Porter et al., 2018). On the other hand, S1P unleashes threatening processes in Müller glial cells and RPE cells, such as secretion of pro- inflammatory cytokines, proliferation, migration and transdifferentiation that promote and/or enhance inflammation and fibrosis (Swaney et al., 2008; Qiao et al., 2012; Simón et al., 2015; Terao et al., 2017). Thus, S1P facilitates the formation of gliotic scars that alter retinal structure and enhance visual dysfunction instead of preventing it.

The central role of S1P in the regulation of the crucial cellular processes that are altered in retinal pathologies turns it into an exceptional therapeutic target for treating these diseases. In order to accomplish this goal, several questions remain to be answered. How to take advantage of S1P protective role on photoreceptors and simultaneously elude the potentially risks for visual function derived from its effects on glial and epithelial cells? The S1P concentration might provide a clue, since the concentration that protects photoreceptors is 5-fold lower than that enhancing glial migration; promoting a controlled intracellular synthesis of S1P and preventing its release might preclude S1P deleterious effects.

Whether S1P dual roles depend on the signaling pathways it activates in each cell type and whether they respond to the microenvironment and/ or the type of injury cells are exposed to are pending questions as well. An attractive hypothesis for the dual role of S1P in retina degeneration is its function as a DAMP, signals that are exposed or released from stressed cells and recognized by and mobilize the immune system. S1P and Cer have been proposed as DAMPs in cancer cells; treating squamous carcinoma cells by photodynamic therapy results in Cer and S1P increases on the cell surface and in S1P release, and both sphingolipids trigger NFκB signaling in macrophages in co-culture (Korbelik et al., 2014). The ubiquitous expression of S1PRs in macrophages supports this proposal (Fischer et al., 2007). Recent research has shown that apoptotic cells release exosome-like vesicles, the biogenesis of which depends on S1P/S1PRs signaling; these vesicles have S1P, S1P1, and S1P3 and induce genes of proinflammatory cytokines and chemokines (Park et al., 2018), highlighting a new pathway for S1P in the pathogenesis of inflammatory diseases. Microglia, as resident retinal macrophages, has a detrimental role and contributes to retinal degeneration; microglia release of harmful factors contributes to Müller glial cell reactivity in *rd10* mice (Peng et al., 2014; Zhao et al., 2015). DAMPs have dual roles in the retina; e.g., fractalkine, which has been reported as a DAMP, is neuroprotective in *rd10* retinas by signaling through its CX3CR1 receptor, preventing microglia-induced damage (Roche et al., 2016). Stressed photoreceptors release DAMPs early in degeneration to induce neuroprotective responses in retinal glial cells by interacting with receptors as Toll-like receptor 2, a DAMP receptor that increases in Müller glial cells during degeneration (Hooper et al., 2018). S1P promotes migration in Müller glial cells and RPE cells (Swaney et al., 2008; Simón et al., 2015), which might release it to the retina milieu to act as an autocrine signal and promote a fibrotic process and/or to act as a paracrine signal in photoreceptors, promoting neuroprotection. Whether S1P is a DAMP released by retinal cells to either promote inflammation or neuroprotection is an exciting question to be explored in the sphingolipid field.

Finding answers to these questions would provide crucial understanding of the puzzling behavior of S1P and new insight to design effective therapeutic for the treatment of retinopathies.

SEARCHING FOR CERAMIDE-1-PHOSPHATE FUNCTIONS IN THE RETINA

C1P Synthesis and Functions

Ceramide-1-phosphate is a later incorporation to the sphingolipid family, now established as a pleiotropic bioactive sphingolipid with multiple cellular roles. CerK was first identified in brain synaptic vesicles and shown to synthesize a molecule identified as C1P (Bajjalieh et al., 1989). C1P existence and its synthesis from Cer were then demonstrated in the human pro-myelocytic leukemia cell line HL-60 (Dressler et al., 1992). Cer phosphorylation by CerK is the only mechanism for C1P generation established in mammals, although the presence of a small pool of C1P in CerK-/CerK- mutants suggests an alternative biosynthetic mechanism must exist (Bornancin, 2011). C1P is synthesized in the *trans* Golgi and a specific C1P transfer protein transports it to the plasma membrane, where it can be released for autocrine or paracrine signaling (Lamour et al., 2007; Simanshu et al., 2013). CerK is present in the brain and brain synaptic vesicles (Bajjalieh et al., 1989; Bajjalieh and Batchelor, 2000; Hannun et al., 2001) whereas cerebellar granule cells generate C1P from newly synthesized Cer, formed through SM degradation and Sph recycling (Riboni et al., 2002).

First thought as an intermediate in the complex sphingolipid metabolism, C1P functions began to be unraveled when it was shown to promote proliferation, in fibroblasts and macrophages (Gomez-Muñoz et al., 1995, 1997; Gangoiti et al., 2008), myoblasts and cancer cells (Mitra et al., 2007; Gangoiti et al., 2008). C1P is now known to be antiapoptotic (Gómez-Muñoz et al., 2004; Granado et al., 2009), to promote cell migration in different cell types (Granado et al., 2009; Arana et al., 2012), and to regulate the production of TNF-α (Lamour et al., 2011). Although mostly known for its pro-inflammatory actions, both C1P and CerK have been shown to exert either pro- or anti-inflammatory actions depending on the cell type (Presa et al., 2016). C1P has been proposed to be relevant for cancer progression, promoting tumor cell survival, growth and migration (Mitra et al., 2007; Rivera et al., 2016).

Ceramide-1-phosphate is also an intracellular and an extracellular messenger. In most cases, it acts as an intracellular signal, but it can be released to the extracellular milieu in specific circumstances or upon cell damage (Boath et al., 2008; Kim et al., 2012; Schneider et al., 2013). The Gomez-Muñoz laboratory demonstrated that exogenous C1P stimulates migration of macrophages independently of intracellular C1P synthesis by activating a G-protein coupled membrane receptor for C1P, partially identified and different from S1PRs (Granado et al., 2009). In contrast, C1P mitogenic effect on macrophages depends on its action as an intracellular messenger, as C1P effect can be mimicked by a photolabile caged-C1P analog, which activates cPLA2, PKCα and NADPH oxidase, generating ROS that promote proliferation (Arana et al., 2012).

Ceramide-1-phosphate activates multiple signaling pathways. To enhance proliferation, C1P activates the PI3K and the ERK/MAPK pathways, Jun N terminal kinase (JNK), nuclear factor NF-κB (NF-κB) and glucogen synthase kinase 3 (GSK3) (Gangoiti et al., 2010). C1P promotes survival of macrophages in the absence of trophic factors by inhibiting caspases and blocking Cer synthesis (Gómez-Muñoz et al., 2004; Granado et al., 2009). Activation of PI3K, NF-κB, increases in Bcl-2, decreases in Bax levels and inhibition of caspases 9 and 3 also participate in its survival effects (Gómez-Muñoz et al., 2005; Gomez-Muñoz, 2018). The findings by the Chalfant laboratory that C1P is a direct activator of cPLA2 provided the link between this sphingolipid and inflammation (Pettus et al., 2004). C1P interacts with cPLA2, promoting its translocation and association to membranes, and its subsequent activation, producing inflammatory mediators such as eicosanoids (Lamour et al., 2009; Hoeferlin et al., 2013; Simanshu et al., 2013).

Mounting evidence points to different roles for C1P in the nervous system. A 5-fold increase in C1P levels in the subventricular zone in Huntington disease patients has been reported, with no associated changes in Cer levels; this increase might represent a response to the chronic brain damage in these patients and might either reflect an attempt at neuroprotection and enhanced neurogenesis or contribute to neuroinflammation and neurodegeneration (Hunter et al., 2018). C1P has neuroprotective effects in the nervous system. Upregulation of CerK by Peroxisome proliferator-activated receptors protects neurons and astrocytes against Cer-induced death (Aleshin and Reiser, 2014) and promotes survival of cochlear hair cells during ototoxicity (Tabuchi and Hara, 2018). C1P might also be involved in neurotransmitter release; C1P promotes dopamine release from PC12 cells (Jeon et al., 2005), which is consistent with the ability of C1P to promote phagolysosome formation and with CerK presence in synaptic vesicles (Bajjalieh et al., 1989; Hinkovska-Galcheva et al., 1998).

C1P in the Retina

Little is known regarding C1P and CerK roles in the eye (**Table 2**). Pioneer work from Acharya's group in *Drosophila* eye revealed an indirect effect of *Drosophila* ceramide kinase (DCerK) in phototransduction. DCerK is an integral membrane protein that phosphorylates Cer, thus decreasing its levels (Dasgupta et al., 2009). DCerK mutants show severe photoreceptor degeneration and do not respond to light. The absence of DCerK increases Cer levels, and leads to proteolysis of NORPA, a critical effector of phototransduction. The degradation of this phospholipase C homolog leads to a consequent loss of activity, and failure in light signal transduction (Dasgupta et al., 2009). Thus, modulation of Cer levels by DCerK is essential for phototransduction. Noteworthy, C1P is involved in light-dependent regulation of other enzymes of lipid metabolism, such as diacylglycerol lipase and lipid phosphatases, in photoreceptor rod OS (Pasquaré and Giusto, 2008; Pasquaré et al., 2008), suggesting its role in phototransduction might also extend to the mammalian retina.

The finding that mutations in a CerKL gene are associated to a variant of autosomal recessive retinitis pigmentosa (Tuson et al., 2004), and to Cone-rod dystrophy (Littink et al., 2010; Birtel et al., 2018) brought huge expectations to the field, as it associated sphingolipid metabolism and retinal degeneration. CerKL has been further connected with retinitis pigmentosa in numerous studies (Auslender et al., 2007; Avila-Fernandez et al., 2008; Avela et al., 2018). However, the physiological functions of CerKL and its contribution to degeneration are still unclear. CerKL has no kinase activity neither on lipids nor on proteins in spite of having a diacylglycerol kinase domain (Tuson et al., 2004, 2009; Bornancin et al., 2005) and it interacts with several calcium sensor proteins in the retina (Nevet et al., 2012). A targeted deletion of CerKL in mouse leads to a mild retinal phenotype, with increased gliosis and mild functional alterations of the ganglion cell layer but no gross morphological alterations (Garanto et al., 2012). In contrast, CerKL knockdown causes retinal degeneration in zebrafish, with failure in the development of photoreceptor OS and increased apoptosis (Riera et al., 2013). CerKL might have antioxidant functions in the retina. Its overexpression protects retinal cells from oxidative stress-induced death, whereas its downregulation renders cells sensitive to this damage; CerKL deficiency causes zebrafish retinal degeneration and photoreceptor apoptosis through increased oxidative damage (Tuson et al., 2009; Li et al., 2014). CerKL is prominently localized in RPE cells, ganglion cells, inner nuclear layer and photoreceptor inner segments and its expression increases in light-stressed retinas (Mandal et al., 2013). An alteration in OS phagocytosis in a zebrafish CerKL knockout suggests a role for CerKL in RPE cell phagocytosis, leading to rod-cone dystrophy (Yu et al., 2017). Recent miRNA analysis of RPE cells exposed to oxidative stress shows that CerKL is a target of five altered miRNA (Donato et al., 2018). Existing evidence thus points to a role for CerKL in retina protection from oxidative stress-induced damage, and not related to Cer phosphorylation.

Ceramide kinase is ubiquitously and highly expressed in the retina (Mandal et al., 2013). $CerK^{-}/-$ retinas show decreased C1P and increased Cer; on the contrary, CerKL−/− retinas have normal C1P and Cer levels, supporting CerK as the major and probably unique responsible for C1P synthesis in the retina (Graf et al., 2008). RPE cells express CerK, among other enzymes involved in sphingolipid metabolism (Zhu et al., 2010) and no C1P is detected in these cells in $CerK^{-}/-$ retinas (Graf et al., 2008). Our group has shown that exogenous C1P promotes the proliferation of cultured photoreceptor progenitors and advances their differentiation as photoreceptors, enhancing the expression of opsin and peripherin and promoting the formation of rudimentary OS (Miranda et al., 2011). Notably, overexpression of CerK inhibits all-trans retinoic acid (ATRA)-induced differentiation of a human neuroblastoma cell line, SH-SY5Y (Murakami et al., 2010), suggesting that the effect of C1P on differentiation might be cell or context dependent. C1P also stimulates the survival of cultured photoreceptors, preventing their degeneration; this protection involves the preservation of mitochondrial potential, suggesting that C1P activates pathways upstream of mitochondrial depolarization (Miranda et al., 2011). Consistently, whereas a pan-caspase inhibitor decreases photoreceptor death in controls, it promotes no further reduction in photoreceptor death in C1P-supplemented cultures, suggesting C1P might prevent caspase activation (Miranda et al., 2011). Inhibiting the *de novo* synthesis of Cer prevents photoreceptor cell death in culture (German et al., 2006). Since C1P prevents macrophage apoptosis by impeding Cer accumulation, either by inhibiting its *de novo* synthesis or acid SMase activity (Gómez-Muñoz et al., 2004; Granado et al., 2009), C1P might also block Cer synthesis in photoreceptors, thus promoting their survival (**Figures 3, 4**).

Higher levels of C12-, C16- and C24-C1P, and of C16- and C18-Cer have been found in retinas in a rat model of endotoxin-induced uveitis, together with increases in TNF-α and IL-6 levels, suggesting these sphingolipids might participate in the inflammation process (Wang and Bieberich, 2018). Ongoing work in our laboratory suggests that C1P might promote the migration of retina Müller glial cells *in vitro*, which, together with glial proliferation, contributes to the progression of proliferative retinopathies (Vera et al., unpublished data).

Ceramide-1-phosphate functions in the retina are just starting to be uncovered. Existing evidence points to a crucial role of C1P in photoreceptor functionality, promoting their proliferation, survival and advancing differentiation. It might also be involved in modulation of phototransduction. Its contribution to inflammatory and proliferative pathologies of the retina has to be further explored.

DIHYDROCERAMIDE, A NEWCOMER PLAYER IN RETINA CELL DEATH?

Dihydroceramide, the immediate precursor of Cer in the *de novo* synthetic pathway, had long been considered as an inactive sphingolipid, since its exogenous addition had little effect on cell death (Ahn and Schroeder, 2010). However, cumulative evidence during the last decade supports a signaling role for endogenous DHCer and for other dihydrosphingolipids as well. Its accumulation has been implicated in autophagy regulation. Noteworthy, DHCer increase has been shown to induce cytotoxic autophagy in cancer cells and an impairment of autophagic flux and increase in fibrosis markers in liver cells (Hernández-Tiedra et al., 2016; Lee et al., 2017). DHCer also triggers cell cycle arrest and cell death (reviewed in Siddique et al., 2015). Therefore, it is now thought that DHCer is the principal Cer-mediated autophagy regulator (Siddique et al., 2015; Hannun and Obeid, 2018).

In the eye, early work showed distinct effects between Cer and DHCer. Cer induces cell death in cultured rat photoreceptors and amacrine neurons, in human RPE cells, in human corneal stromal fibroblasts and in lens epithelial cells, whereas addition of DHCer has no deleterious effect in these cell types (Barak et al., 2001; German et al., 2006; Samadi, 2007; Rizvi et al., 2011). However, recent evidence suggests a noxious role for

DHCer in the eye. DHCer content increases during aging in human lens and might be related to changes in the permeability barrier properties (Deeley et al., 2010). Both Cer and DHCer content increase in light-induced photoreceptor degeneration in albino rats, and preventing these increases protects retinal function and structure (Chen et al., 2013; Huang et al., 2014). DHCer desaturase catalyzes the conversion of DHCer to Cer and its modulation is crucial for the signaling pathways regulated by both sphingolipids. Loss of DHCer desaturase in *Drosophila* eye leads to DHCer accumulation, increased ROS production and loss of photoreceptor functionality and viability; in turn, blocking DHCer synthesis preserves their viability (Jung et al., 2017). Further work will establish whether DHCer is a member of the club of deadly sphingolipid messengers and whether it contributes to retinal pathologies.

Unraveling the Sphingolipid Network in the Retina

Sphingolipids emerge as crucial mediators in the activation of numerous pathways that might either activate neuroprotective mechanisms or whose dysregulation might lead to retina dysfunction. Cer stands out as a key messenger in the onset of degeneration in photoreceptors induced by oxidative stress and in numerous models of retina neurodegeneration; its increase through *de novo* synthesis or by SM breakdown activates different downstream pathways leading to cell death. Cer buildup, due to an activation or increased expression of SMases is also crucial in the onset of RPE cell death and inflammation. Preventing Cer increase through the inhibition or modulation of different enzymes of its intricate metabolism has been shown to effectively prevent photoreceptor and RPE cell death, both *in vivo* and *in vitro*, and preserve visual function. These findings underscore both the relevance of imbalances in Cer levels as inducers of RPE and photoreceptor cell death and the significance of modulation of the sphingolipid metabolism as a therapeutic strategy for the treatment of retina neurodegenerations. Having an integral picture of the functions of Cer in the retina and of the effects of preventing its accretion demands establishing the processes regulated by Cer in glial cells and its potential role in their gliotic response. Several questions remain to be answered in order to accomplish the fine tuning of the highly interconnected sphingolipid metabolism, which is crucial for the development of new treatments for retinal pathologies. The complexity of this metabolism makes its modulation a powerful approach for preserving vision function but might also be an Achilles' heel, jeopardizing strategies based on the inhibition of one of the metabolic pathways leading to Cer synthesis. Being Cer the central molecule in sphingolipid metabolism, the effects of blocking a single pathway established as crucial in generating Cer accumulation in a particular pathological circumstance should be explored. This inhibition might efficiently reduce cell death but impair other key, Cer-dependent, retinal processes or affect them indirectly, through the increase in bioactive sphingolipid metabolites. As blocking a certain biosynthetic pathway for Cer has been shown to provide a transient protection, it is critical to explore whether altering the flux through the network activates alternative Cer biosynthetic pathways and/or leads to the accumulation of bioactive sphingolipids, such as Sph or DHCer, which might trigger cell death. Further research aimed at understanding these balances and connections in a comprehensive molecular way might contribute to devising successful treatments based in new or already established drugs or suggest the necessity of combining different drugs in order to simultaneously modulate these metabolic processes.

Modulation of the sphingolipid rheostat might provide clues for preventing the death of photoreceptors (**Figure 4**). Nevertheless, S1P functions remain enigmatic. S1P, either exogenous or generated intracellularly, promotes survival of these cells; notably, photoreceptor trophic factors enhance S1P synthesis to exert their functions. A pending question is determining whether increasing S1P intracellular levels, either by promoting its synthesis and/or or blocking its degradation can prevent degeneration of photoreceptors and preserve their functionality in diseased retinas. Even if this is the case, taking advantage of S1P neuroprotective effect on photoreceptors still requires uncovering the clues to prevent or overcome S1P deleterious effects on other retinal cells, as glial, epithelial and endothelial cells, that may turn on fibrosis, neovascularization and inflammation. Similarly, the actions of S1P and Cer are critical for the pathogeneses of proliferative diseases, such as diabetic retinopathy and AMD. Both sphingolipids drive forward the crucial events leading to the progression of these diseases, with S1P inducing fibrosis and pro-inflammatory changes and Cer triggering cell death. Given the cross-conversions of sphingolipids, it is necessary to find out how to simultaneously balance their levels to avoid the onset of lethal processes in the retina. As stated above, this requires unraveling the intricate network of metabolic and signaling pathways to obtain the cues for refining the adjustment of the sphingolipid network. At least part of these cues might lie in the differential cellular expression of S1PRs and/or the molecular pathways activated by S1P. Uncovering the myriad of potential combinations of S1PRs and downstream signaling pathways, either activatory or inhibitory, might explain the variety of the responses triggered by S1P in different retinal cell types. In order to make use of the S1P axis as a tool for the treatment of retinal diseases, the precise mechanisms by which S1P achieves its effects should be clarified. Current evidence suggests that the expression pattern of S1PRs in the retina is modified in particular pathologies. Further studies are now required to establish whether photoreceptors, glial and epithelial cells differ in their S1PR expression pattern, and if and how are these patterns differentially modulated in each cell type by the environmental context, i.e., healthy or diseased retina and by extracellular cues, such as starvation, light damage, or oxidative stress. In addition, it is essential to understand the roles of S1P, and also establish those of C1P, in controlling neovascularization and fibrotic changes and whether they exhibit pro or anti-inflammatory actions in different pathological environments. Advancing our understanding of the multiple roles of sphingolipids and of the fine detail and regulation of their complex metabolic network will contribute to achieve much-needed therapies for retina pathologies.

AUTHOR CONTRIBUTIONS

MS wrote and edited the manuscript and contributed to the design of the figures. FPS wrote and edited the manuscript and contributed to the design of the figures. MV wrote the manuscript. NR designed the manuscript and figures and wrote and edited the manuscript.

FUNDING

Funding from the National Agency for Science and Technology (ANPCYT) (PICT-2015-0284 to NR); National Research Council of Argentina (CONICET) (PIP 11220-1101-00827, to NR); and PGI 24/B254 from the Secretary of Science and Technology, Universidad Nacional del Sur (to NR).

ACKNOWLEDGMENTS

NR is a principal researcher from the National Research Council of Argentina (CONICET), and Professor of Biological Chemistry from the Universidad Nacional del Sur (UNS). MS is an Assistant Researcher from CONICET and a Teaching Assistant from UNS. FPS is a Teaching Assistant from UNS and MV is a CONICET Doctoral Research fellow.

REFERENCES

Aarthi, J. J., Darendeliler, M. A., and Pushparaj, P. N. (2011). Dissecting the role of the S1P/S1PR axis in health and disease. *J. Dent. Res.* 90, 841–854. doi: 10.1177/0022034510389178

Abrahan, C. E., Miranda, G. E., Agnolazza, D. L., Politi, L. E., and Rotstein, N. P. (2010). Synthesis of sphingosine is essential for oxidative stress-induced apoptosis of photoreceptors. *Invest. Ophthalmol. Vis. Sci.* 51, 1171–1180. doi: 10.1167/iovs.09-3909

Abu El-Asrar, A. M., Nawaz, M. I., Mohammad, G., Siddiquei, M. M., Alam, K., Mousa, A., et al. (2014). Expression of bioactive lysophospholipids and processing enzymes in the vitreous from patients with proliferative diabetic retinopathy. *Lipids Health Dis.* 13:187. doi: 10.1186/1476-511X-13-187

Acharya, J. K., Dasgupta, U., Rawat, S. S., Yuan, C., Sanxaridis, P. D., Yonamine, I., et al. (2008). Cell-nonautonomous function of ceramidase in photoreceptor homeostasis. *Neuron* 57, 69–79. doi: 10.1016/j.neuron.2007.10.041

Acharya, U., Patel, S., Koundakjian, E., Nagashima, K., Han, X., and Acharya, J. K. (2003). Modulating sphingolipid biosynthetic pathway rescues photoreceptor degeneration. *Science* 299, 1740–1743. doi: 10.1126/science.1080549

Agudo-Barriuso, M., Lahoz, A., Nadal-Nicolás, F. M., Sobrado-Calvo, P., Piquer-Gil, M., Díaz-Llopis, M., et al. (2013). Metabolomic changes in the rat retina after optic nerve crush. *Invest. Ophthalmol. Vis. Sci.* 54, 4249–4259. doi: 10.1167/iovs.12-11451

Ahn, E. H., and Schroeder, J. J. (2010). Induction of apoptosis by sphingosine, sphinganine, and C(2)-ceramide in human colon cancer cells, but not by C(2)-dihydroceramide. *Anticancer Res.* 30, 2881–2884.

Aleshin, S., and Reiser, G. (2014). Peroxisome proliferator-activated receptor β/δ (PPARβ/δ) protects against ceramide-induced cellular toxicity in rat brain astrocytes and neurons by activation of ceramide kinase. *Mol. Cell. Neurosci.* 59, 127–134. doi: 10.1016/j.mcn.2014.01.008

Allende, M. L., and Proia, R. L. (2002). Sphingosine-1-phosphate receptors and the development of the vascular system. *Biochim. Biophys. Acta* 1582, 222–227. doi: 10.1016/s1388-1981(02)00175-0

Al-Zamil, W., and Yassin, S. (2017). Recent developments in age-related macular degeneration: a review. *Clin. Interv. Aging* 12, 1313–1330. doi: 10.2147/CIA.S143508

Aoki, M., Aoki, H., Ramanathan, R., Hait, N. C., and Takabe, K. (2016). Sphingosine-1-phosphate signaling in immune cells and inflammation: roles and therapeutic potential. *Mediators Inflamm.* 2016:8606878. doi: 10.1155/2016/8606878

Arana, L., Gangoiti, P., Ouro, A., Rivera, I.-G., Ordoñez, M., Trueba, M., et al. (2012). Generation of reactive oxygen species (ROS) is a key factor for stimulation of macrophage proliferation by ceramide 1-phosphate. *Exp. Cell Res.* 318, 350–360. doi: 10.1016/j.yexcr.2011.11.013

Arango-Gonzalez, B., Trifunović, D., Sahaboglu, A., Kranz, K., Michalakis, S., Farinelli, P., et al. (2014). Identification of a common non-apoptotic cell death mechanism in hereditary retinal degeneration. *PLoS One* 9:e112142. doi: 10.1371/journal.pone.0112142

Auslender, N., Sharon, D., Abbasi, A. H., Garzozi, H. J., Banin, E., and Ben-Yosef, T. (2007). A common founder mutation of CERKL underlies autosomal recessive retinal degeneration with early macular involvement among Yemenite Jews. *Invest. Ophthalmol. Vis. Sci.* 48, 5431–5438. doi: 10.1167/iovs.07-0736

Avela, K., Sankila, E.-M., Seitsonen, S., Kuuluvainen, L., Barton, S., Gillies, S., et al. (2018). A founder mutation in CERKL is a major cause of retinal dystrophy in Finland. *Acta Ophthalmol.* 96, 183–191. doi: 10.1111/aos.13551

Aveldaño, M. I., and Sprecher, H. (1987). Very long chain (C24 to C36) polyenoic fatty acids of the n-3 and n-6 series in dipolyunsaturated phosphatidylcholines from bovine retina. *J. Biol. Chem.* 262, 1180–1186.

Avila-Fernandez, A., Riveiro-Alvarez, R., Vallespin, E., Wilke, R., Tapias, I., Cantalapiedra, D., et al. (2008). CERKL mutations and associated phenotypes in seven Spanish families with autosomal recessive retinitis pigmentosa. *Invest. Ophthalmol. Vis. Sci.* 49, 2709–2713. doi: 10.1167/iovs.07-0865

Awad, A. S., Rouse, M. D., Khutsishvili, K., Huang, L., Bolton, W. K., Lynch, K. R., et al. (2011). Chronic sphingosine 1-phosphate 1 receptor activation attenuates early-stage diabetic nephropathy independent of lymphocytes. *Kidney Int.* 79, 1090–1098. doi: 10.1038/ki.2010.544

Bajjalieh, S., and Batchelor, R. (2000). Ceramide kinase. *Methods Enzymol.* 311, 207–215.

Bajjalieh, S. M., Martin, T. F., and Floor, E. (1989). Synaptic vesicle ceramide kinase. A calcium-stimulated lipid kinase that co-purifies with brain synaptic vesicles. *J. Biol. Chem.* 264, 14354–14360.

Bandhuvula, P., and Saba, J. D. (2007). Sphingosine-1-phosphate lyase in immunity and cancer: silencing the siren. *Trends Mol. Med.* 13, 210–217. doi: 10.1016/j.molmed.2007.03.005

Barak, A., Goldkorn, T., and Morse, L. S. (2005). Laser induces apoptosis and ceramide production in human retinal pigment epithelial cells. *Investig. Opthalmol. Vis. Sci.* 46, 2587. doi: 10.1167/iovs.04-0920

Barak, A., Morse, L. S., and Goldkorn, T. (2001). Ceramide: a potential mediator of apoptosis in human retinal pigment epithelial cells. *Invest. Ophthalmol. Vis. Sci.* 42, 247–254.

Bartke, N., and Hannun, Y. A. (2009). Bioactive sphingolipids: metabolism and function. *J. Lipid Res.* 50, S91–S96. doi: 10.1194/jlr.R800080-JLR200

Bazan, N. G. (2018). Docosanoids and elovanoids from omega-3 fatty acids are pro-homeostatic modulators of inflammatory responses, cell damage and neuroprotection. *Mol. Aspects Med.* 64, 18–33. doi: 10.1016/j.mam.2018.09.003

Berdyshev, E. V., Gorshkova, I., Skobeleva, A., Bittman, R., Lu, X., Dudek, S. M., et al. (2009). FTY720 inhibits ceramide synthases and up-regulates dihydrosphingosine 1-phosphate formation in human lung endothelial cells. *J. Biol. Chem.* 284, 5467–5477. doi: 10.1074/jbc.M805186200

Bian, G., Yu, C., Liu, L., Fang, C., Chen, K., Ren, P., et al. (2018). Sphingosine 1-phosphate stimulates eyelid closure in the developing rat by stimulating EGFR signaling. *Sci. Signal.* 11:eaat1470. doi: 10.1126/scisignal.aat1470

Birtel, J., Eisenberger, T., Gliem, M., Müller, P. L., Herrmann, P., Betz, C., et al. (2018). Clinical and genetic characteristics of 251 consecutive patients with macular and cone/cone-rod dystrophy. *Sci. Rep.* 8:4824. doi: 10.1038/s41598-018-22096-0

Boath, A., Graf, C., Lidome, E., Ullrich, T., Nussbaumer, P., and Bornancin, F. (2008). Regulation and traffic of ceramide 1-phosphate produced by ceramide kinase: comparative analysis to glucosylceramide and sphingomyelin. *J. Biol. Chem.* 283, 8517–8526. doi: 10.1074/jbc.M707107200

Bode, H., Bourquin, F., Suriyanarayanan, S., Wei, Y., Alecu, I., Othman, A., et al. (2016). HSAN1 mutations in serine palmitoyltransferase reveal a close structure-function-phenotype relationship. *Hum. Mol. Genet.* 25, 853–865. doi: 10.1093/hmg/ddv611

Bornancin, F. (2011). Ceramide kinase: the first decade. *Cell. Signal.* 23, 999–1008. doi: 10.1016/j.cellsig.2010.11.012

Bornancin, F., Mechtcheriakova, D., Stora, S., Graf, C., Wlachos, A., Dévay, P., et al. (2005). Characterization of a ceramide kinase-like protein. *Biochim. Biophys. Acta* 1687, 31–43. doi: 10.1016/j.bbalip.2004.11.012

Bringmann, A., and Wiedemann, P. (2009). Involvement of Müller glial cells in epiretinal membrane formation. *Graefes Arch. Clin. Exp. Ophthalmol.* 247, 865–883. doi: 10.1007/s00417-009-1082-x

Brinkmann, V., Billich, A., Baumruker, T., Heining, P., Schmouder, R., Francis, G., et al. (2010). Fingolimod (FTY720): discovery and development of an oral drug to treat multiple sclerosis. *Nat. Rev. Drug Discov.* 9, 883–897. doi: 10.1038/nrd3248

Brownstein, S., Carpenter, S., Polomeno, R. C., and Little, J. M. (1980). Sandhoff's disease (GM2 gangliosidosis type 2). Histopathology and ultrastructure of the eye. *Arch. Ophthalmol.* 98, 1089–1097.

Brownstein, S., Meagher-Villemure, K., Polomeno, R. C., and Little, J. M. (1978). Optic nerve in globoid leukodystrophy (Krabbe's disease). Ultrastructural changes. *Arch. Ophthalmol.* 96, 864–870.

Brush, R. S., Tran, J.-T. A., Henry, K. R., McClellan, M. E., Elliott, M. H., and Mandal, M. N. A. (2010). Retinal sphingolipids and their very-long-chain fatty acid–containing species. *Investig. Opthalmol. Vis. Sci.* 51, 4422. doi: 10.1167/iovs.09-5134

Busik, J. V., Esselman, W. J., and Reid, G. E. (2012). Examining the role of lipid mediators in diabetic retinopathy. *Clin. Lipidol.* 7, 661–675. doi: 10.2217/clp.12.68

Caballero, S., Swaney, J., Moreno, K., Afzal, A., Kielczewski, J., Stoller, G., et al. (2009). Anti-sphingosine-1-phosphate monoclonal antibodies inhibit angiogenesis and sub-retinal fibrosis in a murine model of laser-induced choroidal neovascularization. *Exp. Eye Res.* 88, 367–377. doi: 10.1016/j.exer.2008.07.012

Canals, D., Salamone, S., and Hannun, Y. A. (2018). Visualizing bioactive ceramides. *Chem. Phys. Lipids* 216, 142–151. doi: 10.1016/j.chemphyslip.2018.09.013

Castro, B. M., Prieto, M., and Silva, L. C. (2014). Ceramide: a simple sphingolipid with unique biophysical properties. *Prog. Lipid Res.* 54, 53–67. doi: 10.1016/j.plipres.2014.01.004

Chakravarthy, H., Navitskaya, S., O'Reilly, S., Gallimore, J., Mize, H., Beli, E., et al. (2016). Role of acid sphingomyelinase in shifting the balance between proinflammatory and reparative bone marrow cells in diabetic retinopathy. *Stem Cells* 34, 972–983. doi: 10.1002/stem.2259

Chalfant, C. E., Kishikawa, K., Mumby, M. C., Kamibayashi, C., Bielawska, A., and Hannun, Y. A. (1999). Long chain ceramides activate protein phosphatase-1 and protein phosphatase-2A. *J. Biol. Chem.* 274, 20313–20317. doi: 10.1074/jbc.274.29.20313

Chang, G. Q., Hao, Y., and Wong, F. (1993). Apoptosis: final common pathway of photoreceptor death in rd, rds, and rhodopsin mutant mice. *Neuron* 11, 595–605. doi: 10.1016/0896-6273(93)90072-y

Chaurasia, B., and Summers, S. A. (2015). Ceramides – lipotoxic inducers of metabolic disorders. *Trends Endocrinol. Metab.* 26, 538–550. doi: 10.1016/j.tem.2015.07.006

Chen, H., Chan, A. Y., Stone, D. U., and Mandal, N. A. (2014). Beyond the cherry-red spot: Ocular manifestations of sphingolipid-mediated neurodegenerative and inflammatory disorders. *Surv. Ophthalmol.* 59, 64–76. doi: 10.1016/j.survophthal.2013.02.005

Chen, H., Tran, J.-T. A., Eckerd, A., Huynh, T.-P., Elliott, M. H., Brush, R. S., et al. (2013). Inhibition of de novo ceramide biosynthesis by FTY720 protects rat retina from light-induced degeneration. *J. Lipid Res.* 54, 1616–1629. doi: 10.1194/jlr.M035048

Choi, J. W., Gardell, S. E., Herr, D. R., Rivera, R., Lee, C.-W., Noguchi, K., et al. (2011). FTY720 (fingolimod) efficacy in an animal model of multiple sclerosis requires astrocyte sphingosine 1-phosphate receptor 1 (S1P1) modulation. *Proc. Natl. Acad. Sci. U.S.A.* 108, 751–756. doi: 10.1073/pnas.1014154108

Chun, J., and Hartung, H.-P. (2010). Mechanism of action of oral fingolimod (FTY720) in multiple sclerosis. *Clin. Neuropharmacol.* 33, 91–101. doi: 10.1097/WNF.0b013e3181cbf825

Connor, T. B., Roberts, A. B., Sporn, M. B., Danielpour, D., Dart, L. L., Michels, R. G., et al. (1989). Correlation of fibrosis and transforming growth factor-beta type 2 levels in the eye. *J. Clin. Invest.* 83, 1661–1666. doi: 10.1172/JCI114065

Crousillac, S., Colonna, J., McMains, E., Dewey, J. S., and Gleason, E. (2009). Sphingosine-1-phosphate elicits receptor-dependent calcium signaling in retinal amacrine cells. *J. Neurophysiol.* 102, 3295–3309. doi: 10.1152/jn.00119.2009

Cuvillier, O. (2002). Sphingosine in apoptosis signaling. *Biochim. Biophys. Acta* 1585, 153–162. doi: 10.1016/s1388-1981(02)00336-0

Cuvillier, O., Edsall, L., and Spiegel, S. (2000). Involvement of sphingosine in mitochondria-dependent Fas-induced apoptosis of type II Jurkat T cells. *J. Biol. Chem.* 275, 15691–15700. doi: 10.1074/jbc.M000280200

Cuvillier, O., Nava, V. E., Murthy, S. K., Edsall, L. C., Levade, T., Milstien, S., et al. (2001). Sphingosine generation, cytochrome c release, and activation of caspase-7 in doxorubicin-induced apoptosis of MCF7 breast adenocarcinoma cells. *Cell Death Differ.* 8, 162–171. doi: 10.1038/sj.cdd.4400793

Cuvillier, O., Pirianov, G., Kleuser, B., Vanek, P. G., Cosot, O. A., Gutkind, J. S., et al. (1996). Suppression of ceramide-mediated programmed cell death by sphingosine- 1-phosphate. *Nature* 381, 800–803. doi: 10.1038/381800a0

Cyster, J. G., and Schwab, S. R. (2012). Sphingosine-1-phosphate and lymphocyte egress from lymphoid organs. *Annu. Rev. Immunol.* 30, 69–94. doi: 10.1146/annurev-immunol-020711-075011

Czubowicz, K., and Strosznajder, R. (2014). Ceramide in the molecular mechanisms of neuronal cell death. The role of sphingosine-1-phosphate. *Mol. Neurobiol.* 50, 26–37. doi: 10.1007/s12035-013-8606-4

Dany, M., and Ogretmen, B. (2015). Ceramide induced mitophagy and tumor suppression. *Biochim. Biophys. Acta* 1853, 2834–2845. doi: 10.1016/j.bbamcr.2014.12.039

Dasgupta, U., Bamba, T., Chiantia, S., Karim, P., Tayoun, A. N. A., Yonamine, I., et al. (2009). Ceramide kinase regulates phospholipase C and phosphatidylinositol 4, 5, bisphosphate in phototransduction. *Proc. Natl. Acad. Sci. U.S.A.* 106, 20063–20068. doi: 10.1073/pnas.0911028106

Davaille, J., Li, L., Mallat, A., and Lotersztajn, S. (2002). Sphingosine 1-phosphate triggers both apoptotic and survival signals for human hepatic myofibroblasts. *J. Biol. Chem.* 277, 37323–37330. doi: 10.1074/jbc.M202798200

David, K. K., Andrabi, S. A., Dawson, T. M., and Dawson, V. L. (2009). Parthanatos, a messenger of death. *Front. Biosci.* 14, 1116–1128.

Deeley, J. M., Hankin, J. A., Friedrich, M. G., Murphy, R. C., Truscott, R. J. W., Mitchell, T. W., et al. (2010). Sphingolipid distribution changes with age in the human lens. *J. Lipid Res.* 51, 2753–2760. doi: 10.1194/jlr.M007716

Donato, L., Bramanti, P., Scimone, C., Rinaldi, C., D'Angelo, R., and Sidoti, A. (2018). miRNAexpression profile of retinal pigment epithelial cells under oxidative stress conditions. *FEBS Open Biol.* 8, 219–233. doi: 10.1002/2211-5463.12360

Dressler, K. A., Mathias, S., and Kolesnick, R. N. (1992). Tumor necrosis factor-alpha activates the sphingomyelin signal transduction pathway in a cell-free system. *Science* 255, 1715–1718. doi: 10.1126/science.1313189

Durham, J. T., Dulmovits, B. M., Cronk, S. M., Sheets, A. R., and Herman, I. M. (2015). Pericyte chemomechanics and the angiogenic switch: insights into the pathogenesis of proliferative diabetic retinopathy? *Invest. Ophthalmol. Vis. Sci.* 56, 3441–3459. doi: 10.1167/iovs.14-13945

Eresch, J., Stumpf, M., Koch, A., Vutukuri, R., Ferreirós, N., Schreiber, Y., et al. (2018). Sphingosine kinase 2 modulates retinal neovascularization in the mouse model of oxygen-induced retinopathy. *Invest. Ophthalmol. Vis. Sci.* 59, 653–661. doi: 10.1167/iovs.17-22544

Fabiani, C., Zulueta, A., Bonezzi, F., Casas, J., Ghidoni, R., Signorelli, P., et al. (2017). 2-Acetyl-5-tetrahydroxybutyl imidazole (THI) protects 661W cells against oxidative stress. *Naunyn. Schmiedebergs Arch. Pharmacol.* 390, 741–751. doi: 10.1007/s00210-017-1374-3

Fahy, E., Subramaniam, S., Brown, H. A., Glass, C. K., Merrill, A. H., Murphy, R. C., et al. (2005). A comprehensive classification system for lipids. *J. Lipid Res.* 46, 839–862. doi: 10.1194/jlr.E400004-JLR200

Fan, J., Wu, B. X., and Crosson, C. E. (2016). Suppression of acid sphingomyelinase protects the retina from ischemic injury. *Investig. Opthalmol. Vis. Sci.* 57, 4476. doi: 10.1167/iovs.16-19717

Fang, C., Bian, G., Ren, P., Xiang, J., Song, J., Yu, C., et al. (2018). S1p transporter spns2 regulates proper postnatal retinal morphogenesis. *FASEB J.* 32, 3597–3613. doi: 10.1096/fj.201701116R

Fischer, H., Ellström, P., Ekström, K., Gustafsson, L., Gustafsson, M., and Svanborg, C. (2007). Ceramide as a TLR4 agonist; a putative signalling intermediate between sphingolipid receptors for microbial ligands and TLR4. *Cell. Microbiol.* 9, 1239–1251. doi: 10.1111/j.1462-5822.2006.00867.x

Fliesler, S. J., and Bretillon, L. (2010). The ins and outs of cholesterol in the vertebrate retina. *J. Lipid Res.* 51, 3399–3413. doi: 10.1194/jlr.R010538

Fox, T. E., Han, X., Kelly, S., Merrill, A. H., Martin, R. E., Anderson, R. E., et al. (2006). Diabetes alters sphingolipid metabolism in the retina: a potential mechanism of cell death in diabetic retinopathy. *Diabetes* 55, 3573–3580. doi: 10.2337/db06-0539

Friedman, J. S., Chang, B., Krauth, D. S., Lopez, I., Waseem, N. H., Hurd, R. E., et al. (2010). Loss of lysophosphatidylcholine acyltransferase 1 leads to photoreceptor degeneration in rd11 mice. *Proc. Natl. Acad. Sci. U.S.A.* 107, 15523–15528. doi: 10.1073/pnas.1002897107

Galadari, S., Rahman, A., Pallichankandy, S., and Thayyullathil, F. (2015). Tumor suppressive functions of ceramide: evidence and mechanisms. *Apoptosis* 20, 689–711. doi: 10.1007/s10495-015-1109-1

Gamulescu, M.-A., Chen, Y., He, S., Spee, C., Jin, M., Ryan, S. J., et al. (2006). Transforming growth factor beta2-induced myofibroblastic differentiation of human retinal pigment epithelial cells: regulation by extracellular matrix proteins and hepatocyte growth factor. *Exp. Eye Res.* 83, 212–222. doi: 10.1016/j.exer.2005.12.007

Ganesan, V., Perera, M. N., Colombini, D., Datskovskiy, D., Chadha, K., and Colombini, M. (2010). Ceramide and activated Bax act synergistically to permeabilize the mitochondrial outer membrane. *Apoptosis* 15, 553–562. doi: 10.1007/s10495-009-0449-0

Gangoiti, P., Granado, M. H., Arana, L., Ouro, A., and Gomez-Muñoz, A. (2010). Activation of protein kinase C-α is essential for stimulation of cell proliferation by ceramide 1-phosphate. *FEBS Lett.* 584, 517–524. doi: 10.1016/j.febslet.2009.11.086

Gangoiti, P., Granado, M. H., Wang, S. W., Kong, J. Y., Steinbrecher, U. P., and Gómez-Muñoz, A. (2008). Ceramide 1-phosphate stimulates macrophage proliferation through activation of the PI3-kinase/PKB, JNK and ERK1/2 pathways. *Cell. Signal.* 20, 726–736. doi: 10.1016/j.cellsig.2007.12.008

Garanto, A., Vicente-Tejedor, J., Riera, M., de la Villa, P., Gonzàlez-Duarte, R., Blanco, R., et al. (2012). Targeted knockdown of Cerkl, a retinal dystrophy gene, causes mild affectation of the retinal ganglion cell layer. *Biochim. Biophys. Acta* 1822, 1258–1269. doi: 10.1016/j.bbadis.2012.04.004

García-Ruiz, C., Colell, A., Marí, M., Morales, A., and Fernández-Checa, J. C. (1997). Direct effect of ceramide on the mitochondrial electron transport chain leads to generation of reactive oxygen species. Role of mitochondrial glutathione. *J. Biol. Chem.* 272, 11369–11377. doi: 10.1074/jbc.272.17.11369

Gellings Lowe, N., Swaney, J. S., Moreno, K. M., and Sabbadini, R. A. (2009). Sphingosine-1-phosphate and sphingosine kinase are critical for transforming growth factor-beta-stimulated collagen production by cardiac fibroblasts. *Cardiovasc. Res.* 82, 303–312. doi: 10.1093/cvr/cvp056

Geoffroy, K., Troncy, L., Wiernsperger, N., Lagarde, M., and El Bawab, S. (2005). Glomerular proliferation during early stages of diabetic nephropathy is associated with local increase of sphingosine-1-phosphate levels. *FEBS Lett.* 579, 1249–1254. doi: 10.1016/j.febslet.2004.12.094

German, O. L., Miranda, G. E., Abrahan, C. E., and Rotstein, N. P. (2006). Ceramide is a mediator of apoptosis in retina photoreceptors. *Invest. Ophthalmol. Vis. Sci.* 47, 1658–1668. doi: 10.1167/iovs.05-1310

Gomez-Muñoz, A. (2018). "The role of ceramide 1-phosphate in tumor cell survival and dissemination," in *Advances in Cancer Research*, eds C. E. Chalfant and P. Fisher (Cambridge, MA: Academic Press), 217–234. doi: 10.1016/bs.acr.2018.04.012

Gomez-Muñoz, A., Duffy, P. A., Martin, A., O'Brien, L., Byun, H. S., Bittman, R., et al. (1995). Short-chain ceramide-1-phosphates are novel stimulators of DNA synthesis and cell division: antagonism by cell-permeable ceramides. *Mol. Pharmacol.* 47, 833–839.

Gomez-Muñoz, A., Frago, L. M., Alvarez, L., and Varela-Nieto, I. (1997). Stimulation of DNA synthesis by natural ceramide 1-phosphate. *Biochem. J.* 325(Pt 2), 435–440. doi: 10.1042/bj3250435

Gómez-Muñoz, A., Kong, J. Y., Parhar, K., Wang, S. W., Gangoiti, P., González, M., et al. (2005). Ceramide-1-phosphate promotes cell survival through activation of the phosphatidylinositol 3-kinase/protein kinase B pathway. *FEBS Lett.* 579, 3744–3750. doi: 10.1016/j.febslet.2005.05.067

Gómez-Muñoz, A., Kong, J. Y., Salh, B., and Steinbrecher, U. P. (2004). Ceramide-1-phosphate blocks apoptosis through inhibition of acid sphingomyelinase in macrophages. *J. Lipid Res.* 45, 99–105. doi: 10.1194/jlr.M300158-JLR200

Gómez-Muñoz, A., Waggoner, D. W., O'Brien, L., and Brindley, D. N. (1995). Interaction of ceramides, sphingosine, and sphingosine 1-phosphate in regulating DNA synthesis and phospholipase D activity. *J. Biol. Chem.* 270, 26318–26325. doi: 10.1074/jbc.270.44.26318

Graf, C., Niwa, S., Müller, M., Kinzel, B., and Bornancin, F. (2008). Wild-type levels of ceramide and ceramide-1-phosphate in the retina of ceramide kinase-like-deficient mice. *Biochem. Biophys. Res. Commun.* 373, 159–163. doi: 10.1016/j.bbrc.2008.06.002

Granado, M. H., Gangoiti, P., Ouro, A., Arana, L., González, M., Trueba, M., et al. (2009). Ceramide 1-phosphate (C1P) promotes cell migration. *Cell. Signal.* 21, 405–412. doi: 10.1016/j.cellsig.2008.11.003

Grassme, H., Jekle, A., Riehle, A., Schwarz, H., Berger, J., Sandhoff, K., et al. (2001). CD95 signaling via ceramide-rich membrane rafts. *J. Biol. Chem.* 276, 20589–20596. doi: 10.1074/jbc.M101207200

Grassmé, H., Schwarz, H., and Gulbins, E. (2001). Molecular mechanisms of ceramide-mediated CD95 clustering. *Biochem. Biophys. Res. Commun.* 284, 1016–1030. doi: 10.1006/bbrc.2001.5045

Gulbins, E., and Kolesnick, R. (2003). Raft ceramide in molecular medicine. *Oncogene* 22, 7070–7077. doi: 10.1038/sj.onc.1207146

Güntert, T., Hänggi, P., Othman, A., Suriyanarayanan, S., Sonda, S., Zuellig, R. A., et al. (2016). 1-Deoxysphingolipid-induced neurotoxicity involves N-methyl- d -aspartate receptor signaling. *Neuropharmacology* 110, 211–222. doi: 10.1016/j.neuropharm.2016.03.033

Hait, N. C., Allegood, J., Maceyka, M., Strub, G. M., Harikumar, K. B., Singh, S. K., et al. (2009). Regulation of histone acetylation in the nucleus by sphingosine-1-phosphate. *Science* 325, 1254–1257. doi: 10.1126/science.1176709

Hait, N. C., Oskeritzian, C. A., Paugh, S. W., Milstien, S., and Spiegel, S. (2006). Sphingosine kinases, sphingosine 1-phosphate, apoptosis and diseases. *Biochim. Biophys. Acta* 1758, 2016–2026. doi: 10.1016/j.bbamem.2006.08.007

Hait, N. C., Wise, L. E., Allegood, J. C., O'Brien, M., Avni, D., Reeves, T. M., et al. (2014). Active, phosphorylated fingolimod inhibits histone deacetylases and facilitates fear extinction memory. *Nat. Neurosci.* 17, 971–980. doi: 10.1038/nn.3728

Hammer, S. S., and Busik, J. V. (2017). The role of dyslipidemia in diabetic retinopathy. *Vision Res.* 139, 228–236. doi: 10.1016/j.visres.2017.04.010

Hanada, K., Kumagai, K., Tomishige, N., and Yamaji, T. (2009). CERT-mediated trafficking of ceramide. *Biochim. Biophys. Acta* 1791, 684–691. doi: 10.1016/j.bbalip.2009.01.006

Hannun, Y. A., and Bell, R. M. (1989). Functions of sphingolipids and sphingolipid breakdown products in cellular regulation. *Science* 243, 500–507. doi: 10.1126/science.2643164

Hannun, Y. A., Loomis, C. R., Merrill, A. H., and Bell, R. M. (1986). Sphingosine inhibition of protein kinase C activity and of phorbol dibutyrate binding in vitro and in human platelets. *J. Biol. Chem.* 261, 12604–12609.

Hannun, Y. A., and Luberto, C. (2004). Lipid metabolism: ceramide transfer protein adds a new dimension. *Curr. Biol.* 14, R163–R165.

Hannun, Y. A., Luberto, C., and Argraves, K. M. (2001). Enzymes of sphingolipid metabolism: from modular to integrative signaling. *Biochemistry* 40, 4893–4903. doi: 10.1021/bi002836k

Hannun, Y. A., and Obeid, L. M. (2008). Principles of bioactive lipid signalling: lessons from sphingolipids. *Nat. Rev. Mol. Cell Biol.* 9, 139–150. doi: 10.1038/nrm2329

Hannun, Y. A., and Obeid, L. M. (2011). Many ceramides. *J. Biol. Chem.* 286, 27855–27862. doi: 10.1074/jbc.R111.254359

Hannun, Y. A., and Obeid, L. M. (2018). Sphingolipids and their metabolism in physiology and disease. *Nat. Rev. Mol. Cell Biol.* 19, 175–191. doi: 10.1038/nrm.2017.107

Harcourt, B., and Ashton, N. (1973). Ultrastructure of the optic nerve in Krabbe's leucodystrophy. *Br. J. Ophthalmol.* 57, 885–891. doi: 10.1136/bjo.57.12.885

Harmon, J. M., Bacikova, D., Gable, K., Gupta, S. D., Han, G., Sengupta, N., et al. (2013). Topological and functional characterization of the ssSPTs, small activating subunits of serine palmitoyltransferase. *J. Biol. Chem.* 288, 10144–10153. doi: 10.1074/jbc.M113.451526

Hernández-Corbacho, M. J., Canals, D., Adada, M. M., Liu, M., Senkal, C. E., Yi, J. K., et al. (2015). Tumor necrosis factor-α (TNFα)-induced ceramide generation via ceramide synthases regulates loss of focal adhesion kinase (FAK) and programmed cell death. *J. Biol. Chem.* 290, 25356–25373. doi: 10.1074/jbc.M115.658658

Hernández-Tiedra, S., Fabriàs, G., Dávila, D., Salanueva, ÍJ., Casas, J., Montes, L. R., et al. (2016). Dihydroceramide accumulation mediates cytotoxic autophagy of cancer cells via autolysosome destabilization. *Autophagy* 12, 2213–2229. doi: 10.1080/15548627.2016.1213927

Hinkovska-Galcheva, V. T., Boxer, L. A., Mansfield, P. J., Harsh, D., Blackwood, A., and Shayman, J. A. (1998). The formation of ceramide-1-phosphate during neutrophil phagocytosis and its role in liposome fusion. *J. Biol. Chem.* 273, 33203–33209. doi: 10.1074/jbc.273.50.33203

Hla, T., Lee, M. J., Ancellin, N., Paik, J. H., and Kluk, M. J. (2001). Lysophospholipids - receptor revelations. *Science* 294, 1875–1878. doi: 10.1126/science.1065323

Hoeferlin, L. A., Wijesinghe, D. S., and Chalfant, C. E. (2013). The role of ceramide-1-phosphate in biological functions. *Handb. Exp. Pharmacol* 215, 153–166. doi: 10.1007/978-3-7091-1368-4_8

Holopainen, J. M., Angelova, M. I., and Kinnunen, P. K. (2000). Vectorial budding of vesicles by asymmetrical enzymatic formation of ceramide in giant liposomes. *Biophys. J.* 78, 830–838. doi: 10.1016/S0006-3495(00)76640-9

Hooper, M. J., Wang, J., Browning, R., and Ash, J. D. (2018). Damage-associated molecular pattern recognition is required for induction of retinal neuroprotective pathways in a sex-dependent manner. *Sci. Rep.* 8:9115. doi: 10.1038/s41598-018-27479-x

Hornemann, T., Penno, A., Rütti, M. F., Ernst, D., Kivrak-Pfiffner, F., Rohrer, L., et al. (2009). The SPTLC3 subunit of serine palmitoyltransferase generates short chain sphingoid bases. *J. Biol. Chem.* 284, 26322–26330. doi: 10.1074/jbc.M109.023192

Huang, K., Huang, J., Chen, C., Hao, J., Wang, S., Huang, J., et al. (2014). AP-1 regulates sphingosine kinase 1 expression in a positive feedback manner in glomerular mesangial cells exposed to high glucose. *Cell. Signal.* 26, 629–638. doi: 10.1016/j.cellsig.2013.12.002

Hunter, M., Demarais, N. J., Faull, R. L. M., Grey, A. C., and Curtis, M. A. (2018). Subventricular zone lipidomic architecture loss in Huntington's disease. *J. Neurochem.* 146, 613–630. doi: 10.1111/jnc.14468

Huwiler, A., Kolter, T., Pfeilschifter, J., and Sandhoff, K. (2000). Physiology and pathophysiology of sphingolipid metabolism and signaling. *Biochim. Biophys. Acta* 1485, 63–99.

Insua, M. F., Garelli, A., Rotstein, N. P., German, O. L., Arias, A., and Politi, L. E. (2003). Cell cycle regulation in retinal progenitors by glia-derived neurotrophic factor and docosahexaenoic acid. *Investig. Ophthalmol. Vis. Sci.* 44, 2235–2244.

Jain, A., Beutel, O., Ebell, K., Korneev, S., and Holthuis, J. C. M. (2017). Diverting CERT-mediated ceramide transport to mitochondria triggers Bax-dependent apoptosis. *J. Cell Sci.* 130, 360–371. doi: 10.1242/jcs.194191

Jenkins, R. W., Canals, D., and Hannun, Y. A. (2009). Roles and regulation of secretory and lysosomal acid sphingomyelinase. *Cell. Signal.* 21, 836–846. doi: 10.1016/j.cellsig.2009.01.026

Jeon, H. J., Lee, D. H., Kang, M. S., Lee, M.-O., Jung, K. M., Jung, S. Y., et al. (2005). Dopamine release in PC12 cells is mediated by Ca^{2+}-dependent production of ceramide via sphingomyelin pathway. *J. Neurochem.* 95, 811–820. doi: 10.1111/j.1471-4159.2005.03403.x

Jiménez-Rojo, N., Sot, J., Busto, J. V., Shaw, W. A., Duan, J., Merrill, A. H., et al. (2014). Biophysical properties of novel 1-deoxy-(dihydro)ceramides occurring in mammalian cells. *Biophys. J.* 107, 2850–2859. doi: 10.1016/j.bpj.2014.10.010

Joly, S., and Pernet, V. (2016). Sphingosine 1-phosphate receptor 1 is required for retinal ganglion cell survival after optic nerve trauma. *J. Neurochem.* 138, 571–586. doi: 10.1111/jnc.13701

Jun, B., Mukherjee, P. K., Asatryan, A., Kautzmann, M.-A., Heap, J., Gordon, W. C., et al. (2017). Elovanoids are novel cell-specific lipid mediators necessary for neuroprotective signaling for photoreceptor cell integrity. *Sci. Rep.* 7:5279. doi: 10.1038/s41598-017-05433-7

Jung, W.-H., Liu, C.-C., Yu, Y.-L., Chang, Y.-C., Lien, W.-Y., Chao, H.-C., et al. (2017). Lipophagy prevents activity-dependent neurodegeneration due to dihydroceramide accumulation in vivo. *EMBO Rep.* 18, 1150–1165. doi: 10.15252/embr.201643480

Kady, N. M., Liu, X., Lydic, T. A., Syed, M. H., Navitskaya, S., Wang, Q., et al. (2018). ELOVL4-mediated production of very long-chain ceramides stabilizes tight junctions and prevents diabetes-induced retinal vascular permeability. *Diabetes* 67, 769–781. doi: 10.2337/db17-1034

Kannan, R., Jin, M., Gamulescu, M.-A., and Hinton, D. R. (2004). Ceramide-induced apoptosis: role of catalase and hepatocyte growth factor. *Free Radic. Biol. Med.* 37, 166–175. doi: 10.1016/j.freeradbiomed.2004.04.011

Kaur, G., Tan, L. X., Rathnasamy, G., La Cunza, N., Germer, C. J., Toops, K. A., et al. (2018). Aberrant early endosome biogenesis mediates complement activation in the retinal pigment epithelium in modelsof macular degeneration. *Proc. Natl. Acad. Sci. U.S.A* 115, 9014–9019. doi: 10.1073/pnas.1805039115

Kawahara, A., Nishi, T., Hisano, Y., Fukui, H., Yamaguchi, A., and Mochizuki, N. (2009). The sphingolipid transporter Spns2 functions in migration of zebrafish myocardial precursors. *Science* 323, 524–527. doi: 10.1126/science.1167449

Kim, C. H., Wu, W., Wysoczynski, M., Abdel-Latif, A., Sunkara, M., Morris, A., et al. (2012). Conditioning for hematopoietic transplantation activates the complement cascade and induces a proteolytic environment in bone marrow: a novel role for bioactive lipids and soluble C5b-C9 as homing factors. *Leukemia* 26, 106–116. doi: 10.1038/leu.2011.185

Kisseleva, T., and Brenner, D. A. (2008). Mechanisms of Fibrogenesis. *Exp. Biol. Med.* 233, 109–122. doi: 10.3181/0707-MR-190

Kitatani, K., Idkowiak-Baldys, J., and Hannun, Y. A. (2008). The sphingolipid salvage pathway in ceramide metabolism and signaling. *Cell. Signal.* 20, 1010–1018. doi: 10.1016/j.cellsig.2007.12.006

Klein, R., Klein, B. E., Jensen, S. C., Cruickshanks, K. J., Lee, K. E., Danforth, L. G., et al. (2001). Medication use and the 5-year incidence of early age-related maculopathy: the Beaver Dam Eye Study. *Arch. Ophthalmol.* 119, 1354–1359.

Knapp, M. (2011). Cardioprotective role of sphingosine-1-phosphate. *J. Physiol. Pharmacol.* 62, 601–607. doi: 10.1016/S0040-4020(99)00597-9

Ko, J., Chae, M. K., Lee, J. H., Lee, E. J., and Yoon, J. S. (2017). Sphingosine-1-phosphate mediates fibrosis in orbital fibroblasts in Graves' Orbitopathy. *Investig. Opthalmol. Vis. Sci.* 58, 2544. doi: 10.1167/iovs.16-20684

Kolesnick, R. N. (1987). 1,2-Diacylglycerols but not phorbol esters stimulate sphingomyelin hydrolysis in GH3 pituitary cells. *J. Biol. Chem.* 262, 16759–16762.

Kono, Y., Nishiuma, T., Nishimura, Y., Kotani, Y., Okada, T., Nakamura, S.-I., et al. (2007). Sphingosine kinase 1 regulates differentiation of human and mouse lung fibroblasts mediated by TGF-beta1. *Am. J. Respir. Cell Mol. Biol.* 37, 395–404. doi: 10.1165/rcmb.2007-0065OC

Korbelik, M., Banáth, J., Sun, J., Canals, D., Hannun, Y. A., and Separovic, D. (2014). Ceramide and sphingosine-1-phosphate act as photodynamic therapy-elicited damage-associated molecular patterns: cell surface exposure. *Int. Immunopharmacol.* 20, 359–365. doi: 10.1016/j.intimp.2014.03.016

Kremser, C., Klemm, A.-L., van Uelft, M., Imgrund, S., Ginkel, C., Hartmann, D., et al. (2013). Cell-type-specific expression pattern of ceramide synthase 2 protein in mouse tissues. *Histochem. Cell Biol.* 140, 533–547. doi: 10.1007/s00418-013-1091-z

Kucuksayan, E., Konuk, E. K., Demir, N., Mutus, B., and Aslan, M. (2014). Neutral sphingomyelinase inhibition decreases ER stress-mediated apoptosis and inducible nitric oxide synthase in retinal pigment epithelial cells. *Free Radic. Biol. Med.* 72, 113–123. doi: 10.1016/j.freeradbiomed.2014.04.013

Kurz, J., Parnham, M. J., Geisslinger, G., and Schiffmann, S. (2018). Ceramides as novel disease biomarkers. *Trends Mol. Med.* 52, 20–32. doi: 10.1016/j.molmed.2018.10.009

Lahiri, S., and Futerman, A. H. (2007). The metabolism and function of sphingolipids and glycosphingolipids. *Cell. Mol. Life Sci.* 64, 2270–2284. doi: 10.1007/s00018-007-7076-0

Lamour, N. F., Stahelin, R. V., Wijesinghe, D. S., Maceyka, M., Wang, E., Allegood, J. C., et al. (2007). Ceramide kinase uses ceramide provided by ceramide transport protein: localization to organelles of eicosanoid synthesis. *J. Lipid Res.* 48, 1293–1304. doi: 10.1194/jlr.M700083-JLR200

Lamour, N. F., Subramanian, P., Wijesinghe, D. S., Stahelin, R. V., Bonventre, J. V., and Chalfant, C. E. (2009). Ceramide 1-phosphate is required for the translocation of group IVA cytosolic phospholipase A2 and prostaglandin synthesis. *J. Biol. Chem.* 284, 26897–26907. doi: 10.1074/jbc.M109.001677

Lamour, N. F., Wijesinghe, D. S., Mietla, J. A., Ward, K. E., Stahelin, R. V., and Chalfant, C. E. (2011). Ceramide kinase regulates the production of tumor necrosis factor α (TNFα) via inhibition of TNFα-converting enzyme. *J. Biol. Chem.* 286, 42808–42817. doi: 10.1074/jbc.M111.310169

Laviad, E. L., Albee, L., Pankova-Kholmyansky, I., Epstein, S., Park, H., Merrill, A. H., et al. (2008). Characterization of ceramide synthase 2: tissue distribution, substrate specificity, and inhibition by sphingosine 1-phosphate. *J. Biol. Chem.* 283, 5677–5684. doi: 10.1074/jbc.M707386200

Lee, A. Y., Lee, J. W., Kim, J.-E., Mock, H. J., Park, S., Kim, S., et al. (2017). Dihydroceramide is a key metabolite that regulates autophagy and promotes fibrosis in hepatic steatosis model. *Biochem. Biophys. Res. Commun.* 494, 460–469. doi: 10.1016/j.bbrc.2017.10.110

Lei, H., Hovland, P., Velez, G., Haran, A., Gilbertson, D., Hirose, T., et al. (2007). A potential role for PDGF-C in experimental and clinical proliferative vitreoretinopathy. *Invest. Ophthalmol. Vis. Sci.* 48, 2335–2342. doi: 10.1167/iovs.06-0965

Lépine, S., Lakatos, B., Courageot, M.-P., Le Stunff, H., Sulpice, J.-C., and Giraud, F. (2004). Sphingosine contributes to glucocorticoid-induced apoptosis of thymocytes independently of the mitochondrial pathway. *J. Immunol.* 173, 3783–3790. doi: 10.4049/jimmunol.173.6.3783

Levy, M., and Futerman, A. H. (2010). Mammalian ceramide synthases. *IUBMB Life* 62, 347–356. doi: 10.1002/iub.319

Li, C., Wang, L., Zhang, J., Huang, M., Wong, F., Liu, X., et al. (2014). CERKL interacts with mitochondrial TRX2 and protects retinal cells from oxidative stress-induced apoptosis. *Biochim. Biophys. Acta* 1842, 1121–1129. doi: 10.1016/j.bbadis.2014.04.009

Li, C., Zheng, S., You, H., Liu, X., Lin, M., Yang, L., et al. (2011). Sphingosine 1-phosphate (S1P)/S1P receptors are involved in human liver fibrosis by action on hepatic myofibroblasts motility. *J. Hepatol.* 54, 1205–1213. doi: 10.1016/j.jhep.2010.08.028

Littink, K. W., Koenekoop, R. K., van den Born, L. I., Collin, R. W. J., Moruz, L., Veltman, J. A., et al. (2010). Homozygosity mapping in patients with cone-rod dystrophy: novel mutations and clinical characterizations. *Invest. Ophthalmol. Vis. Sci.* 51, 5943–5951. doi: 10.1167/iovs.10-5797

Liu, X., Yue, S., Li, C., Yang, L., You, H., and Li, L. (2011). Essential roles of sphingosine 1-phosphate receptor types 1 and 3 in human hepatic stellate cells motility and activation. *J. Cell. Physiol.* 226, 2370–2377. doi: 10.1002/jcp.22572

Lou, H., Kang, D., Yang, Q., Lian, C., Zhang, C., Li, Z., et al. (2017). Erythropoietin protects retina against ceramide 2-induced damage in rat. *Curr. Mol. Med.* 17, 699–706. doi: 10.2174/1566524018666180322161252

Lukowski, Z. L., Min, J., Beattie, A. R., Meyers, C. A., Levine, M. A., Stoller, G., et al. (2013). Prevention of ocular scarring after glaucoma filtering surgery using the monoclonal antibody LT1009 (Sonepcizumab) in a rabbit model. *J. Glaucoma* 22, 145–151. doi: 10.1097/IJG.0b013e31822e8c83

Lv, M., Zhang, D., Dai, D., Zhang, W., and Zhang, L. (2016). Sphingosine kinase 1/sphingosine-1-phosphate regulates the expression of interleukin-17A in activated microglia in cerebral ischemia/reperfusion. *Inflamm. Res.* 65, 551–562. doi: 10.1007/s00011-016-0939-9

Maceyka, M., Harikumar, K. B., Milstien, S., and Spiegel, S. (2012). Sphingosine-1-phosphate signaling and its role in disease. *Trends Cell Biol.* 22, 50–60. doi: 10.1016/j.tcb.2011.09.003

Maceyka, M., Sankala, H., Hait, N. C., Le Stunff, H., Liu, H., Toman, R., et al. (2005). SphK1 and SphK2, sphingosine kinase isoenzymes with opposing functions in sphingolipid metabolism. *J. Biol. Chem.* 280, 37118–37129. doi: 10.1074/jbc.M502207200

Mandal, N. A., Tran, J.-T. A., Saadi, A., Rahman, A. K., Huynh, T.-P., Klein, W. H., et al. (2013). Expression and localization of CERKL in the mammalian retina, its response to light-stress, and relationship with NeuroD1 gene. *Exp. Eye Res.* 106, 24–33. doi: 10.1016/j.exer.2012.10.014

Mandala, S. M. (2001). Sphingosine-1-phosphate phosphatases. *Prostaglandins Other Lipid Mediat.* 64, 143–156. doi: 10.1016/S0090-6980(01)00111-3

Mandon, E. C., Ehses, I., Rother, J., van Echten, G., and Sandhoff, K. (1992). Subcellular localization and membrane topology of serine palmitoyltransferase, 3-dehydrosphinganine reductase, and sphinganine N-acyltransferase in mouse liver. *J. Biol. Chem.* 267, 11144–11148.

Marchesini, N., and Hannun, Y. A. (2004). Acid and neutral sphingomyelinases: roles and mechanisms of regulation. *Biochem. Cell Biol.* 82, 27–44. doi: 10.1139/o03-091

Martin, R. E., Elliott, M. H., Brush, R. S., and Anderson, R. E. (2005). Detailed characterization of the lipid composition of detergent-resistant membranes from photoreceptor rod outer segment membranes. *Invest. Ophthalmol. Vis. Sci.* 46, 1147–1154. doi: 10.1167/iovs.04-1207

McGuire, P. G., Rangasamy, S., Maestas, J., and Das, A. (2011). Pericyte-derived sphingosine 1-phosphate induces the expression of adhesion proteins and modulates the retinal endothelial cell barrier. *Arterioscler. Thromb. Vasc. Biol.* 31, e107–e115. doi: 10.1161/ATVBAHA.111.235408

Merrill, A. H., Hannun, Y. A., and Bell, R. M. (1993). Introduction: sphingolipids and their metabolites in cell regulation. *Adv. Lipid Res.* 25, 1–24.

Merrill, A. H., Nimkar, S., Menaldino, D., Hannun, Y. A., Loomis, C., Bell, R. M., et al. (1989). Structural requirements for long-chain (sphingoid) base inhibition of protein kinase C in vitro and for the cellular effects of these compounds. *Biochemistry* 28, 3138–3145. doi: 10.1021/bi00434a004

Milara, J., Navarro, R., Juan, G., Peiró, T., Serrano, A., Ramón, M., et al. (2012). Sphingosine-1-phosphate is increased in patients with idiopathic pulmonary fibrosis and mediates epithelial to mesenchymal transition. *Thorax* 67, 147–156. doi: 10.1136/thoraxjnl-2011-200026

Miranda, G. E., Abrahan, C. E., Agnolazza, D. L., Politi, L. E., and Rotstein, N. P. (2011). Ceramide-1-phosphate, a new mediator of development and survival in retina photoreceptors. *Invest. Ophthalmol. Vis. Sci.* 52, 6580–6588. doi: 10.1167/iovs.10-7065

Miranda, G. E., Abrahan, C. E., Politi, L. E., and Rotstein, N. P. (2009). Sphingosine-1-phosphate is a key regulator of proliferation and differentiation in retina photoreceptors. *Investig. Ophthalmol. Vis. Sci.* 50, 4416–4428. doi: 10.1167/iovs.09-3388

Mitra, P., Maceyka, M., Payne, S. G., Lamour, N., Milstien, S., Chalfant, C. E., et al. (2007). Ceramide kinase regulates growth and survival of A549 human lung adenocarcinoma cells. *FEBS Lett.* 581, 735–740. doi: 10.1016/j.febslet.2007.01.041

Mitra, P., Oskeritzian, C. A., Payne, S. G., Beaven, M. A., Milstien, S., and Spiegel, S. (2006). Role of ABCC1 in export of sphingosine-1-phosphate from mast cells. *Proc. Natl. Acad. Sci. U.S.A.* 103, 16394–16399. doi: 10.1073/pnas.0603734103

Murakami, M., Ito, H., Hagiwara, K., Yoshida, K., Sobue, S., Ichihara, M., et al. (2010). ATRA inhibits ceramide kinase transcription in a human neuroblastoma cell line, SH-SY5Y cells: the role of COUP-TFI. *J. Neurochem.* 112, 511–520. doi: 10.1111/j.1471-4159.2009.06486.x

Nagahashi, M., Yamada, A., Aoyagi, T., Allegood, J., Wakai, T., Spiegel, S., et al. (2016). Sphingosine-1-phosphate in the lymphatic fluid determined by novel methods. *Heliyon* 2:e00219. doi: 10.1016/j.heliyon.2016.e00219

Nava, V. E., Cuvillier, O., Edsall, L. C., Kimura, K., Milstien, S., Gelmann, E. P., et al. (2000). Sphingosine enhances apoptosis of radiation-resistant prostate cancer cells. *Cancer Res.* 60, 4468–4474.

Nayak, D., Huo, Y., Kwang, W. X. T., Pushparaj, P. N., Kumar, S. D., Ling, E.-A., et al. (2010). Sphingosine kinase 1 regulates the expression of proinflammatory cytokines and nitric oxide in activated microglia. *Neuroscience* 166, 132–144. doi: 10.1016/j.neuroscience.2009.12.020

Nevet, M. J., Vekslin, S., Dizhoor, A. M., Olshevskaya, E. V., Tidhar, R., Futerman, A. H., et al. (2012). Ceramide kinase-like (CERKL) interacts with neuronal calcium sensor proteins in the retina in a cation-dependent manner. *Invest. Ophthalmol. Vis. Sci* 53, 4565–4574. doi: 10.1167/iovs.12-9770

Newton, J., Lima, S., Maceyka, M., and Spiegel, S. (2015). Revisiting the sphingolipid rheostat: Evolving concepts in cancer therapy. *Exp. Cell Res.* 333, 195–200. doi: 10.1016/j.yexcr.2015.02.025

Nicholas, S. E., Rowsey, T. G., Priyadarsini, S., Mandal, N. A., and Karamichos, D. (2017). Unravelling the interplay of sphingolipids and TGF-β signaling in the human corneal stroma. *PLoS One* 12:e0182390. doi: 10.1371/journal.pone.0182390

Norsworthy, M. W., Bei, F., Kawaguchi, R., Wang, Q., Tran, N. M., Li, Y., et al. (2017). Sox11 expression promotes regeneration of some retinal ganglion cell types but kills others. *Neuron* 94, 1112–1120.e4. doi: 10.1016/j.neuron.2017.05.035

Novgorodov, S. A., Wu, B. X., Gudz, T. I., Bielawski, J., Ovchinnikova, T. V., Hannun, Y. A., et al. (2011). Novel pathway of ceramide production in mitochondria: thioesterase and neutral ceramidase produce ceramide from sphingosine and acyl-CoA. *J. Biol. Chem.* 286, 25352–25362. doi: 10.1074/jbc.M110.214866

Obeid, L. M., Linardic, C. M., Karolak, L. A., and Hannun, Y. A. (1993). Programmed cell death induced by ceramide. *Science* 259, 1769–1771. doi: 10.1126/science.8456305

Ogretmen, B., and Hannun, Y. A. (2004). Biologically active sphingolipids in cancer pathogenesis and treatment. *Nat. Rev. Cancer* 4, 604–616. doi: 10.1038/nrc1411

Ohta, H., Sweeney, E. A., Masamune, A., Yatomi, Y., Hakomori, S., and Igarashi, Y. (1995). Induction of apoptosis by sphingosine in human leukemic HL-60 cells: a possible endogenous modulator of apoptotic DNA fragmentation occurring during phorbol ester-induced differentiation. *Cancer Res.* 55, 691–697.

Okazaki, T., Bell, R. M., and Hannun, Y. A. (1989). Sphingomyelin turnover induced by vitamin D3 in HL-60 cells. Role in cell differentiation. *J. Biol. Chem.* 264, 19076–19080.

Olivera, A., Allende, M. L., and Proia, R. L. (2013). Shaping the landscape: Metabolic regulation of S1P gradients. *Biochim. Biophys. Acta* 1831, 193–202. doi: 10.1016/j.bbalip.2012.06.007

Opreanu, M., Lydic, T. A., Reid, G. E., McSorley, K. M., Esselman, W. J., and Busik, J. V. (2010). Inhibition of cytokine signaling in human retinal endothelial cells through downregulation of sphingomyelinases by docosahexaenoic acid. *Invest. Ophthalmol. Vis. Sci.* 51, 3253–3263. doi: 10.1167/iovs.09-4731

Opreanu, M., Tikhonenko, M., Bozack, S., Lydic, T. A., Reid, G. E., McSorley, K. M., et al. (2011). The unconventional role of acid sphingomyelinase in regulation of retinal microangiopathy in diabetic human and animal models. *Diabetes* 60, 2370–2378. doi: 10.2337/db10-0550

Oresti, G. M., Luquez, J. M., Furland, N. E., and Aveldaño, M. I. (2011). Uneven distribution of ceramides, sphingomyelins and glycerophospholipids between heads and tails of rat spermatozoa. *Lipids* 46, 1081–1090. doi: 10.1007/s11745-011-3601-x

Osborne, N., Brand-Arzamendi, K., Ober, E. A., Jin, S. W., Verkade, H., Holtzman, N. G., et al. (2008). The spinster homolog, two of hearts, is required for sphingosine 1-phosphate signaling in zebrafish. *Curr. Biol.* 18, 1882–1888. doi: 10.1016/j.cub.2008.10.061

Park, J.-W., and Pewzner-Jung, Y. (2013). Ceramide synthases: reexamining longevity. *Handb. Exp. Pharmacol.* 215, 89–107. doi: 10.1007/978-3-7091-1368-4_5

Park, S. J., Kim, J. M., Kim, J., Hur, J., Park, S., Kim, K., et al. (2018). Molecular mechanisms of biogenesis of apoptotic exosome-like vesicles and their roles as damage-associated molecular patterns. *Proc. Natl. Acad. Sci. U.S.A.* 115, E11721–E11730. doi: 10.1073/pnas.1811432115

Pasquaré, S. J., and Giusto, N. M. (2008). Diacylglyceride lipase activity in rod outer segments depends on the illumination state of the retina. *Neurochem. Int.* 53, 382–388. doi: 10.1016/j.neuint.2008.09.007

Pasquaré, S. J., Salvador, G. A., and Giusto, N. M. (2008). Involvement of lysophosphatidic acid, sphingosine 1-phosphate and ceramide 1-phosphate in the metabolization of phosphatidic acid by lipid phosphate phosphatases in bovine rod outer segments. *Neurochem. Res.* 33, 1205–1215. doi: 10.1007/s11064-007-9569-5

Paugh, B. S., Bryan, L., Paugh, S. W., Wilczynska, K. M., Alvarez, S. M., Singh, S. K., et al. (2009). Interleukin-1 regulates the expression of sphingosine kinase 1 in glioblastoma cells. *J. Biol. Chem.* 284, 3408–3417. doi: 10.1074/jbc.M807170200

Paugh, S. W., Payne, S. G., Barbour, S. E., Milstien, S., and Spiegel, S. (2003). The immunosuppressant FTY720 is phosphorylated by sphingosine kinase type 2. *FEBS Lett.* 554, 189–193. doi: 10.1016/s0014-5793(03)01168-2

Pchejetski, D., Foussal, C., Alfarano, C., Lairez, O., Calise, D., Guilbeau-Frugier, C., et al. (2012). Apelin prevents cardiac fibroblast activation and collagen production through inhibition of sphingosine kinase 1. *Eur. Heart J.* 33, 2360–2369. doi: 10.1093/eurheartj/ehr389

Peng, B., Xiao, J., Wang, K., So, K.-F., Tipoe, G. L., and Lin, B. (2014). Suppression of microglial activation is neuroprotective in a mouse model of human retinitis pigmentosa. *J. Neurosci.* 34, 8139–8150. doi: 10.1523/JNEUROSCI.5200-13.2014

Penno, A., Reilly, M. M., Houlden, H., Laurá, M., Rentsch, K., Niederkofler, V., et al. (2010). Hereditary sensory neuropathy type 1 is caused by the accumulation of two neurotoxic sphingolipids. *J. Biol. Chem.* 285, 11178–11187. doi: 10.1074/jbc.M109.092973

Pettus, B. J., Bielawska, A., Subramanian, P., Wijesinghe, D. S., Maceyka, M., Leslie, C. C., et al. (2004). Ceramide 1-phosphate is a direct activator of cytosolic phospholipase A2. *J. Biol. Chem.* 279, 11320–11326. doi: 10.1074/jbc.M309262200

Phillips, D. C., Martin, S., Doyle, B. T., and Houghton, J. A. (2007). Sphingosine-induced apoptosis in rhabdomyosarcoma cell lines is dependent on pre-mitochondrial Bax activation and post-mitochondrial caspases. *Cancer Res.* 67, 756–764. doi: 10.1158/0008-5472.can-06-2374

Piano, I., Novelli, E., Gasco, P., Ghidoni, R., Strettoi, E., and Gargini, C. (2013). Cone survival and preservation of visual acuity in an animal model of retinal degeneration. *Eur. J. Neurosci.* 37, 1853–1862. doi: 10.1111/ejn.12196

Politi, L. E., Rotstein, N. P., and Carri, N. G. (2001). Effect of GDNF on neuroblast proliferation and photoreceptor survival: additive protection with docosahexaenoic acid. *Investig. Ophthalmol. Vis. Sci.* 42, 3008–3015.

Porter, H., Qi, H., Prabhu, N., Grambergs, R., McRae, J., Hopiavuori, B., et al. (2018). Characterizing sphingosine kinases and sphingosine 1-phosphate receptors in the mammalian eye and retina. *Int. J. Mol. Sci.* 19:E3885. doi: 10.3390/ijms19123885

Portera-Cailliau, C., Sung, C. H., Nathans, J., and Adler, R. (1994). Apoptotic photoreceptor cell death in mouse models of retinitis pigmentosa. *Proc. Natl. Acad. Sci. U.S.A.* 91, 974–978. doi: 10.1073/pnas.91.3.974

Prado Spalm, F. H., Vera, M. S., Dibo, M. J., Simón, M. V., Politi, L. E., and Rotstein, N. P. (2018). Ceramide induces the death of retina photoreceptors through activation of parthanatos. *Mol. Neurobiol.* doi: 10.1007/s12035-018-1402-4 [Epub ahead of print].

Presa, N., Gomez-Larrauri, A., Rivera, I.-G., Ordoñez, M., Trueba, M., and Gomez-Muñoz, A. (2016). Regulation of cell migration and inflammation by ceramide 1-phosphate. *Biochim. Biophys. Acta-Mol. Cell Biol. Lipids* 1861, 402–409. doi: 10.1016/j.bbalip.2016.02.007

Pujol-Lereis, L. M., Liebisch, G., Schick, T., Lin, Y., Grassmann, F., Uchida, K., et al. (2018). Evaluation of serum sphingolipids and the influence of genetic risk factors in age-related macular degeneration. *PLoS One* 13:e0200739. doi: 10.1371/journal.pone.0200739

Puranam, K., Qian, W. H., Nikbakht, K., Venable, M., Obeid, L., Hannun, Y., et al. (1997). Upregulation of Bcl-2 and elevation of ceramide in Batten disease. *Neuropediatrics* 28, 37–41. doi: 10.1055/s-2007-973664

Pyne, S., Lee, S. C., Long, J., and Pyne, N. J. (2009). Role of sphingosine kinases and lipid phosphate phosphatases in regulating spatial sphingosine 1-phosphate signalling in health and disease. *Cell. Signal.* 21, 14–21. doi: 10.1016/j.cellsig.2008.08.008

Qiao, Y., Hu, R., Wang, Q., Qi, J., Yang, Y., Kijlstra, A., et al. (2012). Sphingosine 1-phosphate elicits proinflammatory responses in ARPE-19 cells. *Invest. Ophthalmol. Vis. Sci.* 53, 8200–8207. doi: 10.1167/iovs.12-10965

Raas-Rothschild, A., Pankova-Kholmyansky, I., Kacher, Y., and Futerman, A. H. (2004). Glycosphingolipidoses: beyond the enzymatic defect. *Glycoconj. J.* 21, 295–304. doi: 10.1023/B:GLYC.0000046272.38480.ef

Rajagopalan, V., Canals, D., Luberto, C., Snider, J., Voelkel-Johnson, C., Obeid, L. M., et al. (2015). Critical determinants of mitochondria-associated neutral sphingomyelinase (MA-nSMase) for mitochondrial localization. *Biochim. Biophys. Acta* 1850, 628–639. doi: 10.1016/j.bbagen.2014.11.019

Ranty, M.-L., Carpentier, S., Cournot, M., Rico-Lattes, I., Malecaze, F., Levade, T., et al. (2009). Ceramide production associated with retinal apoptosis after retinal detachment. *Graefes Arch. Clin. Exp. Ophthalmol.* 247, 215–224. doi: 10.1007/s00417-008-0957-6

Riboni, L., Bassi, R., Anelli, V., and Viani, P. (2002). Metabolic formation of ceramide-1-phosphate in cerebellar granule cells: evidence for the phosphorylation of ceramide by different metabolic pathways. *Neurochem. Res.* 27, 711–716.

Riera, M., Burguera, D., Garcia-Fernàndez, J., and Gonzàlez-Duarte, R. (2013). CERKL knockdown causes retinal degeneration in zebrafish. *PLoS One* 8:e64048. doi: 10.1371/journal.pone.0064048

Rivera, I.-G., Ordoñez, M., Presa, N., Gangoiti, P., Gomez-Larrauri, A., Trueba, M., et al. (2016). Ceramide 1-phosphate regulates cell migration and invasion of human pancreatic cancer cells. *Biochem. Pharmacol.* 102, 107–119. doi: 10.1016/j.bcp.2015.12.009

Rizvi, F., Heimann, T., Herrnreiter, A., and O'Brien, W. J. (2011). Mitochondrial dysfunction links ceramide activated HRK expression and cell death. *PLoS One* 6:e18137. doi: 10.1371/journal.pone.0018137

Roche, S. L., Wyse-Jackson, A. C., Gómez-Vicente, V., Lax, P., Ruiz-Lopez, A. M., Byrne, A. M., et al. (2016). Progesterone attenuates microglial-driven retinal degeneration and stimulates protective fractalkine-CX3CR1 signaling. *PLoS One* 11:e0165197. doi: 10.1371/journal.pone.0165197

Rotstein, N. P., Aveldaño, M. I., Barrantes, F. J., and Politi, L. E. (1996). Docosahexaenoic acid is required for the survival of rat retinal photoreceptors in vitro. *J. Neurochem.* 66, 1851–1859. doi: 10.1046/j.1471-4159.1996.66051851.x

Rotstein, N. P., Aveldaño, M. I., Barrantes, F. J., Roccamo, A. M., and Politi, L. E. (1997). Apoptosis of retinal photoreceptors during development in vitro: protective effect of docosahexaenoic acid. *J. Neurochem.* 69, 504–513. doi: 10.1046/j.1471-4159.1997.69020504.x

Rotstein, N. P., Miranda, G. E., Abrahan, C. E., and German, O. L. (2010). Regulating survival and development in the retina: key roles for simple sphingolipids. *J. Lipid Res.* 51, 1247–1262. doi: 10.1194/jlr.R003442

Ruvolo, P. P. (2003). Intracellular signal transduction pathways activated by ceramide and its metabolites. *Pharmacol. Res.* 47, 383–392. doi: 10.1016/s1043-6618(03)00050-1

Saba, J. D., and Hla, T. (2004). Point-counterpoint of sphingosine 1-phosphate metabolism. *Circ. Res.* 94, 724–734. doi: 10.1161/01.RES.0000122383.60368.24

Sahaboglu, A., Sharif, A., Feng, L., Secer, E., Zrenner, E., and Paquet-Durand, F. (2017). Temporal progression of PARP activity in the Prph2 mutant rd2 mouse: neuroprotective effects of the PARP inhibitor PJ34. *PLoS One* 12:e0181374. doi: 10.1371/journal.pone.0181374

Saika, S. (2006). TGFbeta pathobiology in the eye. *Lab. Invest.* 86, 106–115. doi: 10.1038/labinvest.3700375

Saika, S., Yamanaka, O., Sumioka, T., Miyamoto, T., Miyazaki, K., Okada, Y., et al. (2008). Fibrotic disorders in the eye: targets of gene therapy. *Prog. Retin. Eye Res.* 27, 177–196. doi: 10.1016/j.preteyeres.2007.12.002

Samadi, A. (2007). Ceramide-induced cell death in lens epithelial cells. *Mol. Vis.* 13, 1618–1626.

Sancho-Pelluz, J., Arango-Gonzalez, B., Kustermann, S., Romero, F. J., Van Veen, T., Zrenner, E., et al. (2008). Photoreceptor cell death mechanisms in inherited retinal degeneration. *Mol. Neurobiol.* 38, 253–269. doi: 10.1007/s12035-008-8045-9

Sanvicens, N., and Cotter, T. G. (2006). Ceramide is the key mediator of oxidative stress-induced apoptosis in retinal photoreceptor cells. *J. Neurochem.* 98, 1432–1444. doi: 10.1111/j.1471-4159.2006.03977.x

Sato, K., Malchinkhuu, E., Horiuchi, Y., Mogi, C., Tomura, H., Tosaka, M., et al. (2007). Critical role of ABCA1 transporter in sphingosine 1-phosphate release from astrocytes. *J. Neurochem.* 103, 2610–2619. doi: 10.1111/j.1471-4159.2007.04958.x

Scarlatti, F., Bauvy, C., Ventruti, A., Sala, G., Cluzeaud, F., Vandewalle, A., et al. (2004). Ceramide-mediated macroautophagy involves inhibition of protein kinase B and up-regulation of beclin 1. *J. Biol. Chem.* 279, 18384–18391. doi: 10.1074/jbc.M313561200

Schneider, G., Bryndza, E., Abdel-Latif, A., Ratajczak, J., Maj, M., Tarnowski, M., et al. (2013). Bioactive lipids S1P and C1P are prometastatic factors in human rhabdomyosarcoma, and their tissue levels increase in response to radio/chemotherapy. *Mol. Cancer Res.* 11, 793–807. doi: 10.1158/1541-7786.MCR-12-0600

Siddique, M. M., Li, Y., Chaurasia, B., Kaddai, V. A., and Summers, S. A. (2015). Dihydroceramides: from bit players to lead actors. *J. Biol. Chem.* 290, 15371–15379. doi: 10.1074/jbc.R115.653204

Simanshu, D. K., Kamlekar, R. K., Wijesinghe, D. S., Zou, X., Zhai, X., Mishra, S. K., et al. (2013). Non-vesicular trafficking by a ceramide-1-phosphate transfer protein regulates eicosanoids. *Nature* 500, 463–467. doi: 10.1038/nature12332

Simón, M. V., Prado Spalm, F. H., Politi, L. E., and Rotstein, N. P. (2015). Sphingosine-1-phosphate is a crucial signal for migration of retina Müller Glial cells. *Invest. Ophthalmol. Vis. Sci.* 56, 5808–5815. doi: 10.1167/iovs.14-16195

Skoura, A., Sanchez, T., Claffey, K., Mandala, S. M., Proia, R. L., and Hla, T. (2007). Essential role of sphingosine 1-phosphate receptor 2 in pathological angiogenesis of the mouse retina. *J. Clin. Invest.* 117, 2506–2516. doi: 10.1172/JCI31123

Snider, A. J., Orr Gandy, K. A., and Obeid, L. M. (2010). Sphingosine kinase: role in regulation of bioactive sphingolipid mediators in inflammation. *Biochimie* 92, 707–715. doi: 10.1016/j.biochi.2010.02.008

Sorensen, S. D., Nicole, O., Peavy, R. D., Montoya, L. M., Lee, C. J., Murphy, T. J., et al. (2003). Common signaling pathways link activation of murine PAR-1, LPA, and S1P receptors to proliferation of astrocytes. *Mol. Pharmacol.* 64, 1199–1209. doi: 10.1124/mol.64.5.1199

Spiegel, S., and Milstien, S. (2002). Sphingosine 1-phosphate, a key cell signaling molecule. *J. Biol. Chem.* 277, 25851–25854. doi: 10.1074/jbc.R200007200

Spiegel, S., Maczis, M. A., Maceyka, M., and Milstien, S. (2019). New insights into functions of the sphingosine-1-phosphate transporter SPNS2. *J. Lipid Res.* 60, 484–489. doi: 10.1194/jlr.S091959

Sreekumar, P. G., Ding, Y., Ryan, S. J., Kannan, R., and Hinton, D. R. (2009). Regulation of thioredoxin by ceramide in retinal pigment epithelial cells. *Exp. Eye Res.* 88, 410–417. doi: 10.1016/j.exer.2008.10.009

Stancevic, B., and Kolesnick, R. (2010). Ceramide-rich platforms in transmembrane signaling. *FEBS Lett.* 584, 1728–1740. doi: 10.1016/j.febslet.2010.02.026

Stiles, M., Qi, H., Sun, E., Tan, J., Porter, H., Allegood, J., et al. (2016). Sphingolipid profile alters in retinal dystrophic P23H-1 rats and systemic FTY720 can delay retinal degeneration. *J. Lipid Res.* 57, 818–831. doi: 10.1194/jlr.M063719

Strettoi, E., Gargini, C., Novelli, E., Sala, G., Piano, I., Gasco, P., et al. (2010). Inhibition of ceramide biosynthesis preserves photoreceptor structure and function in a mouse model of retinitis pigmentosa. *Proc. Natl. Acad. Sci. U.S.A.* 107, 18706–18711. doi: 10.1073/pnas.1007644107

Strochlic, L., Dwivedy, A., van Horck, F. P. G., Falk, J., and Holt, C. E. (2008). A role for S1P signalling in axon guidance in the Xenopus visual system. *Development* 135, 333–342. doi: 10.1242/dev.009563

Strub, G. M., Paillard, M., Liang, J., Gomez, L., Allegood, J. C., Hait, N. C., et al. (2011). Sphingosine-1-phosphate produced by sphingosine kinase 2 in mitochondria interacts with prohibitin 2 to regulate complex IV assembly and respiration. *FASEB J.* 25, 600–612. doi: 10.1096/fj.10-167502

Sugano, E., Edwards, G., Saha, S., Wilmott, L., Grambergs, R. C., Mondal, K., et al. (2018). Overexpression of acid-Ceramidase (ASAH1) Protects Retinal Cells (ARPE19) from Oxidative Stress. *J. Lipid Res.* 60, 30–43. doi: 10.1194/jlr.M082198

Suzuki, E., Handa, K., Toledo, M. S., and Hakomori, S. (2004). Sphingosine-dependent apoptosis: a unified concept based on multiple mechanisms operating in concert. *Proc. Natl. Acad. Sci. U.S.A.* 101, 14788–14793. doi: 10.1073/pnas.0406536101

Swaney, J. S., Moreno, K. M., Gentile, A. M., Sabbadini, R. A., and Stoller, G. L. (2008). Sphingosine-1-phosphate (S1P) is a novel fibrotic mediator in the eye. *Exp. Eye Res.* 87, 367–375. doi: 10.1016/j.exer.2008.07.005

Sweeney, E. A., Sakakura, C., Shirahama, T., Masamune, A., Ohta, H., Hakomori, S., et al. (1996). Sphingosine and its methylated derivative N,N-dimethylsphingosine (DMS) induce apoptosis in a variety of human cancer cell lines. *Int. J. Cancer* 66, 358–366. doi: 10.1002/(sici)1097-0215(19960503)66%3A3%3C358%3A%3Aaid-ijc16%3E3.0.co%3B2-7

Tabasinezhad, M., Samadi, N., Ghanbari, P., Mohseni, M., Saei, A. A., Sharifi, S., et al. (2013). Sphingosin 1-phosphate contributes in tumor progression. *J. Cancer Res. Ther.* 9, 556–563. doi: 10.4103/0973-1482.126446

Tabuchi, K., and Hara, A. (2018). Impact of sphingolipid mediators on the determination of cochlear survival in ototoxicity. *Curr. Mol. Pharmacol.* 11, 279–284. doi: 10.2174/1874467211666180516101111

Tafesse, F. G., Ternes, P., and Holthuis, J. C. M. (2006). The multigenic sphingomyelin synthase family. *J. Biol. Chem.* 281, 29421–29425. doi: 10.1074/jbc.R600021200

Taha, T. A., Hannun, Y. A., and Obeid, L. M. (2006). Sphingosine kinase: biochemical and cellular regulation and role in disease. *J. Biochem. Mol. Biol.* 39, 113–131. doi: 10.5483/bmbrep.2006.39.2.113

Takabe, K., Kim, R. H., Allegood, J. C., Mitra, P., Ramachandran, S., Nagahashi, M., et al. (2010). Estradiol induces export of sphingosine 1-phosphate from breast cancer cells via ABCC1 and ABCG2. *J. Biol. Chem.* 285, 10477–10486. doi: 10.1074/jbc.M109.064162

Takabe, K., Paugh, S. W., Milstien, S., and Spiegel, S. (2008). Inside-Out" signaling of sphingosine-1-phosphate: therapeutic targets. *Pharmacol. Rev.* 60, 181–195. doi: 10.1124/pr.107.07113

Takuwa, Y., Ikeda, H., Okamoto, Y., Takuwa, N., and Yoshioka, K. (2013). Sphingosine-1-phosphate as a mediator involved in development of fibrotic diseases. *Biochim. Biophys. Acta* 1831, 185–192. doi: 10.1016/j.bbalip.2012.06.008

Terao, R., Honjo, M., and Aihara, M. (2017). Apolipoprotein M inhibits angiogenic and inflammatory response by sphingosine 1-phosphate on retinal pigment epithelium cells. *Int. J. Mol. Sci.* 19:112. doi: 10.3390/ijms19010112

Tikhonenko, M., Lydic, T. A., Wang, Y., Chen, W., Opreanu, M., Sochacki, A., et al. (2010). Remodeling of retinal fatty acids in an animal model of diabetes: a decrease in long-chain polyunsaturated fatty acids is associated with a decrease in fatty acid Elongases Elovl2 and Elovl4. *Diabetes* 59, 219–227. doi: 10.2337/db09-0728

Toman, R. E., Payne, S. G., Watterson, K. R., Maceyka, M., Lee, N. H., Milstien, S., et al. (2004). Differential transactivation of sphingosine-1-phosphate receptors modulates NGF-induced neurite extension. *J. Cell Biol.* 166, 381–392. doi: 10.1083/jcb.200402016

Tomita, H., Abe, T., and Tamai, M. (2000). Ceramide-induced cell death in cultured rat retinal pigment epithelial cells. *Tohoku J. Exp. Med.* 190, 223–229. doi: 10.1620/tjem.190.223

Toops, K. A., Tan, L. X., Jiang, Z., Radu, R. A., and Lakkaraju, A. (2015). Cholesterol-mediated activation of acid sphingomyelinase disrupts autophagy in the retinal pigment epithelium. *Mol. Biol. Cell* 26, 1–14. doi: 10.1091/mbc.e14-05-1028

Trayssac, M., Hannun, Y. A., and Obeid, L. M. (2018). Role of sphingolipids in senescence: implication in aging and age-related diseases. *J. Clin. Invest.* 128, 2702–2712. doi: 10.1172/JCI97949

Tuson, M., Garanto, A., Gonzàlez-Duarte, R., and Marfany, G. (2009). Overexpression of CERKL, a gene responsible for retinitis pigmentosa in humans, protects cells from apoptosis induced by oxidative stress. *Mol. Vis.* 15, 168–180.

Tuson, M., Marfany, G., and Gonzàlez-Duarte, R. (2004). Mutation of CERKL, a novel human ceramide kinase gene, causes autosomal recessive retinitis pigmentosa (RP26). *Am. J. Hum. Genet.* 74, 128–138. doi: 10.1086/381055

Wang, G., and Bieberich, E. (2018). Sphingolipids in neurodegeneration (with focus on ceramide and S1P). *Adv. Biol. Regul.* 70, 51–64. doi: 10.1016/j.jbior.2018.09.013

Wang, G., Silva, J., Krishnamurthy, K., Tran, E., Condie, B. G., and Bieberich, E. (2005). Direct binding to ceramide activates protein kinase C Cζ before the formation of a pro-apoptotic complex with PAR-4 in differentiating stem cells. *J. Biol. Chem.* 280, 26415–26424. doi: 10.1074/jbc.M501492200

Wang, Q., Navitskaya, S., Chakravarthy, H., Huang, C., Kady, N., Lydic, T. A., et al. (2016). Dual anti-inflammatory and anti-angiogenic action of miR-15a in diabetic retinopathy. *EBioMedicine* 11, 138–150. doi: 10.1016/j.ebiom.2016.08.013

Wang, H.-Y., Wang, Y., Zhang, Y., Wang, J., Xiong, S.-Y., and Sun, Q. (2018). Crosslink between lipids and acute uveitis: a lipidomic analysis. *Int. J. Ophthalmol.* 11, 736–746. doi: 10.18240/ijo.2018.05.05

Wattenberg, B. W., Pitson, S. M., and Raben, D. M. (2006). The sphingosine and diacylglycerol kinase superfamily of signaling kinases: localization as a key to signaling function. *J. Lipid Res.* 47, 1128–1139. doi: 10.1194/jlr.R600003-JLR200

Wegner, M.-S., Schiffmann, S., Parnham, M. J., Geisslinger, G., and Grösch, S. (2016). The enigma of ceramide synthase regulation in mammalian cells. *Prog. Lipid Res.* 63, 93–119. doi: 10.1016/j.plipres.2016.03.006

Wijesinghe, D. S., Massiello, A., Subramanian, P., Szulc, Z., Bielawska, A., and Chalfant, C. E. (2005). Substrate specificity of human ceramide kinase. *J. Lipid Res.* 46, 2706–2716. doi: 10.1194/jlr.M500313-JLR200

Wu, B. X., Clarke, C. J., and Hannun, Y. A. (2010). Mammalian neutral sphingomyelinases: regulation and roles in cell signaling responses. *Neuromolecular Med.* 12, 320–330. doi: 10.1007/s12017-010-8120-z

Wu, B. X., Fan, J., Boyer, N. P., Jenkins, R. W., Koutalos, Y., Hannun, Y. A., et al. (2015). Lack of acid sphingomyelinase induces age-related retinal degeneration. *PLoS One* 10:e0133032. doi: 10.1371/journal.pone.0133032

Wynn, T. A. (2007). Common and unique mechanisms regulate fibrosis in various fibroproliferative diseases. *J. Clin. Invest.* 117, 524–529. doi: 10.1172/JCI31487

Yamanaka, M., Shegogue, D., Pei, H., Bu, S., Bielawska, A., Bielawski, J., et al. (2004). Sphingosine kinase 1 (SPHK1) is induced by transforming growth factor-beta and mediates TIMP-1 up-regulation. *J. Biol. Chem.* 279, 53994–54001. doi: 10.1074/jbc.M410144200

Yao, J., Bi, H.-E., Sheng, Y., Cheng, L.-B., Wendu, R.-L., Wang, C.-H., et al. (2013). Ultraviolet (UV) and hydrogen peroxide activate ceramide-ER stress-AMPK signaling axis to promote retinal pigment epithelium (RPE) cell apoptosis. *Int. J. Mol. Sci.* 14, 10355–10368. doi: 10.3390/ijms140510355

You, Y., Gupta, V. K., Li, J. C., Al-Adawy, N., Klistorner, A., and Graham, S. L. (2014). FTY720 protects retinal ganglion cells in experimental glaucoma. *Investig. Ophthalmol. Vis. Sci.* 55, 3060–3066. doi: 10.1167/iovs.13-13262

Young, M. M., Kester, M., and Wang, H.-G. (2013). Sphingolipids: regulators of crosstalk between apoptosis and autophagy. *J. Lipid Res.* 54, 5–19. doi: 10.1194/jlr.R031278

Yu, F. P., Sajdak, B., Sikora, J., Salmon, A. E., Nagree, M. S., Gurka, J., et al. (2018). Acid ceramidase deficiency in mice leads to severe ocular pathology and visual impairment. *Am. J. Pathol.* 189, 320–338. doi: 10.1016/j.ajpath.2018.10.018

Yu, S., Li, C., Biswas, L., Hu, X., Liu, F., Reilly, J., et al. (2017). CERKL gene knockout disturbs photoreceptor outer segment phagocytosis and causes rod-cone dystrophy in zebrafish. *Hum. Mol. Genet.* 26, 2335–2345. doi: 10.1093/hmg/ddx137

Yu, Y., Reynolds, R., Fagerness, J., Rosner, B., Daly, M. J., and Seddon, J. M. (2011). Association of variants in the LIPC and ABCA1 genes with intermediate and large drusen and advanced age-related macular degeneration. *Invest. Ophthalmol. Vis. Sci.* 52, 4663–4670. doi: 10.1167/iovs.10-7070

Zarbin, M. A., Green, W. R., Moser, A. B., and Tiffany, C. (1988). Increased levels of ceramide in the retina of a patient with Farber's disease. *Arch. Ophthalmol.* 106:1163. doi: 10.1001/archopht.1988.01060140323008

Zhao, L., Zabel, M. K., Wang, X., Ma, W., Shah, P., Fariss, R. N., et al. (2015). Microglial phagocytosis of living photoreceptors contributes to inherited retinal degeneration. *EMBO Mol. Med.* 7, 1179–1197. doi: 10.15252/emmm.201505298

Zhu, D., Sreekumar, P. G., Hinton, D. R., and Kannan, R. (2010). Expression and regulation of enzymes in the ceramide metabolic pathway in human retinal pigment epithelial cells and their relevance to retinal degeneration. *Vision Res.* 50, 643–651. doi: 10.1016/j.visres.2009.09.002

5

Fatty Acid Signaling Mechanisms in Neural Cells: Fatty Acid Receptors

Lisandro Jorge Falomir-Lockhart[1,2], Gian Franco Cavazzutti[1,2], Ezequiel Giménez[1,3] and Andrés Martín Toscani[1,3]*

[1] *Instituto de Investigaciones Bioquímicas de La Plata (INIBIOLP), Centro Científico Tecnológico – La Plata, Consejo Nacional de Investigaciones Científicas y Técnicas (CONICET), La Plata, Argentina,* [2] *Facultad de Ciencias Exactas, Universidad Nacional de La Plata (UNLP), La Plata, Argentina,* [3] *Facultad de Ciencias Médicas, Universidad Nacional de La Plata (UNLP), La Plata, Argentina*

Correspondence:
Lisandro Jorge Falomir-Lockhart
lfalomir@conicet.gov.ar;
ljfalomir@biol.unlp.edu.ar

Fatty acids (FAs) are typically associated with structural and metabolic roles, as they can be stored as triglycerides, degraded by β-oxidation or used in phospholipids' synthesis, the main components of biological membranes. It has been shown that these lipids exhibit also regulatory functions in different cell types. FAs can serve as secondary messengers, as well as modulators of enzymatic activities and substrates for cytokines synthesis. More recently, it has been documented a direct activity of free FAs as ligands of membrane, cytosolic, and nuclear receptors, and cumulative evidence has emerged, demonstrating its participation in a wide range of physiological and pathological conditions. It has been long known that the central nervous system is enriched with poly-unsaturated FAs, such as arachidonic (C20:4ω-6) or docosohexaenoic (C22:6ω-3) acids. These lipids participate in the regulation of membrane fluidity, axonal growth, development, memory, and inflammatory response. Furthermore, a whole family of low molecular weight compounds derived from FAs has also gained special attention as the natural ligands for cannabinoid receptors or key cytokines involved in inflammation, largely expanding the role of FAs as precursors of signaling molecules. Nutritional deficiencies, and alterations in lipid metabolism and lipid signaling have been associated with developmental and cognitive problems, as well as with neurodegenerative diseases. The molecular mechanism behind these effects still remains elusive. But in the last two decades, different families of proteins have been characterized as receptors mediating FAs signaling. This review focuses on different receptors sensing and transducing free FAs signals in neural cells: (1) membrane receptors of the family of G Protein Coupled Receptors known as Free Fatty Acid Receptors (FFARs); (2) cytosolic transport Fatty Acid-Binding Proteins (FABPs); and (3) transcription factors Peroxisome Proliferator-Activated Receptors (PPARs). We discuss how these proteins modulate and mediate direct regulatory functions of free FAs in neural cells. Finally, we briefly discuss the advantages of evaluating them as potential targets for drug design in order to manipulate lipid signaling. A thorough characterization of lipid receptors of the nervous system could provide a framework for a better understanding of their roles in neurophysiology and, potentially, help for the development of novel drugs against aging and neurodegenerative processes.

Keywords: lipid sensing, neuronal differentiation and development, signal transduction, free fatty acid receptor, fatty acid binding protein, peroxisome proliferator activated receptor, docosahexaenoic acid, arachidonic acid

INTRODUCTION

The central nervous system (CNS) is an intricate network of a variety of cell types, with a wide range of distinct properties and functions. Notoriously, lipids represent a larger proportion of mass than in most other tissues, second only after adipose tissue (Etschmaier et al., 2011). The main difference is that, whereas in adipocytes lipids are mainly stored as energy reserve in lipid droplets, in the CNS lipids fulfill multiple functions; such as forming large extensions of membranes necessary for crosstalk between neural cells. This is not limited only to the inner and plasma membranes of neurons, comprising axons, dendrites, and spines; astrocytes, oligodendrocytes, and microglia also have highly complex cellular shapes and, hence, extensive surface areas defined largely by lipids, and their functions in the healthy brain are integrated both physically and metabolically (von Bernhardi et al., 2016). Brain membranes are constituted by proteins, cholesterol (on average, 21.5% mol/mol lipids), sphingomyelin (1.9%), gangliosides (1.4%) and phospholipids (75.1%) (Scandroglio et al., 2008), where the lipids were typically constrained to structural or support functions for the first ones. Lipid distribution is not equivalent for all cell types or brain regions, and neurons are usually enriched in polyunsaturated glycerolipids and cholesterol (Scandroglio et al., 2008; Chan et al., 2012; Arai et al., 2015; Ingolfsson et al., 2017). These lipids are essential for many cellular processes in CNS. For example, the brain is the richest tissue in cholesterol with up to 20 mg/g of tissue, 10-time more than the rest, and it is mainly synthesized *in situ* (Dietschy and Turley, 2001, 2004). Therefore, its levels are independent from circulating cholesterol, highlighting its pivotal role in multiple brain functions such as signal transduction, synaptic transmission, and cell differentiation by modulation of lipid rafts organization and segregation of membrane proteins, as well as in several pathological conditions, either directly by its self or through its metabolism into neurosteroids and oxysterols (Reddy, 2010; Leoni and Caccia, 2011; Orth and Bellosta, 2012; Vance, 2012).

Lipid signaling has attracted increasing attention as different families of lipids have been shown to exhibit important regulatory functions through highly specific receptors (Fernandis and Wenk, 2007; Sunshine and Iruela-Arispe, 2017). Polyunsaturated fatty acids (PUFAs) are of particular relevance because they can also be transformed into much more potent derivatives, such as eicosanoids and docosanoids, from arachidonic (C20:4ω-6, ARA) and docosahexanoic (C22:6ω-3, DHA) acids, respectively (Serhan, 2014; Dennis and Norris, 2015). In the last decades, different families of proteins have been identified and characterized to mediate signaling processes triggered directly by lipids *per se*, including free FAs (Im, 2004; Kostenis, 2004; Wolfrum, 2007). The interest on how these proteins mediate FAs regulatory functions increased as they have been demonstrated to be targets and/or essential carriers for the therapeutic actions of certain drugs (Wolfrum et al., 2001; Landrier et al., 2004; Martin et al., 2013).

Fatty acids regulatory functions are most probably defined by the group of specific receptors expressed in a particular cell-type and, therefore, they are dynamically modulated throughout the cell life-span, the developmental stage, and its differentiation process. This review resumes part of the present understanding on FAs regulatory functions in pathophysiology of neural tissues and three families of proteins involved in these roles. Noteworthy, other proteins involved in lipid signaling with more promiscuous selectivity of ligands, such as FA Translocase (FAT/CD36) or Toll-like Receptor 4 (TLR4), were not included in this manuscript, and their roles could be consulted elsewhere (Pepino et al., 2014; Magnan et al., 2015; Rocha et al., 2016).

PHYSIOLOGICAL FUNCTIONS AND PARTICIPATION OF FATTY ACIDS IN NEURONAL PATHOLOGIES

Fatty acids are typically considered as a source of energy through β-oxidation, and, as part of phospholipids, either as membrane building blocks or reservoir of second messengers and substrates for cytokines synthesis. They can also induce multiple cellular responses, ranging from cell motility and changes in cell morphology (Kamata et al., 2007; Brown et al., 2014), to regulation of gene expression (Kitajka et al., 2004), modulation of hormones secretion or their effects (Wang and Chan, 2015). But several distinctions must be made when referring to FAs in general, because saturated FAs (SFAs) have a clear different origin, metabolism, and functions compared to essential ω-3 and ω-6 PUFAs. Brain SFAs, such as palmitate (16:0, PA) or stearic (18:0, SA), are known to be generated *in situ* as much as being imported into the brain, whereas PUFAs are elongated and further unsaturated mainly in the liver and then transported through the bloodstream and imported into the neural tissue as non-esterified FAs (Edmond et al., 1998; Chen et al., 2008). Only a small fraction of PUFAs is actually synthesized locally from linoleic (C18:2ω-6) and α-linolenic (C18:3ω-3, ALA) acids; and, due to enzymatic restrictions and competition between ω-3 and ω-6 PUFAS for the same enzymes, less than 5% of total ALA assimilated from diet can be transformed into DHA

(Dyall and Michael-Titus, 2008). Both, endogenous and blood-derived PUFAs, accumulate preferentially in neurons as part of phospholipids.

Neurogenesis includes three contiguous phases, namely proliferation, migration and differentiation, and maturation and integration of the precursor cells; with PUFAs having inherence in all of these stages (Chalon, 2006). Therefore, PUFAs are critical for pre- and post-natal brain development, as well as in adulthood or during natural aging (Uauy and Dangour, 2006; Rombaldi Bernardi et al., 2012). For example, ALA maternal restriction during gestation and lactation impairs hippocampal neuronal differentiation, thus compromising neuronal maturation and related brain functions, such as learning and memory (Bhatia et al., 2011; Niculescu et al., 2011). DHA is the most abundant PUFA and accumulates in the immature brain during perinatal life all through the grey matter expansion; and it can reach over 10% of total FAs in human adult brains (McNamara and Carlson, 2006). Actually, preterm-born adolescents, who skipped the fetal DHA accumulation in the CNS during the last weeks of gestation and usually also lactation during the early life, exhibit deficits in cognitive functions associated to attention, including increased risk for attention-deficit/hyperactivity disorder (ADHD) and schizophrenia (McNamara and Carlson, 2006). That is why dietary deficiencies commonly stimulate a more tightened retention of essential FAs in the brain.

Docosahexanoic acid is particularly important for proper neuronal development in cerebral cortex, retina, and hippocampus, where it promotes neurogenesis and neuronal differentiation (Cao et al., 2009; Gharami et al., 2015). It also boosts synaptogenesis by promoting neurite outgrowth and synapsis formation, accompanied by an increase in the expression of neuronal and synaptic proteins. Particularly, in rat neuronal stem cells, DHA stimulates neuronal differentiation by two mechanisms: (1) a decrease in expression levels of basic Helix-loop-Helix transcription factors (NeuroD, Mash1, Hes1, etc.); and (2) an extension of the expression of cyclin-dependent kinase inhibitor p27 (kip1). This results in an increase in the number of positive cells for the neuronal markers TUBB3 and MAP2 and in a reduction of the percentage of cells in S-phase, suggesting an exit from the cell cycle (Katakura et al., 2009). In aged mice, DHA also prevents neuroinflammation and apoptosis, whereas improving memory (Labrousse et al., 2012). DHA can prevent many of the lipopolysaccharide (LPS) deleterious effects on both neurons and microglia, including loss of dendritic spines or production of nitric oxide as biomarkers of neuroinflammation (Chang et al., 2015). Actually, multiple animal and *in vitro* models of neuroinflammation consistently show a marked anti-inflammatory effect of DHA and other ω-3 PUFAs, presumably by reducing the production of proinflammatory cytokines and/or promoting the secretion of anti-inflammatory cytokines (reviewed in Orr et al., 2013). PUFAs can also directly modify neurotransmitter production, accumulation, release, and re-uptake. Dopamine's content, storage in presynaptic vesicles and tyramine-stimulated release, for example, significantly decrease in rat frontal cortex after chronic ω-3 PUFAs deficiency (Delion et al., 1996; Zimmer et al., 1998, 2000). Contrarily, supplementation with ω-3 PUFAs increases dopamine levels in the same area (Chalon et al., 1998).

Fatty acids have been implicated in neuropathological conditions, including neurodegenerative diseases, mental disorders, stroke, and trauma. Severe dietary restriction of essential FAs usually correlates with anxiety-like behavior and deficit in cognitive functions, including memory and learning. However, imbalance between ω-3 and ω-6 PUFAs during gestation also leads to alterations in brain development. In adults, an imbalance in the PUFAs ratio in brain membranes is believed to be a risk factor active during the pathogenesis of neurological and psychiatric disorders (Chalon, 2006). For example, an increase in ARA is known to promote α-Synuclein aggregation. However, it is not clear which is the most relevant cause affecting secretion of dopamine and serotonin, the greater availability of ARA, the deficiency of DHA or the imbalance between them (Chalon, 2006). During normal aging, there is a common cognitive decline and an increasing risk of dementia. High ω-3 PUFAs intake slows down this decline (Johnson and Schaefer, 2006; van Gelder et al., 2007), suggesting that they may have neuroprotective action in the aging brain and even therapeutic potential. Aging is also characterized by increased oxidative stress and neuroinflammation together with altered energy metabolism (reviewed in Prolla and Mattson, 2001). Beside changes in FA composition that favor monounsaturated FAs (MUFAs) over ω-3 and ω-6 PUFAs with time in rodents, the aging brain is also prone to lipid oxidation due to its large content of PUFAs (Favrelere et al., 2000). In humans, the decrease of PUFAs, though subtler during normal aging, is quite evident in neurodegenerative pathologies, including Alzheimer Disease (AD), Parkinson's Disease (PD), Schizophrenia and depression (reviewed in Hussain et al., 2013). Nevertheless, PUFAs are known to promote α-Synuclein pathological aggregation (Yakunin et al., 2012). On the other hand, the anterior cingulate cortex of depressive patients shows reduced quantities of SFAs and PUFAs (Conklin et al., 2010). The deficiency of ω-3 PUFAs also impairs the normal signaling of endocannabinoid in prelimbic prefrontal cortex and accumbens, leading to abnormal emotional behavior (Lafourcade et al., 2011). The reduction in total PUFAs in erythrocyte's membranes of patients with early onset schizophrenia correlates with the degree of demyelination in brain white matter (Peters et al., 2009). Finally, PUFAs also serve as anti-depressants and anti-convulsants, confer protection against traumatic insults, and enhance repairing processes. For example, numerous animal models of epilepsy support the anticonvulsant properties of PUFAs, like the greater resistance to pentylenetetrazol-induced seizures in ω-3 PUFAs fed rats (Taha et al., 2009).

Arachidonic acid is particularly enriched in phosphatidylinositol (PI), whereas DHA is a major component of brain phosphatidylethanolamine (PE) and phosphatidylserine (PS). Both PUFAs are highly enriched in the phospholipids of the synaptic plasma membrane and synaptic vesicles (Glomset, 2006). ARA is also particularly rich in membranes of leukocytes, presumably because it serves as a precursor of a myriad of cytokines (Innes and Calder, 2018). PUFAs are almost exclusively found in position 2 of the glycerol moiety within any phospholipid and, therefore, their release is catalyzed by phospholipases A_2 (PLA_2). Noteworthy, ARA and eicosapentaenoic acid (20:5ω-3, EPA) are released preferentially by cytoplasmic PLA_2 ($cPLA_2$), whereas DHA is released by Ca^{+2}-independent PLA_2 ($iPLA_2$) (Dyall and Michael-Titus, 2008). These three PUFAs can be converted into more potent cytokines than the free FAs, including prostaglandins, leukotrienes, thromboxanes, protectins and resolvins, and their effects differ from one other (Calder, 2015; Dyall, 2017).

Neuroinflammation is a common denominator for several neuropathologies. SFAs are known to promote the inflammatory phenotype of microglia, stimulating the secretion of TNF-α and IL-6 through TLR4. Furthermore, PA exposure of astrocytes leads to Caspase-3 activation and alters Bax/Bcl-2 ratio, both effects promoting apoptosis (Gupta et al., 2012). On the contrary, ω-3 PUFAs usually have a marked antiinflammatory effect by blocking microglia activation and stimulating the secretion of neurotrophic factors. However, some deleterious effects have also been reported, such as the worsening of neuritic injury and astrocytosis in PD-mice model (Hussain et al., 2013). ARA is the precursor for potent proinflammatory eicosanoids. On the other hand, compounds derived from DHA and EPA, known as resolvins and protectins, show strong anti-inflammatory effects and mediate the end of an ongoing inflammatory response (Hussain et al., 2013). These compounds are just an example of those derived from FAs that have important roles in brain pathophysiology. A special mention should be given to endocannabinoids, such as arachidonoylethanolamine (also known as anandamide), arachidonylglycerol or oleoylethanolamine, just to name a few (Freitas et al., 2017). Nevertheless, the role of free FAs has a renewed interest since the identification of multiple receptors that can couple their signaling to diverse cellular responses. The next section focusses on three families of proteins that recognize FAs and could be modulating FAs regulatory functions.

RECEPTORS FOR FATTY ACIDS SIGNALING

Originally, lipid signaling was limited to steroid hormones and its binding to cytosolic receptors, or to cytokines derived from ARA (leukotrienes and thromboxanes) that bind to specific membrane receptors. As of today, three families of proteins have been identified to be able to sense the presence and type of FAs whether in the extracellular medium, the cytosol or the nuclear matrix. At the plasma membrane, FAs can activate G Protein-coupled receptors known as Free Fatty Acid Receptors (FFARs) (Hara et al., 2013; Offermanns, 2013); while in the cytosol they can be taken by Fatty Acid Binding Proteins (FABPs) and targeted to specific subcellular structures or metabolic pathways (Veerkamp and Zimmerman, 2001; Storch and Corsico, 2008). Finally, nuclear receptors Peroxisome Proliferator-Activated Receptors (PPARs) mediate FAs regulatory functions in the nucleus (Zolezzi et al., 2017). The specific spatio-temporal pattern of expression and the co-expression of more than one isoform from each family of proteins in a single cell suggest a platform for sensing and modulating the cellular response to the bioavailability of the different FAs, for example, adapting the cell to developmental or functional requirements. Therefore, the regulatory and signaling roles of free FAs are gaining importance in physiological and pathological processes as these receptors are better characterized.

We describe bellow some of the known characteristics of each family of FAs receptors selected for this review, including expression patterns, structural features, and specific functions in the CNS. Noteworthy, when the source of expression data is not specified, it was taken from The Human Protein Atlas website[1] (Uhlen et al., 2015), based on Genotype-Tissue Expression (GTEx) project (The GTEx Consortium, 2013), or from the Allen Mouse Brain Atlas[2] (Lein et al., 2007).

Plasma Membrane Receptors

A large number of putative genes coding for GPCRs was identified based on genome sequences, and their deorphanization is still in progress (Civelli, 2005; Diaz et al., 2018; Laschet et al., 2018). Particularly, a cluster of 4 sequences (*GPR40, GPR41, GPR42* and *GPR43*) was identified in chromosome 19 (Sawzdargo et al., 1997) and FAs were proved to work as their specific endogenous ligands (Briscoe et al., 2003; Brown et al., 2003), dubbing this subfamily of GPCRs as FFARs (Offermanns, 2013). Later on, two other receptors activated by FAs were described, GPR84 and GPR120, located in chromosome 12 and 10, respectively; as well as many others activated by diverse lipids derived from FAs, including lysophosphatidic acid (termed LPARs), endocannabinoids (CBs) and hydroxycarboxylic acids (HCAs) (Offermanns, 2013; Audet and Stevens, 2019).

Within the superfamily of GPCRs, FFARs belong to the largest subfamily of Class A/1 (rhodopsin-like) receptors, constituted by a motif of 7 transmembrane segments (TMs) and at least one longer cytosolic domain that serves as binding site for signaling machinery assembly (Dorsam and Gutkind, 2007; Heldin et al., 2016). The ligand recognition site is defined within the transmembrane helix bundle (**Figure 1A**). The original cluster of FFARs was deorphanized by heterologous expression and ligand screening through monitoring cytosolic Ca^{+2} levels (Briscoe et al., 2003). FAs-triggered Ca^{+2} release from the endoplasmic reticulum is PI3K-dependent. However, some of these receptors can also transduce FAs signal through inhibition of cAMP synthesis, CREB, Akt/PKB, and/or Erk phosphorylation, as well as by β-Arrestin recruitment (Kimura et al., 2011; Zamarbide et al., 2014). Each FFAR shows specific patterns of expression and distinctive ligand selectivity. Their functions have been better studied in peripheral tissues, including the promotion of hormone secretion by the pancreas, lipid taste sensing and the activation of immune cells as a preliminary response toward a putative growing infection. Their participation in the CNS had less attention, although recent results suggest that some isoforms could participate in brain development, neuronal differentiation (Ma et al., 2010) and could be potential drug targets against several neuropathies,

[1] www.proteinatlas.org (accessed January 3, 2019)
[2] http://portal.brain-map.org (accessed January 3, 2019)

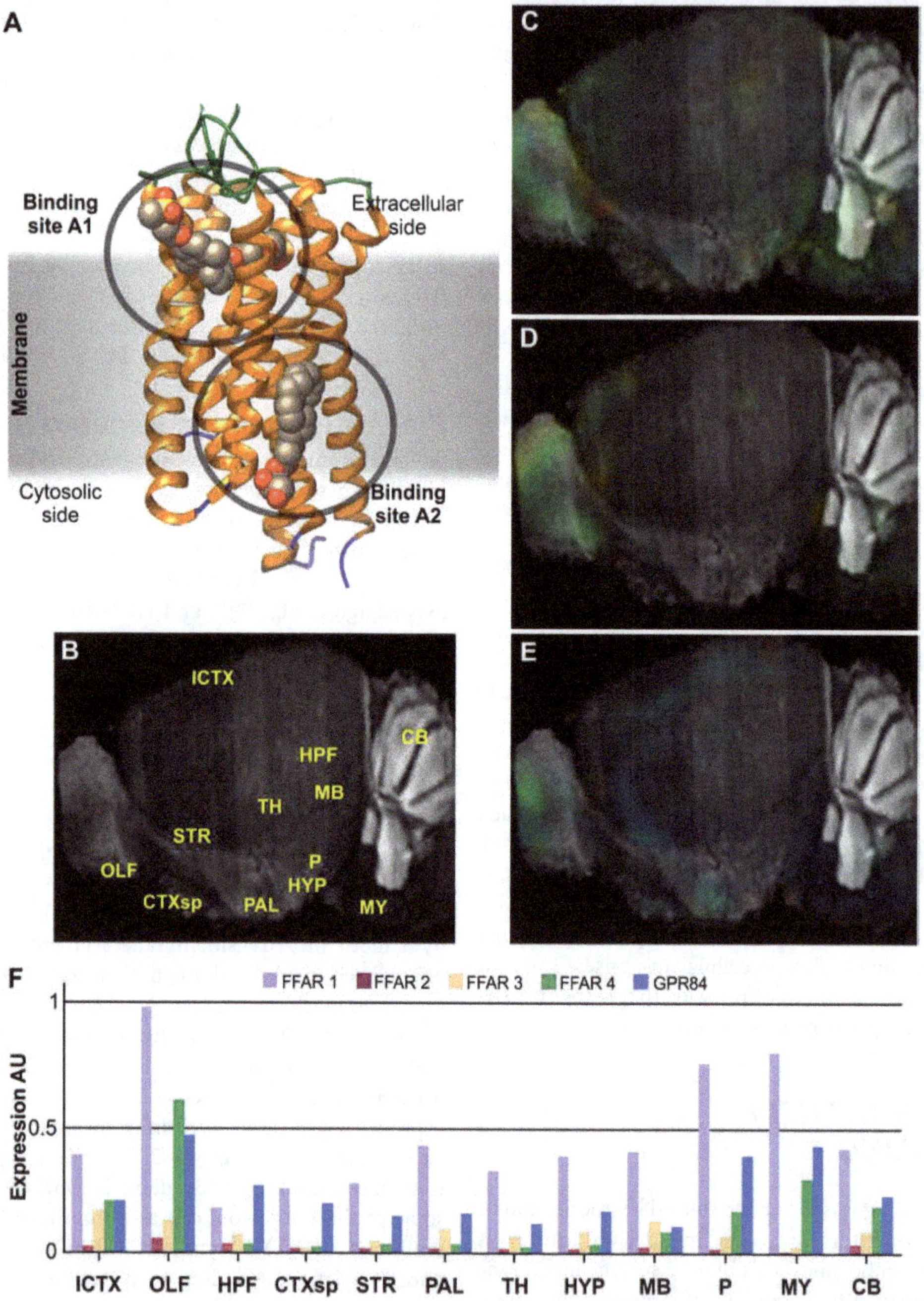

FIGURE 1 | Structure and brain expression patterns of FFARs. **(A)** Cartoon based on FFAR1 crystal structure (PDB-ID: 4PHU) (Srivastava et al., 2014), highlighting membrane orientation and two ligand binding sites in opposite sides of the membrane. **(B)** Central brain section of 8-weeks, male mouse (C57BL/6J) indicating reference regions. **(C–E)** Brain left hemisphere sagittal projection showing expression of FFAR1, FFAR4 and GPR84, respectively, based on *in situ* hybridization (ISH) data. FFAR2 and FFAR3 are not shown due to its lower expression levels. **(F)** Quantification of relative expression from ISH data for all FFARs isoforms. AU: Arbitrary units; ICTX: Isocortex; OLF: Olfactory areas; HPF: Hyppocampal formation; CTXsp: Cortical subplate; STR: Striatum; PAL: Pallidum; TH: Thalamus; HYP: Hypothalamus; MB: Midbrain; P: Pons; MY: Medulla; and CB: Cerebellum. Image credit for panels **C–E**: Allen Institute © 2007 Allen Institute for Brain Science. Allen Mouse Brain Atlas. Available from: http://mouse.brain-map.org/search/. Panels **B** and **F** were constructed from data available through Allen Mouse Brain Atlas website.

such as neuropathic pain and epilepsy (Yoshimura et al., 2015; Yang et al., 2018).

Each isoform presents distinct body expression profiles and different affinity for FAs (Brown et al., 2005; Hara et al., 2013; Offermanns, 2013). There are two FFARs with prominent levels of expression in neural tissues: FFAR1 (also known as GPR40) and FFAR4 (GPR120 or O3FAR). Nevertheless, all isoforms have been detected, though weakly, in some restricted brain region.

We review bellow some of the most recent findings about this novel family of GPCRs activated by FAs.

FFAR1 (GPR40)

The genes that code for FFAR1, FFAR2 and FFAR3, originally named *GPR40*, *GPR43* and *GPR41*, respectively, were identified in 1997 as a group of tandemly encoded genes located on human chromosome 19q13.1. FFAR1 is a 300 amino acids membrane protein of 31.45 kDa. As the product of the single exon gene *GPR40*, it is most abundantly expressed in pancreas and brain of primates (Briscoe et al., 2003; Brown et al., 2005). Other tissues with significant expression include small intestine, spleen, testis, ovaries, and Fallopian tubes. According to GTEx data, within the CNS, higher expression levels of FFAR1 mRNA are found in hippocampus, caudate nucleus, hypothalamus, and cerebral cortex, presumably mainly in neurons but also in glial cells. On the other hand, qPCR targeted experiments showed a wider expression of FFAR1 in neuronal tissues, with higher expression levels in medulla oblongata, *substantia nigra* and spinal cord, followed by putamen, locus cereleus, globus palidus, and amygdala (Briscoe et al., 2003), while western blot analysis showed higher expression in pons, dentate gyrus, pituitary gland, *substantia nigra* and spinal cord, followed by subgranular and subventricular zones, CA1, medulla oblongata, and cerebral cortex, with minor expression in cerebellum (Ma et al., 2007). *In situ* hybridization (ISH) of mice brain sagittal sections indicated discrete preferential FFAR1 expression in olfactory bulb, pons, and medulla (**Figures 1C,F**), while coronal sections highlighted hippocampus and cerebral cortex (Zamarbide et al., 2014). Its levels are weaker than in primates and, hence, it has been suggested that is not essential. Actually, FFAR1-KO mice manifested no evident alteration of social or motor behavior, although they showed a reduction anxiety-like responses (Mancini et al., 2015). An increase in noradrenaline was also observed in FFAR1-KO mice brain regions were the expression of the receptor was shown to be higher, suggesting a role in anxiety and depression symptoms.

This receptor is the only FFAR with solved crystal structures (PDB-ID: 5KW2, 4PHU, 5TZR and 5TZY), as different fusions to Lysozyme, and in complex with different partial and full synthetic agonists, such as TAK-875, MK-8666 or the novel compound (3~{S})-3-cyclopropyl-3-[2-[1-[2-[2,2-dimethylpropyl-(6-methylpyridin-2-yl) carbamoyl]-5-methoxy-phenyl]piperidin-4-yl]-1-benzofuran-6-yl] propanoic acid (Srivastava et al., 2014; Lu et al., 2017; Ho et al., 2018). Noteworthy, the different structures identified two putative binding sites in opposite sides of the transmembrane region, A1 in the extracellular side and A2 in the cytosolic one (**Figure 1A**). Only the occupancy of the latter by synthetic or natural ligands promotes full agonistic response and structure of intracellular loop IC2 located between transmembrane regions TM3 and TM4, which is believed to be necessary for G-protein interaction. The extracellular loop located between TM4 and TM5 is stabilized by a disulfide bond formed between Cys^{79} and Cys^{170}. Residues participating in ligand recognition have been mapped to include Arg^{183}, Asn^{244} and Arg^{258} that work as anchors for the carboxylic head of the FAs. Residues Tyr^{12}, Tyr^{91}, His^{137}, and Leu^{186} were also identified as relevant for receptor activation; while His^{86}, Tyr^{91}, His^{137} and the anchoring positions seem to be critical for the binding and activation by the synthetic agonist GW9508 (Sum et al., 2007; Tikhonova et al., 2007).

FFAR1 has approximately the same high affinity (EC_{50} 5-60 μM) for medium and long chain saturated FAs ranging from C6 (caproic acid) to C23 (tricosanoic acid), with FAs between C10 to C18 being the preferred endogenous agonists; but it is not active in the presence of acetate, propionate, butyrate, or pentanoate (valerate). It also shows the same range of high affinities for both MUFAs and PUFAs, with ARA (C20:4ω-6), EPA (C22:5ω-3), and DHA (22:6ω-3) exhibiting the highest potencies (Briscoe et al., 2003; Offermanns, 2013). Noteworthy, retinoids can also activate FFAR1 with similar affinities, and, particularly, all-trans-retinoic acid, a well-known factor required for neuronal differentiation (Yu et al., 2012; Janesick et al., 2015), shows one of the highest affinities, EC_{50} < 5 μM (Briscoe et al., 2003).

In pancreas, its activation stimulates insulin secretion from β-cells (Itoh et al., 2003), involving signaling by both $G\alpha_{q/11}$ subunit and β-Arrestin2 (Mancini et al., 2015), what does have an impact on systemic metabolism control. Diverse functions have been proposed for FFAR1 in the CNS or the peripheral sensory system. Cartoni et al. (2010) described the expression of FFAR1 in type I cells of the taste buds, along with FFAR4 in type II cells, both participating in the oral perception of fats. FFAR1 has also been associated to neurogenesis and linked to cognitive functions such as memory, space orientation and learning (Ma et al., 2008; Yamashima, 2008; Boneva et al., 2011; Zamarbide et al., 2014). Although these effects are probably mediated mainly by phosphorylation of CREB, its signaling pathway is still not well understood. Since $G\alpha_s$ proteins do not seem to be activated by FFAR1, an alternative phosphorylation of CERB via Erk has been proposed (Yamashima, 2012). Differentiation and maturation of cultures of rat neuronal stem cells overexpressing FFAR1 can be stimulated by DHA, promoting neurite outgrowth and branching, even at concentrations as low as 1,5 μM (Ma et al., 2010). FFAR1 has also been proved to mediate the antinociceptive activities of DHA via induction of secretion of μ and δ opioid peptides, but not κ opioid peptides (Nakamoto et al., 2012). In the hypothalamus FFAR1 is expressed in NPY and POMC expressing neurons linked to satiety and control of food intake, and its activation by its synthetic agonist TUG905 increase POMC (anorexigenic precursor) secretion that leads to body weight loss (Dragano et al., 2017).

High fat diet in mice and PA-albumin complex in neuroblastome derived cells in culture were shown to stimulate synthesis of amyloid precursor protein (APP) and β-site APP cleaving enzyme 1 (BACE1), promoting the release of Aβ peptides in hippocampus and brain cortex, similarly to Akt pathways activation by GW9508 agonist of FFAR1 (Kim et al., 2017). This effect can be blocked in SK-N-MC cells *in vitro* if FFAR1 is pharmacologically inhibited with GW1100, knocked down by siRNA or delocalized from lipid rafts when membranes are depleted from cholesterol with methyl-β-cyclodextrin. However, GW9508 activation of FFAR1 in a mouse model of AD, based on Aβ intracerebroventricular (icv) injection, leads to significant improvement in cognitive and behavioral tests, what seems to be mediated by CREB phosphorylation and the concomitant increase in expression of NGF and BDNF neurotrophic factors. These effects were not observed when the inhibitor GW1100 was co-administered with the synthetic agonist (Khan et al., 2016). As these opposing effects originate from divergent signaling pathways from a single receptor, exploitation of FFAR1 synthetic agonists or inhibitors for treating neuropathologies may be a task worth pursuing. But first, it is imperative to fully characterize the signal transduction mechanisms active in the CNS, as well as to develop specific drugs that can selectively activate only those promoting neuroprotection, neuronal differentiation, and maturation. During the last decades, an increasing amount of evidence was collected linking the etiology and pathology of AD with Type-2 Diabetes Mellitus (Benedict and Grillo, 2018; Ferreira et al., 2018; Chornenkyy et al., 2019). Considering the wide range of synthetic agonist of FFAR1 being developed to treat Diabetes, it became an interesting possibility to evaluate their repurposing for treating AD as well (Li et al., 2016; Chen et al., 2019). For example, two different mouse models of diabesity (diabetes and obesity), based on high fat diet or db/db mice, present a decrease in FFAR1 and BDNF expression in the hippocampus and brain cortex, that can be reverted by chronic administration of DHA or GW9608 (Sona et al., 2018). Since it can be inhibited by Erk and MAPK inhibitors, BDNF expression depends on FFAR1-pErk pathway.

FFAR2 (GPR43)

Although the gene structure of GPR43 is not yet fully defined, FFAR2 was described to be encoded as a 330 amino acids protein (37.14 kDa) in a single exon. Its structure is predicted to have a topology very similar to FFAR1, where the extra 30 amino acids would correspond mainly to a longer C-terminal tail. However, FFAR2 preferential endogenous ligands are limited to acetate, propionate, butyrate, and pentanoate (with EC_{50} somewhat an order of magnitude larger than those for FFAR1), and this receptor does not respond to ligands with chain length above C6 (Brown et al., 2003; Offermanns, 2013). Its activation has been describe to be coupled both to pertussis toxin sensitive ($G\alpha_i$) and insensitive ($G\alpha_q$) proteins (Brown et al., 2003; Stoddart et al., 2008). In the first pathway, FFAR2 activation leads to a decrease in cAMP production by adenylate cyclase (AC) and, therefore, to a reduction in protein kinase cAMP-activated (PKA) activity. On the other hand, $G\alpha_q$ activates phospholipase C (PLC) that cleaves phosphatidylinositol bisphosphates (PIP_2) into inositol-triphosphate (IP_3) and diacylglycerol. IP_3 binds to IP_3R receptor in the endoplasmic reticulum and induces the internal release of Ca^{+2} to the cytosol, which then activates Ca^{+2}-dependent protein kinase C (PKC). DAG attracts certain PKC isoforms to the plasma membrane and helps to direct its activity to a subset of potential target substrates.

FFAR2 is most abundantly expressed in spleen, bone marrow, and lung, followed by adipose tissue, breast, and all the digestive tract. Its expression is mainly consistent with a leukocyte markers expression pattern, with higher presence in macrophages and leukocyte germ line (Brown et al., 2003). The low level, but widespread FFAR2 expression may be due to its presence in immune cells, such as infiltrating neutrophils and macrophages. Its expression in CNS is rather low compared to other FFARs (**Figure 1F**) and limited to glia and neurons of the caudate, but FFAR2 can also be detected in cortical neurons and pituitary gland. However, the participation of FFAR2 in neuronal processes still needs further analysis.

FFAR3 (GPR41)

FFAR3 is the product of the gene *GPR41*, only 6.62 kb downstream of *GPR40* promoter, but it lacks a formal promoter of its own. Although 3 sites of transcription initiation can be predicted in putative exons upstream *GPR41*, none of them could be confirmed. Contrarily, *GPR41* may be expressed as the result of the skipping of a termination sequence immediately downstream FFAR1 stop codon. Bahar Halpern et al. (2012) demonstrated that *GPR40* and *GPR41* are transcribed as a single bicistronic mRNA thanks to the action of an H2R enhancer, and that a tissue-specific internal ribosome entry site controls the translation of *GPR41* into FFAR3 in pancreatic β-cells. FFAR3 is also coded in a single exon, as a 346 amino acids protein (38.,65 kDa). *GPR40*-common origin is inferred from the relatively high sequence similarity/identity (31/34%), compared to other GPCRs. Like FFAR2, its structure is believed to be similar to FFAR1, with the extra 46 amino acids mainly corresponding to an extension of the cytosolic C-terminal tail; and its activation is mainly due to the binding of the same short chain FAs (Brown et al., 2003). The difference is that pentanoate is more potent than acetate for FFAR3, while it is quite the opposite for FFAR2. FFAR3 activation has been described to be coupled only to $G\alpha i$ subunits. Its activation by β-hydroxy-butirate negatively regulates the activity of Cav2.2 N-type Ca^{+2} channel (Won et al., 2013; Colina et al., 2018).

High-throughput RNAseq screening analysis of FFAR3 expression indicated a widespread, but weak pattern, with higher levels observed in adipose tissue, breast, spleen, and digestive tract. Neural expression is scarce (**Figure 1F**) and only very weakly detected in the pituitary gland in GTEx (The GTEx Consortium, 2013). A GPR41-mRFP transgenic mice model published by Nohr et al. (2013) showed FFAR3 expression in the digestive tract intimately associated to the enteroendocrine system, mainly in enteric neurons of the submucosal and myenteric ganglia, and in several of the postganglionic sympathetic and sensory neurons, both in autonomic and somatic peripheral nervous system (PNS). But this model showed no expression in the brain or spinal cord. FFAR3 enteroendocrine expression links signaling of short FAs from the microbiota with enteric hormone secretion (Samuel et al., 2008). Its activation by short chain FAs and β-hydroxy-butirate in sympathetic neurons also inhibited $Ca_V2.2$ currents, linking the functions of the PNS to the metabolic state (Won et al., 2013).

FFAR4 (GPR120)

The gene that codes for FFAR4, originally called *GPR120*, was described in 2003 to have four exons that are located on human chromosome 10q23.33 (Fredriksson et al., 2003). It is expressed, at least, as two variants generated by alternative splicing that leads to exon 3 skipping, *GPR120S* (coding for a 361 amino acids peptide, 40,49 kDa) and *GPR120L* (377 amino acids, 42,24 kDa). Predicted transmembrane regions leave N- and C-terminal segments longer than in previous FFARs, but the most notorious difference is the cytoplasmic loop between TM5 and TM6, where the *GPR120S* lacks 16 amino acids (from 233 to 248) compared to the longer variant *GPR120L*. Activation of FFAR4 signals through $G\alpha_{q/11}$.

Highest expression of FFAR4 includes lower digestive tract, brain, adipose tissue, lung, testis, breast, and adrenal glands. Within the CNS, FFAR4 is found mainly in glial and neuronal cells of hippocampus, cerebral cortex, hypothalamus, and cerebellum (only granular layer and Purkinje cells), with a particularly high expression in pituitary gland (The GTEx Consortium, 2013). ISH of mice brain sections show FFAR4 preferential expression in medulla, pons and olfactory bulb, followed by hypothalamus and cerebellum (**Figures 1D,F**).

FFAR4 natural ligands include saturated FAs of C14, C16 and C18, with affinities around EC_{50} = 30, 52 and 18 μM, respectively. When overexpressed in HEK293 cells, both agonist-stimulated GPR120S and GPR120L receptors recruit β-Arrestin2 and undergo internalization, but the longer variant shows much less Ca^{+2} mobilization and average cellular response (Watson et al., 2012). Two Arg residues on the outer edge of TM2 (Arg^{99}) and TM4 (Arg^{178}) have been mapped to be responsible for FAs binding (Watson et al., 2012), unlike the other FFARs members that have two conserved Arg residues on the outer edge of TM5 and TM7 (Sum et al., 2007; Stoddart et al., 2008), showing once more the evolutionary divergence of FFAR4 from the rest of the GPCRs activated by FAs. Other residues involved in ligand binding and activation of the receptor included four aromatic residues Phe^{115}, Phe^{211}, Trp^{277}, and Phe^{304} that, when mutated, essentially eliminated responsiveness to agonists (Hudson et al., 2014).

FFAR4 has been more thoroughly studied in adipocytes and intestine where it promotes insulin sensitizing and anti-inflammatory effects, respectively (Song et al., 2017). In enteroendocrine cells it helps controlling the secretion of hormones, promoting glucagon-like peptide 1 release but inhibiting ghrelin secretion (Hirasawa et al., 2005; Engelstoft et al., 2013); whereas, in adipocytes, oleic acid stimulates lipid droplet formation by activation of this receptor, which signals through $G\alpha_q$, PI3K-Akt, and PLC pathways (Rohwedder et al., 2014; Villegas-Comonfort et al., 2017). However, it has a greater affinity for PUFAs, particularly those from the ω-3 series. In Caco-2 cells, EPA, DHA, and ARA elicit the same signaling events through FFAR4, but with different kinetics and efficiency (Mobraten et al., 2013). Basal and heterologous phosphorylation of Thr^{347}, Ser^{350}, and Ser^{357} in the C-terminal tail (GPR120S) mediates receptor internalization (Burns et al., 2014; Sanchez-Reyes et al., 2014). Hypothalamic expression of FFAR4 corresponds to microglia and its activation ameliorates neuroinflammatory response by decreasing the production of proinflammatory cytokines (TNFα and IL-1β) and promoting those with anti-inflammatory action (IL-6 and IL-10) (Dragano et al., 2017).

GPR84

This isoform was identified, through an EST library, in B cells encoded in a single exon (exon2) (Wittenberger et al., 2001), but it was the last one to be deorphanized (Wang et al., 2006). Therefore, GPR84 is the least studied isoform of the FFARs and has not yet been assigned with the "FFAR5" name. Its expression was confirmed by Northern-blot in brain, colon, thymus, spleen, kidney, liver, intestine, placenta, lung, leukocytes, heart, and muscle. Regarding CNS expression, it is most abundantly found in medulla and spinal cord, but also significantly in amygdala, *substantia nigra*, thalamus, and *corpus callosum*, whereas only weakly detected in other brain regions such as the cerebellum (Wittenberger et al., 2001) (**Figures 1E,F**). GPR84 is activated only by medium length acyl chain FAs (C9 to C14) and does not recognize longer or shorter chain carboxylic acids, promoting Ca^{+2} mobilization and inhibiting cAMP production, mainly through the activation of $G\alpha_{i/o}$ (Wang et al., 2006). Its expression is augmented in monocytes by incubation with LPS, and its activation by medium chain FAs exacerbates the production of proinflammatory cytokines, highlighting GPR84 role in immune responses (Wang et al., 2006; Muller et al., 2017). Alternatively to endogenous ligands, GPR84 can also be activated by hidroxylated medium chain FAs and synthetic drugs like ZQ16 (2-(hexylthio)pyrimidine-4,6-diol), diindolylmethane or 6-n-octylaminouracil (Suzuki et al., 2013; Nikaido et al., 2015; Zhang et al., 2016).

When activated, GPR84 expressed in mouse primary cultures of microglia stimulates membrane ruffling, modifies its morphology, and promotes motility, but it does not promote an inflammatory response, including the secretion proinflammatory cytokines (Wei et al., 2017). Different FAs are known to be released after diverse brain injuries, from traumatic lesions to neurodegenerative diseases and neuroinflammatory conditions, and they may function as chemo-attractants for microglia, especially short and middle chain FAs that exhibit higher solubility and that can be recognized by FFAR2, FFAR3, and GPR84. This suggests that GPR84 could be a valid therapeutic target in microglia-associated diseases, such as AD or Multiple Sclerosis.

Citosolic Receptors

Due to their low solubility, free FAs need to be bound to proteins in order to diffuse through the aqueous medium of the cytosol. Since the 1970s, the proteins known as FABPs have been studied and proved to help overcome this problem. They are small (15 kDa) intracellular soluble proteins that reversibly bind FAs and other hydrophobic ligands, trafficking them to different intracellular compartments, such as mitochondria, peroxisome, endoplasmic reticulum or the nucleus. Even with as low as 30% identity of amino acids sequence, they share a highly conserved structure (**Figures 2A,B**), consisting in a barrel of 10 β-strands enclosing the binding cavity, and a helix-turn-helix motif capping this barrel. The latter regulates both ligand entry and exit, as well as origin and destiny points of traffic (Banaszak et al., 1994; Thompson et al., 1999; Storch and Corsico, 2008; Storch and Thumser, 2010). These proteins have been

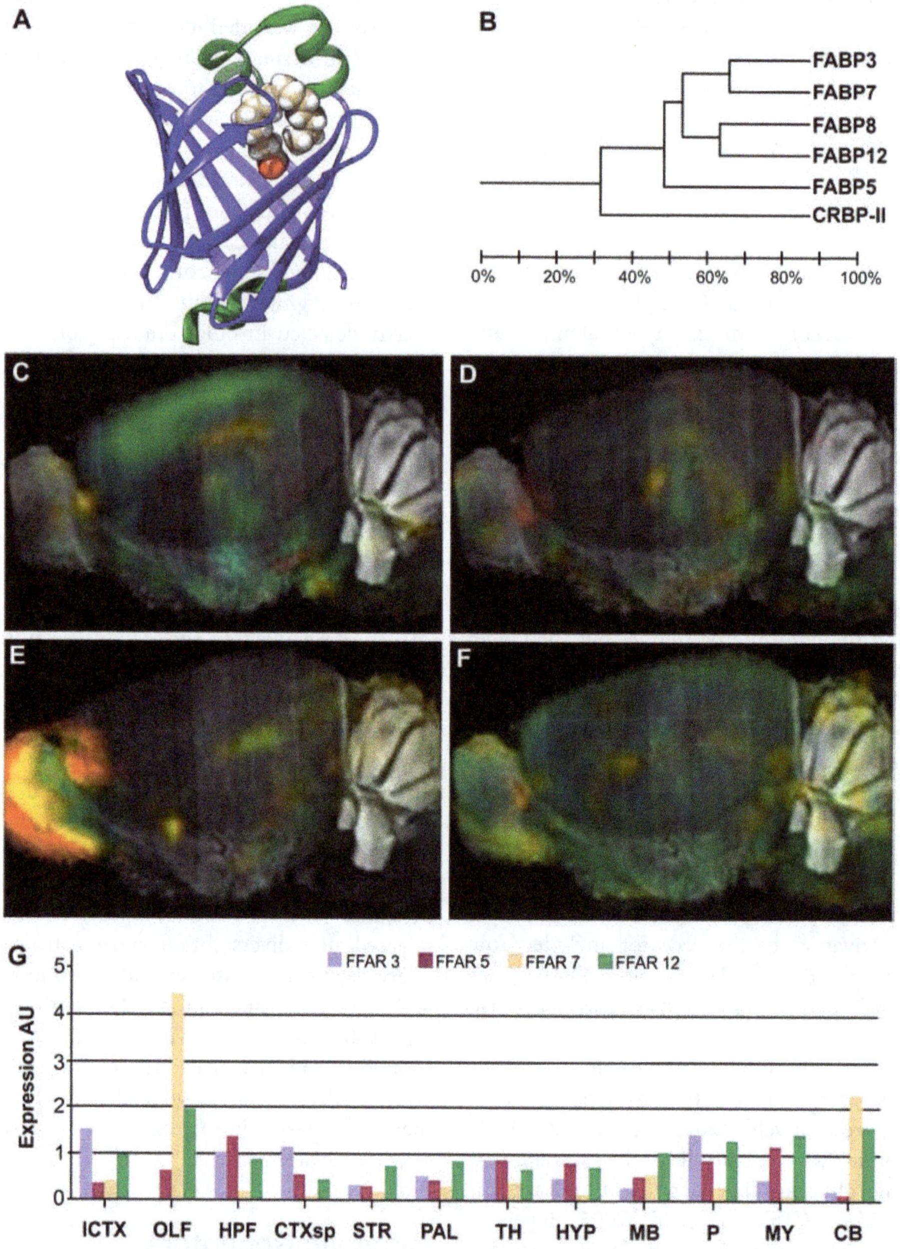

FIGURE 2 | Structure and brain expression patterns of FABPs. **(A)** Cartoon based on crystal structure of human FABP3 complex with palmitic acid (PDB-ID: 6AQ1) (Yan et al., 2018). The β-barrel, array of 10 antiparallel β-strands, is shown in blue, and the helix-tur-helix motif cap is shown in green, with the palmitic acid (in filled-balls model) adopting a U-shaped conformation inside. **(B)** Dendrogram showing relationship between identity of sequence between FABPs expressed in neural tissues. Also belonging to the same folding, CRBP-II was included as and outlier. **(C–F)** Brain left hemisphere sagittal projection showing expression of FABP3, FABP5, FABP7 and FABP12, respectively, based on ISH data. FABP8 expression in mice brain is not significant. **(G)** Quantification of relative brain expression from ISH data for neural FABPs isoforms. AU: Arbitrary units. For brain regions references see legend of **Figure 1**. Image credit for panels **C–F**: Allen Institute. © 2007 Allen Institute for Brain Science. Allen Mouse Brain Atlas. Available from: http://mouse.brain-map.org/search/. Panel **G** was constructed from data available through Allen Mouse Brain Atlas website.

extensively characterized *in vitro*, including its three-dimensional structures by NMR and X-ray Crystallography, with and without any cargo, natural or synthetic (Sacchettini et al., 1987; Xu et al., 1991; Ory et al., 1997; Balendiran et al., 2000; Hanhoff et al., 2002; Rademacher et al., 2002; Reese and Banaszak, 2004). They can uptake FAs from model phospholipid vesicles and transfer its cargo to other membranes, according to the properties of each isoform (Herr et al., 1996; Storch and Thumser, 2000; Veerkamp and Zimmerman, 2001; Liou et al., 2002; Storch et al., 2002; Falomir-Lockhart et al., 2006). It has been demonstrated that some isoforms interact better with membranes in the apo-form, presumably looking for ligand uptake; whereas others are dominated mainly by electrostatic interaction between the holo-protein and the phospholipid's headgroups (Falomir-Lockhart et al., 2006, 2011).

FABPs were originally named after the tissue where each isoform was firstly identified, and intestinal enterocytes were the exception that expressed large quantities of two isoforms, FABP1 and FABP2. Nowadays, the numbered nomenclature is preferred over tissue-related names in order to avoid misinterpretations derived from the fact that most cell types can express more than one member of the FABP family, and their level of expression responds to metabolic conditions, external stimuli, or development stages. Therefore, most FABPs show distinctive expression patterns in different organs and cell types. No isoform shows a high degree of selectivity for a particular FA, although it is usually found a higher affinity for saturated compared to unsaturated FAs (Richieri et al., 2000). The affinity for FAs of each isoform depends on chain length and number of double bonds, but isoforms FABP1 and FABP5 show significant affinity for a wider range of hydrophobic ligands. A total of 9 FABP isoforms with high affinity for long chain FAs (between C12 and C22) are described in mammals, plus 4 more members that show specificity for retinoid ligands (CRBP-I, CRBP-II, CRABP1 and CRABP2) and one extra for bile acids (FABP6, I-BABP or ILBP).

There are five FABP isoforms with relevant levels of expression in neural tissues: FABP3 (commonly known also as Heart-FABP), FABP5 (Epidermal-FABP), FABP7 (Brain-FABP), FABP8 (Myelin-FABP or PMP2), and FABP12 (Retinal-FABP). Each of them presents distinct spatio-temporal expression patterns (Owada et al., 1996; Liu et al., 2000). Many of them are significantly expressed in the brain, whereas FABP8 is apparently exclusive of PNS. Bellow there is a resume of the most prominent information available about each neural isoform.

FABP3

Significant expression of FABP3 is not detected in embryonic stages of rodent or in fetal human brains (Cheon et al., 2003; Saino-Saito et al., 2009). Perinatal FABP3 expression increases gradually, mainly confined to gray matter in rodents. In adult individuals, FABP3 is stably expressed in the neuronal layers of hippocampus, the cerebral neocortex, interneurons of the retina and the olfactory mitral cell layer, particularly in CA1 and CA2 portions (Owada, 2008; Saino-Saito et al., 2009). Its mRNA can also be detected in Purkinje and granulate cells of the cerebellum (Owada, 2008). ISH of mice brain slices localizes FABP3 expression in isocortex, cortex, pons and hippocampus (**Figures 2C,G**).

FABP3 shows somewhat preferential binding of ω-6 PUFAs, but affinities for all FAs range from 0.8 to 5 μM. FABP3 is thought to help to consolidate and maintain the differentiated status of neurons in adult brains through the utilization of PUFAs. Actually, brain ARA assimilation and its incorporation into phospholipids correlate with FABP3 expression levels, which is also necessary to maintain an optimal balance between ω-6 and ω-3 PUFAs in adult neurons (Murphy et al., 2005). FABP3 could also modulate dopamine signaling, since it is highly expressed in acetylcholinergic and terminals of glutamatergic neurons of dorsal *striatum*, and it can interact physically and modulate dopamine D2 receptors (D2R) in mice (Shioda et al., 2010). This was confirmed by dysfunctional response of D2R to amphetamines and to D2R-specific agonist Haloperidol in FABP3$^{-/-}$ mice; whereas response to D1R-specific agonist SCH23390 was not impaired. The expression of FABP3 in dopaminergic neurons is still controversial, even between the same authors (Shioda et al., 2010, 2014). On the other hand, FABP3 can be found in the cochlea, as well as FABP7, not involved in sensing but present in different support cells, suggesting a non-redundant function of these proteins in modulation of the hearing process (Saino-Saito et al., 2010).

Regarding pathological conditions, FABP3 was found to be significantly decreased in frontal, occipital, and parietal cortices of patients suffering Down Syndrome; and it was also elevated in temporal cortex of patients with AD (Cheon et al., 2003; Sanchez-Font et al., 2003; Watanabe et al., 2007). FABP3 expression in dopaminergic neurons may promote MPTP and ARA-induced α-Synuclein aggregation (Shioda et al., 2014), the main component of the characteristic Lewy Bodies present in PD and related neurodegenerative diseases. Furthermore, aberrant expression of FABP3 may affect PUFA enrichment and alter membrane fluidity and signal transduction. Consequently, this deficiency could lead to cellular dysfunction in neurodegenerative disorders.

FABP5

FABP5 is the most ubiquitously expressed FABP. During midterm embryonic stages, it is particularly present in the ventricular germinal zone and the cerebral cortex, as well as in the stem cells differentiating into motor neurons or astrocytes. But its expression progressively decreases after birth until it is only weakly detected in the adult brain (Liu et al., 2010). This moderate expression is shared, with varying intensity in different brain regions, by neurons and glia (**Figures 2D,G**). Regarding mouse retina, FABP5 is found in the retinal ganglion cells, up to E14 strictly localized in the soma, but progressively migrating into axons of optic nerve by E18 and until P10 (Allen et al., 2001; Saino-Saito et al., 2009). This suggests that FABP5 may have a role in neurite outgrowth and axon development by supplying LCFA for phospholipid synthesis. FABP5 also shows high affinity for retinoic acid (RA) and, therefore, it is associated to neuronal survival and differentiation by activation of PPARβ/δ, not only through FAs but RA signaling as well. Actually, the latter depends on the distribution ratio between CRABP2 and FABP5, and it may be as well modulated by displacement from either protein by FAs, and particularly by DHA (Schug et al., 2007, 2008; Yu et al., 2012). Recent publications also link FABP5 to regulatory functions of estrogen receptors (Senga et al., 2018), which could be related to its heterodimerization to Retinoid X Receptors (RXRs), similarly to PPARs.

FABP5 expression is induced under pathological or stress conditions, for example, after axonal injury in peripheral nerves (De Leon et al., 1996), but not in Down Syndrome, AD or Bipolar Disorder (Cheon et al., 2003). Under oxidative stress conditions, FABP5 has been proved to work as a scavenging system of 4-Hydroxynonenal lipid peroxidation subproduct (Bennaars-Eiden et al., 2002). Altogether, we can summarize that FABP5 is expressed when the fate of the neural cell differentiation must be decided or when it has to adapt to stress or pathological conditions.

FABP7

In embryonic brains, FABP7 is highly expressed in the radial glia, in the ventricular and subventricular zones. After birth, the expression remains strongly positive in gray and white matter (Kurtz et al., 1994). In the neonatal brain, its expression is more evident in the olfactory nerve fiber layers, hippocampal dentate gyrus, and the cerebellar Purkinje cell layer. Finally, in adulthood, the expression decreases although it remains in the Schwann cells of olfactory nerve, in the radial glia of dentate gyrus, and in the glial cells located adjacent to the cerebellar Purkinje cells (Kurtz et al., 1994). Its mRNA expression in 8 weeks-old mice is evident only in olfactory bulb and the cerebellum (**Figures 2E,G**). FABP7 was proposed to be downstream regulator of Pax6 participating in the maintenance of pre-neurogenesis neuroepithelia, while its knock-down promotes neuronal differentiation (Arai et al., 2005). FABP7 and FABP3 are usually expressed in the same regions of the brain, with the later usually showing 10-time higher levels, although local concentration may vary (Pelsers et al., 2004). As mentioned before, both proteins are present in different support cells of the cochlea, suggesting a regulatory function of hearing signals (Saino-Saito et al., 2010). FABP7 is also expressed by glial progenitor cells located in the foregut and midgut during enteric nervous system development (Sasselli et al., 2012).

FABP7 preferentially binds ω-3 PUFAs and oleic acid (18:1n-9, OA) over ω-6 PUFAs, and shows lower affinity for SFAs (Xu et al., 1996; Balendiran et al., 2000; Hanhoff et al., 2002). Therefore, null mice display decreased DHA incorporation into PLs, with an increase in AA and PA instead (Owada, 2008). Its up-regulation during embryonic stages of development (and, probably, FABP5's as well) is likely related to the proliferation and initial differentiation of neural stem cells and progenitorse, with an increasing demand of PUFAs, rather than to their maturation and integration (Liu et al., 2010). Actually, the fluorescent probe CDr3 was identified as a specific ligand for FABP7 in neural stem cells (Yun et al., 2012) and successfully employed for its flow cytometry isolation from both adult and embryonic mouse brains (Leong et al., 2013).

Regarding pathological conditions, FABP7 has been shown to be significantly increased in occipital cortex of patients with Down Syndrome, although no changes were detected in fetal brain (Cheon et al., 2003). Gene allele association studies showed correlation of FABP7 expression with schizophrenia and bipolar disorder (Saino-Saito et al., 2010).

FABP8

FABP8 can be abundantly and exclusively found, although unevenly distributed, in the myelin sheaths and Schwann cells of peripheral nerves, for example, in the human *nervus suralis*. It can represent up to 15% of total protein of bovine PNS myelin (Greenfield et al., 1973). In mice, mRNA levels increase gradually and the protein is detectable after P4 (Zenker et al., 2014). FABP8 is present only in minor amounts in CNS white matter, being more abundant in spinal cord and brain stem myelin. The expression levels of FABP8 vary both in intensity and distribution between different regions of a single nerve as well as between nerves (DeArmond et al., 1980).

FABP8 has a unique function in the organization and stabilization of myelin multilayers as it is capable of stacking phospholipid membranes synergistically with Myelin Basic Protein (Greenfield et al., 1973). Its higher expression during the early postnatal life also suggests a role in FAs uptake and lipid metabolism toward myelination of axons (Zenker et al., 2014). Notably, knock-out of one or both proteins does not affect myelin structure, and its only consequence is a minor retardation in motor nerve conduction (Zenker et al., 2014). However, several point mutations of FABP8 have been associated to the inherited neuropathy known as Charcot-Marie-Tooth disease (Motley et al., 2016; Punetha et al., 2018).

FABP12

The *FABP12* gene was the last one to be identified to code for a member of this family of proteins (Liu et al., 2008) and, hence, has not yet been thoroughly studied like other members. Its mRNA was found at high levels mainly in the retina and testis, and to a lesser extent in the cerebral cortex, kidney and epididymis of rat and mouse tissues (Smathers and Petersen, 2011). ISH of mouse brain sections shows a ubiquitous expression (**Figures 2F,G**). Under oxidative stress conditions, FABP12 protects retinal rod cells from peroxidation mediated by LCFA hydroperoxides (Guajardo et al., 2002).

Nuclear Receptors-Transcription Factors

In many tissues, FAs induce changes in gene expression through nuclear receptors of the PPARs family of transcription factors, ligand-activated nuclear receptors subfamily 1 group C (Capelli et al., 2016). PPARs structure consists of a variable N-terminal region, a conserved DNA binding domain, a variable hinge region, a conserved ligand binding domain, and a variable C-terminal region (Mangelsdorf et al., 1995). Heterodimerization of PPARs with Retinoid-X Receptor (RXR) depends on ligand and DNA binding, being affected also by posttranslational modifications (Berrabah et al., 2011; Anbalagan et al., 2012; Brunmeir and Xu, 2018). The DNA binding domain includes two segments with Zn-fingers motifs, which recognizes its target sequence or Response Element (RE). The N- and C-terminal regions include the Activation-Function 1 (AF1) and 2 (AF2), respectively, essential for interaction with coregulators and transcription modulation functions (**Figure 3A**). PPAR–RXR complexes recognize a direct repeat of the consensus sequence AGGTCA with a single nucleotide in between, also referred to as PPRE: AGGTCA-N_1-AGGTCA. These features have been corroborated by the crystal structures available (PDB-IDs: 3E00, 3DZU, 3DZY) (**Figure 3A**) (Chandra et al., 2008). PPARs are thought to be permanently bound to PPREs as heterodimers with one of the three RXR isoforms (RXRα, RXRβ, or RXRγ). The lack of ligand bound to them promotes their repressor activity through association with corepressors, such as Nuclear Receptor Corepressor (NCoR) or the Silencing Mediator of Retinoid and Thyroid hormone receptor (SMART). Upon ligand binding, corepressors are released and co-activators recruited, including

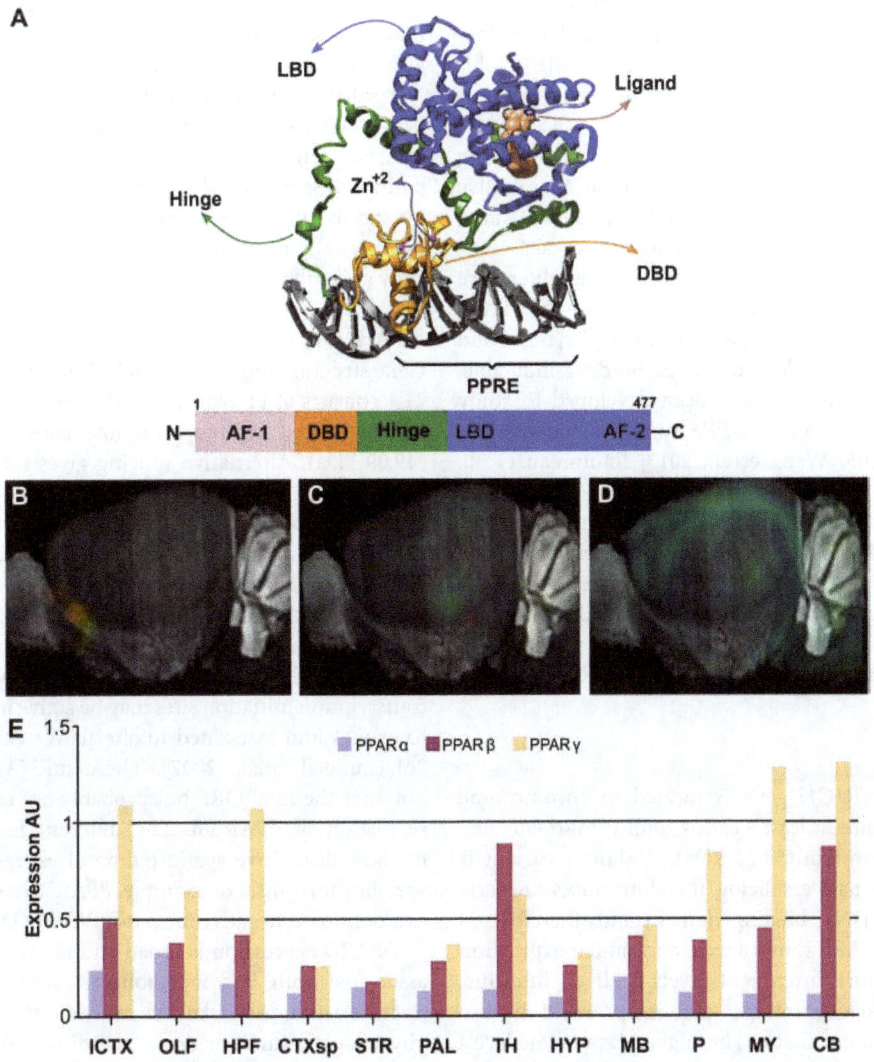

FIGURE 3 | Structure and brain expression patterns of PPARs. **(A)** Cartoon based on crystal structure (PDB-ID: 3DZY) of the full-length PPARγ in a complex with RXRα and two accessory 13-amino acids peptides of Nuclear receptor coactivator 2 and a dsDNA containing the PPRE (Chandra et al., 2008). For clarity, only PPARγ, its synthetic agonist Rosiglitazone and the dsDNA are shown. N-terminal region of PPARγ is not visible because it was not determined due to high flexibility. **(B–D)** Brain left hemisphere sagittal projection showing expression of PPARα, PPARβ and PPARγ, respectively based on ISH data. **(E)** Quantification of relative brain expression from ISH data for neural FABPs isoforms. AU: Arbitrary units. For brain regions references see legend of **Figure 1**. Image credit for panels **B–D**: Allen Institute. © 2007 Allen Institute for Brain Science. Allen Mouse Brain Atlas. Available from: http://mouse.brain-map.org/search/. Panel **E** was constructed from data available through Allen Mouse Brain Atlas website.

p300, CREB-binding protein, or Steroid Receptor Coactivator 1 (SRC1); promoting transcriptional activation of their target genes (Zoete et al., 2007).

PPARα was first identified as a new member of the steroid hormone receptor superfamily and proved to mediate the effects of hypolipidemic drugs commonly used in hyperlipidemias. These drugs were known as peroxisome proliferators, dubbing this receptor PPARs (Issemann and Green, 1990). Parallel identification of multiple isoforms in mammals and *Xenopus* sp. led to some controversy regarding their nomenclature, but nowadays it is accepted that three isoforms are present, comprising PPARα, PPARβ/δ, and PPARγ (Echeverria et al., 2016; Brunmeir and Xu, 2018). Besides FAs, PPARs have also been reported to be activated by other endogenous lipidic compounds, such as endocannabinoids (oleylethanolamide, arachidonylethanolamide, 2-arachidonyl-glycerol, etc.) and by RA (O'Sullivan, 2007; Schug et al., 2007). Unfortunately, little progress has been made identifying natural endogenous ligands which are specific or preferential for any of the PPARs isoforms due to their rather low affinity and similar specificities.

As mentioned above, the activation of PPARs modulates directly the expression of genes near the bound PPER. But a second mechanism of action has been proposed for certain isoforms, blocking or preventing the interaction of other transcription factors. The better studied example corresponds to the ligand-dependent SUMOylation of activated PPARγ that gets displaced from its PPRE and blocks NFκB interaction with its own response elements and, hence, limiting the inflammatory response (Ricote and Glass, 2007; Glass and Saijo, 2010). This mechanism is known as transrepression and may be a putative target for handling neuroinflmammation.

All PPARs isoforms were detected in the CNS employing multiple techniques, such as reverse transcription-quantitative PCR (RT-qPCR), immunohistochemistry (IHC), and ISH (Kainu et al., 1994; Braissant et al., 1996; Cullingford et al., 1998; Warden et al., 2016). However, despite the vast literature available, there is still some controversy regarding PPARs expression patterns. They are essential for embryonic and fetal development in mammals and, therefore, drug-inducible, tissue specific knockout models have been developed to study their specific roles, particularly for PPARγ null mice which is lethal (Gray et al., 2005; Wang et al., 2013; Rautureau et al., 2017). Double neuronal conditional knockout of PPARβ/δ and PPARγ exacerbates cytotoxicity of 1-methyl-4-phenyl-1,2,3,6-tetrahydropyridine (MPTP) on striatum dopaminergic neurons (Mounsey et al., 2015). Noteworthy, it is not rare to find co-expression of PPARs within a single cell. Some details are offered below about protein expression levels, together with mRNA and protein variants, and the connections of PPARs with brain pathophysiology.

PPARα

Human *PPARA* (or *NR1C1*) gene is located in chromosome 22q12-q13.1 and contains at least 9 exons, with PPARα encoded as a 468 amino acid protein (52.23 kDa). A shorter variant is also described by alternative splicing that introduces an early stop codon after the DNA binding domain and, therefore, is not ligand-sensitive. PPARα shows a wide and similar expression in all tissues, with more prominent levels in liver, intestine, kidney, heart, and skeletal muscle; and its presence is also reported in brown adipose tissue. The higher expression levels of PPARα in these tissues correlate with their high capacities for FAs oxidation, and its main function seems to be related to the control of energy expenditure through lipid catabolism and the adaptation to different nutritional states, such as the postprandial period or fasting. Regarding CNS expression, the GTEx project detected similar levels of *PPARA* mRNA in caudate, pituitary gland, hypothalamus, hippocampus, cerebral cortex, and cerebellum. Furthermore, ISH of brain section showed very similar expression throughout regions and weaker than other isoforms (**Figures 3B,E**). Targeted expression analysis of PPARα reported it in olfactory bulb, retina, cerebellum, and hippocampus (Braissant et al., 1996; Moreno et al., 2004; Rivera et al., 2014). PPARα has been localized in neurons (Cristiano et al., 2001; Santos et al., 2005), oligodendrocytes (Kainu et al., 1994), microglia (Warden et al., 2016), and specially in astrocytes (Cristiano et al., 2001; Chistyakov et al., 2015).

PPARα shows relatively higher affinities for FAs compared to alternative endogenous agonists (eicosanoids and endocannabinoids), and it can be activated also by hypolimidemic drugs, but generally not or only weakly by non-steroidal anti-inflammatory drugs (NSAIDs) and anti-diabetic thiazolidinediones (Corton et al., 2000). PPARα functions in the CNS are still unclear. Its proposed functions include the regulation of sleep process (Murillo-Rodriguez, 2017), also have an impact on learning and memory consolidation. Nevertheless, it has been shown that PPARα agonists such as Wy-14643 reduce Aβ-derived oxidative damage by increasing catalase activity, and activate the Wnt/β-Catenin survival pathway (Santos et al., 2005). Furthermore, PPARα activation by statins is responsible for boosting BDNF production, that mediates cognitive improvement in another mouse mode of AD (Roy and Pahan, 2015).

PPARβ/δ

Gene structure of *PPARD* (*NR1C2*) gene in chromosome 6p21.2-21.1 consists of 11 exons, with the ORF spanning from exon 4 to exon 9 and coding for a 441 amino acids protein termed PPARδ1 (49,09 kDa). Alternative splicing gives rise to shorter isoforms: 80 amino acids shorter isoform 2 (PPARδ2) is the product of an early stop signal due to overtranscription of the 3'-end of exon 8 that introduces an in-frame non-sense codon; variant 4 lacks 98 amino acids (44 to 141) due to exon skipping; while variant 3 is the result of an alternative transcription initiation site with three new N-terminal amino acids instead of the first 43 residues of PPARδ1 (coded by exon 4). Another four alternative transcription initiation sites may be active in *PPARD* downstream to exon 1 and associated to alternative exon 2 (2a′, 2c, 2c′ and 2e) (Lundell et al., 2007). These mRNA 5′-UTR variants do not alter the final ORF but probably are related to translational regulation of PPARβ/δ. The different isoforms are suspected to show distinctive spatio-temporal expression patterns and/or specific functions. For example, PPARδ2 has been proposed to act as a dominant negative form of PPARδ1 (Dickey et al., 2016).

PPARD expression is broad and is particularly high in tissues associated with FAs metabolism, such as the gastrointestinal tract, heart, kidney, skeletal muscle, fat, and skin. Its systemic physiological function is to coordinate and balance the usage levels of FAs and glucose in muscle and liver. However, PPARβ/δ is also the most predominant PPARs isoform in the human CNS and has a ubiquitous expression in the rat brain (**Figures 3C,E**). Despite, all PPARs are co-expressed in developing CNS, PPARβ/δ remains with high expression levels in adult rats (Braissant et al., 1996), suggesting a role in brain development, mielynation, and neuronal function. It was localized in olfactory bulb, cerebral cortex, basal ganglia, hippocampus, hypothalamus, cerebellum, and spinal cord, among others brain areas (Xing et al., 1995; Braissant et al., 1996; Moreno et al., 2004). In mouse models, PPARβ/δ is widely distributed and has been found in neurons of the prefrontal cortex, nucleus accumbens, amydala, cerebellum, hypothalamus, and spinal cord, at mRNA and protein expression levels (Woods et al., 2003; Warden et al., 2016). Regarding cell types, PPARβ/δ is mainly expressed in neurons (Hall et al., 2008), but it has also been found in oligondendrocytes of the corpus callosum (Moreno et al., 2004), and in primary cultures of cortical and cerebral astrocytes (Cristiano et al., 2001). Among the glial cells, PPARβ/δ only co-localized with oligondendrocytes of the corpus callosum (Woods et al., 2003), but no with astrocytes and microglia. *In vitro*, agonists of PPARβ/δ induce the differentiation of SH-SY5Y cells (Di Loreto et al., 2007).

PPARβ/δ shows preferentially affinities for PUFAs, compared to other FAs and eicosanoids, and is selectively activated by bezafibrate (hypolipidemic drug), GW2433 and L-65041 (NSAIDs) among synthetic agonists (Corton et al., 2000). Regarding its pathological links, PPARβ/δ is repressed in patients with Huntington Disease (HD) and its pharmacological activation improves motor function, reduces neurodegeneration, and increases neuronal survival in a HD mice and cellular models (Dickey et al., 2016). The novel PPARβ/δ agonist gemfibrozil is believed to promote oligodentrocyte differentiation by increasing the expression of genes required for myelin formation (Jana et al., 2012) and could potentially be employed against demyelination-related pathologies.

PPARγ

PPARG (*NR1C3*) gene is located in chromosome 3p25. At least four transcriptional start sites actively transcribe different mRNAs with functional cDNAs coding for PPARγ isoforms. While variants 1, 3 and 4 code for the same PPARγ1 isoform (477 amino acids, 54.68 kDa), mRNA variant 2 codes for PPARγ2 which has an additional 28 amino acids at the N-terminus (505 amino acids, 57,62 kDA). PPARγ1 is expressed in a broad variety of cells including immune and brain cells, whereas PPARγ2 is highly abundant in adipose tissue and is considered the master regulator of adipocyte differentiation, where it controls FAs uptake and storage in lipid droplets as triglycerides. Within the CNS, PPARγ was found to show a more discrete pattern of expression than PPARβ/δ, and to be slightly enriched in the hippocampus, being identified both in neurons and glial cells, including microglia, (Bernardo et al., 2000; Roth et al., 2003; Heneka and Landreth, 2007; Sarruf et al., 2009; Warden et al., 2016; Villapol, 2018). Expression analysis in mice brain by ISH showed hippocampus, isocortex, cerebellum and medulla higher levels of *PPARG* mRNAs (**Figures 3D,E**). In the neuroblastome cell line SH-SY5Y, the activation of PPARγ by synthetic agonists promotes neurite outgrowth and neuronal differentiation (Miglio et al., 2009).

PPARγ shows higher affinities for PUFAs than for MUFAs, and it cannot be activated by SFAs, and its response to eicosanoids, hipolipidemic and NSAIDs is diverse, but it is generally activated by thiazolidinediones (Corton et al., 2000). PPARγ is probably the most studied isoform regarding its functions in immune cells, and its interest in neuropathological processes points toward its strong anti-inflammatory effects (Corona and Duchen, 2015). PPARγ activation can induce differentiation of oligodendrocytes and protects them from TNFα toxicity (Bernardo et al., 2009, 2017; De Nuccio et al., 2015). Furthermore, natural and synthetic agonists PPARγ can control brain inflammation processes by shutting-down proinflammatory phenotype of activated microglia, and inhibiting the expression of surface antigens or the synthesis of proinflammatory signals, such as prostaglandins and nitric oxide (Bernardo and Minghetti, 2006). PPARγ can be either positively or negatively modulated by phosphorylation, according to the residue that is modified (Shao et al., 1998; Anbalagan et al., 2012; Brunmeir and Xu, 2018), and can be sent for degradation via the Ubiquitine-Proteasome pathway. PPARγ ability to transrepress NFκB inhibits, or at least limits, the inflammatory response, a regulatory mechanism activated by SUMOylation of its N-terminal region (Ricote and Glass, 2007; Diezko and Suske, 2013; Glass and Saijo, 2010). This could be a putative target for minimizing the neuroinflammatory condition characteristic of many neurodegenerative diseases, such as PAD and AD. Actually, multiple drugs designed as agonist of PPARγ have been and tested in AD models showed to reduce the β-amyloid accumulation, its cytotoxicity and stimulation of inflammatory cytokines (Combs et al., 2000; Sastre et al., 2006; Zolezzi and Inestrosa, 2013; Bonet-Costa et al., 2016).

FUTURE PERSPECTIVES

Fatty acids participate in essential and diverse cellular processes involving neurons and glial cells, ranging from embryonic and perinatal development of tissues, including the CNS, to cognitive functions such as memory and learning. Therefore, they are unavoidably involved in neuropathological processes, including traumatic brain injury and neurodegenerative diseases. But, due to its rather simple chemical structures and low solubility, FAs require specific proteins that could recognize them and mediate its regulatory or signaling functions. Membrane receptors FFARs, cytosolic transport proteins FABPs and nuclear transcription factors PPARs are the preferential mediators of FAs functions. Taken together, and considering that almost all cell types express at least one member of each of these three families of proteins, we could hypothesize that they may be working as a complex, but coordinated sensory system for FAs. Actually, functional interaction of FABPs and PPARs has already been proved in hepatocytes and adipocytes (Smith et al., 2008; Hostetler et al., 2009). The identification of two possible ligand binding sites in FFAR1 structures in opposite sides of the membrane opens the possibility that they could be regulated and/or activated by intracellular lipids as well as by external lipokines, for example released by PLA_2 enzymes, but also by interaction with FABPs. FABP-FFAR interaction, though not yet proved, could be understood either by unloading FAs cargo from the FABPs to activate the FFARs, or as a termination mechanism of FFAR signaling by retrieval of ligands by the FABPs from the FFARs. This is an interesting possibility that would integrate all FAs receptors (**Figure 4**), and its better understanding would definitely help in the design of new drugs with increased specificity and selectivity for its primary targets, avoiding undesired adverse effects.

Fatty acids signaling effects are usually mixed with those displayed by their multiple derivatives, adding a new layer of complexity to distinguish direct cellular responses free FAs signaling. Although specific receptors have been identified for endocannabinoids, eicosanoids, resolvins, protectines, lysophosphatidic acids, monoacylglycerols, N-acylethanolamines, and so on, crosstalk between the different receptors should not be neglected or discarded. Cellular responses are the result of the integration of a myriad of external and internal signals, as evidenced by the convergence of signaling pathways. Particularly, a functional interaction between FFAR2 and FFAR3 to form an heteromeric receptor

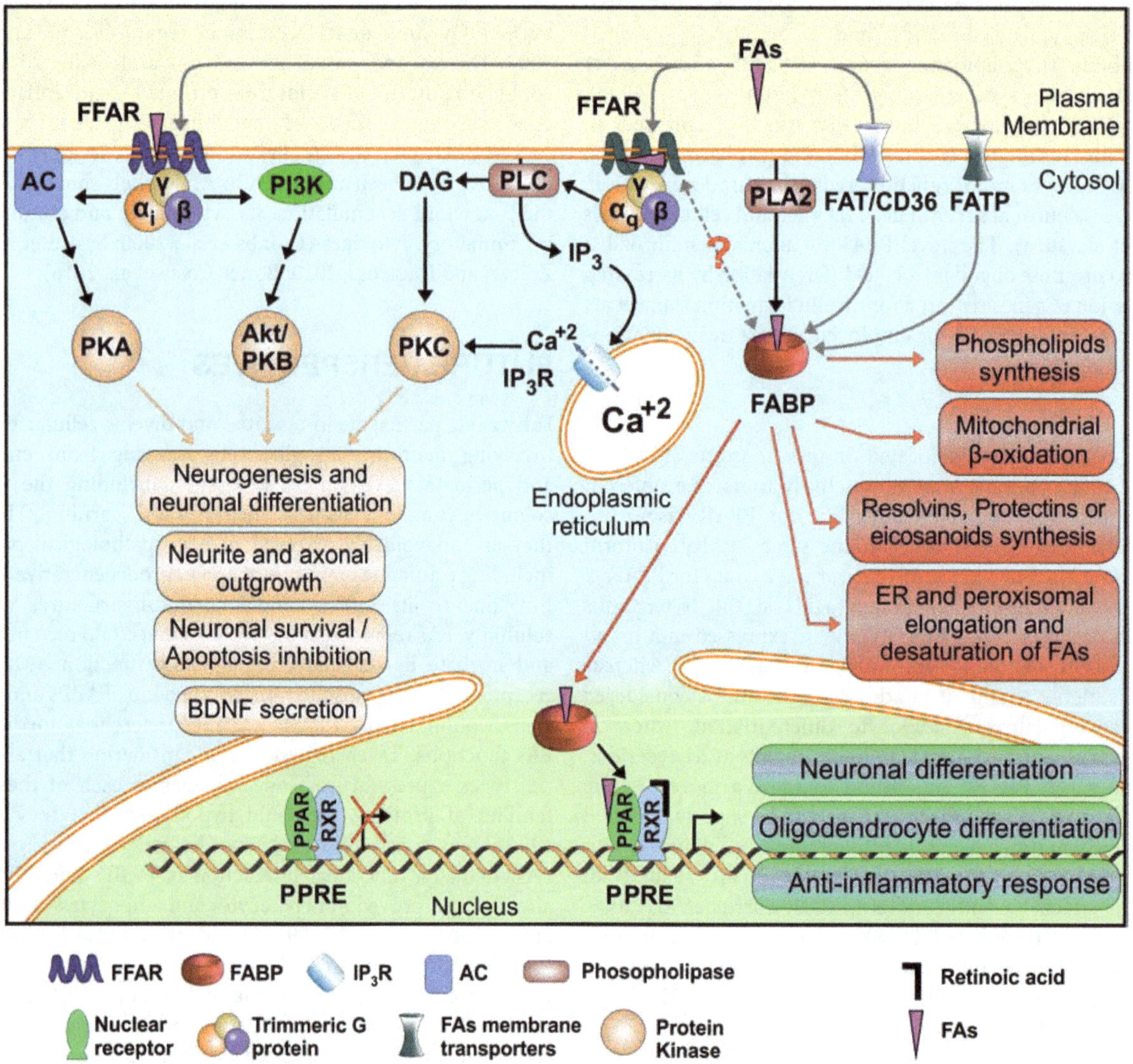

FIGURE 4 | Schematic mechanism proposed for integration of the FAs Receptors System. Alternative FAs receptors are shown along with their demonstrated or putative interactions and their better characterized cellular effects. FFAR: Free Fatty Acid Receptor; FABP: Fatty Acid Binding Protein; PPAR: Peroxisome Proliferator-Activated Receptor; RXR: Retinoid X Receptor; FA: Fatty Acid; PPRE: PPAR Response Element. AC: Adenylate Cyclase; DAG: Diacylglycerol; FATP: FAT/CD36: Fatty Acid Translocase; Fatty Acid Transport Protein; IP3: Inositol (1,4,5)-Trisphosphate; IP_3R: Inositol trisphosphate Receptor; PI3K: Phosphatidyl Inositol (3,4,5)-Trisphosphate Kinase; PLA2: Phospholipase A2; PLC: Phospholipase C; PKA: Protein Kinase A; PKAB/Akt: Protein Kinase B; PKC: Protein Kinase C.

has been proposed in primary monocytes and macrophages, and during heterologous expression in HEK293 cells (Ang et al., 2018). Considering that the origin of the short chain carboxylic acids available in mammals' bloodstream is exclusive from the microbiota colonizing their body, FFAR2 and FFAR3 may act as a remote sensory system to prevent infections, activating the proliferation and modulating the reactivity of immune cells in preparation against a growing focus of bacteria (Ulven, 2012).

Signaling of PUFAs is intimately related to RA signaling, as mentioned above by the similar activation of FFAR1. Furthermore, and similarly to what happens with FABP5 and CRABP2, PPARγ has been described to be activated by RA, as well as RXRs by DHA. In this case, FABP5 translocate its ligand, either DHA or RA, to the nucleus and unload it to the PPARβ/δ (Noy, 2016). Similarly, CRABP2 would do the same to RXR. Therefore, FABP/CRABP2 biological interaction with PPAR/RXXR is not only direct but they also compete for the same ligands, increasing the possibilities of diverse responses mounted and the subset of target genes affected. Regarding this, one must remember that many nuclear receptors heterodimerize with RXRs and, therefore the final cellular response observed is also affected by their presence and ligands (Zhang et al., 2015).

Another utility for FABPs is their detection as early biomarkers of tissue injuries, and increasing evidence is being recorded for the early or differential diagnosis of diverse pathologies (Pelsers et al., 2004, 2005; Wunderlich et al., 2005). Their main advantages are related to their fast release, as close as 30 min to the injurious event, and their relatively fast clearance. Consequently,

FABPs presence in plasma or cephaloraquidean liquid reports for recent trauma, allowing for the differentiation of consecutive events separated by less than 24 h. Neural FABPs detection has been correlated with traumatic brain injury and certain gliomas overexpressing FABP5 or FABP7 (De Rosa et al., 2012; Walder et al., 2013).

Finally, the increasing complexity of the lipid-sensing system available in humans raises the question if the regulatory and signaling functions of FAs can be individually discriminated and specifically targeted for the treatment of pathological conditions. Significant effort is being invested in the development of new drugs that would allow for their precise manipulation and the better treatment of brain injuries, neurological or neurodegenerative diseases by taking advantage of the neuroprotective and anti-inflammatory properties, particularly of PUFAs, employing either FFARs, FABPs, or PPARs as drug targets (Holliday et al., 2012; Wang et al., 2016; Zhou et al., 2016; Li et al., 2018a,b,c, 2019; Shang et al., 2018). Specificity will come together with our better understanding of how these proteins work. For example, an important step forward in this direction is the recent variation analysis of the PPRE sequence for PPARα/RXRα complex that resulted in the ideal sequence WAWVT-RGGBBA-H-RGKTYA (where W = A or T; V = not T; R = A or G; B = not A; H = not G; K = G or T; Y = T or C) as an optimized DNA sequence for PPARα (underlined) and RXRα binding (not underlined) (Tzeng et al., 2015). Noteworthy, although stronger DNA binding of RXRα to PPRE led to higher transcription rates, this is not always the case for PPARα. New candidate target genes have been identified employing this optimized sequence to screen genomic databases as being regulated by PPARα, and that could not be recognized by the consensus sequence for PPRE, improving our understanding of PPARs isoform specific functions. This could also help to development of drugs that could selectively affect only one PPAR isoform and/or only its functions regarding a certain subset of genes under its control.

Another elements that must be considered are non-coding microRNAs (miRs), which act usually as negative regulators of gene expression in the CNS, and several of them have been reported to participate in the regulation exhibited by lipids (Wnuk and Kajta, 2017). For example, the expression levels of miR-21 are decreased by DHA treatment of SH-SY5Y neuroblastome cells, showing an inverse correlation with PPARα levels (Fu et al., 2017). The miR-21 is thought to destabilize PPARα mRNAs and reduce its translation (Chen et al., 2017). Treatment with DHA plus salicylic acid promotes PPARα-RXRα heterodimer formation that correlates with a reduction of miR-21. Together, they promote PSD-95, BDNF and GDNF neuronal differentiation markers and reduce NFκB, COX-2, caspase 3 levels proinflammatory markers (Fu et al., 2017). Similarly, miR-499a negatively regulates the level of expression of PPARγ in microglia cells, promoting the expression of proinflammatory markers, such as iba-1, TNFα and IL-1β (Yu et al., 2018). Finally, PPARs can be activated by valproic acid and its short/medium-chain derivatives, a long time used family of anticonvulsants to treat epilepsy, that has also showed beneficial effects against autism, maniac and bipolar disorders (Lampen et al., 2001; Hunsberger et al., 2013; Hirsch et al., 2018). Its beneficial effects as a promoter of neuroregeneration, neurodifferentiation and neuroprotection (Liu et al., 2012; Foti et al., 2013; Oikawa and Sng, 2016) may come from the modulation of the expression of multiple miRs through PPARs, either by their transrepression or transactivation (Dharap et al., 2015). FFARs may also participate of miRs expression, such as miR-143 that is controlled in adipocytes by both PPARγ and FFAR4 activation (Bae et al., 2017). These line of evidence has recently pushed miRs to be evaluated as novel therapeutic targets against neurodegenerative diseases, such as PD o AD.

Drug discovery strategies focused on FFARs, FABPs and PPARs have already started aiming at neurological and also other pathologies like diabetes, obesity, leukemia, cancer, and so on (Kaczocha et al., 2014; Nikaido et al., 2015; Corona and Duchen, 2016; Wang et al., 2016; Cheng et al., 2019), paving the way for new developments and facilitating drug repurposing, what may save years of research and development. Noteworthy, in the case of FFARs with multiple signal transduction pathways, the concept of biased signaling is of particular interest, where a partial agonistic ligand may only and selectively activate a single pathway over the others available for that receptor. For example, FFARs partial agonist could activate β-Arrestin-mediated but not G protein-mediated signaling (Mancini et al., 2015). This kind of developments has attracted substantial attention for its potential to model molecular differences in receptors functionality that could yield enhanced therapeutic strategies, with improved efficacy and reduced adverse effects (Whalen et al., 2011; Kenakin and Christopoulos, 2013; Correll and McKittrick, 2014).

AUTHOR CONTRIBUTIONS

All authors listed have made a substantial, direct and intellectual contribution to the work, and approved it for publication.

FUNDING

This work was supported by funds from the Consejo Nacional de Investigaciones Científicas y Tecnológicas (CONICET, Argentina, grant PIP2014-618), Agencia Nacional de Promoción Científica y Tecnológica (ANPCyT, Argentina, grants PICT2014-2019 and PICT2016-3776) to LJF-L. AMT was recipient of CONICET postdoctoral fellowship. EG was recipient of CONICET doctoral fellowship and of Bunge & Born Foundation-Max Planck Society-Williams Foundations doctoral research fellowship. GFC was recipient of Consejo Interuniversitario Nacional (CIN, Argentina) undergraduate and of Universidad Nacional de La Plata (UNLP, Argentina) doctoral fellowships.

ACKNOWLEDGMENTS

We are grateful with Rosana del Cid for use-of-English revision, and with Mario R. Ramos for graphic design support. We apologize to all researchers whose work is also relevant to this manuscript but, in interest of space, was not included.

REFERENCES

Allen, G. W., Liu, J., Kirby, M. A., and De Leon, M. (2001). Induction and axonal localization of epithelial/epidermal fatty acid-binding protein in retinal ganglion cells are associated with axon development and regeneration. *J. Neurosci. Res.* 66, 396–405. doi: 10.1002/jnr.1232

Anbalagan, M., Huderson, B., Murphy, L., and Rowan, B. G. (2012). Post-translational modifications of nuclear receptors and human disease. *Nucl. Recept. Signal.* 10:e001. doi: 10.1621/nrs.10001

Ang, Z., Xiong, D., Wu, M., and Ding, J. L. (2018). FFAR2-FFAR3 receptor heteromerization modulates short-chain fatty acid sensing. *FASEB J.* 32, 289–303. doi: 10.1096/fj.201700252RR

Arai, Y., Funatsu, N., Numayama-Tsuruta, K., Nomura, T., Nakamura, S., and Osumi, N. (2005). Role of Fabp7, a downstream gene of Pax6, in the maintenance of neuroepithelial cells during early embryonic development of the rat cortex. *J. Neurosci.* 25, 9752–9761. doi: 10.1523/JNEUROSCI.2512-05.2005

Arai, Y., Sampaio, J. L., Wilsch-Brauninger, M., Ettinger, A. W., Haffner, C., and Huttner, W. B. (2015). Lipidome of midbody released from neural stem and progenitor cells during mammalian cortical neurogenesis. *Front. Cell. Neurosci.* 9:325. doi: 10.3389/fncel.2015.00325

Audet, M., and Stevens, R. C. (2019). Emerging structural biology of lipid G protein-coupled receptors. *Protein Sci.* 28, 292–304. doi: 10.1002/pro.3509

Bae, I.-S., Park, P. J., Lee, J. H., Cho, E.-G., Lee, T. R., and Kim, S. H. (2017). PPARgamma-mediated G-protein coupled receptor 120 signaling pathway promotes transcriptional activation of miR-143 in adipocytes. *Gene* 626, 64–69. doi: 10.1016/j.gene.2017.05.016

Bahar Halpern, K., Veprik, A., Rubins, N., Naaman, O., and Walker, M. D. (2012). GPR41 gene expression is mediated by internal ribosome entry site (IRES)-dependent translation of bicistronic mRNA encoding GPR40 and GPR41 proteins. *J. Biol. Chem.* 287, 20154–20163. doi: 10.1074/jbc.M112.358887

Balendiran, G. K., Schnutgen, F., Scapin, G., Borchers, T., Xhong, N., Lim, K., et al. (2000). Crystal structure and thermodynamic analysis of human brain fatty acid-binding protein. *J. Biol. Chem.* 275, 27045–27054. doi: 10.1074/jbc.M003001200

Banaszak, L., Winter, N., Xu, Z. H., Bernlohr, D. A., Cowan, S., and Jones, T. A. (1994). Lipid-binding proteins - a family of fatty-acid and retinoid transport proteins. *Adv. Protein Chem.* 45, 89–151. doi: 10.1016/S0065-3233(08)60639-7

Benedict, C., and Grillo, C. A. (2018). Insulin resistance as a therapeutic target in the treatment of Alzheimer's disease: a state-of-the-art review. *Front. Neurosci.* 12:215. doi: 10.3389/fnins.2018.00215

Bennaars-Eiden, A., Higgins, L., Hertzel, A. V., Kapphahn, R. J., Ferrington, D. A., and Bernlohr, D. A. (2002). Covalent modification of epithelial fatty acid-binding protein by 4-hydroxynonenal in vitro and in vivo. Evidence for a role in antioxidant biology. *J. Biol. Chem.* 277, 50693–50702. doi: 10.1074/jbc.M209493200

Bernardo, A., Bianchi, D., Magnaghi, V., and Minghetti, L. (2009). Peroxisome proliferator-activated receptor-gamma agonists promote differentiation and antioxidant defenses of oligodendrocyte progenitor cells. *J. Neuropathol. Exp. Neurol.* 68, 797–808. doi: 10.1097/NEN.0b013e3181aba2c1

Bernardo, A., Giammarco, M. L., De Nuccio, C., Ajmone-Cat, M. A., Visentin, S., De Simone, R., et al. (2017). Docosahexaenoic acid promotes oligodendrocyte differentiation via PPAR-gamma signalling and prevents tumor necrosis factor-alpha-dependent maturational arrest. *Biochim. Biophys. Acta* 1862, 1013–1023. doi: 10.1016/j.bbalip.2017.06.014

Bernardo, A., Levi, G., and Minghetti, L. (2000). Role of the peroxisome proliferator-activated receptor-gamma (PPAR-gamma) and its natural ligand 15-deoxy-Delta12, 14-prostaglandin J2 in the regulation of microglial functions. *Eur. J. Neurosci.* 12, 2215–2223. doi: 10.1046/j.1460-9568.2000.00110.x

Bernardo, A., and Minghetti, L. (2006). PPAR-gamma agonists as regulators of microglial activation and brain inflammation. *Curr. Pharm. Des.* 12, 93–109. doi: 10.2174/138161206780574579

Berrabah, W., Aumercier, P., Lefebvre, P., and Staels, B. (2011). Control of nuclear receptor activities in metabolism by post-translational modifications. *FEBS Lett.* 585, 1640–1650. doi: 10.1016/j.febslet.2011.03.066

Bhatia, H. S., Agrawal, R., Sharma, S., Huo, Y.-X., Ying, Z., and Gomez-Pinilla, F. (2011). Omega-3 fatty acid deficiency during brain maturation reduces neuronal and behavioral plasticity in adulthood. *PLoS One* 6:e28451. doi: 10.1371/journal.pone.0028451

Bonet-Costa, V., Herranz-Perez, V., Blanco-Gandia, M., Mas-Bargues, C., Ingles, M., Garcia-Tarraga, P., et al. (2016). Clearing amyloid-beta through PPARgamma/ApoE activation by Genistein is a treatment of experimental Alzheimer's disease. *J. Alzheimers Dis.* 51, 701–711. doi: 10.3233/JAD-151020

Boneva, N. B., Kaplamadzhiev, D. B., Sahara, S., Kikuchi, H., Pyko, I. V., Kikuchi, M., et al. (2011). Expression of fatty acid-binding proteins in adult hippocampal neurogenic niche of postischemic monkeys. *Hippocampus* 21, 162–171. doi: 10.1002/hipo.20732

Braissant, O., Foufelle, F., Scotto, C., Dauca, M., and Wahli, W. (1996). Differential expression of peroxisome proliferator-activated receptors (PPARs): tissue distribution of PPAR-alpha, -beta, and -gamma in the adult rat. *Endocrinology* 137, 354–366. doi: 10.1210/endo.137.1.8536636

Briscoe, C. P., Tadayyon, M., Andrews, J. L., Benson, W. G., Chambers, J. K., Eilert, M. M., et al. (2003). The orphan G protein-coupled receptor GPR40 is activated by medium and long chain fatty acids. *J. Biol. Chem.* 278, 11303–11311. doi: 10.1074/jbc.M211495200

Brown, A. J., Goldsworthy, S. M., Barnes, A. A., Eilert, M. M., Tcheang, L., Daniels, D., et al. (2003). The Orphan G protein-coupled receptors GPR41 and GPR43 are activated by propionate and other short chain carboxylic acids. *J. Biol. Chem.* 278, 11312–11319. doi: 10.1074/jbc.M211609200

Brown, A. J., Jupe, S., and Briscoe, C. P. (2005). A family of fatty acid binding receptors. *DNA Cell Biol.* 24, 54–61. doi: 10.1089/dna.2005.24.54

Brown, M., Roulson, J.-A., Hart, C. A., Tawadros, T., and Clarke, N. W. (2014). Arachidonic acid induction of Rho-mediated transendothelial migration in prostate cancer. *Br. J. Cancer* 110, 2099–2108. doi: 10.1038/bjc.2014.99

Brunmeir, R., and Xu, F. (2018). Functional regulation of PPARs through post-translational modifications. *Int. J. Mol. Sci.* 19:E1738. doi: 10.3390/ijms19061738

Burns, R. N., Singh, M., Senatorov, I. S., and Moniri, N. H. (2014). Mechanisms of homologous and heterologous phosphorylation of FFA receptor 4 (GPR120): GRK6 and PKC mediate phosphorylation of Thr(3)(4)(7), Ser(3)(5)(0), and Ser(3)(5)(7) in the C-terminal tail. *Biochem. Pharmacol.* 87, 650–659. doi: 10.1016/j.bcp.2013.12.016

Calder, P. C. (2015). Marine omega-3 fatty acids and inflammatory processes: effects, mechanisms and clinical relevance. *Biochim. Biophys. Acta* 1851, 469–484. doi: 10.1016/j.bbalip.2014.08.010

Cao, D., Kevala, K., Kim, J., Moon, H.-S., Jun, S. B., Lovinger, D., et al. (2009). Docosahexaenoic acid promotes hippocampal neuronal development and synaptic function. *J. Neurochem.* 111, 510–521. doi: 10.1111/j.1471-4159.2009.06335.x

Capelli, D., Cerchia, C., Montanari, R., Loiodice, F., Tortorella, P., Laghezza, A., et al. (2016). Structural basis for PPAR partial or full activation revealed by a novel ligand binding mode. *Sci. Rep.* 6:34792. doi: 10.1038/srep34792

Cartoni, C., Yasumatsu, K., Ohkuri, T., Shigemura, N., Yoshida, R., Godinot, N., et al. (2010). Taste preference for fatty acids is mediated by GPR40 and GPR120. *J. Neurosci.* 30, 8376–8382. doi: 10.1523/JNEUROSCI.0496-10.2010

Chalon, S. (2006). Omega-3 fatty acids and monoamine neurotransmission. *Prostaglandins Leukot. Essent. Fatty Acids* 75, 259–269. doi: 10.1016/j.plefa.2006.07.005

Chalon, S., Delion-Vancassel, S., Belzung, C., Guilloteau, D., Leguisquet, A. M., Besnard, J. C., et al. (1998). Dietary fish oil affects monoaminergic neurotransmission and behavior in rats. *J. Nutr.* 128, 2512–2519. doi: 10.1093/jn/128.12.2512

Chan, R. B., Oliveira, T. G., Cortes, E. P., Honig, L. S., Duff, K. E., Small, S. A., et al. (2012). Comparative lipidomic analysis of mouse and human brain with Alzheimer disease. *J. Biol. Chem.* 287, 2678–2688. doi: 10.1074/jbc.M111.274142

Chandra, V., Huang, P., Hamuro, Y., Raghuram, S., Wang, Y., Burris, T. P., et al. (2008). Structure of the intact PPAR-gamma-RXR- nuclear receptor complex on DNA. *Nature* 456, 350–356. doi: 10.1038/nature07413

Chang, P. K.-Y., Khatchadourian, A., McKinney, R. A., and Maysinger, D. (2015). Docosahexaenoic acid (DHA): a modulator of microglia activity and dendritic spine morphology. *J. Neuroinflammation* 12:34. doi: 10.1186/s12974-015-0244-5

Chen, C. T., Green, J. T., Orr, S. K., and Bazinet, R. P. (2008). Regulation of brain polyunsaturated fatty acid uptake and turnover. *Prostaglandins Leukot. Essent. Fatty Acids* 79, 85–91. doi: 10.1016/j.plefa.2008.09.003

Chen, J.-J., Gong, Y.-H., and He, L. (2019). Role of GPR40 in pathogenesis and treatment of Alzheimer's disease and type 2 diabetic dementia. *J. Drug Target.* 27, 347–354. doi: 10.1080/1061186X.2018.1491979

Chen, Q., Qiu, F., Zhou, K., Matlock, H. G., Takahashi, Y., Rajala, R. V. S., et al. (2017). Pathogenic role of microRNA-21 in diabetic retinopathy through downregulation of PPARalpha. *Diabetes* 66, 1671–1682. doi: 10.2337/db16-1246

Cheng, A., Shinoda, Y., Yamamoto, T., Miyachi, H., and Fukunaga, K. (2019). Development of FABP3 ligands that inhibit arachidonic acid-induced alpha-synuclein oligomerization. *Brain Res.* 1707, 190–197. doi: 10.1016/j.brainres.2018.11.036

Cheon, M. S., Kim, S. H., Fountoulakis, M., and Lubec, G. (2003). "Heart type fatty acid binding protein (H-FABP) is decreased in brains of patients with Down syndrome and Alzheimer's disease," in *Advances in Down Syndrome Research. Journal of Neural Transmission Supplement 67*, ed. G. Lubec (Vienna: Springer), 225–234. doi: 10.1007/978-3-7091-6721-2_20

Chistyakov, D. V., Aleshin, S. E., Astakhova, A. A., Sergeeva, M. G., and Reiser, G. (2015). Regulation of peroxisome proliferator-activated receptors (PPAR) α and -γ Of rat brain astrocytes in the course of activation by toll-like receptor agonists. *J. Neurochem.* 134, 113–124. doi: 10.1111/jnc.13101

Chornenkyy, Y., Wang, W.-X., Wei, A., and Nelson, P. T. (2019). Alzheimer's disease and type 2 diabetes mellitus are distinct diseases with potential overlapping metabolic dysfunction upstream of observed cognitive decline. *Brain Pathol.* 29, 3–17. doi: 10.1111/bpa.12655

Civelli, O. (2005). GPCR deorphanizations: the novel, the known and the unexpected transmitters. *Trends Pharmacol. Sci.* 26, 15–19. doi: 10.1016/j.tips.2004.11.005

Colina, C., Puhl, H. L. III, and Ikeda, S. R. (2018). Selective tracking of FFAR3-expressing neurons supports receptor coupling to N-type calcium channels in mouse sympathetic neurons. *Sci. Rep.* 8:17379. doi: 10.1038/s41598-018-35690-z

Combs, C. K., Johnson, D. E., Karlo, J. C., Cannady, S. B., and Landreth, G. E. (2000). Inflammatory mechanisms in Alzheimer's disease: inhibition of beta-amyloid-stimulated proinflammatory responses and neurotoxicity by PPARgamma agonists. *J. Neurosci.* 20, 558–567. doi: 10.1523/JNEUROSCI.20-02-00558.2000

Conklin, S. M., Runyan, C. A., Leonard, S., Reddy, R. D., Muldoon, M. F., and Yao, J. K. (2010). Age-related changes of n-3 and n-6 polyunsaturated fatty acids in the anterior cingulate cortex of individuals with major depressive disorder. *Prostaglandins Leukot. Essent. Fatty Acids* 82, 111–119. doi: 10.1016/j.plefa.2009.12.002

Corona, J. C., and Duchen, M. R. (2015). PPAR c and PGC-1 a as Therapeutic Targets in Parkinson ' s. *Neurochem. Res.* 40, 308–316. doi: 10.1007/s11064-014-1377-0

Corona, J. C., and Duchen, M. R. (2016). PPARgamma as a therapeutic target to rescue mitochondrial function in neurological disease. *Free Radic. Biol. Med.* 100, 153–163. doi: 10.1016/j.freeradbiomed.2016.06.023

Correll, C. C., and McKittrick, B. A. (2014). Biased ligand modulation of seven transmembrane receptors (7TMRs): functional implications for drug discovery. *J. Med. Chem.* 57, 6887–6896. doi: 10.1021/jm401677g

Corton, J. C., Anderson, S. P., and Stauber, A. (2000). Central role of peroxisome proliferator-activated receptors in the actions of peroxisome proliferators. *Annu. Rev. Pharmacol. Toxicol.* 40, 491–518. doi: 10.1146/annurev.pharmtox.40.1.491

Cristiano, L., Bernardo, A., and Cerù, M. P. (2001). Peroxisome proliferator-activated receptors (PPARs) and peroxisomes in rat cortical and cerebellar astrocytes. *J. Neurocytol.* 30, 671–683. doi: 10.1023/A:1016525716209

Cullingford, T. E., Bhakoo, K., Peuchen, S., Dolphin, C. T., Patel, R., and Clark, J. B. (1998). Distribution of mRNAs encoding the peroxisome proliferator-activated receptor alpha, beta, and gamma and the retinoid X receptor α, β, and γ in rat central nervous system. *J. Neurochem.* 70, 1366–1375. doi: 10.1046/j.1471-4159.1998.70041366.x

De Leon, M., Welcher, A. A., Nahin, R. H., Liu, Y., Ruda, M. A., Shooter, E. M., et al. (1996). Fatty acid binding protein is induced in neurons of the dorsal root ganglia after peripheral nerve injury. *J. Neurosci. Res.* 44, 283–292. doi: 10.1002/(sici)1097-4547(19960501)44:3<283::aid-jnr9>3.0.co;2-c

De Nuccio, C., Bernardo, A., Cruciani, C., De Simone, R., Visentin, S., and Minghetti, L. (2015). Peroxisome proliferator activated receptor-gamma agonists protect oligodendrocyte progenitors against tumor necrosis factor-alpha-induced damage: effects on mitochondrial functions and differentiation. *Exp. Neurol.* 271, 506–514. doi: 10.1016/j.expneurol.2015.07.014

De Rosa, A., Pellegatta, S., Rossi, M., Tunici, P., Magnoni, L., Speranza, M. C., et al. (2012). A radial glia gene marker, fatty acid binding protein 7 (FABP7), is involved in proliferation and invasion of glioblastoma cells. *PLoS One* 7:e52113. doi: 10.1371/journal.pone.0052113PONE-D-12-11234

DeArmond, S. J., Deibler, G. E., Bacon, M., Kies, M. W., and Eng, L. F. (1980). A neurochemical and immunocytochemical study of P2 protein in human and bovine nervous systems. *J. Histochem. Cytochem.* 28, 1275–1285. doi: 10.1177/28.12.6785343

Delion, S., Chalon, S., Guilloteau, D., Besnard, J. C., and Durand, G. (1996). alpha-Linolenic acid dietary deficiency alters age-related changes of dopaminergic and serotoninergic neurotransmission in the rat frontal cortex. *J. Neurochem.* 66, 1582–1591. doi: 10.1046/j.1471-4159.1996.66041582.x

Dennis, E. A., and Norris, P. C. (2015). Eicosanoid storm in infection and inflammation. *Nat. Rev. Immunol.* 15, 511–523. doi: 10.1038/nri3859

Dharap, A., Pokrzywa, C., Murali, S., Kaimal, B., and Vemuganti, R. (2015). Mutual induction of transcription factor PPARgamma and microRNAs miR-145 and miR-329. *J. Neurochem.* 135, 139–146. doi: 10.1111/jnc.13220

Di Loreto, S., D'Angelo, B., D'Amico, M. A., Benedetti, E., Cristiano, L., Cinque, B., et al. (2007). PPARbeta agonists trigger neuronal differentiation in the human neuroblastoma cell line SH-SY5Y. *J. Cell. Physiol.* 211, 837–847. doi: 10.1002/jcp.20996

Diaz, C., Angelloz-Nicoud, P., and Pihan, E. (2018). Modeling and Deorphanization of Orphan GPCRs. *Methods Mol. Biol.* 1705, 413–429. doi: 10.1007/978-1-4939-7465-8_21

Dickey, A. S., Pineda, V. V., Tsunemi, T., Liu, P. P., Miranda, H. C., Gilmore-Hall, S. K., et al. (2016). PPAR-delta is repressed in Huntington's disease, is required for normal neuronal function and can be targeted therapeutically. *Nat. Med.* 22, 37–45. doi: 10.1038/nm.4003

Dietschy, J. M., and Turley, S. D. (2001). Cholesterol metabolism in the brain. *Curr. Opin. Lipidol.* 12, 105–112.

Dietschy, J. M., and Turley, S. D. (2004). Thematic review series: brain Lipids. Cholesterol metabolism in the central nervous system during early development and in the mature animal. *J. Lipid Res.* 45, 1375–1397. doi: 10.1194/jlr.R400004-JLR200

Diezko, R., and Suske, G. (2013). Ligand binding reduces SUMOylation of the peroxisome proliferator-activated receptor gamma (PPARgamma) activation function 1 (AF1) domain. *PLoS One* 8:e66947. doi: 10.1371/journal.pone.0066947

Dorsam, R. T., and Gutkind, J. S. (2007). G-protein-coupled receptors and cancer. *Nat. Rev. Cancer* 7, 79–94. doi: 10.1038/nrc2069

Dragano, N. R. V., Solon, C., Ramalho, A. F., de Moura, R. F., Razolli, D. S., Christiansen, E., et al. (2017). Polyunsaturated fatty acid receptors, GPR40 and GPR120, are expressed in the hypothalamus and control energy homeostasis and inflammation. *J. Neuroinflammation* 14:91. doi: 10.1186/s12974-017-0869-7

Dyall, S. C. (2017). Interplay between n-3 and n-6 long-chain polyunsaturated fatty acids and the endocannabinoid system in brain protection and repair. *Lipids* 52, 885–900. doi: 10.1007/s11745-017-4292-8

Dyall, S. C., and Michael-Titus, A. T. (2008). Neurological benefits of omega-3 fatty acids. *Neuromolecular Med.* 10, 219–235. doi: 10.1007/s12017-008-8036-z

Echeverria, F., Ortiz, M., Valenzuela, R., and Videla, L. A. (2016). Long-chain polyunsaturated fatty acids regulation of PPARs, signaling: Relationship to tissue development and aging. *Prostaglandins Leukot. Essent. Fatty Acids* 114, 28–34. doi: 10.1016/j.plefa.2016.10.001

Edmond, J., Higa, T. A., Korsak, R. A., Bergner, E. A., and Lee, W. N. (1998). Fatty acid transport and utilization for the developing brain. *J. Neurochem.* 70, 1227–1234. doi: 10.1046/j.1471-4159.1998.70031227.x

Engelstoft, M. S., Park, W.-M., Sakata, I., Kristensen, L. V., Husted, A. S., Osborne-Lawrence, S., et al. (2013). Seven transmembrane G protein-coupled receptor repertoire of gastric ghrelin cells. *Mol. Metab.* 2, 376–392. doi: 10.1016/j.molmet.2013.08.006

Etschmaier, K., Becker, T., Eichmann, T. O., Schweinzer, C., Scholler, M., Tam-Amersdorfer, C., et al. (2011). Adipose triglyceride lipase affects triacylglycerol metabolism at brain barriers. *J. Neurochem.* 119, 1016–1028. doi: 10.1111/j.1471-4159.2011.07498.x

Falomir-Lockhart, L. J., Franchini, G. R., Guerbi, M. X., Storch, J., and Córsico, B. (2011). Interaction of enterocyte FABPs with phospholipid membranes: clues for specific physiological roles. *Biochim. Biophys. Acta* 1811, 452–459. doi: 10.1016/j.bbalip.2011.04.005

Falomir-Lockhart, L. J., Laborde, L., Kahn, P. C., Storch, J., Córsico, B., Falomir Lockhart, L. J., et al. (2006). Protein-membrane interaction and fatty acid transfer from intestinal fatty acid-binding protein to membranes. Support for a multistep process. *J. Biol. Chem.* 281, 13979–13989. doi: 10.1074/jbc.M511943200

Favrelere, S., Stadelmann-Ingrand, S., Huguet, F., De Javel, D., Piriou, A., Tallineau, C., et al. (2000). Age-related changes in ethanolamine glycerophospholipid fatty acid levels in rat frontal cortex and hippocampus. *Neurobiol. Aging* 21, 653–660. doi: 10.1016/S0197-4580(00)00170-6

Fernandis, A. Z., and Wenk, M. R. (2007). Membrane lipids as signaling molecules. *Curr. Opin. Lipidol.* 18, 121–128. doi: 10.1097/MOL.0b013e328082e4d5

Ferreira, L. S. S., Fernandes, C. S., Vieira, M. N. N., and De Felice, F. G. (2018). Insulin Resistance in Alzheimer's Disease. *Front. Neurosci.* 12:830. doi: 10.3389/fnins.2018.00830

Foti, S. B., Chou, A., Moll, A. D., and Roskams, A. J. (2013). HDAC inhibitors dysregulate neural stem cell activity in the postnatal mouse brain. *Int. J. Dev. Neurosci.* 31, 434–447. doi: 10.1016/j.ijdevneu.2013.03.008

Fredriksson, R., Höglund, P. J., Gloriam, D. E., Lagerström, M. C., and Schiöth, H. B. (2003). Seven evolutionarily conserved human rhodopsin G protein-coupled receptors lacking close relatives. *FEBS Lett.* 554, 381–388. doi: 10.1016/S0014-5793(03)01196-7

Freitas, H. R., Isaac, A. R., Malcher-Lopes, R., Diaz, B. L., Trevenzoli, I. H., and De Melo Reis, R. A. (2017). Polyunsaturated fatty acids and endocannabinoids in health and disease. *Nutr. Neurosci.* 21, 695–714. doi: 10.1080/1028415X.2017.1347373

Fu, Y., Zhen, J., and Lu, Z. (2017). Synergetic neuroprotective effect of docosahexaenoic acid and aspirin in SH-Y5Y by inhibiting miR-21 and activating RXRalpha and PPARalpha. *DNA Cell Biol.* 36, 482–489. doi: 10.1089/dna.2017.3643

Gharami, K., Das, M., and Das, S. (2015). Essential role of docosahexaenoic acid towards development of a smarter brain. *Neurochem. Int.* 89, 51–62. doi: 10.1016/j.neuint.2015.08.014

Glass, C. K., and Saijo, K. (2010). Nuclear receptor transrepression pathways that regulate inflammation in macrophages and T cells. *Nat. Rev. Immunol.* 10, 365–376. doi: 10.1038/nri2748

Glomset, J. A. (2006). Role of docosahexaenoic acid in neuronal plasma membranes. *Sci. STKE* 2006:pe6. doi: 10.1126/stke.3212006pe6

Gray, S. L., Dalla Nora, E., and Vidal-Puig, A. J. (2005). Mouse models of PPAR-gamma deficiency: dissecting PPAR-gamma's role in metabolic homoeostasis. *Biochem. Soc. Trans.* 33, 1053–1058. doi: 10.1042/BST20051053

Greenfield, S., Brostoff, S., Eylar, E. H., and Morell, P. (1973). Protein composition of myelin of the peripheral nervous system. *J. Neurochem.* 20, 1207–1216. doi: 10.1111/j.1471-4159.1973.tb00089.x

Guajardo, M. H., Terrasa, A. M., and Catala, A. (2002). Retinal fatty acid binding protein reduce lipid peroxidation stimulated by long-chain fatty acid hydroperoxides on rod outer segments. *Biochim. Biophys. Acta* 1581, 65–74. doi: 10.1016/S1388-1981(02)00121-X

Gupta, S., Knight, A. G., Gupta, S., Keller, J. N., and Bruce-Keller, A. J. (2012). Saturated long-chain fatty acids activate inflammatory signaling in astrocytes. *J. Neurochem.* 120, 1060–1071. doi: 10.1111/j.1471-4159.2012.07660.x

Hall, M. G., Quignodon, L., and Desvergne, B. (2008). Peroxisome proliferator-activated receptor β/δ in the brain: Facts and hypothesis. *PPAR Res.* 2008:780452. doi: 10.1155/2008/780452

Hanhoff, T., Lücke, C., and Spener, F. (2002). Insights into binding of fatty acids by fatty acid binding proteins. *Mol. Cell. Biochem.* 239, 45–54. doi: 10.1023/A:1020502624234

Hara, T., Kimura, I., Inoue, D., Ichimura, A., and Hirasawa, A. (2013). Free fatty acid receptors and their role in regulation of energy metabolism. *Rev. Physiol. Biochem. Pharmacol.* 164, 77–116. doi: 10.1007/112_2013_13

Heldin, C., Lu, B., Evans, R., and Gutkind, J. S. (2016). Signals and receptors. *Cold Spring Harb. Perspect. Biol.* 8:a005900. doi: 10.1101/cshperspect.a005900

Heneka, M. T., and Landreth, G. E. (2007). PPARs in the brain. *Biochim. Biophys. Acta* 1771, 1031–1045. doi: 10.1016/j.bbalip.2007.04.016

Herr, F. M., Aronson, J., and Storch, J. (1996). Role of portal region lysine residues in electrostatic interactions between heart fatty acid binding protein and phospholipid membranes. *Biochemistry* 35, 1296–1303. doi: 10.1021/bi952204b

Hirasawa, A., Tsumaya, K., Awaji, T., Katsuma, S., Adachi, T., Yamada, M., et al. (2005). Free fatty acids regulate gut incretin glucagon-like peptide-1 secretion through GPR120. *Nat. Med.* 11, 90–94. doi: 10.1038/nm1168

Hirsch, M. M., Deckmann, I., Fontes-Dutra, M., Bauer-Negrini, G., Della-Flora Nunes, G., Nunes, W., et al. (2018). Behavioral alterations in autism model induced by valproic acid and translational analysis of circulating microRNA. *Food Chem. Toxicol.* 115, 336–343. doi: 10.1016/j.fct.2018.02.061

Ho, J. D., Chau, B., Rodgers, L., Lu, F., Wilbur, K. L., Otto, K. A., et al. (2018). Structural basis for GPR40 allosteric agonism and incretin stimulation. *Nat. Commun.* 9:1645. doi: 10.1038/s41467-017-01240-w

Holliday, N. D., Watson, S.-J., and Brown, A. J. H. (2012). Drug discovery opportunities and challenges at g protein coupled receptors for long chain free fatty acids. *Front. Endocrinol.* 2:112. doi: 10.3389/fendo.2011.00112

Hostetler, H. A., McIntosh, A. L., Atshaves, B. P., Storey, S. M., Payne, H. R., Kier, A. B., et al. (2009). L-FABP directly interacts with PPAR alpha in cultured primary hepatocytes. *J. Lipid Res.* 50, 1663–1675. doi: 10.1194/jlr.M900058-JLR200

Hudson, B. D., Shimpukade, B., Milligan, G., and Ulven, T. (2014). The molecular basis of ligand interaction at free fatty acid receptor 4 (FFA4/GPR120). *J. Biol. Chem.* 289, 20345–20358. doi: 10.1074/jbc.M114.561449

Hunsberger, J. G., Fessler, E. B., Chibane, F. L., Leng, Y., Maric, D., Elkahloun, A. G., et al. (2013). Mood stabilizer-regulated miRNAs in neuropsychiatric and neurodegenerative diseases: identifying associations and functions. *Am. J. Transl. Res.* 5, 450–464.

Hussain, G., Schmitt, F., Loeffler, J.-P., and de Aguilar, J.-L. G. (2013). Fatting the brain: a brief of recent research. *Front. Cell. Neurosci.* 7:144. doi: 10.3389/fncel.2013.00144

Im, D.-S. (2004). Discovery of new G protein-coupled receptors for lipid mediators. *J. Lipid Res.* 45, 410–418. doi: 10.1194/jlr.R300006-JLR200

Ingolfsson, H. I., Carpenter, T. S., Bhatia, H., Bremer, P.-T., Marrink, S. J., and Lightstone, F. C. (2017). Computational lipidomics of the neuronal plasma membrane. *Biophys. J.* 113, 2271–2280. doi: 10.1016/j.bpj.2017.10.017

Innes, J. K., and Calder, P. C. (2018). Omega-6 fatty acids and inflammation. *Prostaglandins Leukot. Essent. Fatty Acids* 132, 41–48. doi: 10.1016/j.plefa.2018.03.004

Issemann, I., and Green, S. (1990). Activation of a member of the steroid hormone receptor superfamily by peroxisome proliferators. *Nature* 347, 645–650. doi: 10.1038/347645a0

Itoh, Y., Kawamata, Y., Harada, M., Kobayashi, M., Fujii, R., Fukusumi, S., et al. (2003). Free fatty acids regulate insulin secretion from pancreatic beta cells through GPR40. *Nature* 422, 173–176. doi: 10.1038/nature01478

Jana, M., Mondal, S., Gonzalez, F. J., and Pahan, K. (2012). Gemfibrozil, a lipid-lowering drug, increases myelin genes in human oligodendrocytes via peroxisome proliferator-activated receptor-beta. *J. Biol. Chem.* 287, 34134–34148. doi: 10.1074/jbc.M112.398552

Janesick, A., Wu, S. C., and Blumberg, B. (2015). Retinoic acid signaling and neuronal differentiation. *Cell. Mol. Life Sci.* 72, 1559–1576. doi: 10.1007/s00018-014-1815-9

Johnson, E. J., and Schaefer, E. J. (2006). Potential role of dietary n-3 fatty acids in the prevention of dementia and macular degeneration. *Am. J. Clin. Nutr.* 83, 1494S–1498S. doi: 10.1093/ajcn/83.6.1494S

Kaczocha, M., Rebecchi, M. J., Ralph, B. P., Teng, Y.-H. G., Berger, W. T., Galbavy, W., et al. (2014). Inhibition of fatty acid binding proteins elevates brain anandamide levels and produces analgesia. *PLoS One* 9:e94200. doi: 10.1371/journal.pone.0094200

Kainu, T., Wikstrom, A. C., Gustafsson, J. A., and Pelto-Huikko, M. (1994). Localization of the peroxisome proliferator-activated receptor in the brain. *Neuroreport* 5, 2481–2485.

Kamata, Y., Shiraga, H., Tai, A., Kawamoto, Y., and Gohda, E. (2007). Induction of neurite outgrowth in PC12 cells by the medium-chain fatty acid octanoic acid. *Neuroscience* 146, 1073–1081. doi: 10.1016/j.neuroscience.2007.03.001

Katakura, M., Hashimoto, M., Shahdat, H. M., Gamoh, S., Okui, T., Matsuzaki, K., et al. (2009). Docosahexaenoic acid promotes neuronal differentiation by regulating basic helix-loop-helix transcription factors and cell cycle in neural stem cells. *Neuroscience* 160, 651–660. doi: 10.1016/j.neuroscience.2009.02.057

Kenakin, T., and Christopoulos, A. (2013). Signalling bias in new drug discovery: detection, quantification and therapeutic impact. *Nat. Rev. Drug Discov.* 12, 205–216. doi: 10.1038/nrd3954

Khan, M. Z., Zhuang, X., and He, L. (2016). GPR40 receptor activation leads to CREB phosphorylation and improves cognitive performance in an Alzheimer's disease mouse model. *Neurobiol. Learn. Mem.* 131, 46–55. doi: 10.1016/j.nlm.2016.03.006

Kim, J. Y., Lee, H. J., Lee, S.-J., Jung, Y. H., Yoo, D. Y., Hwang, I. K., et al. (2017). Palmitic acid-BSA enhances amyloid-beta production through GPR40-mediated dual pathways in neuronal cells: Involvement of the Akt/mTOR/HIF-1alpha and Akt/NF-kappaB pathways. *Sci. Rep.* 7:4335. doi: 10.1038/s41598-017-04175-w

Kimura, I., Inoue, D., Maeda, T., Hara, T., Ichimura, A., Miyauchi, S., et al. (2011). Short-chain fatty acids and ketones directly regulate sympathetic nervous system via G protein-coupled receptor 41 (GPR41). *Proc. Natl. Acad. Sci. U.S.A.* 108, 8030–8035. doi: 10.1073/pnas.1016088108

Kitajka, K., Sinclair, A. J., Weisinger, R. S., Weisinger, H. S., Mathai, M., Jayasooriya, A. P., et al. (2004). Effects of dietary omega-3 polyunsaturated fatty acids on brain gene expression. *Proc. Natl. Acad. Sci. U.S.A.* 101, 10931–10936. doi: 10.1073/pnas.0402342101

Kostenis, E. (2004). A glance at G-protein-coupled receptors for lipid mediators: a growing receptor family with remarkably diverse ligands. *Pharmacol. Ther.* 102, 243–257. doi: 10.1016/j.pharmthera.2004.04.005

Kurtz, A., Zimmer, A., Schnutgen, F., Bruning, G., Spener, F., and Muller, T. (1994). The expression pattern of a novel gene encoding brain-fatty acid binding protein correlates with neuronal and glial cell development. *Development* 120, 2637–2649.

Labrousse, V. F., Nadjar, A., Joffre, C., Costes, L., Aubert, A., Gregoire, S., et al. (2012). Short-term long chain omega3 diet protects from neuroinflammatory processes and memory impairment in aged mice. *PLoS One* 7:e36861. doi: 10.1371/journal.pone.0036861

Lafourcade, M., Larrieu, T., Mato, S., Duffaud, A., Sepers, M., Matias, I., et al. (2011). Nutritional omega-3 deficiency abolishes endocannabinoid-mediated neuronal functions. *Nat. Neurosci.* 14, 345–350. doi: 10.1038/nn.2736

Lampen, A., Carlberg, C., and Nau, H. (2001). Peroxisome proliferator-activated receptor delta is a specific sensor for teratogenic valproic acid derivatives. *Eur. J. Pharmacol.* 431, 25–33. doi: 10.1016/s0014-2999(01)01423-6

Landrier, J.-F., Thomas, C., Grober, J., Duez, H., Percevault, F., Souidi, M., et al. (2004). Statin induction of liver fatty acid-binding protein (L-FABP) gene expression is peroxisome proliferator-activated receptor-alpha-dependent. *J. Biol. Chem.* 279, 45512–45518. doi: 10.1074/jbc.M407461200

Laschet, C., Dupuis, N., and Hanson, J. (2018). The G protein-coupled receptors deorphanization landscape. *Biochem. Pharmacol.* 153, 62–74. doi: 10.1016/j.bcp.2018.02.016

Lein, E. S., Hawrylycz, M. J., Ao, N., Ayres, M., Bensinger, A., Bernard, A., et al. (2007). Genome-wide atlas of gene expression in the adult mouse brain. *Nature* 445, 168–176. doi: 10.1038/nature05453

Leong, C., Zhai, D., Kim, B., Yun, S.-W., and Chang, Y.-T. (2013). Neural stem cell isolation from the whole mouse brain using the novel FABP7-binding fluorescent dye, CDr3. *Stem Cell Res.* 11, 1314–1322. doi: 10.1016/j.scr.2013.09.002

Leoni, V., and Caccia, C. (2011). Oxysterols as biomarkers in neurodegenerative diseases. *Chem. Phys. Lipids* 164, 515–524. doi: 10.1016/j.chemphyslip.2011.04.002

Li, Z., Chen, Y., Zhang, Y., Jiang, H., Liu, Y., Chen, Y., et al. (2018a). Structure-based design of free fatty acid receptor 1 agonists bearing non-biphenyl scaffold. *Bioorg. Chem.* 80, 296–302. doi: 10.1016/j.bioorg.2018.06.039

Li, Z., Chen, Y., Zhou, Z., Deng, L., Xu, Y., Hu, L., et al. (2019). Discovery of first-in-class thiazole-based dual FFA1/PPARdelta agonists as potential anti-diabetic agents. *Eur. J. Med. Chem.* 164, 352–365. doi: 10.1016/j.ejmech.2018.12.069

Li, Z., Qiu, Q., Geng, X., Yang, J., Huang, W., and Qian, H. (2016). Free fatty acid receptor agonists for the treatment of type 2 diabetes: drugs in preclinical to phase II clinical development. *Expert Opin. Investig. Drugs* 25, 871–890. doi: 10.1080/13543784.2016.1189530

Li, Z., Xu, X., Hou, J., Wang, S., Jiang, H., and Zhang, L. (2018b). Structure-based optimization of free fatty acid receptor 1 agonists bearing thiazole scaffold. *Bioorg. Chem.* 77, 429–435. doi: 10.1016/j.bioorg.2018.01.039

Li, Z., Zhou, Z., Deng, F., Li, Y., Zhang, D., and Zhang, L. (2018c). Design, synthesis, and biological evaluation of novel pan agonists of FFA1, PPARgamma and PPARdelta. *Eur. J. Med. Chem.* 159, 267–276. doi: 10.1016/j.ejmech.2018.09.071

Liou, H. L., Kahn, P. C., and Storch, J. (2002). Role of the helical domain in fatty acid transfer from adipocyte and heart fatty acid-binding proteins to membranes - Analysis of chimeric proteins. *J. Biol. Chem.* 277, 1806–1815. doi: 10.1074/jbc.M107987200

Liu, R.-Z., Li, X., and Godbout, R. (2008). A novel fatty acid-binding protein (FABP) gene resulting from tandem gene duplication in mammals: transcription in rat retina and testis. *Genomics* 92, 436–445. doi: 10.1016/j.ygeno.2008.08.003

Liu, R. Z., Mita, R., Beaulieu, M., Gao, Z., and Godbout, R. (2010). Fatty acid binding proteins in brain development and disease. *Int. J. Dev. Biol.* 54, 1229–1239. doi: 10.1387/ijdb.092976rl092976rl

Liu, X. S., Chopp, M., Kassis, H., Jia, L. F., Hozeska-Solgot, A., Zhang, R. L., et al. (2012). Valproic acid increases white matter repair and neurogenesis after stroke. *Neuroscience* 220, 313–321. doi: 10.1016/j.neuroscience.2012.06.012

Liu, Y., Longo, L. D., and De Leon, M. (2000). In situ and immunocytochemical localization of E-FABP mRNA and protein during neuronal migration and differentiation in the rat brain. *Brain Res.* 852, 16–27. doi: 10.1016/s0006-8993(99)02158-7

Lu, J., Byrne, N., Wang, J., Bricogne, G., Brown, F. K., Chobanian, H. R., et al. (2017). Structural basis for the cooperative allosteric activation of the free fatty acid receptor GPR40. *Nat. Struct. Mol. Biol.* 24, 570–577. doi: 10.1038/nsmb.3417

Lundell, K., Thulin, P., Hamsten, A., and Ehrenborg, E. (2007). Alternative splicing of human peroxisome proliferator-activated receptor delta (PPAR delta): effects on translation efficiency and trans-activation ability. *BMC Mol. Biol.* 8:70. doi: 10.1186/1471-2199-8-70

Ma, D., Lu, L., Boneva, N. B., Warashina, S., Kaplamadzhiev, D. B., Mori, Y., et al. (2008). Expression of free fatty acid receptor GPR40 in the neurogenic niche of adult monkey hippocampus. *Hippocampus* 18, 326–333. doi: 10.1002/hipo.20393

Ma, D., Tao, B., Warashina, S., Kotani, S., Lu, L., Kaplamadzhiev, D. B., et al. (2007). Expression of free fatty acid receptor GPR40 in the central nervous system of adult monkeys. *Neurosci. Res.* 58, 394–401. doi: 10.1016/j.neures.2007.05.001

Ma, D., Zhang, M., Larsen, C. P., Xu, F., Hua, W., Yamashima, T., et al. (2010). DHA promotes the neuronal differentiation of rat neural stem cells transfected with GPR40 gene. *Brain Res.* 1330, 1–8. doi: 10.1016/j.brainres.2010.03.002

Magnan, C., Levin, B. E., and Luquet, S. (2015). Brain lipid sensing and the neural control of energy balance. *Mol. Cell. Endocrinol.* 418(Pt. 1), 3–8. doi: 10.1016/j.mce.2015.09.019

Mancini, A. D., Bertrand, G., Vivot, K., Carpentier, E., Tremblay, C., Ghislain, J., et al. (2015). beta-Arrestin recruitment and biased agonism at free fatty acid receptor 1. *J. Biol. Chem.* 290, 21131–21140. doi: 10.1074/jbc.M115.644450

Mangelsdorf, D. J., Thummel, C., Beato, M., Herrlich, P., Schutz, G., Umesono, K., et al. (1995). The nuclear receptor superfamily: the second decade. *Cell* 83, 835–839. doi: 10.1016/0092-8674(95)90199-X

Martin, G. G., McIntosh, A. L., Huang, H., Gupta, S., Atshaves, B. P., Landrock, K. K., et al. (2013). The human liver fatty acid binding protein T94A variant alters the structure, stability, and interaction with fibrates. *Biochemistry* 52, 9347–9357. doi: 10.1021/bi401014k

McNamara, R. K., and Carlson, S. E. (2006). Role of omega-3 fatty acids in brain development and function: potential implications for the pathogenesis and prevention of psychopathology. *Prostaglandins Leukot. Essent. Fatty Acids* 75, 329–349. doi: 10.1016/j.plefa.2006.07.010

Miglio, G., Rattazzi, L., Rosa, A. C., and Fantozzi, R. (2009). PPARgamma stimulation promotes neurite outgrowth in SH-SY5Y human neuroblastoma cells. *Neurosci. Lett.* 454, 134–138. doi: 10.1016/j.neulet.2009.03.014

Mobraten, K., Haug, T. M., Kleiveland, C. R., and Lea, T. (2013). Omega-3 and omega-6 PUFAs induce the same GPR120-mediated signalling events, but with different kinetics and intensity in Caco-2 cells. *Lipids Health Dis.* 12:101. doi: 10.1186/1476-511X-12-101

Moreno, S., Farioli-vecchioli, S., and Cerù, M. P. (2004). Immunolocalization of peroxisome proliferator-activated receptors and retinoid X receptors in the adult rat CNS. *Neuroscience* 123, 131–145. doi: 10.1016/j.neuroscience.2003.08.064

Motley, W. W., Palaima, P., Yum, S. W., Gonzalez, M. A., Tao, F., Wanschitz, J. V., et al. (2016). De novo PMP2 mutations in families with type 1 Charcot-Marie-Tooth disease. *Brain* 139, 1649–1656. doi: 10.1093/brain/aww055

Mounsey, R. B., Martin, H. L., Nelson, M. C., Evans, R. M., and Teismann, P. (2015). The effect of neuronal conditional knock-out of peroxisome proliferator-activated receptors in the MPTP mouse model of Parkinson's disease. *Neuroscience* 300, 576–584. doi: 10.1016/j.neuroscience.2015.05.048

Muller, M. M., Lehmann, R., Klassert, T. E., Reifenstein, S., Conrad, T., Moore, C., et al. (2017). Global analysis of glycoproteins identifies markers of endotoxin tolerant monocytes and GPR84 as a modulator of TNFalpha expression. *Sci. Rep.* 7:838. doi: 10.1038/s41598-017-00828-y

Murillo-Rodriguez, E. (2017). The role of nuclear receptor pparalpha in the sleep-wake cycle modulation. A tentative approach for treatment of sleep disorders. *Curr. Drug Deliv.* 14, 473–482. doi: 10.2174/1567201814666161109123803

Murphy, E. J., Owada, Y., Kitanaka, N., Kondo, H., and Glatz, J. F. C. (2005). Brain arachidonic acid incorporation is decreased in heart fatty acid binding protein gene-ablated mice. *Biochemistry* 44, 6350–6360. doi: 10.1021/bi047292r

Nakamoto, K., Nishinaka, T., Matsumoto, K., Kasuya, F., Mankura, M., Koyama, Y., et al. (2012). Involvement of the long-chain fatty acid receptor GPR40 as a novel pain regulatory system. *Brain Res.* 1432, 74–83. doi: 10.1016/j.brainres. 2011.11.012

Niculescu, M. D., Lupu, D. S., and Craciunescu, C. N. (2011). Maternal alpha-linolenic acid availability during gestation and lactation alters the postnatal hippocampal development in the mouse offspring. *Int. J. Dev. Neurosci.* 29, 795–802. doi: 10.1016/j.ijdevneu.2011.09.006

Nikaido, Y., Koyama, Y., Yoshikawa, Y., Furuya, T., and Takeda, S. (2015). Mutation analysis and molecular modeling for the investigation of ligand-binding modes of GPR84. *J. Biochem.* 157, 311–320. doi: 10.1093/jb/mvu075

Nohr, M. K., Pedersen, M. H., Gille, A., Egerod, K. L., Engelstoft, M. S., Husted, A. S., et al. (2013). GPR41/FFAR3 and GPR43/FFAR2 as cosensors for short-chain fatty acids in enteroendocrine cells vs FFAR3 in enteric neurons and FFAR2 in enteric leukocytes. *Endocrinology* 154, 3552–3564. doi: 10.1210/en. 2013-1142

Noy, N. (2016). Non-classical transcriptional activity of retinoic acid. *Subcell. Biochem.* 81, 179–199. doi: 10.1007/978-94-024-0945-1_7

Offermanns, S. (2013). Free fatty acid (FFA) and hydroxy carboxylic acid (HCA) receptors. *Annu. Rev. Pharmacol. Toxicol.* 54, 407–434. doi: 10.1146/annurev-pharmtox-011613-135945

Oikawa, H., and Sng, J. C. G. (2016). Valproic acid as a microRNA modulator to promote neurite outgrowth. *Neural Regen. Res.* 11, 1564–1565. doi: 10.4103/1673-5374.193227

Orr, S. K., Trepanier, M. O., and Bazinet, R. P. (2013). n-3 Polyunsaturated fatty acids in animal models with neuroinflammation. *Prostaglandins Leukot. Essent. Fatty Acids* 88, 97–103. doi: 10.1016/j.plefa.2012.05.008

Orth, M., and Bellosta, S. (2012). Cholesterol: its regulation and role in central nervous system disorders. *Cholesterol* 2012:292598. doi: 10.1155/2012/292598

Ory, J., Kane, C. D., Simpson, M. A., Banaszak, L. J., and Bernlohr, D. A. (1997). Biochemical and crystallographic analyses of a portal mutant of the adipocyte lipid-binding protein. *J. Biol. Chem.* 272, 9793–9801. doi: 10.1074/jbc.272.15. 9793

O'Sullivan, S. E. (2007). Cannabinoids go nuclear: evidence for activation of peroxisome proliferator-activated receptors. *Br. J. Pharmacol.* 152, 576–582. doi: 10.1038/sj.bjp.0707423

Owada, Y. (2008). Fatty acid binding protein: localization and functional significance in the brain. *Tohoku J. Exp. Med.* 214, 213–220. doi: 10.1620/tjem. 214.213

Owada, Y., Yoshimoto, T., and Kondo, H. (1996). Spatio-temporally differential expression of genes for three members of fatty acid binding proteins in developing and mature rat brains. *J. Chem. Neuroanat.* 12, 113–122. doi: 10.1016/s0891-0618(96)00192-5

Pelsers, M. M., Hanhoff, T., Van Der Voort, D., Arts, B., Peters, M., Ponds, R., et al. (2004). Brain- and heart-type fatty acid-binding proteins in the brain: Tissue distribution and clinical utility. *Clin. Chem.* 50, 1568–1575. doi: 10.1373/clinchem.2003.030361

Pelsers, M. M., Hermens, W. T., and Glatz, J. F. C. (2005). Fatty acid-binding proteins as plasma markers of tissue injury. *Clin. Chim. Acta* 352, 15–35. doi: 10.1016/j.cccn.2004.09.001

Pepino, M. Y., Kuda, O., Samovski, D., and Abumrad, N. A. (2014). Structure-function of CD36 and importance of fatty acid signal transduction in fat metabolism. *Annu. Rev. Nutr.* 34, 281–303. doi: 10.1146/annurev-nutr-071812-161220

Peters, B. D., Duran, M., Vlieger, E. J., Majoie, C. B., den Heeten, G. J., Linszen, D. H., et al. (2009). Polyunsaturated fatty acids and brain white matter anisotropy in recent-onset schizophrenia: a preliminary study. *Prostaglandins Leukot. Essent. Fatty Acids* 81, 61–63. doi: 10.1016/j.plefa.2009.04.007

Prolla, T. A., and Mattson, M. P. (2001). Molecular mechanisms of brain aging and neurodegenerative disorders: lessons from dietary restriction. *Trends Neurosci.* 24, S21–S31. doi: 10.1016/S0166-2236(01)00 005-4

Punetha, J., Mackay-Loder, L., Harel, T., Coban-Akdemir, Z., Jhangiani, S. N., Gibbs, R. A., et al. (2018). Identification of a pathogenic PMP2 variant in a multi-generational family with CMT type 1: clinical gene panels versus genome-wide approaches to molecular diagnosis. *Mol. Genet. Metab.* 125, 302–304. doi: 10.1016/j.ymgme.2018.08.005

Rademacher, M., Zimmerman, A. W., Ruterjans, H., Veerkamp, J. H., and Lucke, C. (2002). Solution structure of fatty acid-binding protein from human brain. *Mol. Cell. Biochem.* 239, 61–68. doi: 10.1023/A:1020566909213

Rautureau, Y., Paradis, P., and Schiffrin, E. L. (2017). Generation of a mouse model with smooth muscle cell specific loss of the expression of PPARgamma. *Methods Mol. Biol.* 1527, 381–407. doi: 10.1007/978-1-4939-6625-7_30

Reddy, D. S. (2010). Neurosteroids: endogenous role in the human brain and therapeutic potentials. *Prog. Brain Res.* 186, 113–137. doi: 10.1016/B978-0-444-53630-3.00008-7

Reese, A. J., and Banaszak, L. J. (2004). Specificity determinants for lipids bound to beta-barrel proteins. *J. Lipid Res.* 45, 232–243. doi: 10.1194/jlr.M300113-JLR200

Richieri, G. V., Ogata, R. T., Zimmerman, A. W., Veerkamp, J. H., and Kleinfeld, A. M. (2000). Fatty acid binding proteins from different tissues show distinct patterns of fatty acid interactions. *Biochemistry* 39, 7197–7204. doi: 10.1021/bi000314z

Ricote, M., and Glass, C. K. (2007). PPARs and molecular mechanisms of transrepression. *Biochim. Biophys. Acta* 1771, 926–935. doi: 10.1016/j.bbalip. 2007.02.013

Rivera, P., Arrabal, S., Vargas, A., Blanco, E., Serrano, A., Pavon, F. J., et al. (2014). Localization of peroxisome proliferator-activated receptor alpha (PPARα) and N-acyl phosphatidylethanolamine phospholipase D (NAPE-PLD) in cells expressing the Ca^{2+}-binding proteins calbindin, calretinin, and parvalbumin in the adult rat hippocampus. *Front. Neuroanat.* 8:12. doi: 10.3389/fnana.2014. 00012

Rocha, D. M., Caldas, A. P., Oliveira, L. L., Bressan, J., and Hermsdorff, H. H. (2016). Saturated fatty acids trigger TLR4-mediated inflammatory response. *Atherosclerosis* 244, 211–215. doi: 10.1016/j.atherosclerosis.2015.11.015

Rohwedder, A., Zhang, Q., Rudge, S. A., and Wakelam, M. J. O. (2014). Lipid droplet formation in response to oleic acid in Huh-7 cells is mediated by the fatty acid receptor FFAR4. *J. Cell Sci.* 127, 3104–3115. doi: 10.1242/jcs.145854

Rombaldi Bernardi, J., de Souza Escobar, R., Ferreira, C. F., and Pelufo Silveira, P. (2012). Fetal and neonatal levels of omega-3: effects on neurodevelopment, nutrition, and growth. *ScientificWorldJournal* 2012:202473. doi: 10.1100/2012/202473

Roth, A. D., Leisewitz, A. V., Jung, J. E., Cassina, P., Barbeito, L., Inestrosa, N. C., et al. (2003). PPAR γ activators induce growth arrest and process extension in B12 oligodendrocyte-like cells and terminal differentiation of cultured oligodendrocytes. *J. Neurosci. Res.* 72, 425–435. doi: 10.1002/jnr.10596

Roy, A., and Pahan, K. (2015). PPARalpha signaling in the hippocampus: crosstalk between fat and memory. *J. Neuroimmune Pharmacol.* 10, 30–34. doi: 10.1007/s11481-014-9582-9

Sacchettini, J. C., Meininger, T. A., Lowe, J. B., Gordon, J. I., and Banaszak, L. J. (1987). Crystallization of rat intestinal fatty-acid binding protein - preliminary-x-ray data obtained from protein expressed in *Escherichia*-coli. *J. Biol. Chem.* 262, 5428–5430.

Saino-Saito, S., Nourani, R. M., Iwasa, H., Kondo, H., and Owada, Y. (2009). Discrete localization of various fatty-acid-binding proteins in various cell populations of mouse retina. *Cell Tissue Res.* 338, 191–201. doi: 10.1007/s00441-009-0862-2

Saino-Saito, S., Suzuki, R., Tokuda, N., Abe, H., Kondo, H., and Owada, Y. (2010). Localization of fatty acid binding proteins (FABPs) in the cochlea of mice. *Ann. Anat.* 192, 210–214. doi: 10.1016/j.aanat.2010.06.007

Samuel, B. S., Shaito, A., Motoike, T., Rey, F. E., Backhed, F., Manchester, J. K., et al. (2008). Effects of the gut microbiota on host adiposity are modulated by the short-chain fatty-acid binding G protein-coupled receptor, Gpr41. *Proc. Natl. Acad. Sci. U.S.A.* 105, 16767–16772. doi: 10.1073/pnas.0808567105

Sanchez-Font, M. F., Bosch-Comas, A., Gonzalez-Duarte, R., and Marfany, G. (2003). Overexpression of FABP7 in Down syndrome fetal brains is associated with PKNOX1 gene-dosage imbalance. *Nucleic Acids Res.* 31, 2769–2777. doi: 10.1093/nar/gkg396

Sanchez-Reyes, O. B., Romero-Avila, M. T., Castillo-Badillo, J. A., Takei, Y., Hirasawa, A., Tsujimoto, G., et al. (2014). Free fatty acids and protein kinase C activation induce GPR120 (free fatty acid receptor 4) phosphorylation. *Eur. J. Pharmacol.* 723, 368–374. doi: 10.1016/j.ejphar.2013.11.003

Santos, M. J., Quintanilla, R. A., Toro, A., Grandy, R., Dinamarca, M. C., Godoy, J. A., et al. (2005). Peroxisomal proliferation protects from beta-amyloid neurodegeneration. *J. Biol. Chem.* 280, 41057–41068. doi: 10.1074/jbc.M505160200

Sarruf, D. A., Yu, F., Nguyen, H. T., Williams, D. L., Printz, R. L., Niswender, K. D., et al. (2009). Expression of peroxisome proliferator-activated receptor-γ in key neuronal subsets regulating glucose metabolism and energy homeostasis. *Endocrinology* 150, 707–712. doi: 10.1210/en.2008-0899

Sasselli, V., Pachnis, V., and Burns, A. J. (2012). The enteric nervous system. *Dev. Biol.* 366, 64–73. doi: 10.1016/j.ydbio.2012.01.012

Sastre, M., Klockgether, T., and Heneka, M. T. (2006). Contribution of inflammatory processes to Alzheimer's disease: molecular mechanisms. *Int. J. Dev. Neurosci.* 24, 167–176. doi: 10.1016/j.ijdevneu.2005.11.014

Sawzdargo, M., George, S. R., Nguyen, T., Xu, S., Kolakowski, L. F., and O'dowd, B. F. (1997). A cluster of four novel human g protein-coupled receptor genes occurring in close proximity to CD22 gene on chromosome 19q13.1. *Biochem. Biophys. Res. Commun.* 239, 543–547. doi: 10.1006/bbrc.1997.7513

Scandroglio, F., Venkata, J. K., Loberto, N., Prioni, S., Schuchman, E. H., Chigorno, V., et al. (2008). Lipid content of brain, brain membrane lipid domains, and neurons from acid sphingomyelinase deficient mice. *J. Neurochem.* 107, 329–338. doi: 10.1111/j.1471-4159.2008.05591.x

Schug, T. T., Berry, D. C., Shaw, N. S., Travis, S. N., and Noy, N. (2007). Opposing effects of retinoic acid on cell growth result from alternate activation of two different nuclear receptors. *Cell* 129, 723–733. doi: 10.1016/j.cell.2007.02.050

Schug, T. T., Berry, D. C., Toshkov, I. A., Cheng, L., Nikitin, A. Y., and Noy, N. (2008). Overcoming retinoic acid-resistance of mammary carcinomas by diverting retinoic acid from PPARbeta/delta to RAR. *Proc. Natl. Acad. Sci. U.S.A.* 105, 7546–7551. doi: 10.1073/pnas.0709981105

Senga, S., Kawaguchi, K., Kobayashi, N., Ando, A., and Fujii, H. (2018). A novel fatty acid-binding protein 5-estrogen-related receptor alpha signaling pathway promotes cell growth and energy metabolism in prostate cancer cells. *Oncotarget* 9, 31753–31770. doi: 10.18632/oncotarget.25878

Serhan, C. N. (2014). Pro-resolving lipid mediators are leads for resolution physiology. *Nature* 510, 92–101. doi: 10.1038/nature13479

Shang, J., Brust, R., Mosure, S. A., Bass, J., Munoz-Tello, P., Lin, H., et al. (2018). Cooperative cobinding of synthetic and natural ligands to the nuclear receptor PPARgamma. *eLife* 7:e43320. doi: 10.7554/eLife.43320

Shao, D., Rangwala, S. M., Bailey, S. T., Krakow, S. L., Reginato, M. J., and Lazar, M. A. (1998). Interdomain communication regulating ligand binding by PPAR-gamma. *Nature* 396, 377–380. doi: 10.1038/24634

Shioda, N., Yabuki, Y., Kobayashi, Y., Onozato, M., Owada, Y., and Fukunaga, K. (2014). FABP3 protein promotes alpha-synuclein oligomerization associated with 1-methyl-1,2,3,6-tetrahydropiridine-induced neurotoxicity. *J. Biol. Chem.* 289, 18957–18965. doi: 10.1074/jbc.M113.527341

Shioda, N., Yamamoto, Y., Watanabe, M., Binas, B., Owada, Y., and Fukunaga, K. (2010). Heart-type fatty acid binding protein regulates dopamine D2 receptor function in mouse brain. *J. Neurosci.* 30, 3146–3155. doi: 10.1523/JNEUROSCI.4140-09.2010

Smathers, R. L., and Petersen, D. R. (2011). The human fatty acid-binding protein family: evolutionary divergences and functions. *Hum. Genomics* 5, 170–191.

Smith, A. J., Sanders, M. A., Juhlmann, B. E., Hertzel, A. V., and Bernlohr, D. A. (2008). Mapping of the hormone-sensitive lipase binding site on the adipocyte fatty acid-binding protein (AFABP). Identification of the charge quartet on the AFABP/aP2 helix-turn-helix domain. *J. Biol. Chem.* 283, 33536–33543. doi: 10.1074/jbc.M806732200

Sona, C., Kumar, A., Dogra, S., Kumar, B. A., Umrao, D., and Yadav, P. N. (2018). Docosahexaenoic acid modulates brain-derived neurotrophic factor via GPR40 in the brain and alleviates diabesity-associated learning and memory deficits in mice. *Neurobiol. Dis.* 118, 94–107. doi: 10.1016/j.nbd.2018.07.002

Song, T., Yang, Y., Zhou, Y., Wei, H., and Peng, J. (2017). GPR120: a critical role in adipogenesis, inflammation, and energy metabolism in adipose tissue. *Cell. Mol. Life Sci.* 74, 2723–2733. doi: 10.1007/s00018-017-2492-2

Srivastava, A., Yano, J., Hirozane, Y., Kefala, G., Gruswitz, F., Snell, G., et al. (2014). High-resolution structure of the human GPR40 receptor bound to allosteric agonist TAK-875. *Nature* 513, 124–127. doi: 10.1038/nature13494

Stoddart, L. A., Smith, N. J., Jenkins, L., Brown, A. J., and Milligan, G. (2008). Conserved polar residues in transmembrane domains V, VI, and VII of free fatty acid receptor 2 and free fatty acid receptor 3 are required for the binding and function of short chain fatty acids. *J. Biol. Chem.* 283, 32913–32924. doi: 10.1074/jbc.M805601200

Storch, J., and Corsico, B. (2008). The emerging functions and mechanisms of mammalian fatty acid-binding proteins. *Annu. Rev. Nutr.* 28, 73–95. doi: 10.1146/annurev.nutr.27.061406.093710

Storch, J., and Thumser, A. E. (2010). Tissue-specific functions in the fatty acid-binding protein family. *J. Biol. Chem.* 285, 32679–32683. doi: 10.1074/jbc.R110.135210

Storch, J., and Thumser, A. E. A. (2000). The fatty acid transport function of fatty acid-binding proteins. *Biochim. Biophys. Acta* 1486, 28–44. doi: 10.1016/S1388-1981(00)00046-9

Storch, J., Veerkamp, J. H., and Hsu, K. T. (2002). Similar mechanisms of fatty acid transfer from human anal rodent fatty acid-binding proteins to membranes: liver, intestine, heart muscle, and adipose tissue FABPs. *Mol. Cell. Biochem.* 239, 25–33. doi: 10.1023/A:1020546321508

Sum, C. S., Tikhonova, I. G., Neumann, S., Engel, S., Raaka, B. M., Costanzi, S., et al. (2007). Identification of residues important for agonist recognition and activation in GPR40. *J. Biol. Chem.* 282, 29248–29255. doi: 10.1074/jbc.M705077200

Sunshine, H., and Iruela-Arispe, M. L. (2017). Membrane lipids and cell signaling. *Curr. Opin. Lipidol.* 28, 408–413. doi: 10.1097/MOL.0000000000000443

Suzuki, M., Takaishi, S., Nagasaki, M., Onozawa, Y., Iino, I., Maeda, H., et al. (2013). Medium-chain fatty acid-sensing receptor, GPR84, is a proinflammatory receptor. *J. Biol. Chem.* 288, 10684–10691. doi: 10.1074/jbc.M112.420042

Taha, A. Y., Filo, E., Ma, D. W. L., and McIntyre Burnham, W. (2009). Dose-dependent anticonvulsant effects of linoleic and alpha-linolenic polyunsaturated fatty acids on pentylenetetrazol induced seizures in rats. *Epilepsia* 50, 72–82. doi: 10.1111/j.1528-1167.2008.01731.x

The GTEx Consortium (2013). The genotype-tissue expression (GTEx) project. *Nat. Genet.* 45, 580–585. doi: 10.1038/ng.2653

Thompson, J., Reese-Wagoner, A., and Banaszak, L. (1999). Liver fatty acid binding protein: species variation and the accommodation of different ligands. *Biochim. Biophys. Acta* 1441, 117–130. doi: 10.1016/S1388-1981(99)00146-8

Tikhonova, I. G., Sum, C. S., Neumann, S., Thomas, C. J., Raaka, B. M., Costanzi, S., et al. (2007). Bidirectional, iterative approach to the structural delineation of the functional "chemoprint" in GPR40 for agonist recognition. *J. Med. Chem.* 50, 2981–2989. doi: 10.1021/jm0614782

Tzeng, J., Byun, J., Park, J. Y., Yamamoto, T., Schesing, K., Tian, B., et al. (2015). An Ideal PPAR response element bound to and activated by PPARalpha. *PLoS One* 10:e0134996. doi: 10.1371/journal.pone.0134996

Uauy, R., and Dangour, A. D. (2006). Nutrition in brain development and aging: role of essential fatty acids. *Nutr. Rev.* 64, S24–S33. doi: 10.1111/j.1753-4887.2006.tb00242.x

Uhlen, M., Fagerberg, L., Hallstrom, B. M., Lindskog, C., Oksvold, P., Mardinoglu, A., et al. (2015). Proteomics. Tissue-based map of the human proteome. *Science* 347:1260419. doi: 10.1126/science.1260419

Ulven, T. (2012). Short-chain free fatty acid receptors FFA2/GPR43 and FFA3/GPR41 as new potential therapeutic targets. *Front. Endocrinol.* 3:111. doi: 10.3389/fendo.2012.00111

van Gelder, B. M., Tijhuis, M., Kalmijn, S., and Kromhout, D. (2007). Fish consumption, n-3 fatty acids, and subsequent 5-y cognitive decline in elderly men: the Zutphen Elderly Study. *Am. J. Clin. Nutr.* 85, 1142–1147. doi: 10.1093/ajcn/85.4.1142

Vance, J. E. (2012). Dysregulation of cholesterol balance in the brain: contribution to neurodegenerative diseases. *Dis. Model. Mech.* 5, 746–755. doi: 10.1242/dmm.010124

Veerkamp, J. H., and Zimmerman, A. W. (2001). Fatty acid-binding proteins of nervous tissue. *J. Mol. Neurosci.* 16, 133–137.

Villapol, S. (2018). Roles of peroxisome proliferator-activated receptor gamma on brain and peripheral inflammation. *Cell. Mol. Neurobiol.* 38, 121–132. doi: 10.1007/s10571-017-0554-5

Villegas-Comonfort, S., Takei, Y., Tsujimoto, G., Hirasawa, A., and García-Sáinz, J. A. (2017). Effects of arachidonic acid on FFA4 receptor: signaling, phosphorylation and internalization. *Prostaglandins Leukot. Essent. Fat. Acids* 117, 1–10. doi: 10.1016/j.plefa.2017.01.013

von Bernhardi, R., Eugenin-von Bernhardi, J., Flores, B., and Eugenin Leon, J. (2016). Glial cells and integrity of the nervous system. *Adv. Exp. Med. Biol.* 949, 1–24. doi: 10.1007/978-3-319-40764-7_1

Walder, B., Robin, X., Rebetez, M. M. L., Copin, J.-C., Gasche, Y., Sanchez, J.-C., et al. (2013). The prognostic significance of the serum biomarker heart-fatty acidic binding protein in comparison with s100b in severe traumatic brain injury. *J. Neurotrauma* 30, 1631–1637. doi: 10.1089/neu.2012.2791

Wang, F., Mullican, S. E., DiSpirito, J. R., Peed, L. C., and Lazar, M. A. (2013). Lipoatrophy and severe metabolic disturbance in mice with fat-specific deletion of PPARgamma. *Proc. Natl. Acad. Sci. U.S.A.* 110, 18656–18661. doi: 10.1073/pnas.1314863110

Wang, J., Wu, X., Simonavicius, N., Tian, H., and Ling, L. (2006). Medium-chain fatty acids as ligands for orphan G protein-coupled receptor GPR84. *J. Biol. Chem.* 281, 34457–34464. doi: 10.1074/jbc.M608019200

Wang, X., and Chan, C. B. (2015). n-3 polyunsaturated fatty acids and insulin secretion. *J. Endocrinol.* 224, R97–R106. doi: 10.1530/JOE-14-0581

Wang, Y.-T., Liu, C.-H., and Zhu, H.-L. (2016). Fatty acid binding protein (FABP) inhibitors: a patent review (2012-2015). *Expert Opin. Ther. Pat.* 26, 767–776. doi: 10.1080/13543776.2016.1182500

Warden, A., Truitt, J., Merriman, M., Ponomareva, O., Jameson, K., Ferguson, L. B., et al. (2016). Localization of PPAR isotypes in the adult mouse and human brain. *Sci. Rep.* 6:27618. doi: 10.1038/srep27618

Watanabe, A., Toyota, T., Owada, Y., Hayashi, T., Iwayama, Y., Matsumata, M., et al. (2007). Fabp7 maps to a quantitative trait locus for a schizophrenia endophenotype. *PLoS Biol.* 5:e297. doi: 10.1371/journal.pbio.0050297

Watson, S.-J., Brown, A. J. H., and Holliday, N. D. (2012). Differential signaling by splice variants of the human free fatty acid receptor GPR120. *Mol. Pharmacol.* 81, 631–642. doi: 10.1124/mol.111.077388

Wei, L., Tokizane, K., Konishi, H., Yu, H.-R., and Kiyama, H. (2017). Agonists for G-protein-coupled receptor 84 (GPR84) alter cellular morphology and motility but do not induce pro-inflammatory responses in microglia. *J. Neuroinflammation* 14:198. doi: 10.1186/s12974-017-0970-y

Whalen, E. J., Rajagopal, S., and Lefkowitz, R. J. (2011). Therapeutic potential of beta-arrestin- and G protein-biased agonists. *Trends Mol. Med.* 17, 126–139. doi: 10.1016/j.molmed.2010.11.004

Wittenberger, T., Schaller, H. C., and Hellebrand, S. (2001). An expressed sequence tag (EST) data mining strategy succeeding in the discovery of new G-protein coupled receptors. *J. Mol. Biol.* 307, 799–813. doi: 10.1006/jmbi.2001.4520

Wnuk, A., and Kajta, M. (2017). Steroid and xenobiotic receptor signalling in apoptosis and autophagy of the nervous system. *Int. J. Mol. Sci.* 18:E2394. doi: 10.3390/ijms18112394

Wolfrum, C. (2007). Cytoplasmic fatty acid binding protein sensing fatty acids for peroxisome proliferator activated receptor activation. *Cell. Mol. Life Sci.* 64, 2465–2476. doi: 10.1007/s00018-007-7279-4

Wolfrum, C., Borrmann, C. M., Borchers, T., and Spener, F. (2001). Fatty acids and hypolipidemic drugs regulate peroxisome proliferator-activated receptors alpha - and gamma-mediated gene expression via liver fatty acid binding protein: a signaling path to the nucleus. *Proc. Natl. Acad. Sci. U.S.A.* 98, 2323–2328. doi: 10.1073/pnas.051619898

Won, Y.-J., Lu, V. B., Puhl, H. L. III, and Ikeda, S. R. (2013). beta-Hydroxybutyrate modulates N-type calcium channels in rat sympathetic neurons by acting as an agonist for the G-protein-coupled receptor FFA3. *J. Neurosci.* 33, 19314–19325. doi: 10.1523/JNEUROSCI.3102-13.2013

Woods, J. W., Tanen, M., Figueroa, D. J., Biswas, C., Zycband, E., Moller, D. E., et al. (2003). Localization of PPARδ in murine central nervous system: expression in oligodendrocytes and neurons. *Brain Res.* 975, 10–21. doi: 10.1016/S0006-8993(03)02515-0

Wunderlich, M. T., Hanhoff, T., Goertler, M., Spener, F., Glatz, J. F. C., Wallesch, C. W., et al. (2005). Release of brain-type and heart-type fatty acid-binding proteins in serum after acute ischaemic stroke. *J. Neurol.* 252, 718–724. doi: 10.1007/s00415-005-0725-z

Xing, G., Zhang, L., Zhang, L., Heynen, T., Yoshikawa, T., Smith, M., et al. (1995). Rat PPARgama contains A CGG triplet repeat and is prminently expressed in the thalamic nuclei. *Biochem. Biophys. Res. Commun.* 217, 1015–1025. doi: 10.1006/bbrc.1995.2871

Xu, L. Z., Sanchez, R., Sali, A., and Heintz, N. (1996). Ligand specificity of brain lipid-binding protein. *J. Biol. Chem.* 271, 24711–24719. doi: 10.1074/jbc.271.40.24711

Xu, Z. H., Buelt, M. K., Banaszak, L. J., and Bernlohr, D. A. (1991). Expression, purification, and crystallization of the adipocyte lipid-binding protein. *J. Biol. Chem.* 266, 14367–14370.

Yakunin, E., Loeb, V., Kisos, H., Biala, Y., Yehuda, S., Yaari, Y., et al. (2012). Alpha-synuclein neuropathology is controlled by nuclear hormone receptors and enhanced by docosahexaenoic acid in a mouse model for Parkinson's disease. *Brain Pathol.* 22, 280–294. doi: 10.1111/j.1750-3639.2011.00530.x

Yamashima, T. (2008). A putative link of PUFA, GPR40 and adult-born hippocampal neurons for memory. *Prog. Neurobiol.* 84, 105–115. doi: 10.1016/j.pneurobio.2007.11.002

Yamashima, T. (2012). PUFA-GPR40-CREB signaling hypothesis for the adult primate neurogenesis. *Prog. Lipid Res.* 51, 221–231. doi: 10.1016/j.plipres.2012.02.001

Yan, S., Elmes, M. W., Tong, S., Hu, K., Awwa, M., Teng, G. Y. H., et al. (2018). SAR studies on truxillic acid mono esters as a new class of antinociceptive agents targeting fatty acid binding proteins. *Eur. J. Med. Chem.* 154, 233–252. doi: 10.1016/j.ejmech.2018.04.050

Yang, Y., Tian, X., Xu, D., Zheng, F., Lu, X., Zhang, Y., et al. (2018). GPR40 modulates epileptic seizure and NMDA receptor function. *Sci. Adv.* 4:eaau2357. doi: 10.1126/sciadv.aau2357

Yoshimura, M., Miyata, A., Arita, K., Kurihara, T., Shioda, S., Oyoshi, T., et al. (2015). Attenuation of inflammatory and neuropathic pain behaviors in mice through activation of free fatty acid receptor GPR40. *Mol. Pain* 11:6. doi: 10.1186/s12990-015-0003-8

Yu, S., Levi, L., Siegel, R., and Noy, N. (2012). Retinoic acid induces neurogenesis by activating both retinoic acid receptors (RARs) and peroxisome proliferator-activated receptor beta/delta (PPARbeta/delta). *J. Biol. Chem.* 287, 42195–42205. doi: 10.1074/jbc.M112.410381

Yu, Y., Zhu, M., Zhao, Y., Xu, M., and Qiu, M. (2018). Overexpression of TUSC7 inhibits the inflammation caused by microglia activation via regulating miR-449a/PPAR-gamma. *Biochem. Biophys. Res. Commun.* 503, 1020–1026. doi: 10.1016/j.bbrc.2018.06.111

Yun, S. W., Leong, C., Zhai, D., Tan, Y. L., Lim, L., Bi, X., et al. (2012). Neural stem cell specific fluorescent chemical probe binding to FABP7. *Proc. Natl. Acad. Sci. U.S.A.* 109, 10214–10217. doi: 10.1073/pnas.12008171091200817109

Zamarbide, M., Etayo-Labiano, I., Ricobaraza, A., Martinez-Pinilla, E., Aymerich, M. S., Lanciego, J. L., et al. (2014). GPR40 activation leads to CREB and ERK phosphorylation in primary cultures of neurons from the mouse CNS and in human neuroblastoma cells. *Hippocampus* 24, 733–739. doi: 10.1002/hipo.22263

Zenker, J., Stettner, M., Ruskamo, S., Domenech-Estevez, E., Baloui, H., Medard, J.-J., et al. (2014). A role of peripheral myelin protein 2 in lipid homeostasis of myelinating Schwann cells. *Glia* 62, 1502–1512. doi: 10.1002/glia.22696

Zhang, Q., Yang, H., Li, J., and Xie, X. (2016). Discovery and characterization of a novel small-molecule agonist for medium-chain free fatty acid receptor G protein-coupled receptor 84. *J. Pharmacol. Exp. Ther.* 357, 337–344. doi: 10.1124/jpet.116.232033

Zhang, R., Wang, Y., Li, R., and Chen, G. (2015). Transcriptional factors mediating retinoic acid signals in the control of energy metabolism. *Int. J. Mol. Sci.* 16, 14210–14244. doi: 10.3390/ijms160614210

Zhou, Y., Nie, T., Zhang, Y., Song, M., Li, K., Ding, M., et al. (2016). The discovery of novel and selective fatty acid binding protein 4 inhibitors by virtual screening and biological evaluation. *Bioorg. Med. Chem.* 24, 4310–4317. doi: 10.1016/j.bmc.2016.07.022

Zimmer, L., Delpal, S., Guilloteau, D., Aioun, J., Durand, G., and Chalon, S. (2000). Chronic n-3 polyunsaturated fatty acid deficiency alters dopamine vesicle density in the rat frontal cortex. *Neurosci. Lett.* 284, 25–28. doi: 10.1016/s0304-3940(00)00950-2

Zimmer, L., Hembert, S., Durand, G., Breton, P., Guilloteau, D., Besnard, J. C., et al. (1998). Chronic n-3 polyunsaturated fatty acid diet-deficiency acts on dopamine metabolism in the rat frontal cortex: a microdialysis study. *Neurosci. Lett.* 240, 177–181. doi: 10.1016/s0304-3940(97)00938-5

Zoete, V., Grosdidier, A., and Michielin, O. (2007). Peroxisome proliferator-activated receptor structures: ligand specificity, molecular switch and interactions with regulators. *Biochim. Biophys. Acta* 1771, 915–925. doi: 10.1016/j.bbalip.2007.01.007

Zolezzi, J. M., and Inestrosa, N. C. (2013). Peroxisome proliferator-activated receptors and Alzheimer's disease: hitting the blood-brain barrier. *Mol. Neurobiol.* 48, 438–451. doi: 10.1007/s12035-013-8435-5

Zolezzi, J. M., Santos, M. J., Bastías-Candia, S., Pinto, C., Godoy, J. A., and Inestrosa, N. C. (2017). PPARs in the central nervous system: roles in neurodegeneration and neuroinflammation. *Biol. Rev. Camb. Philos. Soc.* 92, 2046–2069. doi: 10.1111/brv.12320

6

Effects of FGF2/FGFR1 Pathway on Expression of A1 Astrocytes After Infrasound Exposure

Lin-Hui Zou[1,2†], Ya-Jun Shi[1†], Hua He[3†], Shi-Mei Jiang[4], Fang-Fang Huo[5], Xiao-Mu Wang[1], Fan Wu[1] and Lei Ma[1]*

[1] Department of Neurology, Xijing Hospital, Fourth Military Medical University, Xi'an, China, [2] Frontier Medical Training Brigade, Army Medical University, Changji, China, [3] Department of Specific Diagnosis, PLA 986 Hospital, Xi'an, China, [4] Department of Acu-Moxibustion and Tuina, Henan University of Traditional Chinese Medicine, Zhengzhou, China, [5] Department of Medicine, Yulin Yuyang District Hospital of Traditional Chinese Medicine, Yulin, China

Correspondence:
Lei Ma
malei@fmmu.edu.cn

† These authors have contributed equally to this work

Two types of reactive astrocytes, A1 and A2 astrocytes, are induced following neuroinflammation and ischemia. In this study, we evaluated the effects of the fibroblast growth factor (FGF)2/FGF receptor (FGFR)1 pathway on A1 and A2 astrocytes in the rat hippocampus using double-labeling immunofluorescence following infrasound exposure. A1 astrocytes were induced in the CA1 region of the hippocampus after exposure to infrasound for 3 days. The number of microglial cells was also increased, and we investigated if these might be responsible for the reactivity of A1 astrocytes. Accordingly, expression levels of C3 and Iba-1, as markers of A1 astrocytes and microglial cells, respectively, were both up-regulated in rat hippocampus following infrasound exposure, as demonstrated by western blot. We also explored the effect of the FGF2/FGFR1 pathway on A1 astrocyte reactivity by pretreating rats with FGF2 or the specific FGFR1 antagonist, PD173074. A1 astrocytes were gradually down-regulated by activation of the FGF2/FGFR1 pathway and were up-regulated by inhibition of the FGF2/FGFR1 pathway after infrasound damage. These results further our understanding of the role of reactive astrocytes in infrasound-induced central nervous system injury and will thus facilitate the development of new treatments for these injuries.

Keywords: infrasound, hippocampus, A1 astrocyte, microglial cell, FGF2/FGFR1 pathway

INTRODUCTION

Sound waves <20 Hz are referred to as infrasound. Infrasound is generated by numerous environmental factors, including agricultural machinery and industrial processes (Backteman et al., 1983; Bilski, 2017), and has been implicated in various kinds of health damage. For example, infrasound exposure is noted to be harmful in pregnant women (Castelo-Branco and Rodriguez, 1999). Furthermore, human and animal experiments have suggested that prolonged infrasound exposure can damage the central nervous system (CNS), including the hippocampus, cerebellum, limbic-corticular complex, hypothalamus, and cortex (Izmerov et al., 1997; Fei et al., 2000; Yuan et al., 2009; Shi et al., 2013; Cai et al., 2014; Ma et al., 2015). We previously confirmed that infrasound exposure activated astrocytes and induced neuronal apoptosis in the CNS, which subsequently impaired spatial learning and memory abilities (Shi et al., 2013, 2018).

Neuroinflammation and ischemia have been reported to induce two different types of reactive astrocytes, A1 and A2 astrocytes (Zamanian et al., 2012). A1 astrocytes are induced by activated microglia and gain a neurotoxic function, resulting in neuron killing (Liddelow et al., 2017), while A2 astrocytes upregulate many neurotrophic factors and strongly promote neuronal survival and tissue repair (Bush et al., 1999). Double-immunofluorescence labeling with complement component 3 (C3) and glial fibrillary acidic protein (GFAP) had been used to label A1 astrocytes, and double-immunofluorescence labeling with S100a10 and GFAP had been used to label A2 astrocytes (Liddelow et al., 2017).

In this study, we investigated the effects of infrasound on the induction of A1 and A2 astrocytes in the rat hippocampus by double-immunofluorescence labeling with C3 and GFAP, or S100a10 and GFAP, respectively. We also detected microglial cells by immunofluorescence labeling with Iba-1, to investigate their role in the effects of infrasound exposure. We verified the immunofluorescence results by measuring expression levels of C3 and Iba-1 in rat hippocampus.

We previously showed that the fibroblast growth factor (FGF)2/FGF receptor (FGFR)1 pathway inhibited astrocyte-mediated neuroinflammation *in vitro* and *in vivo* after infrasound exposure (Shi et al., 2018), suggesting that the reactivity of A1 astrocytes was related to activation of this pathway. We therefore investigated the role of the FGF2/FGFR1 pathway in infrasound-induced changes of A1 astrocytes in rats pretreated with FGF2 or the selective FGFR1 inhibitor, PD173074 (Mohammadi et al., 1998).

MATERIALS AND METHODS

Infrasound Device

The infrasound radiation laboratory was located at the Center for Radiation, the Fourth Military Medical University, Xi'an, China. The infrasound device included an infrasound chamber and infrasonic signal detection system. Infrasound with a frequency of 16 Hz and a pressure level of 150 dB was used in this study. The frequency and pressure of the infrasound were kept steady during 2 h of animal exposure and monitored using the infrasonic signal detection system.

Animals

Male Sprague-Dawley rats, weighing 220–250 g, were obtained from the Center of Experimental Animals, Fourth Military Medical University. The rats were maintained in an animal laboratory under controlled conditions at 20–25°C, humidity 50–60%, and a 12-h light/dark cycle, and were provided with free access to rodent chow and water.

The rats were divided randomly into groups as described previously (Shi et al., 2018): control group (no infrasound exposure, $n = 6$), infrasound (IS) exposure groups (exposed to 16 Hz, 150 dB of infrasound for 1, 3, 5, or 7 days, $n = 6$ per group), FGF2 groups (treated with FGF2 for 1, 3, 5, or 7 days, $n = 6$ per group), PD groups (treated with PD173074 for 1, 3, 5, or 7 days, $n = 6$ per group), FGF2+IS groups (infrasound-exposed rats treated with FGF2, $n = 6$ per group), and PD + IS groups (infrasound-exposed rats treated with PD173074, $n = 6$ per group). For FGF2 administration, rats were injected intraperitoneally (i.p.) with 0.1 mg/kg FGF2. For PD173074 administration, rats were injected i.p. with 1.5 mg/kg PD173074. FGF2 was dissolved in saline (Graham and Richardson, 2009) and PD173074 was dissolved in saline containing 12.5% Cremophor EL and 2.5% dimethylsulfoxide (Di Marco et al., 2014). FGF2 and PD173074 were injected everyday. The rats were exposed to infrasound of 16 Hz and 150 dB for 2 h a day.

Tissue Preparation

Brain slices were obtained as described previously (Melvin and Sutherland, 2010). After infrasound exposure, the rats were anesthetized with 10% chloral hydrate and then perfused sequentially with 200 ml ice-cold saline via a perfusion pump at 30 rpm, 200 ml 4% ice-cold paraformaldehyde (PFA) at 30 rpm, and 200 ml 4% PFA at 4 rpm. The brains were removed, fixed in 4% PFA for 12 h, dehydrated in 30% sucrose solution, embedded in OCT compound, and sectioned transversely into 35 μm-thick slices using a Leica CM 1900 cryostat. These sections were stored in 60% glycerine at −20°C and used for immunofluorescence.

Primary Astrocyte Culture

Primary cultures of rat hippocampus astrocytes were prepared from neonatal rats. Briefly, hippocampus tissue was minced with forceps and digested with 0.05% trypsin for 5 min. DMEM (Corning, New York, NY, United States) containing 10% fetal bovine serum, 1% glutamine, and 1% penicillin was added to stop the digestion and the supernatant was filtered. After centrifugation at 1000 rpm for 5 min, the cell mass was resuspended in DMEM and streptomycin at 37°C. The culture medium was replaced every 3 days. The purity of the astrocytes was determined by immunostaining with GFAP antibody, as described below. For the experiments, the astrocytes were exposed to infrasound of 16 Hz and 150 dB for 2 h, fixed with 4% PFA for 20 min, and stored for immunofluorescence staining.

Immunofluorescence

Brain sections or cultured astrocytes on coverslips were blocked with 3% bovine serum albumin (BSA) in PBS containing 0.3% Triton X-100 for 1 h at room temperature (RT). The sections or cells were then incubated with primary antibodies overnight at 4°C. Two antibodies were added simultaneously for double-immunofluorescence staining. The following antibodies were used: rabbit anti-S100a10 (1:100; Novus, Colorado Springs, CO, United States), mouse anti-C3 (1:100; Santa Cruz Biotechnology, Santa Cruz, CA, United States), rabbit anti-Iba-1 (1:800; Sigma, United States), mouse anti-GFAP (1:500; Abcam, Cambridge, United Kingdom), and rabbit anti-GFAP (1:500; Abcam). The samples were then incubated with species-specific secondary antibodies conjugated with Alexa Fluor (1:200; Zhuangzhi, Beijing, China) for 2 h at RT, and nuclei were stained with Hoechst-33342 (1:10000, GeneCopoeia, United States). Fluorescent signals were visualized under a confocal laser microscope.

Western Blotting

Rats were killed after each treatment, the hippocampus was collected, and total proteins were extracted using radioimmunoprecipitation assay lysis buffer (Beyotime Biotechnology, China). Protein concentrations were determined by BCA protein assay (Beyotime Biotechnology). Brain tissue extracts from each group were boiled for 5 min and the denatured proteins (40 μg) were separated by 10% sodium dodecyl sulfate-polyacrylamide gel electrophoresis and transferred onto nitrocellulose membranes (Bio-Rad, Hercules, CA, United States). After incubation in blocking buffer (0.1% Tween-20 and 5% non-fat-dried milk in Tris-buffered saline) at RT for 1 h, the membranes were incubated with anti-C3 antibody (1:500; Santa Cruz Biotechnology), anti-Iba-1 antibody (1:1000; Sigma), or anti-β-actin antibody (1:2000; Zhuangzhi). Semi-quantitative analysis of protein expression was carried out using horseradish peroxidase-conjugated secondary antibodies (1:5000; Zhuangzhi) and an electrochemiluminescence system (Bio-Rad).

Statistical Analysis

Fluorescent areas were measured using Image-Pro Plus 6.0 software. All statistical analyses were carried out using SPSS17.0 software and presented as mean ± standard deviation (SD) using GraphPad Prism 6.0 software. Data were analyzed by one-way ANOVA, followed by least significant difference tests for comparisons of three or more samples. Statistical significance was set at $P < 0.05$.

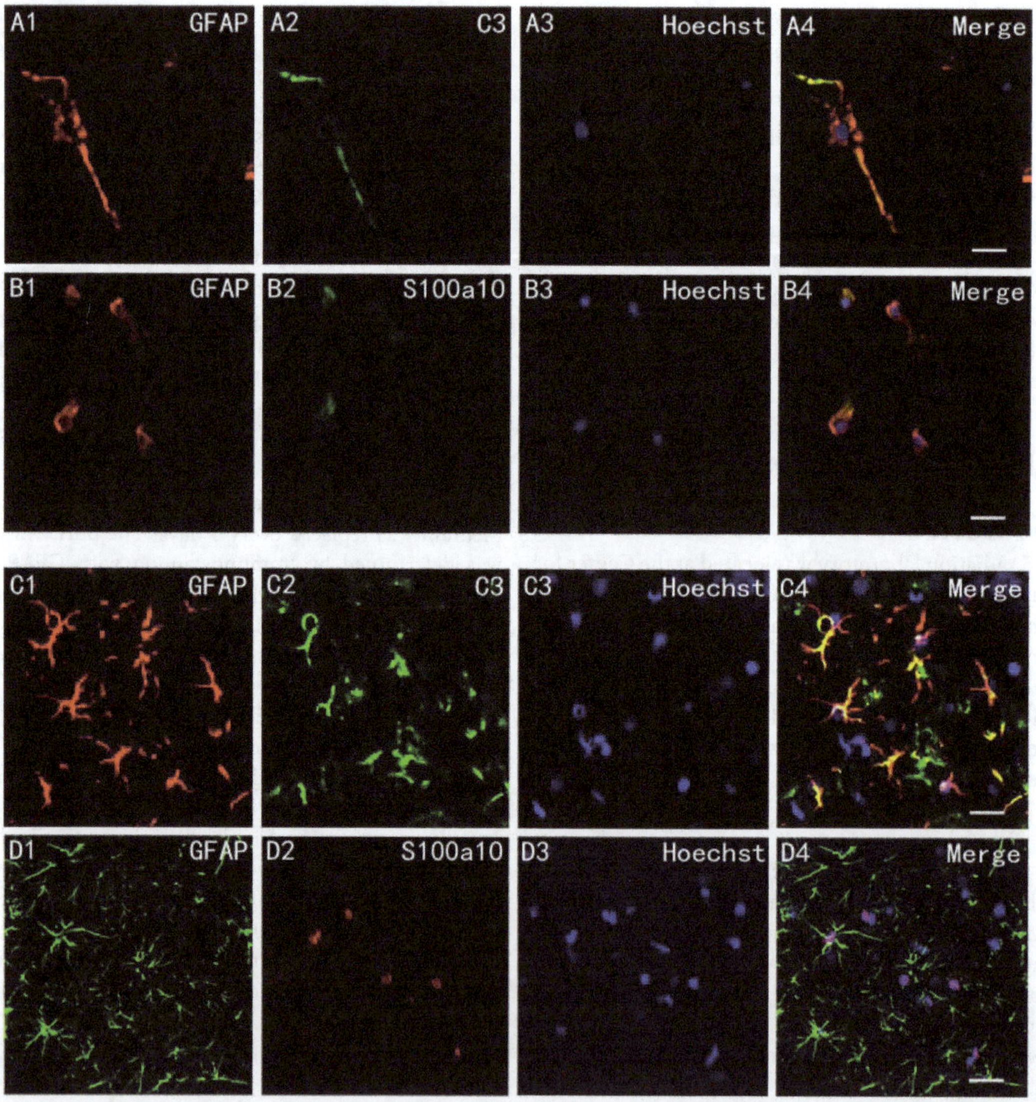

FIGURE 1 | Cell morphology of A1 and A2 astrocytes *in vitro* and *in vivo*. **(A1–A4)** Immunofluorescence staining of cultured astrocytes *in vitro* after exposure to infrasound for 2 h with glial fibrillary acidic protein (GFAP) and component 3 (C3), and **(B1–B4)** with GFAP and S100a10. **(C1–C4)** Immunofluorescence staining of astrocytes in the CA1 region in rats after exposure to infrasound for 3 days with GFAP and C3, and **(D1–D4)** with GFAP and S100a10. Nuclei stained with Hoechst. Scale bar: 25 μm.

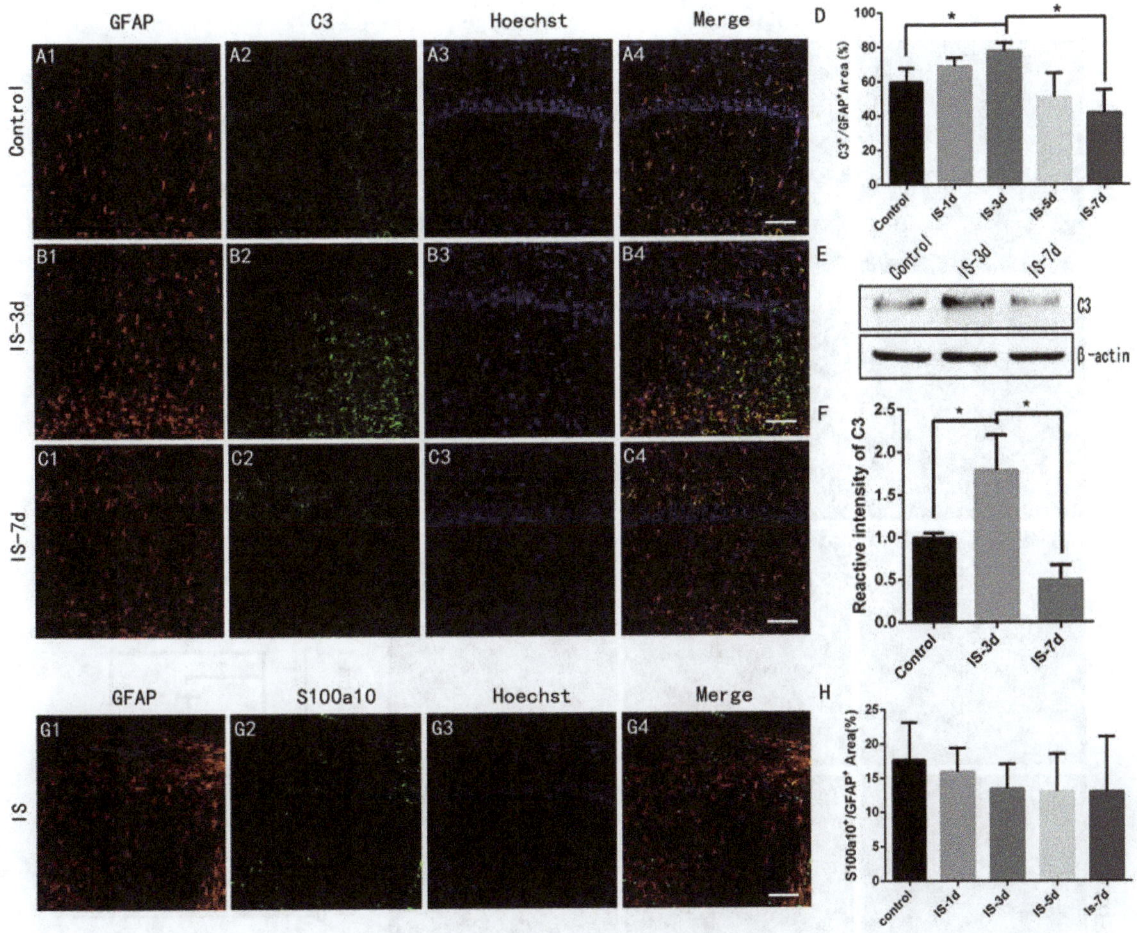

FIGURE 2 | A1 astrocytes were induced in rat hippocampus after 3 days of infrasound exposure. **(A1–A4)** A1 astrocytes in the CA1 region of the rat hippocampus double-labeled by C3 and GFAP in the control group without infrasound exposure, **(B1–B4)** in the group exposed to infrasound (IS) for 3 days (IS-3d), and **(C1–C4)** in the group exposed to infrasound for 7 days (IS-7d). **(D)** Quantitative analysis of percentage of $C3^+/GFAP^+$ area in the CA1 region of rat hippocampus. **(E)** C3 expression in rat hippocampus in control group, IS-3d group, and IS-7d group, by western blotting. **(F)** Semi-quantitative analysis of C3 expression in rat hippocampus in control group, IS-3d group, and IS-7d group. **(G1–G4)** A2 astrocytes in the CA1 region of rat hippocampus double-labeled by S100a10 and GFAP. **(H)** Quantitative analysis of percentage of $S100a10^+/GFAP^+$ area in the CA1 region of rat hippocampus. Nuclei stained with Hoechst. Scale bar: 100 μm. $N = 6–8$ for each experiment. One-way ANOVA. Values are all expressed as mean ± SD. $^*P < 0.05$.

RESULTS

Cell Morphology of A1 and A2 Astrocytes

We cultured rat hippocampus astrocytes *in vitro* and exposed them to infrasound of 16 Hz and 150 dB for 2 h, followed by immunofluorescence staining with S100a10, C3, and GFAP. Fluorescence microscopy showed that $C3^+$ A1 astrocytes had obvious long dendrites (**Figure 1A**), while $S100a10^+$ A2 astrocytes had hypertrophic cell bodies with few dendrites (**Figure 1B**).

In vivo, we pretreated rat by infrasound with a frequency of 16 Hz and a pressure level of 150 dB. Double-immunofluorescence labeling with S100a10, C3, and GFAP was also carried out on brain slices of the rat. Immunofluorescent staining with C3 and GFAP highlighted both the cell bodies and slender processes of A1 astrocytes (**Figure 1C**). But immunofluorescent staining with S100a10 only highlighted the cell bodies of astrocytes (**Figure 1D**).

Infrasound Induced A1 Astrocytes

Then, we used double-immunofluorescent labeling to investigate the effects of infrasound on the activation states of the two types of astrocytes in the CA1 region of the rat hippocampus. The percentage of $C3^+/GFAP^+$ area increased after exposure to infrasound for 3 days ($P < 0.05$) (**Figures 2A–D**). Previous studies demonstrated that GFAP expression increased after infrasound damage (Shi et al., 2013, 2018), and we therefore concluded that A1 astrocytes were activated by infrasound exposure. We also analyzed C3 protein expression levels in rat hippocampus semi-quantitatively by western blotting and confirmed that C3 protein expression levels in the hippocampus were up-regulated after 3 days of infrasound exposure ($P < 0.05$) (**Figures 2E,F**).

There were no significant differences in the percentage of $S100A10^+/GFAP^+$ area between control rats and rats exposed to infrasound for 1, 3, 5, or 7 days ($P > 0.05$) (**Figures 2G,H**).

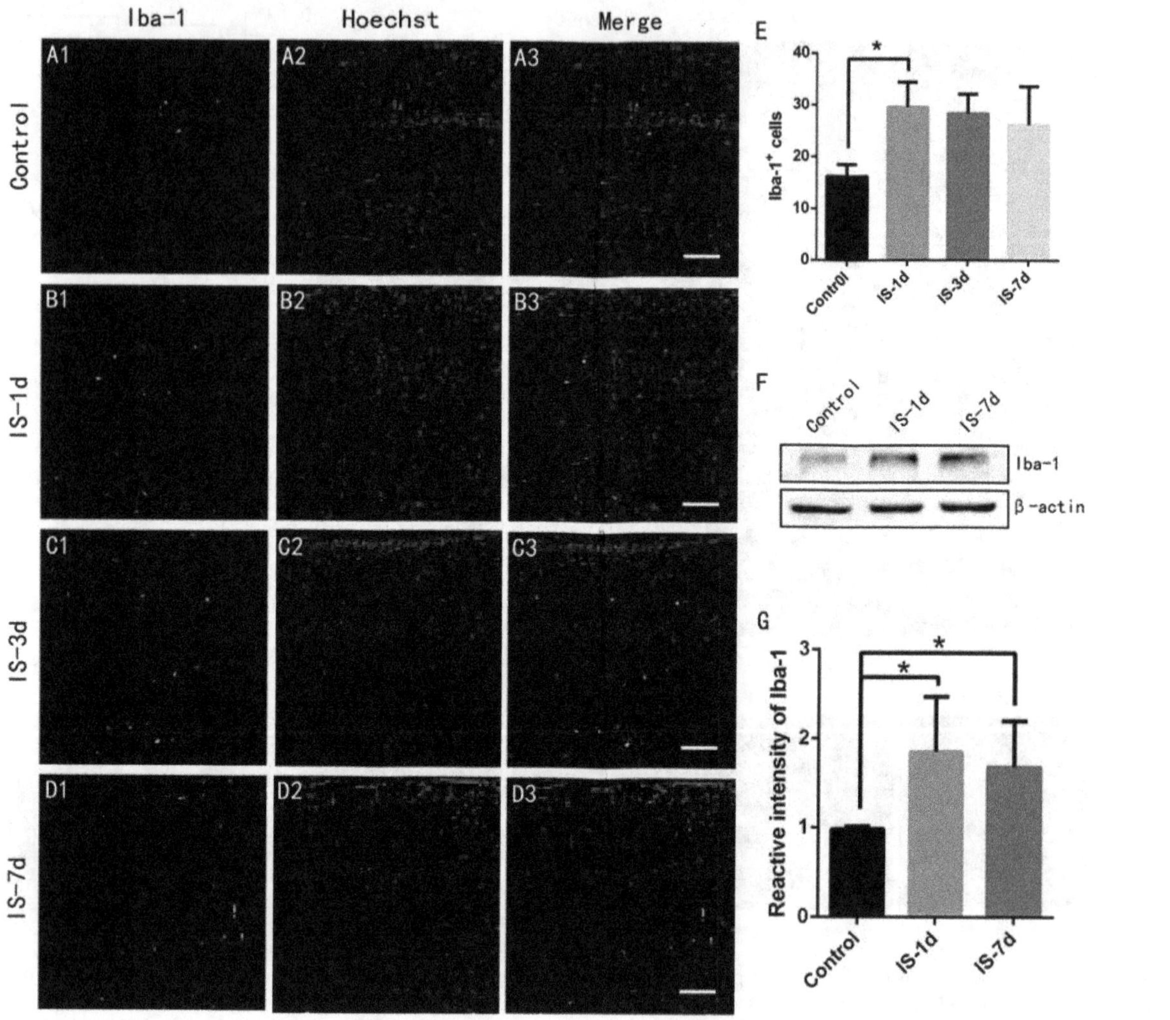

FIGURE 3 | Microglial cells in rat hippocampus increased after 1 day of infrasound exposure. **(A1–A3)** Microglial cells in the CA1 region of the rat hippocampus labeled with Iba-1 in the control group without infrasound exposure, **(B1–B3)** in the IS-1d group (1 day infrasound exposure), **(C1–C3)** IS-3d group (3 days infrasound exposure), and **(D1–D3)** in the IS-7d group (7 days infrasound exposure). **(E)** Quantitative analysis of Iba-1^+ cells per 625 μm × 625 μm in the CA1 region of the rat hippocampus by immunofluorescence staining. **(F)** Iba-1 expression in rat hippocampus in the control group, IS-1d group, and IS-7d group by western blotting. **(G)** Semi-quantitative analysis of Iba-1 expression in rat hippocampus in the control group, IS-1d group, and IS-7d group by western blotting. Nuclei stained with Hoechst. Scale bar: 100 μm. N = 6–8 for each experiment. One-way ANOVA. Values are all expressed as mean ± SD. $^*P < 0.05$.

These results suggested that infrasound induced A1 astrocytes, but not A2 astrocytes.

Microglial Cells Were Reactive Following Infrasound Exposure

Liddelow et al. (2017) demonstrated that reactive microglia induced A1 astrocytes, and we therefore determined if microglial cells were activated by infrasound. We labeled microglial cells by Iba-1 immunofluorescence. The results showed that the number of Iba-1^+ microglial cells in the CA1 region of the rat hippocampus increased after 1 day of infrasound exposure ($P < 0.05$) (**Figures 3A–E**), consistent with the results of a previous study (Xu et al., 2008). Western blotting confirmed that Iba-1 expression in the rat hippocampus increased after 1 day of infrasound exposure. Microglial cells decreased slightly during 1 day and 7 days, but the result was not significant ($P > 0.05$) (**Figures 3E–G**). These results suggested that infrasound exposure for 1 day activated microglial cells in the rat hippocampus.

A1 Astrocytes Were Regulated by the FGF2/FGFR1 Pathway

We initially investigated the role of the FGF2/FGFR1 pathway in A1 astrocyte reactivity by pretreating rats with FGF2 and then exposing them to infrasound. Double-immunofluorescent labeling revealed that the percentage of $C3^+$/$GFAP^+$ area in the CA1 region of the rat hippocampus were decreased during 1 and 7 days of FGF2 treatment and infrasound exposure ($P < 0.05$) (**Figure 4A**). Expression levels of C3 in the rat hippocampus also decreased during 1 and 7 days of treatment, as demonstrated by western blotting ($P < 0.05$) (**Figures 4B,C**).

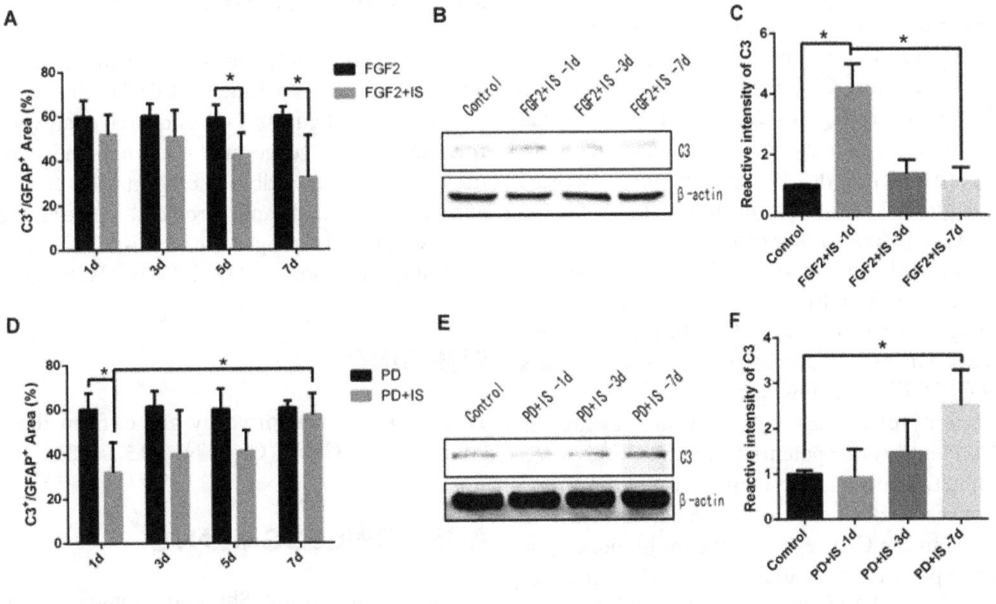

FIGURE 4 | A1 astrocytes were gradually down-regulated by activation of the FGF2/FGFR1 pathway and were up-regulated by inhibition of the FGF2/FGFR1 pathway. **(A,D)** Quantitative analysis of percentage of $C3^+/GFAP^+$ area in the CA1 region of rat hippocampus in different groups, by immunofluorescence staining. **(B,E)** C3 expression in rat hippocampus in different groups by western blotting. **(C,F)** Semi-quantitative analysis of C3 expression in rat hippocampus in different groups. $N = 6–8$ for each experiment. One-way ANOVA. Values expressed as mean ± SD. $^*P < 0.05$.

We then pretreated rats with PD173074 to inhibit activation of the FGF2/FGFR1 pathway. In the CA1 region of the rat hippocampus, the percentage of $C3^+/GFAP^+$ area was increased during 1 and 7 days of PD173074 treatment and infrasound exposure ($P < 0.05$) (**Figure 4D**). C3 expression levels increased gradually as well ($P < 0.05$) (**Figures 4E,F**). In our previous research (Shi et al., 2018), GFAP positive cells were not affected by the FGF2 or PD173074 treatment. Overall, these results suggested that A1 astrocytes were gradually down-regulated by activation of the FGF2/FGFR1 pathway and were up-regulated by inhibition of the FGF2/FGFR1 pathway after infrasound damage.

DISCUSSION

Astrocytes are the main type of glial cells in the brain and spinal cord. Astrocytes undergo astrogliosis during CNS injury and eventually transform into reactive astrocytes (Zamanian et al., 2012; Anderson et al., 2014), as demonstrated for A1 astrocytes in spinal cord injury, CNS brain trauma, and neuroinflammatory and neurodegenerative diseases (Liddelow et al., 2017). Furthermore, we previously demonstrated that infrasound exposure also induced astrocyte and microglial activation (Shi et al., 2013; Cai et al., 2014).

In this study, we examined the activation of microglia and astrocytes to investigate the mechanisms responsible for infrasound-induced neuronal apoptosis in the hippocampus. $C3^+$ and $GFAP^+$ A1 astrocytes in the CA1 region of the rat hippocampus were activated after 3 days of exposure to infrasound, while Iba-1^+ microglial cells were activated after 1 day of exposure, suggesting that microglial cells were activated before A1 astrocyte reactivity. Infrasound-activated microglia have previously been shown to produce a wide range of proinflammatory cytokines, including interleukin (IL)-1β, IL-6, IL-18, and tumor necrosis factor (TNF)-α (Cai et al., 2014). Furthermore, Liddelow et al. (2017) indicated that microglia-derived IL-1α, TNF, and C1q worked together to mediate A1 astrocyte reactivity, while A1 astrocytes exerted powerful neurotoxic effects that killed CNS neurons. Overall, these findings suggest that infrasound exposure initially activated microglial cells in the hippocampus, with subsequent induction of A1 astrocytes and neuronal cell apoptosis, resulting in learning and memory impairments.

The current results also found that FGF2 could restrain the reactivity of A1 astrocytes in the hippocampus after infrasound exposure. This neuroprotective effect of FGF2 against infrasound damage was in accord with previous studies showing that FGF2 could regulate the ability of the newborn hippocampal dentate gyrus, the formation of functional circuits, and the structural plasticity of neurons (Kirby et al., 2013; Pollak et al., 2014). Given that FGF2 could trigger FGFR1 signaling (Sutthiwarotamakun, 2011) and the FGF2/FGFR1 pathway may exert an inhibitory effect on astrocyte-mediated inflammation (Shi et al., 2018), we deduced that the neuroprotective effect involved the inhibition of astrocyte-mediated inflammation via the FGF2/FGFR1 pathway. In contrast, we observed that A1 astrocytes gradually increased in the hippocampus during 7 days of infrasound exposure with PD173074 treatment, thus confirming that inhibition of the FGF2/FGFR1 passageway caused reactivity of A1 astrocytes.

This study had several limitations. We used the method of Liddelow et al. (2017) in the immunofluorescence experiment, but we could not provide enough evidence to verify Liddelow et al.'s (2017) conclusion that the A2-specific marker S100a10 did not co-localize with C3 positive A1 astrocytes. In our experimental results, we found C3 existed in most of astrocytes which were labeled by GFAP (**Figures 2A–C**). It is possible that C3 exist in brain of normal animals (Rong et al., 2007; Fonseca et al., 2011). C3-positive astrocytes is expressed at a low level in normal physiological state, and some brain injury factors may lead to increased pathological expression, thus resulting in neurotoxic effects (Liddelow et al., 2017). We focused on the neurotoxic function of A1 astrocytes in infrasound damage; however, infrasound is a type of noise and might thus also have psychological effects. Furthermore, it is possible that pathways other than the FGF2/FGFR1 pathway might be involved in regulating the reactivity of A1 astrocytes. Further research is therefore needed to identify other potential mechanisms involved in the neurotoxic function of A1 astrocytes in infrasound damage.

In summary, our results demonstrated that A1 astrocytes were induced by microglia in the CA1 region of the rat hippocampus after infrasound exposure, and that these A1 astrocytes were regulated by the FGF2/FGFR1 pathway. Inhibiting A1 astrocytes or activating the FGF2/FGFR1 pathway may thus represent promising targets for the treatment of infrasound-induced CNS injury.

AUTHOR CONTRIBUTIONS

All authors contributed substantially to this work. LM conceived and designed the experiments. L-HZ performed the experiments and drew the figures. Y-JS and HH analyzed the data. S-MJ reviewed the language and grammar and provided reference materials. F-FH contributed reagents and analysis tools. X-MW and FW searched and provided material for writing the manuscript, and arranged the manuscript in accordance with the journal specifications. L-HZ, Y-JS, and HH wrote the manuscript.

FUNDING

This work was supported by grants from the Natural Science Foundation of China (Grant No. 31570848).

ACKNOWLEDGMENTS

We thank Dr. Ming Shi and Dongyun Feng (Department of Neurology, Xijing Hospital, Fourth Military Medical University) for their technical assistance and valuable suggestions. We also thank International Science Editing (http://www.internationalscienceediting.com) for editing a draft of this manuscript.

REFERENCES

Anderson, M., Ao, Y., and Sofroniew, M. (2014). Heterogeneity of reactive astrocytes. *Neurosci. Lett.* 565, 23–29. doi: 10.1016/j.neulet.2013.12.030

Backteman, O., Köhler, J., and Sjöberg, L. (1983). Infrasound-tutorial and review: Part 1.O. Backteman. *J. Low Frequency Noise Vib. Active Control* 3, 1–31.

Bilski, B. (2017). Exposure to infrasonic noise in agriculture. *Ann. Agric. Environ. Med.* 1, 86–89.

Bush, T., Puvanachandra, N., Homer, C., Polito, A., Ostenfeld, T., Svendsen, C., et al. (1999). Leukocyte infiltration, neuronal degeneration, and neurite outgrowth after ablation of scar-forming, reactive astrocytes in adult transgenic mice. *Neuron* 2, 297–308.

Cai, J., Jing, D., Shi, M., Liu, Y., Lin, T., Xie, Z., et al. (2014). Epigallocatechin gallate (EGCG) attenuates infrasound-induced neuronal impairment by inhibiting microglia-mediated inflammation. *J. Nutr. Biochem.* 25, 716–725. doi: 10.1016/j.jnutbio.2014.02.012

Castelo-Branco, N., and Rodriguez, E. (1999). The vibroacoustic disease–an emerging pathology. *Aviat. Space Environ. Med.* 70, 1–6.

Di Marco, S., Reuter, S., Kentrup, D., Grabner, A., Amaral, A., and Fobker, M. (2014). Treatment of established left ventricular hypertrophy with fibroblast growth factor receptor blockade in an animal model of CKD. *Nephrol. Dial. Transplant.* 29, 2028–2035. doi: 10.1093/ndt/gfu190

Fei, Z., Zhang, X., Wang, X., Li, Z., Lu, P., Liu, X., et al. (2000). The changes of rat blood-brain barrier permeability and expression of heat shock protein 70 after infrasonic damage. *J. Low Frequency Noise Vib. Active Control* 2, 93–99.

Fonseca, M., Chu, S., Berci, A., Benoit, M., Peters, D., Kimura, Y., et al. (2011). Contribution of complement activation pathways to neuropathology differs among mouse models of Alzheimer's disease. *J. Neuroinflammation* 8, 4–16.

Graham, B., and Richardson, R. (2009). Acute systemic fibroblast growth factor-2 enhances long-term extinction of fear and reduces reinstatement in rats. *Neuropsychopharmacology* 34, 1875–1882. doi: 10.1038/npp.2009.14

Izmerov, N., Suvorov, G., Kuralesin, N., and Ovakimov, V. (1997). Infrasound: body's effects and hygienic regulation. *Vestn. Ross. Akad. Med. Nauk* 7, 39–46.

Kirby, E., Muroy, S., Sun, W., Covarrubias, D., Leong, M., Barchas, L., et al. (2013). Acute stress enhances adult rat hippocampal neurogenesis and activation of newborn neurons via secreted astrocytic FGF2. *eLife* 2:362. doi: 10.7554/eLife.00362

Liddelow, S., Guttenplan, K., Clarke, L., Bennett, F., Bohlen, C., Schirmer, L., et al. (2017). Neurotoxic reactive astrocytes are induced by activated microglia. *Nature* 541, 481–487. doi: 10.1038/nature21029

Ma, L., He, H., Liu, X., Zhang, G., Li, L., Yan, S., et al. (2015). Involvement of cannabinoid receptors in infrasonic noise-induced neuronal impairment. *Acta Biochim. Biophys. Sin.* 8, 647–653. doi: 10.1093/abbs/gmv049

Melvin, N., and Sutherland, R. (2010). Quantitative caveats of standard immunohistochemical procedures: implications for optical disector-based designs. *J. Histochem. Cytochem.* 58, 577–584. doi: 10.1369/jhc.2009.954164

Mohammadi, M., Froum, S., Hamby, J., Schroeder, M., Panek, R., Lu, G., et al. (1998). Crystal structure of an angiogenesis inhibitor bound to the FGF receptor tyrosine kinase domain. *EMBO J.* 20, 5896–5904.

Pollak, D., Minh, B., Cicvaric, A., and Monje, F. (2014). A novel fibroblast growth factor receptor family member promotes neuronal outgrowth and synaptic plasticity in Aplysia. *Amino Acids* 11, 2477–2488. doi: 10.1007/s00726-014-1803-2

Rong, F., Kelly, D., and William, E. (2007). Induction of complement proteins in a mouse model for cerebral microvascular Aβ deposition. *J. Neuroinflammation* 4, 22–30.

Shi, M., Du, F., Liu, Y., Li, L., Cai, J., Zhang, G., et al. (2013). Glial cell-expressed mechanosensitive channel TRPV4 mediates infrasound-induced neuronal impairment. *Acta Neuropathol.* 5, 725–739. doi: 10.1007/s00401-013-1166-x

Shi, Y., Shi, M., Xiao, L., Zou, L., Li, C., Zhang, Q., et al. (2018). Inhibitive effects of FGF2/FGFR1 pathway on astrocyte-mediated inflammation in vivo and in vitro after infrasound exposure. *Front. Neurosci.* 12:582. doi: 10.3389/fnins.2018.00582

Sutthiwarotamakun, R. (2011). *Perpheral Autoimmunity Induces Central Neuro-Inflammation and Hippocampal Neurogenesis Impairment in a Murine Model of Collagen Induced Rheumatoid Arthritis.* .

Xu, X., Zhao, G., Rao, Z., Du, F., Shi, J., and Liu, J. (2008). The response of microglia in the hypothalamic paraventricular nucleus of rats to infrasound. *Chin. J. Neurosurg. Dis. Res.* 7, 513–516.

Yuan, H., Long, H., Liu, J., Qu, L., Chen, J., and Mou, X. (2009). Effects of infrasound on hippocampus-dependent learning and memory in rats and some underlying mechanisms. *Environ. Toxicol. Pharmacol.* 2, 243–247. doi: 10.1016/j.etap.2009.04.011

Zamanian, J. L., Xu, L., Foo, L., Nouri, N., Zhou, L., Giffard, R., et al. (2012). Genomic analysis of reactive astrogliosis. *J. Neurosci.* 32, 6391–6410. doi: 10.1523/JNEUROSCI.6221-11.2012

7

Lipid Metabolism in Neurons: A Brief Story of a Novel c-Fos-Dependent Mechanism for the Regulation of their Synthesis

*Lucia Rodríguez-Berdini and Beatriz L. Caputto**

Centro de Investigaciones en Química Biológica de Córdoba (Consejo Nacional de Investigaciones Científicas y Técnicas), Departamento de Química Biológica "Ranwel Caputto", Facultad de Ciencias Químicas, Universidad Nacional de Córdoba, Córdoba, Argentina

***Correspondence:**
Beatriz L. Caputto
bcaputto@fcq.unc.edu.ar

The mechanisms that coordinately regulate lipid synthesis in the nervous system together with the high rates of membrane biogenesis needed to support cell growth are largely unknown as are their subcellular site of synthesis. c-Fos, a well-known AP-1 transcription factor, has emerged as a unique protein with the capacity to associate to specific enzymes of the pathway of synthesis of phospholipids at the endoplasmic reticulum and activate their synthesis to accompany genomic decisions of growth. Herein, we discuss this effect of c-Fos in the context of neuronal differentiation and also with respect to pathologies of the nervous system such as the development and growth of tumors. We also provide insights into the sub-cellular sites where this regulation occurs at the endoplasmic reticulum membranes and the molecular mechanism by which c-Fos exerts this activity.

Keywords: nervous system phospholipid synthesis regulation, membrane biogenesis, proliferation and differentiation, brain tumors, endomembrane compartments

INTRODUCTION

Lipids, essential constituent molecules of all organisms, participate in a broad range of cellular processes. Their importance is highlighted by the fact that almost 5% of the human genes are related to their synthesis (van Meer et al., 2008). Particularly, the nervous system has a rich lipid composition, being the brain the second tissue in humans with both the highest lipid content and the highest diversity in their composition (Sastry, 1985; Hamilton et al., 2007; Bozek et al., 2015). Some authors have related this diversity to the cognitive abilities acquired by humans through their evolutionary lineage (Bozek et al., 2015). Among the main functions of lipids in the nervous system, of undoubtable importance is their structural role in biological membranes, their participation as bioactive messengers involved in cell signaling and their contribution to energy supply (Tracey et al., 2018).

The homeostasis of the lipid content of the nervous system is of vital importance, since several neuropathologies have been associated to their abnormal metabolism (Ahmed et al., 2017; Gaspar et al., 2018; Valadas et al., 2018; Yu et al., 2018). Evidence has linked disturbances in cholesterol metabolism to the progressive neurodegeneration observed in Alzheimer patients (Chang et al., 2017; Habchi et al., 2018; Penke et al., 2018) and also to autism spectrum disorders, possibly through lipid rafts disarrangements and the consequent alteration of synaptic functions (Wang, 2014). Elevated ganglioside levels have been related to Parkinson's disease, probably through their influence on α-synuclein aggregation kinetics (Gaspar et al., 2018). Abnormalities in the metabolism of polyphosphoinositides also underlie nervous system diseases such as schizophrenia, bipolar disorder, Friedrich's ataxia, Parkinson's and Down syndrome (Lauwers et al., 2016).

An unbalanced content of fatty acids in the nervous system has also been associated to neurodegenerative diseases. Docosahexaenoic acid (DHA) and arachidonic acid (AA) are the most abundant and biologically active essential fatty acids in brain phospholipids (Sanchez-Mejia and Mucke, 2010). DHA and its derivatives, the docosanoids, are involved in neuronal survival signaling pathways that resolve inflammation and reduce oxidative stress (Farooqui, 2012; Bazan, 2014; Tayebati, 2018). A significant decrease in DHA levels has been observed in cognitive impairment and Alzheimer's disease (AD) (Bazan et al., 2011; Bazan, 2014; Kim et al., 2014). In fact, DHA enriched diets have been proven to be efficient against neurodegeneration and able to prevent AD symptoms (Strokin et al., 2006; Hooijmans et al., 2009; Oster and Pillot, 2010; Tayebati, 2018). In retina neurons, DHA protects cells against oxidative stress and promotes photoreceptor differentiation (Simon et al., 2016). On the other hand, an activated metabolism of AA and its derivatives, the eicosanoids, has been associated to different pathologies, such as multiple sclerosis or AD, probably through the promotion of neuroinflammation and of an increase in neuronal activity and excitotoxicity (Lukiw and Bazan, 2000; Sanchez-Mejia and Mucke, 2010; Palumbo, 2017).

Brain choline metabolism has received much attention due to the important role of acetylcholine transmission in neuronal functions, especially those involved in cognitive abilities (Ferreira-Vieira et al., 2016). Abnormalities in the brain cholinergic system have been observed in AD, Lewy Bodies Dementia, Parkinson's disease and Huntington, among other pathologies (Pepeu and Grazia Giovannini, 2017).

In the case of the neuronal membrane, its lipid composition varies according to the neuronal type and the structural compartment of the neuron (Vance et al., 2000). The first results obtained after addressing the subcellular localization of lipid synthesis in neurons indicated that it was carried out in the neuronal soma (Weiss and Hiscoe, 1948), from where these components were transported by anterograde transport to the growing dendrites and axons during differentiation (Ledeen, 1985). However, it was later suggested that axonal transport was neither fast nor abundant enough to supply the necessary amounts of lipids to support axonal membrane expansion, an event that can reach an increment of up to 20% per day during the peak of neuronal growth (Pfenninger, 2009). So, given the size and architecture of neurons, it seemed reasonable to imagine the existence of a temporal and domain-specific organization. This could regulate lipid synthesis at distal sites of the neuron so as to avoid the sole dependence on axonal transport of these compounds from the soma.

Several reports have demonstrated the presence in axons of endoplasmic reticulum (ER) membranes, the main organelle for lipid synthesis, suggesting that the axon could contain a local functional biosynthetic machinery (Palay, 1958; Tsukita and Ishikawa, 1976; Rambourg and Droz, 1980; Lindsey and Ellisman, 1985; Gonzalez and Couve, 2014; Luarte et al., 2018; Terasaki, 2018). In fact, this seems to be the case: several enzymes of the pathway of lipid synthesis have been shown to be present in axons where they are capable of locally synthetizing phosphatidylcholine, phosphatidylethanolamine, phosphatidylserine, phosphatidylinositol, sphingomyelin and fatty acids (Vance et al., 1991, 1994). For example, 50% of the phosphatidylcholine required for normal axonal elongation has been shown to be locally synthetized in the axonal ER (Posse de Chaves et al., 1995).

These observations posed questions regarding the mechanisms that determine which lipids are synthetized in the axon, the quantitative extent of the domain-specific synthesis of lipids and the regulatory constraints driving this phenomenon. In this regard, many aspects of this metabolism remain unanswered, especially if its influence on neuronal plasticity is considered.

c-FOS: ONE PROTEIN LEADING TO AT LEAST TWO ROADS

The oncogene *fos* codifies for a protein of 380 amino acids called c-Fos that belongs to the *Immediate Early Genes* (IEGs) family (Angel and Karin, 1991). Five different proteins form the Fos family: c-Fos, Fos-B, ΔFos-B, Fra-1, and Fra-2 (Tulchinsky, 2000; Raivich and Behrens, 2006), all of which heterodimerize mainly with proteins of the Jun family thus forming the well-known AP-1 family of transcription factors (Angel and Karin, 1991). c-Fos heterodimerizes with Jun through a leucine zipper domain (LZ) and the resulting heterodimer interacts with a DNA consensus sequence through the basic domains (BD) of both proteins (Glover and Harrison, 1995).

It has been established that AP-1 activity is induced under a wide range of physiological and pathological stimuli including cytokines, growth factors, stress signals, infections and upon oncogenic transformation (Shaulian and Karin, 2001). It has also been proposed that its activity can be regulated through multiple pathways: (a)- via the transcriptional regulation of the proteins that compose each AP-1 dimer; (b)- through the stability of their mRNAs; (c)- via post-transductional modifications; (d)- by regulating the turnover of pre-existing molecules of the proteins or of the newly synthetized ones; (e)- through specific interactions between the different AP-1 subunits; (f)- through interactions with other transcription factors and co-factors (Hess et al., 2004).

Under certain circumstances, c-Fos is capable of inducing cellular transformation (Miller et al., 1984), a role that is usually associated to its function as an AP-1 transcription factor. Evidence has been provided that demonstrates its main role in cell growth and in neoplastic transformation (Tulchinsky, 2000; Shaulian and Karin, 2001; Hess et al., 2004; Milde-Langosch, 2005). Surprisingly, it was shown that, unlike other oncogenes studied, its oncogenic activity does not rely on mutations of its sequence but is rather dependent only on

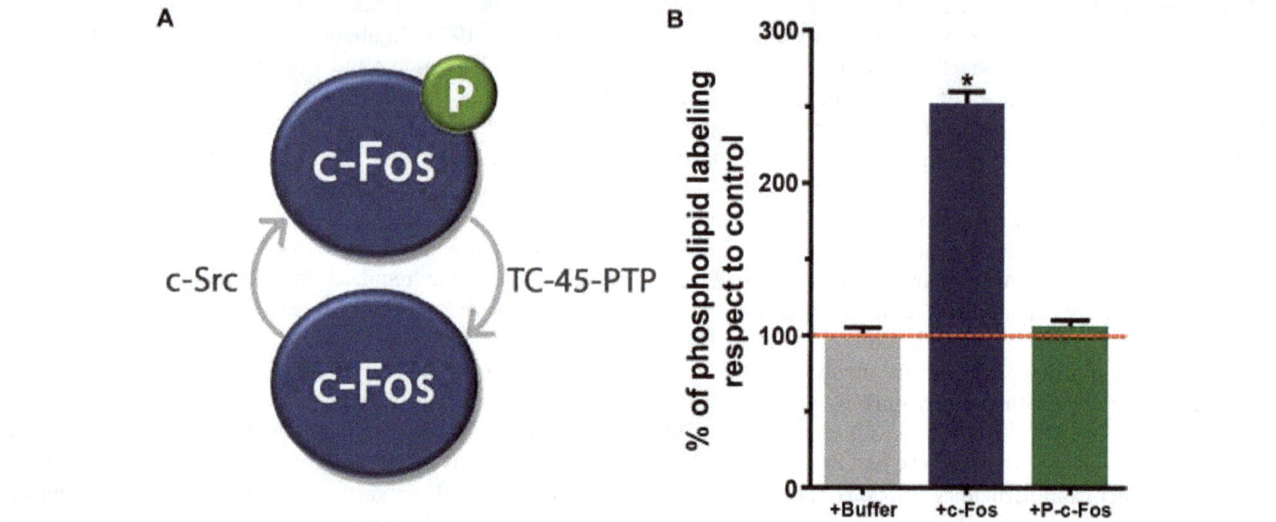

FIGURE 1 | (A) Schematic representation of the phosphorylation/dephosphorylation cycle of the tyrosine residues of c-Fos by the kinase c-Src and the phosphatase TC-45-PTP. Dephosphorylated c-Fos is able to associate to ER membranes whereas phosphorylated c-Fos is not. **(B)** Labeling of total phospholipids in T98G cells homogenates in the presence of recombinant dephosphorylated c-Fos and phosphorylated c-Fos (obtained after incubation with recombinant c-Src). The capacity to incorporate [^{32}P] to phospholipids from [^{32}P]-ATP was measured *in vitro*. The results are the mean ± SD of two experiments performed in triplicate. $^*p < 0.002$ with respect to the control, as determined by Student's two-tailed *t*-test. Adapted from Ferrero et al., 2012.

its over-expression (Miller et al., 1984). In addition, different stress signals such as UV exposure or alkylating agents, that normally provoke cell cycle arrest or cell death, also induce its expression (Buscher et al., 1988; Curran and Franza, 1988; Piechaczyk and Blanchard, 1994; Shaulian and Karin, 2001). Even more, numerous studies pointed out that the outcome of AP-1 activity seems to be cell-type specific: whereas in some cells it promotes apoptosis, in others it is required for survival (Hess et al., 2004). Hence, although the different functions of AP-1 have been exhaustively studied, the complete scenario resulting from its expression/overexpression is complex due to its capacity to exert completely antagonizing functions. This duality can be particularly distinguished in the nervous system where AP-1 is involved in both degenerative and regenerative processes, as a degeneration effector or as a physiological neuroprotective player (Herdegen and Waetzig, 2001).

In the nervous system, c-Fos expression has also been related to processes involving memory and learning (Dragunow, 1996; Grimm and Tischmeyer, 1997; Rosen et al., 1998; Minatohara et al., 2015; Gallo et al., 2018). These findings transformed this protein into a marker of plastic changes that favor the establishment of long term memory and the maintenance of specific neuronal populations (Rosen et al., 1998; Minatohara et al., 2015). In fact, AP-1 inhibition negatively affects memory formation and physiological adaptive processes such as the synchronization of the endogenous clock (Wollnik et al., 1995; Grimm and Tischmeyer, 1997). While all this evidence has reliably demonstrated the importance of c-Fos and the functional consequences of its induction, surely other cellular mechanisms in which this protein participates, remain unknown.

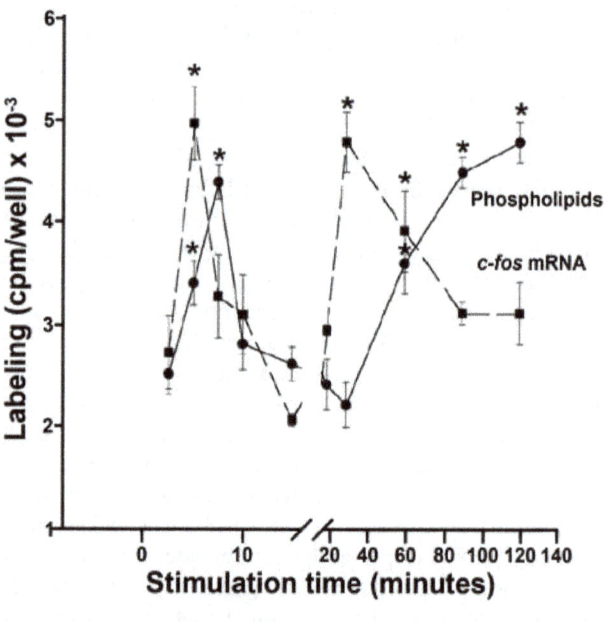

FIGURE 2 | Time curves of phospholipid metabolic labeling (circles, full line) and c-Fos mRNA expression (squares, dashed line) in NIH-3T3 cells stimulated to re-enter cell cycle after quiescence. In all the conditions, phospholipid labeling was determined by pulsing cells with ^{32}P-orthophosphate during 15 min, irrespective of the stimulation status. The results are the mean ± SD of six independent experiments performed in duplicate. $^*p < 0.025$ with respect to time 0 of stimulation. Adapted from Bussolino et al., 2001.

During the last 20 years, our laboratory has accumulated evidence that demonstrates that c-Fos is a moonlighting protein: it is capable of performing two different, apparently autonomous, unrelated functions. In addition to its well-known function as an AP-1 transcription factor, c-Fos associates to the ER where it activates lipid synthetizing enzymes independently of its nuclear function (Guido et al., 1996; Bussolino et al., 1998, 2001; Gil et al., 2004; Crespo et al., 2008; Alfonso Pecchio et al., 2011; Caputto et al., 2014; Cardozo Gizzi et al., 2015). This phenomenon has been observed in animal models with nervous system tumors, in cultured cells derived from the nervous system (PC12 cells, the neuronal tumor cell lines T98G, U87MG, NB41A3, C6, among others) and in non-nervous cells such as breast cancer cells (Gil et al., 2004; Motrich et al., 2013). The association of c-Fos to the ER is essential for lipid synthesis activation to occur and it is regulated by a phosphorylation/dephosphorylation cycle exerted by the enzymes c-Src and TC45-PTP. c-Src phosphorylates the tyrosine residues 10 and 30 of c-Fos determining its dissociation from the ER. By contrast, TC45-PTP is the phosphatase that removes the phosphate groups allowing c-Fos to associate to membranes in its dephosphorylated form (**Figure 1**; Ferrero et al., 2012).

Using different types of cells in culture, we showed that the expression of c-Fos mRNA exhibits two peaks, each of them concordant with a significant increase in the metabolic labeling of lipids (**Figure 2**; Bussolino et al., 2001). Specifically blocking c-Fos expression also blocks activation of lipid synthesis. Even more, in order to obtain an insight on the mechanism for enzyme activation, we performed biochemical assays. We found that at the ER, c-Fos is capable of activating only some particular enzymes of the different lipid synthetizing pathways: CDP-diacylglycerolsynthase-1 (CDS1), Phosphatidylinositol-4-kinase type II α (PI4KIIα) and Lipin-1 are activated by c-Fos, whereas Phosphatidylinositol synthase (PIS1) and Phosphatidylinositol-4-kinase type II β (PI4KIIβ) are not (Alfonso Pecchio et al., 2011; Cardozo Gizzi et al., 2015). As can be seen in the activity assays shown in **Figure 3B**, activation is achieved by increasing their V_{max} without affecting their K_m. Furthermore, for activation to occur, c-Fos interacts with the enzymes it activates but not with those it does not regulate (see FRET experiments in **Figure 3A**). Interestingly, this physical interaction is achieved by the N-terminal domain of c-Fos, where a stretch enriched in basic amino acids (BD domain, 139–159) is of fundamental importance for enzyme activation (Alfonso Pecchio et al., 2011). Surprisingly, c-Fos can also perform this activity in the nucleus, where it promotes transcriptional changes in genes lacking an AP-1 consensus sequence in their promoters by increasing the nuclear content of phosphatidylinositol-4,5-bisphosphate (Ferrero et al., 2014). These findings provide an even more complex scenario regarding the cellular consequences of inducing c-Fos expression and allowed us to propose an additional role for c-Fos as a transcriptional regulator but in an AP-1-independent manner.

A great effort was destined to study this function in the nervous system, where c-Fos-dependent lipid activation has been consistently confirmed. In fact, the first studies that gave the initial evidence of this phenomena in the nervous system were performed in the chicken retina, where we found that during sensory stimulation, the transcription and transduction of c-Fos

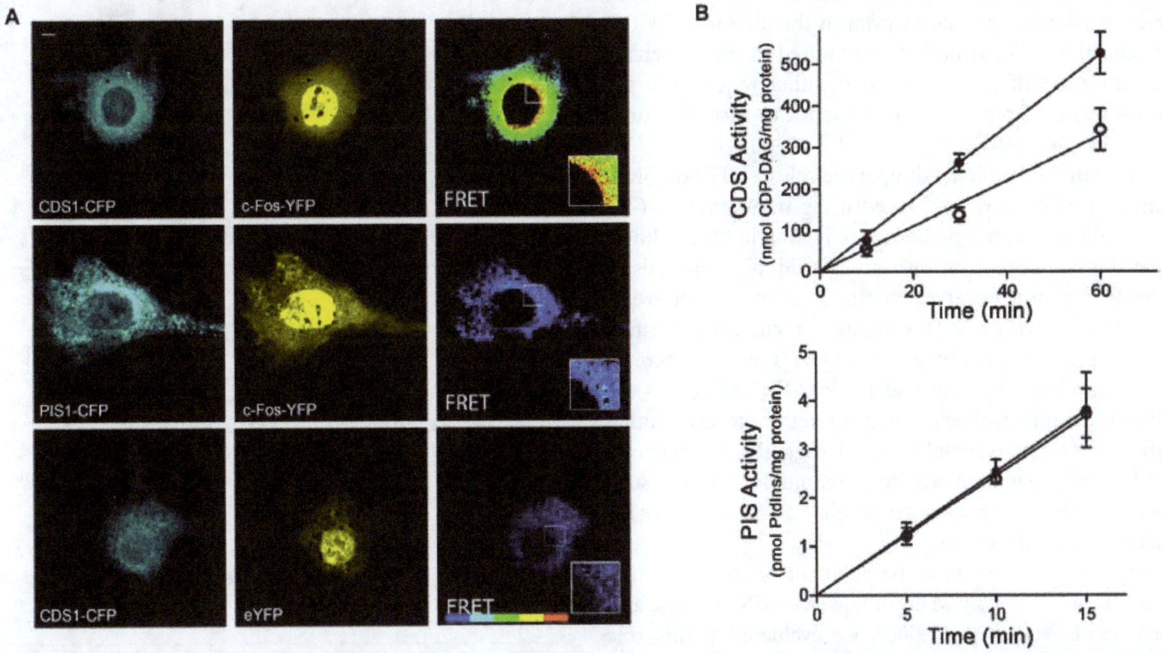

FIGURE 3 | The enzyme CDP-diacylglycerol synthase (CDS) interacts with and is activated by c-Fos, while the enzyme phosphatidylinositol synthase (PIS) neither interacts nor is activated by c-Fos. **(A)** FRET experiments of cells co-transfected to express c-Fos-YFP and CDS1-CFP (first row) or PIS1-CFP (second row) were examined by confocal microscopy using filters for eCFP (left) or for eYFP (middle). FRET efficiency images were obtained and pseudocolored (right). The last row shows control cells co-expressing CDS1-CFP and eYFP. FRET scale goes from no FRET (blue) to maximum FRET (red). Scale bar: 5 μm. **(B)** Effect of c-Fos on CDS and PIS activities. Assays were performed in the presence (black circles) or the absence (open circles) of recombinant c-Fos. Formation of CDP-diacylglycerol (CDP-DAG) was measured in the case of determining CDS activity and phosphatidylinositol (PtdIns) in the case of examining PIS activity. Results are the mean ± SD of at least two experiments performed in triplicate. Adapted from Alfonso Pecchio et al., 2011.

participate in the regulation of glycerophospholipids synthesis: if c-Fos expression is specifically inhibited in photoreceptors and ganglion cells, the differences usually observed in lipid synthesis after the exposure of the animals to light or dark cycles are abolished (Guido et al., 1996; Bussolino et al., 1998).

Later studies showed that this c-Fos-dependent lipid synthesis activation was also present in T98G cells, cells derived from a malignant human glioblastoma: blocking c-Fos expression in these cells promotes a decrease in the metabolic labeling of phospholipids and an impairment in cell proliferation (Portal et al., 2007; Ferrero et al., 2012). Results obtained in PC12 cells, which derive from a pheochromocytoma of the rat adrenal medulla, highlighted the existence of the dual functions of c-Fos as an AP-1 transcription factor and as an activator of lipid synthesis. Normally, the addition of nerve growth factor (NGF) to the cell culture media triggers a genomic differentiation program that drives these cells towards a sympathetic neuron phenotype, a process that is accompanied by an induction of c-Fos expression (Gil et al., 2004). If, together with NGF treatment, the entrance of c-Fos to the nucleus is impaired by blocking AP-1 importation, neuritogenesis and differentiation are inhibited even when c-Fos expression remains at its normal levels. However, if the import of c-Fos into the nucleus is blocked 16 hours after NGF induction, differentiation is normal. This implies that c-Fos is required at early stages of differentiation in the nucleus as AP-1 to trigger the differentiation program. However, once the cells have been induced to differentiate, when c-Fos expression is blocked, there is a decrease in lipid synthesis and neurites not only stop growing, they also begin to retract, a process that can be reverted by the over-expression of only c-Fos even in the absence of NGF. This indicates that c-Fos is no longer required in the nucleus at advanced times of differentiation but is rather required in the cytoplasm activating lipid synthesis at the ER to sustain neurite outgrowth (Gil et al., 2004).

To advance in the understanding of the role of c-Fos on brain development, studies were performed using transgenic *fos* (-/-) mice. These animals show a significant reduction in the thickness of the developing neocortex respect to wild type animals, a phenotype that is still observed at the adult stage (**Figure 4**; Velazquez et al., 2015a,b). This reduction correlates with a decrease in the number of differentiating cells and an increase in apoptosis levels at the ventricular zone. No differences are observed in the number of cells going through mitosis although the mitotic angle found is mainly vertical, suggesting a decreased tendency for the progenitor cells to differentiate. These results probably reflect the initial dependence of c-Fos AP-1 activity for neuronal development to occur.

As c-Fos has been shown to be a potent oncoprotein that induces cell transformation when deregulated (Piechaczyk and Blanchard, 1994; Tulchinsky, 2000), we evaluated if this role could be due to its cytoplasmic lipid-synthetizing function. We found a strong expression of cytoplasmic c-Fos co-localizing with ER markers in 100% of the more than 200 human malignant brain tumor samples examined. This strongly contrasted with the lack of detectable expression of this protein in normal, paired biopsies (Silvestre et al., 2010). In a human glioblastoma multiforme sample, in addition to the increased expression of c-Fos, a > 100% activation of lipid synthesis was observed when assayed *in vitro*, with respect to a paired non-pathological sample. Furthermore, elimination from the assay media of endogenous c-Fos (using high ionic strength followed by centrifugation) reduced the activated levels of lipid synthesis, whereas addition

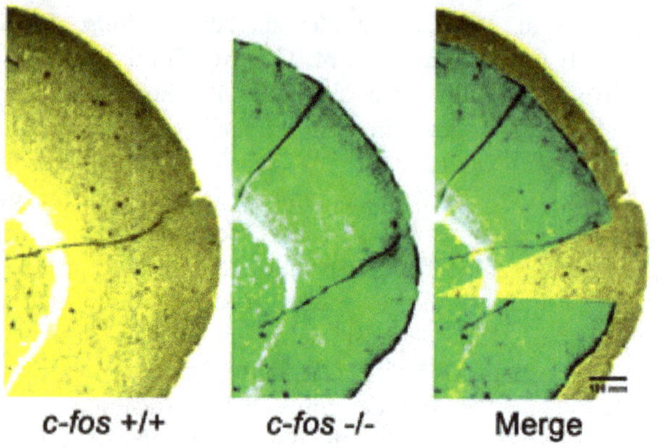

FIGURE 4 | Representative images of brain cortical slices from *fos* (+/+) mice (left, pseudo colored yellow), *fos* (–/–) mice (middle, pseudo colored green) and the merged image (right). Note that in the merged image, part of the *fos* (–/–) image was cropped to better show the superposition of both images. Adapted from Velazquez et al., 2015b.

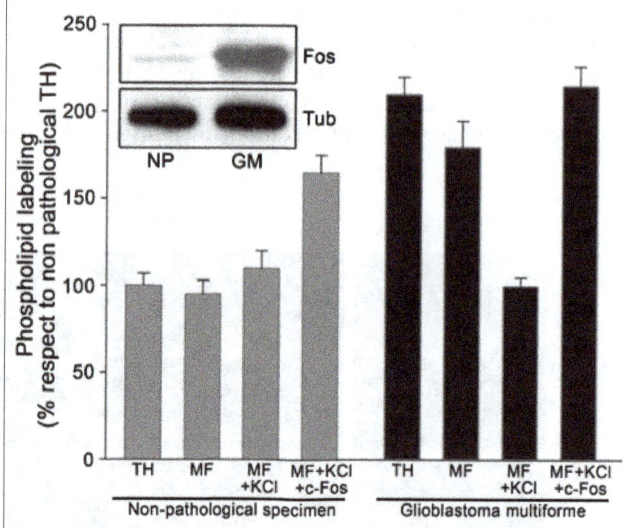

FIGURE 5 | Activation of phospholipid synthesis in membranes from a human glioblastoma multiforme (GM). Homogenates were obtained from a human GM and from adjacent non pathological tissue (NP) excised from the same patient. TH: total homogenate; MF: microsomal membrane fraction; MF+KCl: 1M KCl stripped microsomal membrane fraction; MF+KCl+c-Fos: stripped MF plus recombinant c-Fos. Results are the mean ± SD of three experiments performed in triplicate; non-pathological TH values were taken as 100%. Inset: Western Blot for c-Fos content in the samples assayed; Tubulin staining is used as a loading control. Note the high content of c-Fos in the GM sample as compared to the almost undetectable levels in the NP sample. Adapted from Silvestre et al., 2010.

of recombinant c-Fos to the c-Fos-devoid assay media re-established lipid synthesis levels (**Figure 5**).

Confirmation of the dependence of tumor growth on c-Fos expression was obtained in NPcis mice, a mouse model of the human disease Neurofibromatosis Type 1. These animals spontaneously develop central and peripheral nervous system tumors. In these mice, tumor progression is slowed down or even stopped by blocking c-Fos expression, in concordance with an abrogation of phospholipid synthesis activation in spite that AP-1 content is not substantially affected (Silvestre et al., 2010). Strikingly, NPcis *fos* (−/−) mice do not develop tumors in contrast to their *fos* (+/−) or *fos* (+/+) littermates, in which tumor development was observed in 71% of the animals (Silvestre et al., 2010). These *in vivo* examples of the dependence on c-Fos for nervous system tumors to grow disclose c-Fos as a potential target to control brain cancer.

FINAL COMMENTS

All the above-mentioned results highlight the relevance of c-Fos for the development of the nervous system. The emergence of an AP-1-independent function that relies on the capacity of c-Fos to activate lipid synthesis provides an explanation for many results observed upon the induction of c-Fos expression that remained obscure even though almost 35 years have passed since the first description of this protein. To the best of our knowledge, c-Fos is the first transcription factor with the capacity to regulate lipid synthesis independently of its canonical transcriptional function. The SREBPs transcription factors, for example, are tightly linked to fatty acid and cholesterol synthesis but only through their genomic activity in the nucleus (Eberle et al., 2004; Cheng et al., 2018).

Many questions regarding the cytoplasmic function of c-Fos remain to be elucidated. Clearly, c-Fos expression is related to changes in cell cycle and morphology, controlling different aspects of development (Hess et al., 2004). The fact that c-Fos can act in two different ways, either as an AP-1 transcription factor or activating lipid synthesis, raises the interrogation about how these two functions are coordinated or which are the signals that trigger one or the other function to exert a physiological/pathological role. It has been proposed that AP-1 fulfills a homeostatic role in cells in response to changes in their environment and growth conditions, adjusting gene expression so as to allow the cell to adapt to those changes (Shaulian and Karin, 2001). If we now consider the function of c-Fos as a lipid synthesis activator, the perspective must necessarily be deepened. It seems reasonable to think that the elicited function will depend on the triggering stimulus. In any case, studies must be extended in order to further elucidate this novel mechanism.

c-Fos was the first transcription factor whose induction was shown to be dependent on neuronal activity (Morgan and Curran, 1988; Sagar et al., 1988). As stated previously, this attribute rapidly transformed c-Fos into a marker for neuronal activity. The increase in its expression was observed in the central nervous system after applying learning and memory recovery protocols (Gallo et al., 2018). Interestingly, these changes in c-Fos expression were observed mainly during the first training sessions, indicating that this is probably an adaptive response. Consequently, it seems reasonable to propose that, in light of the above mentioned evidence, this adaptive response might be entailed with neuronal and synaptic plasticity processes that involve the cytoplasmic function of c-Fos: once all the new circuits related to a specific training are formed and established, the cells require a lower amount of lipids just to maintain all the pre-formed contacts. In fact, a reduction in synaptic plasticity mechanisms was found in the hippocampus of a selective *fos* knock-out mouse (Fleischmann et al., 2003).

In any case, all the background information described in the literature regarding the role of c-Fos in the physiology of the nervous system consistently confirmed its importance for cellular plasticity although they have always been associated to changes in gene expression. But, could they be related to changes in lipid homeostasis? This hypothesis seems reasonable given the evidence underlined herein. In this regard, we are currently finishing additional studies on the role of c-Fos in neuronal differentiation, using primary cultures as development models. This will allow us to unravel the mechanisms through which c-Fos participates in normal brain development.

The apparently unrelated functions of c-Fos as a transcription factor or as an activator of lipid synthesis may be related to its structural plasticity given its nature as an Intrinsically Disordered Protein (IDP), a characteristic already described for other proteins (Tompa, 2005). IDPs do not have a tridimensional defined structure in their native states (Dyson and Wright, 2005). This feature gives them the advantage of having conformational plasticity and allows them to recognize and associate with multiple, different targets (Wright and Dyson, 2009). Even though we have described that the N-terminal of c-Fos together with its BD are responsible for its association with different enzymes and their subsequent activation, it is yet to be determined if c-Fos suffers a conformational change to an ordered structure during this process.

It is promising to consider the reaches of this new role of c-Fos in physiological and pathological aspects of the nervous system. It could be involved in controlling neuronal development and in the establishment of correct neuronal circuits, or in regeneration events that require high amounts of lipid synthesis for membrane biogenesis. More importantly, the possible participation of c-Fos in lipid homeostasis in the neurobiology of disease should be approached. Highlighting the importance of lipid synthesis activation by c-Fos is the observation that, by specifically blocking its expression, proliferation and growth of tumor cells of the nervous system are slowed or halted. This discloses the cytoplasmic activity of c-Fos as a potential target for controlling growth of brain carcinomas. Future studies are being driven through this exciting road.

AUTHOR CONTRIBUTIONS

Both authors participated in the preparation of the manuscript.

FUNDING

The authors thank the financial support of the following institutions: the Secretaría de Ciencia y Técnica, Universidad Nacional de Córdoba; the Fondo para la Investigación Científica y Tecnológica, Secretaría de Ciencia, Tecnología e Innovación Productiva, Argentina; and the Instituto Nacional del Cáncer, Ministerio de Salud y Desarrollo Social, Argentina. BC is a member of and LB a fellow of CONICET (Consejo Nacional de Investigaciones Científicas y Tecnológicas), Secretaría de Ciencia, Tecnología e Innovación Productiva, Argentina.

REFERENCES

Ahmed, M. Y., Al-Khayat, A., Al-Murshedi, F., Al-Futaisi, A., Chioza, B. A., Pedro Fernandez-Murray, J., et al. (2017). A mutation of EPT1 (SELENOI) underlies a new disorder of Kennedy pathway phospholipid biosynthesis. *Brain* 140, 547–554. doi: 10.1093/brain/aww318

Alfonso Pecchio, A. R., Cardozo Gizzi, A. M., Renner, M. L., Molina-Calavita, M., and Caputto, B. L. (2011). c-Fos activates and physically interacts with specific enzymes of the pathway of synthesis of polyphosphoinositides. *Mol. Biol. Cell* 22, 4716–4725. doi: 10.1091/mbc.E11-03-0259

Angel, P., and Karin, M. (1991). The role of Jun, Fos and the AP-1 complex in cell-proliferation and transformation. *Biochim. Biophys. Acta* 1072, 129–157. doi: 10.1016/0304-419x(91)90011-9

Bazan, N. G. (2014). Is there a molecular logic that sustains neuronal functional integrity and survival? Lipid signaling is necessary for neuroprotective neuronal transcriptional programs. *Mol. Neurobiol.* 50, 1–5. doi: 10.1007/s12035-014-8897-0

Bazan, N. G., Molina, M. F., and Gordon, W. C. (2011). Docosahexaenoic acid signalolipidomics in nutrition: significance in aging, neuroinflammation, macular degeneration, Alzheimer's, and other neurodegenerative diseases. *Annu. Rev. Nutr.* 31, 321–351. doi: 10.1146/annurev.nutr.012809.104635

Bozek, K., Wei, Y., Yan, Z., Liu, X., Xiong, J., Sugimoto, M., et al. (2015). Organization and evolution of brain lipidome revealed by large-scale analysis of human, chimpanzee, macaque, and mouse tissues. *Neuron* 85, 695–702. doi: 10.1016/j.neuron.2015.01.003

Buscher, M., Rahmsdorf, H. J., Litfin, M., Karin, M., and Herrlich, P. (1988). Activation of the c-fos gene by UV and phorbol ester: different signal transduction pathways converge to the same enhancer element. *Oncogene* 3, 301–311.

Bussolino, D. F., De Arriba Zerpa, G. A., Grabois, V. R., Conde, C. B., Guido, M. E., and Caputto, B. L. (1998). Light affects c-fos expression and phospholipid synthesis in both retinal ganglion cells and photoreceptor cells in an opposite way for each cell type. *Brain Res. Mol. Brain Res.* 58, 10–15. doi: 10.1016/s0169-328x(98)00065-5

Bussolino, D. F., Guido, M. E., Gil, G. A., Borioli, G. A., Renner, M. L., Grabois, V. R., et al. (2001). c-Fos associates with the endoplasmic reticulum and activates phospholipid metabolism. *FASEB J.* 15, 556–558. doi: 10.1096/fj.00-0446fje

Caputto, B. L., Cardozo Gizzi, A. M., and Gil, G. A. (2014). c-Fos: an AP-1 transcription factor with an additional cytoplasmic, non-genomic lipid synthesis activation capacity. *Biochim. Biophys. Acta* 1841, 1241–1246. doi: 10.1016/j.bbalip.2014.05.007

Cardozo Gizzi, A. M., Prucca, C. G., Gaveglio, V. L., Renner, M. L., Pasquare, S. J., and Caputto, B. L. (2015). The catalytic efficiency of lipin 1beta increases by physically interacting with the proto-oncoprotein c-Fos. *J. Biol. Chem.* 290, 29578–29592. doi: 10.1074/jbc.M115.678821

Chang, T. Y., Yamauchi, Y., Hasan, M. T., and Chang, C. (2017). Cellular cholesterol homeostasis and Alzheimer's disease. *J. Lipid Res.* 58, 2239–2254. doi: 10.1194/jlr.R075630

Cheng, C., Geng, F., Cheng, X., and Guo, D. (2018). Lipid metabolism reprogramming and its potential targets in cancer. *Cancer Commun.* 38:27.

Crespo, P. M., Silvestre, D. C., Gil, G. A., Maccioni, H. J., Daniotti, J. L., and Caputto, B. L. (2008). c-Fos activates glucosylceramide synthase and glycolipid synthesis in PC12 cells. *J. Biol. Chem.* 283, 31163–31171. doi: 10.1074/jbc.M709257200

Curran, T., and Franza, B. R. (1988). Fos and Jun: the AP-1 connection. *Cell* 55, 395–397. doi: 10.1016/0092-8674(88)90024-4

Dragunow, M. (1996). A role for immediate-early transcription factors in learning and memory. *Behav. Genet.* 26, 293–299. doi: 10.1007/bf02359385

Dyson, H. J., and Wright, P. E. (2005). Intrinsically unstructured proteins and their functions. *Nat. Rev. Mol. Cell. Biol.* 6, 197–208. doi: 10.1038/nrm1589

Eberle, D., Hegarty, B., Bossard, P., Ferre, P., and Foufelle, F. (2004). SREBP transcription factors: master regulators of lipid homeostasis. *Biochimie* 86, 839–848. doi: 10.1016/j.biochi.2004.09.018

Farooqui, A. A. (2012). Lipid mediators and their metabolism in the nucleous: implications for Alzheimer's disease. *J. Alzheimers Dis.* 30(Suppl. 2), S163–S178. doi: 10.3233/JAD-2011-111085

Ferreira-Vieira, T. H., Guimaraes, I. M., Silva, F. R., and Ribeiro, F. M. (2016). Alzheimer's disease: targeting the cholinergic system. *Curr. Neuropharmacol.* 14, 101–115.

Ferrero, G. O., Renner, M. L., Gil, G. A., Rodriguez-Berdini, L., and Caputto, B. L. (2014). c-Fos-activated synthesis of nuclear phosphatidylinositol 4,5-bisphosphate [PtdIns(4,5)P(2)] promotes global transcriptional changes. *Biochem. J.* 461, 521–530. doi: 10.1042/bj20131376

Ferrero, G. O., Velazquez, F. N., and Caputto, B. L. (2012). The kinase c-Src and the phosphatase TC45 coordinately regulate c-Fos tyrosine phosphorylation and c-Fos phospholipid synthesis activation capacity. *Oncogene* 31, 3381–3391. doi: 10.1038/onc.2011.510

Fleischmann, A., Hvalby, O., Jensen, V., Strekalova, T., Zacher, C., Layer, L. E., et al. (2003). Impaired long-term memory and NR2A-type NMDA receptor-dependent synaptic plasticity in mice lacking c-Fos in the CNS. *J. Neurosci.* 23, 9116–9122. doi: 10.1523/jneurosci.23-27-09116.2003

Gallo, F. T., Katche, C., Morici, J. F., Medina, J. H., and Weisstaub, N. V. (2018). Immediate early genes, memory and psychiatric disorders: focus on c-Fos, Egr1 and Arc. *Front. Behav. Neurosci.* 12:79. doi: 10.3389/fnbeh.2018.00079

Gaspar, R., Pallbo, J., Weininger, U., Linse, S., and Sparr, E. (2018). Ganglioside lipids accelerate alpha-synuclein amyloid formation. *Biochim. Biophys. Acta Proteins Proteom.* doi: 10.1016/j.bbapap.2018.07.004 [Epub ahead of print].

Gil, G. A., Bussolino, D. F., Portal, M. M., Alfonso Pecchio, A., Renner, M. L., Borioli, G. A., et al. (2004). c-Fos activated phospholipid synthesis is required for neurite elongation in differentiating PC12 cells. *Mol. Biol. Cell* 15, 1881–1894. doi: 10.1091/mbc.e03-09-0705

Glover, J. N., and Harrison, S. C. (1995). Crystal structure of the heterodimeric bZIP transcription factor c-Fos-c-Jun bound to DNA. *Nature* 373, 257–261. doi: 10.1038/373257a0

Gonzalez, C., and Couve, A. (2014). The axonal endoplasmic reticulum and protein trafficking: cellular bootlegging south of the soma. *Semin. Cell Dev. Biol.* 27, 23–31. doi: 10.1016/j.semcdb.2013.12.004

Grimm, R., and Tischmeyer, W. (1997). Complex patterns of immediate early gene induction in rat brain following brightness discrimination training and pseudotraining. *Behav. Brain Res.* 84, 109–116. doi: 10.1016/s0166-4328(97)83330-x

Guido, M. E., De Arriba Zerpa, G. A., Bussolino, D. F., and Caputto, B. L. (1996). Immediate early gene c-fos regulates the synthesis of phospholipids but not of gangliosides. *J. Neurosci. Res.* 43, 93–98. doi: 10.1002/jnr.490430112

Habchi, J., Chia, S., Galvagnion, C., Michaels, T. C. T., Bellaiche, M. M. J., Ruggeri, F. S., et al. (2018). Cholesterol catalyses Abeta42 aggregation through a heterogeneous nucleation pathway in the presence of lipid membranes. *Nat. Chem.* 10, 673–683. doi: 10.1038/s41557-018-0031-x

Hamilton, J. A., Hillard, C. J., Spector, A. A., and Watkins, P. A. (2007). Brain uptake and utilization of fatty acids, lipids and lipoproteins: application to neurological disorders. *J. Mol. Neurosci.* 33, 2–11. doi: 10.1007/s12031-007-0060-1

Herdegen, T., and Waetzig, V. (2001). AP-1 proteins in the adult brain: facts and fiction about effectors of neuroprotection and neurodegeneration. *Oncogene* 20, 2424–2437. doi: 10.1038/sj.onc.1204387

Hess, J., Angel, P., and Schorpp-Kistner, M. (2004). AP-1 subunits: quarrel and harmony among siblings. *J. Cell Sci.* 117, 5965–5973. doi: 10.1242/jcs.01589

Hooijmans, C. R., Van Der Zee, C. E., Dederen, P. J., Brouwer, K. M., Reijmer, Y. D., Van Groen, T., et al. (2009). DHA and cholesterol containing diets influence Alzheimer-like pathology, cognition and cerebral vasculature in APPswe/PS1dE9 mice. *Neurobiol. Dis.* 33, 482–498. doi: 10.1016/j.nbd.2008.12.002

Kim, H. Y., Huang, B. X., and Spector, A. A. (2014). Phosphatidylserine in the brain: metabolism and function. *Prog. Lipid Res.* 56, 1–18. doi: 10.1016/j.plipres.2014.06.002

Lauwers, E., Goodchild, R., and Verstreken, P. (2016). Membrane lipids in presynaptic function and disease. *Neuron* 90, 11–25. doi: 10.1016/j.neuron.2016.02.033

Ledeen, R. W. (1985). *Transport, Exchange, and Transfer of Phospholipids in the Nervous System.* New York, NY: John Wiley & Sons Inc.

Lindsey, J. D., and Ellisman, M. H. (1985). The neuronal endomembrane system. III. The origins of the axoplasmic reticulum and discrete axonal cisternae at the axon hillock. *J. Neurosci.* 5, 3135–3144. doi: 10.1523/jneurosci.05-12-03135.1985

Luarte, A., Cornejo, V. H., Bertin, F., Gallardo, J., and Couve, A. (2018). The axonal endoplasmic reticulum: one organelle-many functions in development, maintenance, and plasticity. *Dev. Neurobiol.* 78, 181–208. doi: 10.1002/dneu.22560

Lukiw, W. J., and Bazan, N. G. (2000). Neuroinflammatory signaling upregulation in Alzheimer's disease. *Neurochem. Res.* 25, 1173–1184.

Milde-Langosch, K. (2005). The Fos family of transcription factors and their role in tumourigenesis. *Eur. J. Cancer* 41, 2449–2461. doi: 10.1016/j.ejca.2005.08.008

Miller, A. D., Curran, T., and Verma, I. M. (1984). c-fos protein can induce cellular transformation: a novel mechanism of activation of a cellular oncogene. *Cell* 36, 51–60. doi: 10.1016/0092-8674(84)90073-4

Minatohara, K., Akiyoshi, M., and Okuno, H. (2015). Role of immediate-early genes in synaptic plasticity and neuronal ensembles underlying the memory trace. *Front. Mol. Neurosci.* 8:78. doi: 10.3389/fnmol.2015.00078

Morgan, J. I., and Curran, T. (1988). Calcium as a modulator of the immediate-early gene cascade in neurons. *Cell Calcium* 9, 303–311. doi: 10.1016/0143-4160(88)90011-5

Motrich, R. D., Castro, G. M., and Caputto, B. L. (2013). Old players with a newly defined function: Fra-1 and c-Fos support growth of human malignant breast tumors by activating membrane biogenesis at the cytoplasm. *PLoS One* 8:e53211. doi: 10.1371/journal.pone.0053211

Oster, T., and Pillot, T. (2010). Docosahexaenoic acid and synaptic protection in Alzheimer's disease mice. *Biochim. Biophys. Acta* 1801, 791–798. doi: 10.1016/j.bbalip.2010.02.011

Palay, S. L. (1958). The morphology of synapses in the central nervous system. *Exp Cell Res* 14, 275–293.

Palumbo, S. (2017). "Pathogenesis and progression of multiple sclerosis: the role of arachidonic acid-mediated neuroinflammation," in *Multiple Sclerosis: Perspectives in Treatment and Pathogenesis*, eds I. S. Zagon and P. J. Mclaughlin (Brisbane: Codon Publications).

Penke, B., Paragi, G., Gera, J., Berkecz, R., Kovacs, Z., Crul, T., et al. (2018). The role of lipids and membranes in the pathogenesis of Alzheimer's disease: a comprehensive view. *Curr. Alzheimer Res.* 15, 1191–1212. doi: 10.2174/1567205015666180911151716

Pepeu, G., and Grazia Giovannini, M. (2017). The fate of the brain cholinergic neurons in neurodegenerative diseases. *Brain Res.* 1670, 173–184. doi: 10.1016/j.brainres.2017.06.023

Pfenninger, K. H. (2009). Plasma membrane expansion: a neuron's Herculean task. *Nat. Rev. Neurosci.* 10, 251–261. doi: 10.1038/nrn2593

Piechaczyk, M., and Blanchard, J. M. (1994). c-fos proto-oncogene regulation and function. *Crit. Rev. Oncol. Hematol.* 17, 93–131. doi: 10.1016/1040-8428(94)90021-3

Portal, M. M., Ferrero, G. O., and Caputto, B. L. (2007). N-Terminal c-Fos tyrosine phosphorylation regulates c-Fos/ER association and c-Fos-dependent phospholipid synthesis activation. *Oncogene* 26, 3551–3558. doi: 10.1038/sj.onc.1210137

Posse de Chaves, E., Vance, D. E., Campenot, R. B., and Vance, J. E. (1995). Axonal synthesis of phosphatidylcholine is required for normal axonal growth in rat sympathetic neurons. *J. Cell Biol.* 128, 913–918. doi: 10.1083/jcb.128.5.913

Raivich, G., and Behrens, A. (2006). Role of the AP-1 transcription factor c-Jun in developing, adult and injured brain. *Prog. Neurobiol.* 78, 347–363. doi: 10.1016/j.pneurobio.2006.03.006

Rambourg, A., and Droz, B. (1980). Smooth endoplasmic reticulum and axonal transport. *J. Neurochem.* 35, 16–25. doi: 10.1111/j.1471-4159.1980.tb12484.x

Rosen, J. B., Fanselow, M. S., Young, S. L., Sitcoske, M., and Maren, S. (1998). Immediate-early gene expression in the amygdala following footshock stress and contextual fear conditioning. *Brain Res.* 796, 132–142. doi: 10.1016/s0006-8993(98)00294-7

Sagar, S. M., Sharp, F. R., and Curran, T. (1988). Expression of c-fos protein in brain: metabolic mapping at the cellular level. *Science* 240, 1328–1331. doi: 10.1126/science.3131879

Sanchez-Mejia, R. O., and Mucke, L. (2010). Phospholipase A2 and arachidonic acid in Alzheimer's disease. *Biochim. Biophys. Acta* 1801, 784–790. doi: 10.1016/j.bbalip.2010.05.013

Sastry, P. S. (1985). Lipids of nervous tissue: composition and metabolism. *Prog. Lipid Res.* 24, 69–176. doi: 10.1016/0163-7827(85)90011-6

Shaulian, E., and Karin, M. (2001). AP-1 in cell proliferation and survival. *Oncogene* 20, 2390–2400. doi: 10.1038/sj.onc.1204383

Silvestre, D. C., Gil, G. A., Tomasini, N., Bussolino, D. F., and Caputto, B. L. (2010). Growth of peripheral and central nervous system tumors is supported by cytoplasmic c-Fos in humans and mice. *PLoS One* 5:e9544. doi: 10.1371/journal.pone.0009544

Simon, M. V., Agnolazza, D. L., German, O. L., Garelli, A., Politi, L. E., Agbaga, M. P., et al. (2016). Synthesis of docosahexaenoic acid from eicosapentaenoic acid in retina neurons protects photoreceptors from oxidative stress. *J. Neurochem.* 136, 931–946. doi: 10.1111/jnc.13487

Strokin, M., Chechneva, O., Reymann, K. G., and Reiser, G. (2006). Neuroprotection of rat hippocampal slices exposed to oxygen-glucose deprivation by enrichment with docosahexaenoic acid and by inhibition of hydrolysis of docosahexaenoic acid-containing phospholipids by calcium independent phospholipase A2. *Neuroscience* 140, 547–553. doi: 10.1016/j.neuroscience.2006.02.026

Tayebati, S. K. (2018). Phospholipid and Lipid Derivatives as Potential Neuroprotective Compounds. *Molecules* 23:E2257. doi: 10.3390/molecules23092257

Terasaki, M. (2018). Axonal endoplasmic reticulum is very narrow. *J. Cell Sci.* 131:jcs210450. doi: 10.1242/jcs.210450

Tompa, P. (2005). The interplay between structure and function in intrinsically unstructured proteins. *FEBS Lett.* 579, 3346–3354. doi: 10.1016/j.febslet.2005.03.072

Tracey, T. J., Steyn, F. J., Wolvetang, E. J., and Ngo, S. T. (2018). Neuronal lipid metabolism: multiple pathways driving functional outcomes in health and disease. *Front. Mol. Neurosci.* 11:10. doi: 10.3389/fnmol.2018.00010

Tsukita, S., and Ishikawa, H. (1976). Three-dimensional distribution of smooth endoplasmic reticulum in myelinated axons. *J. Electron. Microsc.* 25, 141–149.

Tulchinsky, E. (2000). Fos family members: regulation, structure and role in oncogenic transformation. *Histol. Histopathol.* 15, 921–928. doi: 10.14670/HH-15.921

Valadas, J. S., Esposito, G., Vandekerkhove, D., Miskiewicz, K., Deaulmerie, L., Raitano, S., et al. (2018). ER lipid defects in neuropeptidergic neurons impair sleep patterns in Parkinson's disease. *Neuron* 98, 1155–1169.e6. doi: 10.1016/j.neuron.2018.05.022

van Meer, G., Voelker, D. R., and Feigenson, G. W. (2008). Membrane lipids: where they are and how they behave. *Nat. Rev. Mol. Cell. Biol.* 9, 112–124. doi: 10.1038/nrm2330

Vance, J. E., Campenot, R. B., and Vance, D. E. (2000). The synthesis and transport of lipids for axonal growth and nerve regeneration. *Biochim. Biophys. Acta* 1486, 84–96. doi: 10.1016/s1388-1981(00)00050-0

Vance, J. E., Pan, D., Campenot, R. B., Bussiere, M., and Vance, D. E. (1994). Evidence that the major membrane lipids, except cholesterol, are made in axons of cultured rat sympathetic neurons. *J. Neurochem.* 62, 329–337. doi: 10.1046/j.1471-4159.1994.62010329.x

Vance, J. E., Pan, D., Vance, D. E., and Campenot, R. B. (1991). Biosynthesis of membrane lipids in rat axons. *J. Cell Biol.* 115, 1061–1068. doi: 10.1083/jcb.115.4.1061

Velazquez, F. N., Caputto, B. L., and Boussin, F. D. (2015a). c-Fos importance for brain development. *Aging* 7, 1028–1029. doi: 10.18632/aging.100862

Velazquez, F. N., Prucca, C. G., Etienne, O., D'astolfo, D. S., Silvestre, D. C., Boussin, F. D., et al. (2015b). Brain development is impaired in c-fos -/- mice. *Oncotarget* 6, 16883–16901.

Wang, H. (2014). Lipid rafts: a signaling platform linking cholesterol metabolism to synaptic deficits in autism spectrum disorders. *Front. Behav. Neurosci.* 8:104. doi: 10.3389/fnbeh.2014.00104

Weiss, P., and Hiscoe, H. B. (1948). Experiments on the mechanism of nerve growth. *J. Exp. Zool.* 107, 315–395. doi: 10.1002/jez.1401070302

Wollnik, F., Brysch, W., Uhlmann, E., Gillardon, F., Bravo, R., Zimmermann, M., et al. (1995). Block of c-Fos and JunB expression by antisense oligonucleotides inhibits light-induced phase shifts of the mammalian circadian clock. *Eur. J. Neurosci.* 7, 388–393. doi: 10.1111/j.1460-9568.1995.tb00334.x

Wright, P. E., and Dyson, H. J. (2009). Linking folding and binding. *Curr. Opin. Struct. Biol.* 19, 31–38. doi: 10.1016/j.sbi.2008.12.003

Yu, Q., He, Z., Zubkov, D., Huang, S., Kurochkin, I., Yang, X., et al. (2018). Lipidome alterations in human prefrontal cortex during development, aging, and cognitive disorders. *Mol. Psychiatry* doi: 10.1038/s41380-018-0200-8 [Epub ahead of print].

8

Phosphatidic Acid: From Pleiotropic Functions to Neuronal Pathology

Emeline Tanguy[1], *Qili Wang*[1], *Hervé Moine*[2] *and Nicolas Vitale*[1]*

[1]*Institut des Neurosciences Cellulaires et Intégratives (INCI), UPR-3212 Centre National de la Recherche Scientifique & Université de Strasbourg, Strasbourg, France,* [2]*Institut de Génétique et de Biologie Moléculaire et Cellulaire (IGBMC), CNRS UMR 7104, INSERM U964, Université de Strasbourg, Illkirch-Graffenstaden, France*

***Correspondence:**
Nicolas Vitale
vitalen@unistra.fr

Among the cellular lipids, phosphatidic acid (PA) is a peculiar one as it is at the same time a key building block of phospholipid synthesis and a major lipid second messenger conveying signaling information. The latter is thought to largely occur through the ability of PA to recruit and/or activate specific proteins in restricted compartments and within those only at defined submembrane areas. Furthermore, with its cone-shaped geometry PA locally changes membrane topology and may thus be a key player in membrane trafficking events, especially in membrane fusion and fission steps, where lipid remodeling is believed to be crucial. These pleiotropic cellular functions of PA, including phospholipid synthesis and homeostasis together with important signaling activity, imply that perturbations of PA metabolism could lead to serious pathological conditions. In this mini-review article, after outlining the main cellular functions of PA, we highlight the different neurological diseases that could, at least in part, be attributed to an alteration in PA synthesis and/or catabolism.

Keywords: lipid signaling, neuron, neuropathology, phosphatidic acid, phospholipase D

INTRODUCTION

Phosphatidic acid (PA) is a low abundant phospholipid of membranes that, nevertheless, constitutes the original building block from which most glycerophospholipids are synthesized, thus plays an important structural task. Interestingly it was later shown that PA also acts to transmit, amplify, and regulate a great number of intracellular signaling pathways and cellular functions. In cells, PA can be synthesized through different enzymatic pathways (Ammar et al., 2014). Structural PA results from two successive acylation reactions (**Figure 1**). Signaling PA instead, results from three biosynthesis alternative pathways. The first pathway includes the phosphorylation of diacylglycerol (DAG) by any of the 10 DAG-kinases (DGKs) in mammals (**Figure 1**). Hydrolysis of the distal phosphodiester bond in phospholipids by phospholipases D (PLD) constitutes the second pathway (**Figure 1**). Although six different PLDs have been identified in mammals, only PLD1/2 and PLD6 have been shown to synthesize PA from phosphatidylcholine (PC) and cardiolipin (CL), respectively (Jang et al., 2012). The third and final biosynthetic pathway involves acylation of lyso-PA by lyso-PA-acyltransferase (LPAAT) enzymes (**Figure 1**).

Chemically, PA is composed of a glycerol backbone esterified with two fatty acyl chains at positions C-1 and C-2, and with a phosphate at position C-3. The latter confers the specific features of PA compared to the other diacyl-glycerophospholipids. Indeed, the small anionic phosphate headgroup provides to PA a combination of unique cone-shaped geometry and negative charge (Jenkins and Frohman, 2005). At the molecular level, these two characteristics enable PA both to

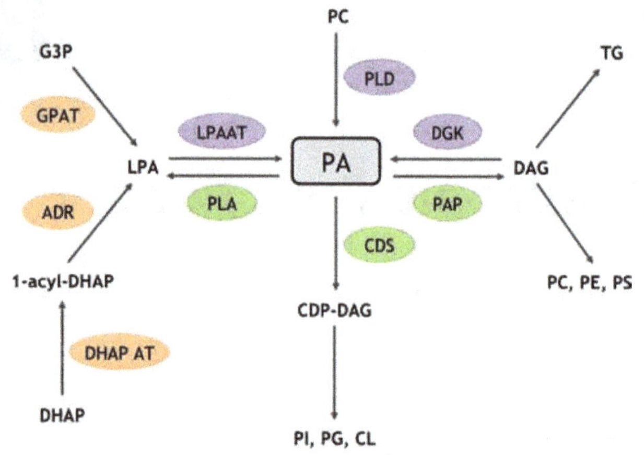

FIGURE 1 | Enzymatic routes for structural and signaling PA metabolism. PA is a major phospholipid for biosynthetic and signaling reactions. Enzymes highlighted in orange are involved in biosynthetic reactions that produce structural PA, whereas enzymes triggering the formation of signaling pools of PA are shown in purple. Enzymes responsible for PA catabolism are shown in green. ADR, Acyldihydroxyacetone-phosphate reductase; CDP, cytidyl phosphatidate; CDS, CDP-diacylglycerol (DAG) synthase; CL, cardiolipin; DHAP, dihydroxyacétone phosphate; DHAP AT, dihydroxyacétone phosphate acyltransferase; G3P, glycerol 3-phosphate; GPAT, glycerol phosphate acyltransferase; PAP, phosphatidic acid phosphatase; PC, phosphatidylcholine; PG, phosphatidylglycerol; PE, phosphatidylethanolamine; PI, phosphatidylinositol; PS, phosphatidylserine; PLA, phospholipase A; TG, triglyceride.

interact with different enzymes to regulate their catalytic activity and/or their association with membrane compartments and also to affect membrane geometry by creating local negative curvatures (Kooijman et al., 2003). As a consequence, PA has been involved in various important cellular functions including membrane trafficking events where membrane rearrangements are necessary (Bader and Vitale, 2009). In this article, we will present some of the most studied PA identified partners, summarize the most well-described cellular processes that require PA and discuss the potential involvement of an alteration in PA synthesis and/or catabolism in different neurological diseases.

PA INTERACTS WITH AND RECRUITS NUMEROUS PROTEINS TO MEMBRANES

Having an overall view of the interaction network of a given molecule is particularly helpful for deciphering the relationships between the constituents of interactomes and characterizing their function in cell signaling. Since the early description of a handful of proteins that bind to PA, at least using the minimal *in vitro* protein-lipid overlay assay, an extensive list of PA interactors has only emerged more recently (Stace and Ktistakis, 2006). For at least some of those, their interaction with PA appears rather specific with little or no interaction with other negatively charged lipids. The position of PA's phosphomonoester headgroup in proximity of the interface of acyl chain headgroup was proposed to be important for binding to specific proteins. Supporting the physiological importance of interactions between PA and proteins, numerous proteins have gained domains that display some level of binding specificity for PA (Jang et al., 2012). Although no clear PA-binding domain can be defined at the three dimensional or secondary structural levels, different factors can influence PA interaction with specific domains in target proteins (Tanguy et al., 2018). For instance, we and others have found that some PA-binding modules possess some levels of specificity for the fatty acyl chains of PA (Kassas et al., 2017). In addition, the local membrane environment surrounding PA also appears to modulate PA binding to these modules (Kassas et al., 2017). Finally, it is most likely that PA-binding domains act first through positively charged residues that initially sample for the negative charge of PA buried within the membrane. This first step is probably followed by a docking state where hydrophobic interaction between hydrophobic residues of the module and the fatty acyl chains of PA stabilize the PA-protein interaction (Potocký et al., 2014; Tanguy et al., 2018). At present, more than 50 different proteins have been shown to directly interact with PA, as extensively reviewed in Jang et al. (2012). Briefly, these PA interactors can be classified in four major families.

Nucleotide-Binding Proteins

Nucleotide (ATP, cAMP, GTP)-binding proteins are important signaling proteins for which the activity is usually regulated by nucleotide binding. Noticeably, the localization and/or activity of many of those proteins are also controlled by PA interaction. This is for instance the case for some of the small GTP-binding proteins of the ADP ribosylation factor (Arf) and Rho (Ras homologous) families that are key players in cytoskeleton remodeling and membrane dynamics. The minimal PA-binding regions of these small GTPases remains however to be defined precisely. Several c-AMP specific phosphodiesterases also interact with PA through their amino-terminal regulatory domains leading to an increase of their enzymatic activity and therefore to a reduction of cAMP levels.

Regulators of GTP-Binding Proteins

The GTPase-activating proteins ArfGAP with GTPase Domain, Ankyrin Repeat and PH domain 1 (AGAP1) and Regulator of G protein Signaling 4 (RGS4) are negative regulators of Arf and Gα GTP-binding proteins, respectively. Intriguingly, while PA stimulates the GTP-hydrolysis activity of AGAP1, it inhibits that of RGS4, highlighting the multiple and sometimes opposite actions of PA on GTP-binding activity. Furthermore, PA has also been shown to recruit and activate different guanine nucleotide-exchange proteins for small GTPases, such as DedicatOr of CytoKinesis 2 (DOCK2) and Son Of Sevenless (SOS), promoting GTP-binding and activation of Rac and Ras, respectively. It is therefore important to have in mind that PA enrichment in particular sub-membrane domains could influence in different and sometimes contradictory manners a given signaling pathway involving GTP-binding proteins by acting at different stages.

Kinases

Protein kinases are among the main signaling regulators with nearly 600 different genes. Among those, protein kinase C (PKC) is one of the largest subgroup and PA modulates the activity of several PKC isoforms. PA also promotes recruitment and activation of the proto-oncogene kinase Raf, acting as a gatekeeper in the ERK1/2 pathway. In addition, PA binding to the FKBP12-rapamycin binding region of mTOR is in competition with FKBP12/rapamycin complex of mTOR and is thus likely to influence nutrient sensing and cell proliferation.

Furthermore, lipid kinases contribute to the great diversity of lipids in cells. Among those, PA is capable to stimulate the action of phosphatidylinositol (PI) 4-phosphate 5-kinase (PI4P5K), to promote the synthesis of PI 4,5-bisphosphate ($PI(4,5)P_2$), a key signaling lipid (Stace and Ktistakis, 2006; Bader and Vitale, 2009). Finally, cytosolic sphingosine kinase that transforms sphingosine into sphingosine-phosphate appears to translocate to the plasma membrane under the control of PA levels, which most likely affects the signaling pathways involving these two lipids. In conclusion, PA binding modules are found in members of the two major kinase families and consequently, the presence of PA in local membrane composition is expected to influence crucial signaling nodes and the various associated key cellular functions.

Phosphatases

In addition to kinases, phosphatases constitute the second important family of signaling proteins that modulate protein activity by removing the phosphate residues added by kinases. The protein-tyrosine phosphatase SHP-1 that negatively modulates signaling pathways involving receptor-tyrosine kinase directly interacts with PA therefore triggering phosphatase activity. Furthermore, PA inhibits the enzymatic activity of protein phosphatase 1 (PP1), involved in many cellular activities such as the metabolism of glycogen, the processing of RNA, and the regulation of cell cycle. In conclusion, although not as well described as for kinases, the regulation of several phosphatases by PA offers the possibility of complex and often paradoxical regulation of signaling pathway by a single lipid family.

THE PLEIOTROPIC CELLULAR FUNCTIONS OF PA

Actin Cytoskeleton Dynamics

Most cellular functions are influenced by precise cell shapes that are under the control of the cytoskeleton proteins network. Among those the dynamics of the cytoskeleton depends on the formation of actin filaments from a pool of cytosolic monomers, and their subsequent association to each other or to cell membranes, pursued by their depolymerization. Most cellular functions actually depend on a permanent remodeling of this actin network and this is orchestrated in large part by actin binding proteins. Interestingly lipids such as phosphoinositides modulate the affinity of these proteins for actin. PA, however, has also been proposed to participate to this regulation (Ammar et al., 2014).

In neurons, the Rho GTPases and related proteins, through the control of the cytoskeleton, modulate various aspects of cell shape including not only neurite outgrowth and differentiation, axonal growth and targeting, but also dendritic spine formation and maintenance (Ammar et al., 2014). As mentioned in the sections "Nucleotide-Binding Proteins" and "Regulators of GTP-Binding Proteins," PA synthesized by either PLD or DGK modulates the activity of some different Rho family of GTPases and their regulators by promoting membrane association and/or through the activation of their regulatory proteins (Chae et al., 2008; Nishikimi et al., 2009; Faugaret et al., 2011; Kurooka et al., 2011; Sanematsu et al., 2013). Alternatively, the p21 activated kinases (PAKs) family that regulates various aspects of neuronal development, through actin cytoskeleton reorganization, is also known for being activated by PA (Daniels et al., 1998; Hayashi et al., 2007). Furthermore, $PI(4,5)P_2$ is a major lipid regulator of the cytoskeleton and PA is an essential building block leading to $PI(4,5)P_2$ synthesis (**Figure 1**). In an alternative pathway, PA stimulates the phospholipid kinase PI4P5K, leading to the phosphorylation of the membrane phospholipid PI(4)P and the formation of $PI(4,5)P_2$ (Honda et al., 1999). In consequence, PA potentially regulates the activity of the three mammalian PI4P5K isozymes that have been described to control actin cytoskeleton reorganization (van den Bout and Divecha, 2009; Roach et al., 2012). Finally, PA levels regulate membrane localization and activity of PKC isoforms α, ε and ζ, all of which are known to affect the morphology of the actin cytoskeleton (Jose Lopez-Andreo et al., 2003).

It is also worth noting that direct interaction of PA with actin-binding proteins has been suggested. Among those potential candidates, the actin-binding protein vinculin known to be involved in neurite outgrowth is a good example (Ito et al., 1982; Johnson and Craig, 1995), but the specificity of these observations remains to be firmly established, since vinculin also binds to other negatively charged lipids, such as $PI(4,5)P_2$.

Membrane Remodeling Events

The secretory pathways have evolved through the establishment of specialized subcellular compartments dedicated to specific biochemical tasks. Membrane trafficking events between these compartments enable particular cells of complex organisms to secrete informative molecules such as hormones, cytokines, and neurotransmitters, for long distance inter-cellular communication. In addition to dedicated and specialized protein machineries, trafficking events of the regulated exocytosis and endocytosis steps also involve remarkable membrane rearrangements that rely on specific lipids (Ammar et al., 2013b). Hence, the first direct molecular data suggesting a role for PLD1-generated PA in hormone release were obtained in chromaffin cells, where overexpression of PLD1, injection of a catalytically-inactive PLD1 mutant (Vitale et al., 2001) or PLD1 silencing (Zeniou-Meyer et al., 2007) affected catecholamine release rates. Using similar approaches, PA synthesized by PLD1 was also shown to govern the regulated secretion of insulin from β-pancreatic cells (Waselle et al., 2005), of von Willebrand factor from endothelial cells (Disse et al., 2009), and acrosomal exocytosis from sperm cells (Lopez et al., 2012; Pelletán et al., 2015). An additional contribution for PA in secretion has been established during the early phase of azurophilic granules release in neutrophils triggered by anti-neutrophil cytoplasmic antibodies (Williams et al., 2007). Ultimately, different enzymes controlling PA metabolism such as PLDs, LPAATs and DGKs have been proposed to regulate neurotransmission in several neuronal models, suggesting that PA regulates synaptic vesicle release and cycle (Humeau et al., 2001; Schwarz et al., 2011; Tabet et al., 2016a,b; Raben and Barber, 2017).

Intense membrane remodeling also occurs in specialized phagocytic cells, such as in macrophages. Indeed, the ingestion of pathogens, cell debris, or any other solid particle through the formation of phagosomes requires plasma membrane extension and either local lipid synthesis, transfer, or vesicular fusion. PA synthesis by PLD2 has been shown to be important for this early step of phagocytosis, while PA synthesis by PLD1 appears to be also important for the later step of phagosome maturation (Corrotte et al., 2006, 2010). Of note, PA transfer from the ER to plasma membrane during "frustrated phagocytosis," a model where macrophages are plated on IgG-coated plates, has also been suggested to occur from experiments using a combination of lipidomic analysis performed on subcellular fractions and novel PA sensors (Kassas et al., 2017). Furthermore, PA is involved in the invasion and exit of infected cells by apicomplexan parasites (Bullen et al., 2016). It was shown that PA is required for the release of adhesins, perforins and proteases from specialized organelles from these parasites called micronemes (Bullen et al., 2016).

Additional intracellular trafficking events involving intense membrane remodeling have also been shown to require modification in PA levels. To cite only a few, we can also mention that PA critically regulates vesicle budding from the Golgi (Yang et al., 2008), autophagy (Holland et al., 2016), and exosome release (Ghossoub et al., 2014). The mechanisms by which PA promotes membrane rearrangements remain however an unsolved issue (**Figure 2**). The first proposed mode of action of PA in membrane remodeling may depends on its ability to induce membrane curvature and promote fusion, but its ability to specifically regulate the activity of different proteins involved in the vesicle docking and/or recruit crucial fusion proteins has also been proposed (Tanguy et al., 2016, 2018). In a simplified model for membrane fusion a mixture of lipids and proteins appear to be crucial at the fusion site (Tanguy et al., 2016). In principle the intrinsic negative curvatures of accumulating cone-shaped lipids, such as PA in the inner (cis) leaflets of contacting bilayers, should facilitate fusion of merging membranes. But it is worth noting that the promotion of membrane fusion through local modification of membrane curvature also appears to hold true for other cone-shaped lipids such as cholesterol and DAG (Tanguy et al., 2016). Reconstituted membrane fusion assays have been valuable to dissect the role of individual components and on this instance it is important to highlight that PA was observed playing a unique role among cone-shaped lipids in a yeast vacuole fusion assay, suggesting a more complex mode of action of this lipid (Mima and Wickner, 2009). Furthermore, PA could locally accumulate and form microdomains highly negatively charged, which potentially serve as membrane retention sites for several proteins key for exocytosis, such as the SNARE protein syntaxin-1 (Lam et al., 2008), or other membrane remodeling processes (Jenkins and Frohman, 2005). Finally, as a precursor for DAG and PI(4,5)P_2, both known to contribute to numerous membrane remodeling events, PA could also have indirect effects. All these potential contributions of PA in membrane fusion have been reviewed elsewhere (Chasserot-Golaz et al., 2010; Ammar et al., 2013b, 2014; Tanguy et al., 2016), but solving the issue of the mechanistic role of PA in a given membrane remodeling process requires probing these different scenarios (**Figure 2**), which is now in need for novel methods and tools.

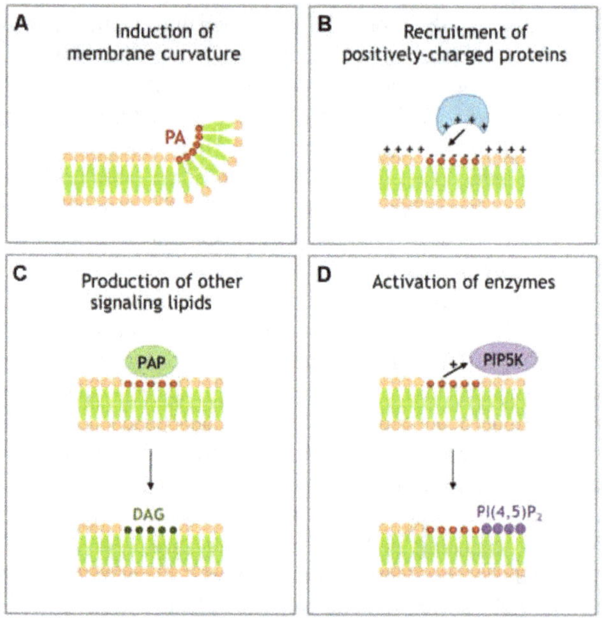

FIGURE 2 | Different models for signaling activity of PA. **(A)** Local accumulation of PA in a single leaflet of membrane generates negative membrane curvature. **(B)** Local accumulation of PA generates local buildup of negative charges that recruit PA effector-containing positively charged domains. **(C)** PAPs transforms PA into DAG, another signaling lipid with specific activity. **(D)** PA stimulates the activity of phosphatidylinositol 4-phosphate 5-kinase (PI4P5K), producing PI 4,5-bisphosphate (PI(4,5)P_2), an additional important signaling lipid.

Apoptosis, Survival, Growth, Proliferation and Migration

Many survival signals including hormones and growth factors activate PA synthesis through the stimulation of PLD activity. Similarly, mitogenic signals trigger cell proliferation, suppression of cell cycle arrest, and prevention of apoptosis. The PLD–PA–Rheb–mTOR and the PLD–PA–MAP kinase pathways are the two main downstream pathways of PLD involved in mitogenic signals and have been described extensively (Foster, 2009). Obviously, future solving of the complex imbrication of these pathways and understanding of the spatiotemporal relationships between PA-generating enzymes, PA-binding partners and PA itself will require development of more specific tools and extensive work.

NEUROLOGICAL DISORDERS POTENTIALLY LINKED TO AN ALTERATION OF PA LEVELS

In all organisms from yeast to mammals, PA was shown to possess signaling activity (Jenkins and Frohman, 2005) and a recent review highlights the apparent mystery of the many roles of PA in plants (Pokotylo et al., 2018). In addition, various PA-generating enzymes were shown to be involved in an increasing number of neuronal pathologies, suggesting a fundamental role of PA in the outcome of these neurodiseases (Tanguy et al., 2018). In the next chapter, we will describe four neuronal pathologies that may be the consequence, at least partially, of an alteration in PA dynamics.

Fetal Alcohol Spectrum Disorders

The damaging effects of alcohol drinking during gestation on the developing fetus are extremely well documented (Ehrhart et al., 2018). Fetal alcohol spectrum disorders (FASDs) is a generic term used to define the birth deficiencies that result from prenatal exposure to alcohol that range from mild to severe. These developmental defects on unborn infants have lifelong physical, behavioral, and cognitive disabilities. As alcohol consumption avoidance during pregnancy is in theory easy to achieve, FASD is in fact considered as one of the largest preventable forms of non-genetic birth disabilities associated with intellectual incapacity.

Although the main effort remains prevention of alcohol consumption during pregnancy, it is also important to understand the underlying pathological mechanisms involved in these effects of ethanol. In addition to the well-recognized ethanol and acetaldehyde toxicity, alcohol intensifies oxidative stress causing consequent effects such as DNA, protein and membrane damages. Additionally, it has been known for over three decades that in the presence of 1%–3% of ethanol, the two best characterized mammalian isoforms PLD1 and PLD2 catalyze a transphosphatidylation reaction. In this case alcohol replaces water during PC hydrolysis, and phosphatidyl alcohols are formed at the expense of PA (Jenkins and Frohman, 2005). Thus, in presence of ethanol, phosphatidylethanol is synthesized while PA is not. Since it is likely that phosphatidylethanol cannot replace PA as a signaling molecule, this was used as a trick to "inhibit" PLD activity (actually prevent PA production), but also in assays to quantify PLD activity (Ammar et al., 2014). It was also shown that ethanol inhibits the mitogenic downstream actions of PA on neuron progenitors (Klein, 2005). Furthermore, it was recently shown that both PLD1 and PLD2 strongly contribute to astroglial proliferation induced by IGF-1 (Burkhardt et al., 2014). Therefore, the perturbation of the IGF1-PLD signaling pathway could, at least in part, explain the teratogenic effects of ethanol observed in FASDs.

Neurological Cancers

Glioblastoma is the most frequent and aggressive brain cancer, with an estimated incidence of near five novel cases per 100,000 persons every year in the USA and Europe. Nearly 200,000 persons die from glioblastoma every year worldwide. It is a relatively difficult cancer to diagnose, as the symptoms are mainly non-specific, including headache and nausea, but leading to alterations of neurological functions such as speech, vision, behavior and memory. Like for many cancer tissues, elevated PLD activity was found in glioblastoma, suggesting that an increase in PA levels is a cause and/or consequence of the pathology (Park et al., 2009). At least part of the survival effect of increased PLD activity on glioblastoma appears to involve the Akt pathway (Bruntz et al., 2014). Interestingly, lipidomic analyses revealed that PA levels are altered in the regions that attract glioblastoma cells, indicating that PA levels control the homing process of glioblastoma (Wildburger et al., 2015). Undoubtedly, a better understanding of the multiple functions of PA in brain tumor development and progression may help to improve treatments and subsequently get a better prognosis for this aggressive cancer.

Intellectual Disability Diseases

Intellectual disability diseases are a common state defined by significant restriction in intellectual capacities and adaptive behavior that happen during childhood, with an overall intelligence quotient bellow 70 together with associated reduction in social, daily living and communication skills. These heterogeneous disease conditions affect 1%–3% of all populations and are thought to result from multiple causes, including environmental, chromosomal and monogenetic alterations. Among the several hundreds of genes involved, some affect brain development, neurogenesis, neuronal migration, or synaptic function (Humeau et al., 2009). Below we will briefly describe the data that support the notion of an alteration of PA levels and/or dynamics in the Fragile-X syndrome (FXS) and the Coffin-Lowry syndrome (CLS).

FXS is a neurodevelopmental pathology accountable for the most common inherited form of intellectual infirmity and autism spectrum disorder. It is generally the consequence of the hypermethylation of CGG expansion repeats (>200) in the 5′ untranslated region of the *FMR1* gene leading to transcription silencing. In a recent study, we pointed DGK kinase-κ (DGKκ) mRNA as the foremost target of Fragile Mental Retardation Protein and found an alteration in PA synthesis in neurons cultured from *Fmr1*-knockout mice after group 1 metabotropic glutamate receptor (mGluRI) stimulation (Tabet et al., 2016a). Silencing DGKκ in CA1 pyramidal neurons modified the immature over mature spine ratio and like in the *Fmr1*-knockout mouse phenotype, reduced LTP and increased LTD (Tabet et al., 2016a). Moreover, the typical *Fmr1*-knockout mouse phenotype on dendritic spine morphology was restored back to normal after overexpression of DGKκ (Tabet et al., 2016a). Finally, DGKκ silencing by shRNA in the mouse reiterated autistic behaviors, such as impaired social interaction, hyperactivity and altered nest-building very much like those seen in the *Fmr1*-knockout mouse model (Tabet et al., 2016a). Based on these observations, it was proposed that a major molecular consequence of the loss of FMRP expression in FXS is to prevent DGKκ translation, leading to an alteration in DAG and PA levels in neurons (Tabet et al., 2016b). A main consequence of this imbalance would be the alteration of the downstream signaling of DAG and PA required for maturation of dendritic spines and establishment of correct synaptic plasticity (Moine and Vitale, 2018).

Loss of function mutations in the gene encoding Ribosomal S6 Kinase 2 (RSK2) lead to CLS, a rare syndromic form of mental retardation that shows X-linked inheritance. However, the molecular bases of the major neuronal alterations of CLS, such as moderate to severe defect in neurodevelopment, remain indefinable. In agreement with the notion that PLD1-generated PA is key to neurite outgrowth, we observed significant delayed in *Pld1* knockout neuron maturation (Ammar et al., 2013a). These observations were as well found in a mouse model for CLS syndrome since *Rsk2* knockout neurons exhibited developmental delay (Ammar et al., 2013a). Furthermore, RSK2 phosphorylates PLD1 at threonine 147 when exocytosis was triggered (Zeniou-Meyer et al., 2008) or during neurite outgrowth (Ammar et al., 2013a) in PC12 cells. A specific sensor for PA revealed an increase in PA levels at the tips of growing neurites in neurons resulting from PLD1 activation (Ammar et al., 2013a). Interestingly, PLD1 was found to be associated with BDNF positive endosomes (Ammar et al., 2015) and with vesicular structures derived from the trans Golgi, co-labeled by the vesicular SNARE VAMP-7/TiVAMP (Ammar et al., 2013a). The fusion efficiency of these PLD1/VAMP-7 vesicles in the growth cone was severely impaired by RSK2 and PLD1 inhibitors, suggesting that both PLD1 and RSK2 are necessary for membrane provision needed during neurite outgrowth (Ammar et al., 2013a). Accordingly, co-immunoprecipitation and confocal colocalization experiments indicated that RSK2 and PLD1 are found in a complex at the tip end of growing neurites, supporting the observation of an increased PA level at this location (Ammar et al., 2013a). Altogether, these results have highlighted the importance of PA-mediated membrane trafficking in neurite outgrowth and a key role of RSK2 in PA synthesis during this process, by phosphorylation and subsequent activation of PLD1. In consequence, it has been proposed that at least some of the clinical consequences of the CLS might result from an inadequate PA production during neuronal development and function (Zeniou-Meyer et al., 2010).

Neurodegeneration

It is becoming more and more evident that human neurodegenerative diseases such as Alzheimer disease (AD) also have a critical lipidic feature in their outcome. This aspect has been first pointed out by the susceptibility of the ApoE4 allele to AD, but more recently PLDs have also been proposed to contribute to the development of the pathology. It was first shown that PLD1 is involved in the vesicular trafficking of βAPP (Cai et al., 2006) and later that increased expression of APP promoted PLD activity in human astroglioma cells (Jin et al., 2007). Although highly debated, the observation that a rare variant of PLD3 gene confers susceptibility to AD has put PLD and PA on the spotlight (Cruchaga et al., 2014; Heilmann et al., 2015; Lambert et al., 2015; van der Lee et al., 2015). The most compelling evidence that defects in PA production by PLDs are involved in AD comes from an elegant study combining detailed lipidomics with behavioral tests in mouse models. In this study, the authors found that PLD2 knockout fully rescued AD-related synaptic dysfunction and cognitive deficits in a model of AD (Oliveira et al., 2010). The exact nature of the PA imbalance in AD awaits however to be fully defined and the possibility to interfere with AD condition by correcting this imbalance is probably very far from reach.

CONCLUSION

The diversity of mechanisms of PA signaling and physiological functions mostly relies on the fact that PA is synthesized by a complex set of different enzymes involved in diverse array of pathways. PLDs, DGKs, and LPAATs each constitute a big collection of isoenzymes differently localized within cells and displaying cell type specificity. In fact, the specific subcellular distribution, regulation, and/or substrate preferences of these enzymes probably account for the heterogeneity of PA composition in membranes. These aspects, altogether with the capacity of PA-binding modules in proteins to sense the local membrane environment and the type of PA species, offer a hub for the functional diversity of PA from molecular and cellular to physiological functions. There is no doubt that advanced lipidomics in combination with novel imaging tools to follow PA's dynamics will help to gain a better understanding of the apparent paradox of the abundance of function of this simple lipid. Further understanding of the biophysical side of PA's action on membranes is also critically needed to provide novel ideas for the treatment of the growing number of neuronal pathologies linked to the alterations of PA metabolism.

AUTHOR CONTRIBUTIONS

All authors listed have made a substantial, direct and intellectual contribution to the work, and approved it for publication.

FUNDING

This work was supported by Fondation pour la Recherche Médicale and by Fondation Jérôme Lejeune funding to HM.

REFERENCES

Ammar, M. R., Humeau, Y., Hanauer, A., Nieswandt, B., Bader, M. F., and Vitale, N. (2013a). The Coffin-Lowry syndrome-associated protein RSK2 regulates neurite outgrowth through phosphorylation of phospholipase D1 (PLD1) and synthesis of phosphatidic acid. *J. Neurosci.* 33, 19470–19479. doi: 10.1523/JNEUROSCI.2283-13.2013

Ammar, M. R., Kassas, N., Chasserot-Golaz, S., Bader, M. F., and Vitale, N. (2013b). Lipids in regulated exocytosis: what are they doing? *Front. Endocrinol.* 4:125. doi: 10.3389/fendo.2013.00125

Ammar, M. R., Kassas, N., Bader, M. F., and Vitale, N. (2014). Phosphatidic acid in neuronal development: a node for membrane and cytoskeleton rearrangements. *Biochimie* 107, 51–57. doi: 10.1016/j.biochi.2014.07.026

Ammar, M. R., Thahouly, T., Hanauer, A., Stegner, D., Nieswandt, B., and Vitale, N. (2015). PLD1 participates in BDNF-induced signalling in cortical neurons. *Sci. Rep.* 5:14778. doi: 10.1038/srep14778

Bader, M. F., and Vitale, N. (2009). Phospholipase D in calcium-regulated exocytosis: lessons from chromaffin cells. *Biochim. Biophys. Acta* 1791, 936–941. doi: 10.1016/j.bbalip.2009.02.016

Bruntz, R. C., Taylor, H. E., Lindsley, C. W., and Brown, H. A. (2014). Phospholipase D2 mediates survival signaling through direct regulation of Akt in glioblastoma cells. *J. Biol. Chem.* 289, 600–616. doi: 10.1074/jbc.M113.532978

Bullen, H. E., Jia, Y., Yamaryo-Botté, Y., Bisio, H., Zhang, O., Jemelin, N. K., et al. (2016). Phosphatidic acid-mediated signaling regulates microneme secretion in toxoplasma. *Cell Host Microbe* 19, 349–360. doi: 10.1016/j.chom.2016.02.006

Burkhardt, U., Wojcik, B., Zimmermann, M., and Klein, J. (2014). Phospholipase D is a target for inhibition of astroglial proliferation by ethanol. *Neuropharmacology* 79, 1–9. doi: 10.1016/j.neuropharm.2013.11.002

Cai, D., Zhong, M., Wang, R., Netzer, W. J., Shields, D., Zheng, H., et al. (2006). Phospholipase D1 corrects impaired βAPP trafficking and neurite outgrowth in familial Alzheimer's disease-linked presenilin-1 mutant neurons. *Proc. Natl. Acad. Sci. U S A* 103, 1936–1940. doi: 10.1073/pnas.0510710103

Chae, Y. C., Kim, J. H., Kim, K. L., Kim, H. W., Lee, H. Y., Heo, W. D., et al. (2008). Phospholipase D activity regulates integrin-mediated cell spreading and migration by inducing GTP-Rac translocation to the plasma membrane. *Mol. Biol. Cell* 19, 3111–3123. doi: 10.1091/mbc.E07-04-0337

Chasserot-Golaz, S., Coorssen, J. R., Meunier, F. A., and Vitale, N. (2010). Lipid dynamics in exocytosis. *Cell. Mol. Neurobiol.* 30, 1335–1342. doi: 10.1007/s10571-010-9577-x

Corrotte, M., Chasserot-Golaz, S., Huang, P., Du, G., Ktistakis, N. T., Frohman, M. A., et al. (2006). Dynamics and function of phospholipase D and phosphatidic acid during phagocytosis. *Traffic* 7, 365–377. doi: 10.1111/j.1600-0854.2006.00389.x

Corrotte, M., Nyguyen, A. P., Harlay, M. L., Vitale, N., Bader, M. F., and Grant, N. J. (2010). Ral isoforms are implicated in Fcγ R-mediated phagocytosis: activation of phospholipase D by RalA. *J. Immunol.* 185, 2942–2950. doi: 10.4049/jimmunol.0903138

Cruchaga, C., Karch, C. M., Jin, S. C., Benitez, B. A., Cai, Y., Guerreiro, R., et al. (2014). Rare coding variants in the phospholipase D3 gene confer risk for Alzheimer's disease. *Nature* 505, 550–554. doi: 10.1038/nature12825

Daniels, R. H., Hall, P. S., and Bokoch, G. M. (1998). Membrane targeting of p21-activated kinase 1 (PAK1) induces neurite outgrowth from PC12 cells. *EMBO J.* 17, 754–764. doi: 10.1093/emboj/17.3.754

Disse, J., Vitale, N., Bader, M. F., and Gerke, V. (2009). Phospholipase D1 is specifically required for regulated secretion of von Willebrand factor from endothelial cells. *Blood* 113, 973–980. doi: 10.1182/blood-2008-06-165282

Ehrhart, F., Roozen, S., Verbeek, J., Koek, G., Kok, G., van Kranen, H., et al. (2018). Review and gap analysis: molecular pathways leading to fetal alcohol spectrum disorders. *Mol. Psychiatry* 24, 10–17. doi: 10.1038/s41380-018-0095-4

Faugaret, D., Chouinard, F. C., Harbour, D., El azreq, M. A., and Bourgoin, S. G. (2011). An essential role for phospholipase D in the recruitment of vesicle amine transport protein-1 to membranes in human neutrophils. *Biochem. Pharmacol.* 81, 144–156. doi: 10.1016/j.bcp.2010.09.014

Foster, D. A. (2009). Phosphatidic acid signaling to mTOR: signals for the survival of human cancer cells. *Biochim. Biophys. Acta* 1791, 949–949. doi: 10.1016/j.bbalip.2009.02.009

Ghossoub, R., Lembo, F., Rubio, A., Gaillard, C. B., Bouchet, J., Vitale, N., et al. (2014). Syntenin-ALIX exosome biogenesis and budding into multivesicular bodies are controlled by ARF6 and PLD2. *Nat. Commun.* 5:3477. doi: 10.1038/ncomms4477

Hayashi, K., Ohshima, T., Hashimoto, M., and Mikoshiba, K. (2007). Pak1 regulates dendritic branching and spine formation. *Dev. Neurobiol.* 67, 655–669. doi: 10.1002/dneu.20363

Heilmann, S., Drichel, D., Clarimon, J., Fernández, V., Lacour, A., Wagner, H., et al. (2015). PLD3 in non-familial Alzheimer's disease. *Nature* 520, E3–E5. doi: 10.1038/nature14039

Holland, P., Knævelsrud, H., Søreng, K., Mathai, B. J., Lystad, A. H., Pankiv, S., et al. (2016). HS1BP3 negatively regulates autophagy by modulation of phosphatidic acid levels. *Nat. Commun.* 7:13889. doi: 10.1038/ncomms13889

Honda, A., Nogami, M., Yokozeki, T., Yamazaki, M., Nakamura, H., Watanabe, H., et al. (1999). Phosphatidylinositol 4-phosphate 5-kinase α is a downstream effector of the small G protein ARF6 in membrane ruffle formation. *Cell* 99, 521–532. doi: 10.1016/s0092-8674(00)81540-8

Humeau, Y., Gambino, F., Chelly, J., and Vitale, N. (2009). X-linked mental retardation: focus on synaptic function and plasticity. *J. Neurochem.* 109, 1–14. doi: 10.1111/j.1471-4159.2009.05881.x

Humeau, Y., Vitale, N., Chasserot-Golaz, S., Dupont, J. L., Du, G., Frohman, M. A., et al. (2001). A role for phospholipase D1 in neurotransmitter release. *Proc. Natl. Acad. Sci. U S A* 98, 15300–15305. doi: 10.1073/pnas.261358698

Ito, S., Richert, N., and Pastan, I. (1982). Phospholipids stimulate phosphorylation of vinculin by the tyrosine-specific protein kinase of Rous sarcoma virus. *Proc. Natl. Acad. Sci. U S A* 79, 4628–4631. doi: 10.1073/pnas.79.15.4628

Jang, J.-H., Lee, C. S., Hwang, D., and Ryu, S. H. (2012). Understanding of the roles of phospholipase D and phosphatidic acid through their binding partners. *Prog. Lipid Res.* 51, 71–81. doi: 10.1016/j.plipres.2011.12.003

Jenkins, G. M., and Frohman, M. A. (2005). Phospholipase D: a lipid centric review. *Cell. Mol. Life Sci.* 62, 2305–2316. doi: 10.1007/s00018-005-5195-z

Jin, J.-K., Ahn, B.-H., Na, Y.-J., Kim, J.-I., Kim, Y.-S., Choi, E.-K., et al. (2007). Phospholipase D1 is associated with amyloid precursor protein in Alzheimer's disease. *Neurobiol. Aging* 28, 1015–1027. doi: 10.1016/j.neurobiolaging.2006.05.022

Johnson, R. P., and Craig, S. W. (1995). The carboxy-terminal tail domain of vinculin contains a cryptic binding site for acidic phospholipids. *Biochem. Biophys. Res. Commun.* 210, 159–164. doi: 10.1006/bbrc.1995.1641

Jose Lopez-Andreo, M., Gomez-Fernandez, J. C., and Corbalan-Garcia, S. (2003). The simultaneous production of phosphatidic acid and diacylglycerol is essential for the translocation of protein kinase Cε to the plasma membrane in RBL-2H3 cells. *Mol. Biol. Cell* 14, 4885–4895. doi: 10.1091/mbc.e03-05-0295

Kassas, N., Tanguy, E., Thahouly, T., Fouillen, L., Heintz, D., Chasserot-Golaz, S., et al. (2017). Comparative characterization of phosphatidic acid sensors and their localization during frustrated phagocytosis. *J. Biol. Chem.* 292, 4266–4279. doi: 10.1074/jbc.m116.742346

Klein, J. (2005). Functions and pathophysiological roles of phospholipase D in thebrain. *J. Neurochem.* 94, 1473–1487. doi: 10.1111/j.1471-4159.2005.03315.x

Kooijman, E. E., Chupin, V., de Kruijff, B., and Burger, K. N. (2003). Modulation of membrane curvature by phosphatidic acid and lysophosphatidic acid. *Traffic* 4, 162–174. doi: 10.1034/j.1600-0854.2003.00086.x

Kurooka, T., Yamamoto, Y., Takai, Y., and Sakisaka, T. (2011). Dual regulation of RA-RhoGAP activity by phosphatidic acid and Rap1 during neurite outgrowth. *J. Biol. Chem.* 286, 6832–6843. doi: 10.1074/jbc.m110.183772

Lam, A. D., Tryoen-Toth, P., Tsai, B., Vitale, N., and Stuenkel, E. L. (2008). SNARE-catalyzed fusion events are regulated by Syntaxin1A-lipid interactions. *Mol. Biol. Cell* 19, 485–497. doi: 10.1091/mbc.e07-02-0148

Lambert, J. C., Grenier-Boley, B., Bellenguez, C., Pasquier, F., Campion, D., Dartigues, J. F., et al. (2015). PLD3 and sporadic Alzheimer's disease risk. *Nature* 520:E1. doi: 10.1038/nature14036

Lopez, C. I., Pelletán, L. E., Suhaiman, L., De Blas, G. A., Vitale, N., Mayorga, L. S., et al. (2012). Diacylglycerol stimulates acrosomal exocytosis by feeding into a PKC- and PLD1-dependent positive loop that continuously supplies phosphatidylinositol 4,5-bisphosphate. *Biochim. Biophys. Acta* 1821, 1186–1199. doi: 10.1016/j.bbalip.2012.05.001

Mima, J., and Wickner, W. (2009). Complex lipid requirements for SNARE- and SNARE chaperone-dependent membrane fusion. *J. Biol. Chem.* 284, 27114–27122. doi: 10.1074/jbc.m109.010223

Moine, H., and Vitale, N. (2018). Of local translation control and lipid signaling in neurons. *Adv. Biol. Regul.* doi: 10.1016/j.jbior.2018.09.005 [Epub ahead of print].

Nishikimi, A., Fukuhara, H., Su, W., Hongu, T., Takasuga, S., Mihara, H., et al. (2009). Sequential regulation of DOCK2 dynamics by two phospholipids during neutrophil chemotaxis. *Science* 324, 384–387. doi: 10.1126/science.1170179

Oliveira, T. G., Chan, R. B., Tian, H., Laredo, M., Shui, G., Staniszewski, A., et al. (2010). Phospholipase d2 ablation ameliorates Alzheimer's disease-linked synaptic dysfunction and cognitive deficits. *J. Neurosci.* 30, 16419–16428. doi: 10.1523/JNEUROSCI.3317-10.2010

Park, M. H., Ahn, B. H., Hong, Y. K., and Min do, S. (2009). Overexpression of phospholipase D enhances matrix metalloproteinase-2 expression and glioma cell invasion via protein kinase C and protein kinase A/NF-κB/Sp1-mediated signaling pathways. *Carcinogenesis* 30, 356–365. doi: 10.1093/carcin/bgn287

Pelletán, L. E., Suhaiman, L., Vaquer, C. C., Bustos, M. A., De Blas, G. A., Vitale, N., et al. (2015). ADP ribosylation factor 6 (ARF6) promotes acrosomal exocytosis by modulating lipid turnover and Rab3A activation. *J. Biol. Chem.* 290, 9823–9841. doi: 10.1074/jbc.m114.629006

Pokotylo, I., Kravets, V., Martinec, J., and Ruelland, E. (2018). The phosphatidic acid paradox: too many actions for one molecule class? Lessons from plants. *Prog. Lipid Res.* 71, 43–53. doi: 10.1016/j.plipres.2018.05.003

Potocký, M., Pleskot, R., Pejchar, P., Vitale, N., Kost, B., and Zárský, V. (2014). Live-cell imaging of phosphatidic acid dynamics in pollen tubes visualized by Spo20p-derive biosensor. *New Phytol.* 203, 483–494. doi: 10.1111/nph.12814

Raben, D. M., and Barber, C. N. (2017). Phosphatidic acid and neurotransmission. *Adv. Biol. Regul.* 63, 15–21. doi: 10.1016/j.jbior.2016.09.004

Roach, A. N., Wang, Z., Wu, P., Zhang, F., Chan, R. B., Yonekubo, Y., et al. (2012). Phosphatidic acid regulation of PIPKI is critical for actin cytoskeletal reorganization. *J. Lipid Res.* 53, 2598–2609. doi: 10.1194/jlr.m028597

Sanematsu, F., Nishikimi, A., Watanabe, M., Hongu, T., Tanaka, Y., Kanaho, Y., et al. (2013). Phosphatidic acid-dependent recruitment and function of the Rac activator DOCK1 during dorsal ruffle formation. *J. Biol. Chem.* 288, 8092–8100. doi: 10.1074/jbc.m112.410423

Schwarz, K., Natarajan, S., Kassas, N., Vitale, N., and Schmitz, F. (2011). The synaptic ribbon is a site of phosphatidic acid generation in ribbon synapses. *J. Neurosci.* 31, 15996–16011. doi: 10.1523/JNEUROSCI.2965-11.2011

Stace, C. L., and Ktistakis, N. T. (2006). Phosphatidic acid- and phosphatidylserine-binding proteins. *Biochim. Biophys. Acta* 1761, 913–926. doi: 10.1016/j.bbalip.2006.03.006

Tabet, R., Moutin, E., Becker, J. A., Heintz, D., Fouillen, L., Flatter, E., et al. (2016a). Fragile X Mental Retardation Protein (FMRP) controls diacylglycerol kinase activity in neurons. *Proc. Natl. Acad. Sci. U S A* 113, E3619–E3628. doi: 10.1073/pnas.1522631113

Tabet, R., Vitale, N., and Moine, H. (2016b). Fragile X syndrome: are signaling lipids the missing Culprits? *Biochimie* 130, 188–194. doi: 10.1016/j.biochi.2016.09.002

Tanguy, E., Carmon, O., Wang, Q., Jeandel, L., Chasserot-Golaz, S., Montero-Hadjadje, M., et al. (2016). Lipids implicated in the journey of a secretory granule: from biogenesis to fusion. *J. Neurochem.* 137, 904–912. doi: 10.1111/jnc.13577

Tanguy, E., Kassas, N., and Vitale, N. (2018). Protein-phospholipid interaction motifs: a focus on phosphatidic acid. *Biomolecules* 8:E20. doi: 10.3390/biom8020020

van den Bout, I., and Divecha, N. (2009). PIP5K-driven PtdIns(4,5)P2 synthesis: regulation and cellular functions. *J. Cell Sci.* 122, 3837–3850. doi: 10.1242/jcs.056127

van der Lee, S. J., Holstege, H., Wong, T. H., Jakobsdottir, J., Bis, J. C., Chouraki, V., et al. (2015). PLD3 variants in population studies. *Nature* 520, E2–E3. doi: 10.1038/nature14038

Vitale, N., Caumont, A. S., Chasserot-Golaz, S., Du, G., Wu, S., Sciorra, V. A., et al. (2001). Phospholipase D1: a key factor for the exocytotic machinery in neuroendocrine cells. *EMBO J.* 20, 2424–2434. doi: 10.1093/emboj/20.10.2424

Waselle, L., Gerona, R. R., Vitale, N., Martin, T. F., Bader, M. F., and Regazzi, R. (2005). Role of phosphoinositide signaling in the control of insulin exocytosis. *Mol. Endocrinol.* 19, 3097–3106. doi: 10.1210/me.2004-0530

Wildburger, N. C., Wood, P. L., Gumin, J., Lichti, C. F., Emmett, M. R., Lang, F. F., et al. (2015). ESI-MS/MS and MALDI-IMS localization reveal alterations in phosphatidic acid, diacylglycerol, and DHA in glioma stem cell xenografts. *J. Proteome Res.* 14, 2511–2519. doi: 10.1021/acs.jproteome.5b00076

Williams, J. M., Pettitt, T. R., Powell, W., Grove, J., Savage, C. O., and Wakelam, M. J. (2007). Antineutrophil cytoplasm antibody-stimulated neutrophil adhesion depends on diacylglycerol kinase-catalyzed phosphatidic acid formation. *J. Am. Soc. Nephrol.* 18, 1112–1120. doi: 10.1681/asn.2006090973

Yang, J. S., Gad, H., Lee, S. Y., Mironov, A., Zhang, L., Beznoussenko, G. V., et al. (2008). A role for phosphatidic acid in COPI vesicle fission yields insights into Golgi maintenance. *Nat. Cell Biol.* 10, 1146–1153. doi: 10.1038/ncb1774

Zeniou-Meyer, M., Gambino, F., Ammar, M. R., Humeau, Y., and Vitale, N. (2010). The Coffin-Lowry syndrome-associated protein RSK2 and neurosecretion. *Cell. Mol. Neurobiol.* 30, 1401–1406. doi: 10.1007/s10571-010-9578-9

Zeniou-Meyer, M., Liu, Y., Béglé, A., Olanich, M. E., Hanauer, A., Becherer, U., et al. (2008). The Coffin-Lowry syndrome-associated protein RSK2 is implicated in calcium-regulated exocytosis through the regulation of PLD1. *Proc. Natl. Acad. Sci. U S A* 105, 8434–8439. doi: 10.1073/pnas.0710676105

Zeniou-Meyer, M., Zabari, N., Ashery, U., Chasserot-Golaz, S., Haeberlé, A. M., Demais, V., et al. (2007). Phospholipase D1 production of phosphatidic acid at the plasma membrane promotes exocytosis of large dense-core granules at a late stage. *J. Biol. Chem.* 282, 21746–21757. doi: 10.1074/jbc.m702968200

9

Inhibition of SIRT2 by Targeting GSK3β-Mediated Phosphorylation Alleviates SIRT2 Toxicity in SH-SY5Y Cells

Shuhu Liu*†, *Zhihua Zhou*†, *Ling Zhang, Siying Meng, Shuji Li and Xuemin Wang*

Key Laboratory of Mental Health of the Ministry of Education, Guangdong Province Key Laboratory of Psychiatric Disorders, Department of Neurobiology, School of Basic Medical Sciences, Southern Medical University, Guangzhou, China

***Correspondence:**
Xuemin Wang
xmwang@fimmu.com

†*These authors have contributed equally to this work*

Sirtuin 2 (SIRT2) is thought to be important in the pathogenesis of Parkinson's disease (PD), and the inhibition of SIRT2 rescues α-synuclein toxicity in a cellular model of PD. Recent studies have focused on identifying inhibitors of SIRT2, but little is known about the processes that directly regulate its function. GSK3β is a serine/threonine protein kinase that affects a wide range of biological functions, and it is localized in Lewy bodies (LBs). Therefore, we investigated whether SIRT2 is regulated by GSK3β and enhances cell death in PD. In the present study, Western blot showed that total SIRT2 levels did not change noticeably in a cellular model of PD but that SIRT2 phosphorylation was increased, and GSK3β activity was elevated. In addition, mass spectrometry (MS) studies indicated that SIRT2 was phosphorylated by GSK3β at three specific sites. Phospho- or dephospho-mimicking studies demonstrated that this postmodification (phosphorylation) increased SIRT2 toxicity in SH-SY5Y cells. Collectively, our findings identify a posttranslational mechanism that controls SIRT2 function in PD and provide evidence for a novel regulatory pathway involving GSK3β, SIRT2, and α-synuclein.

Keywords: SIRT2, GSK3β, 6-OHDA, PD, neuroprotection

INTRODUCTION

Parkinson's disease (PD) is a long-term neurodegenerative disorder that mainly affects the motor system. Since it was first reported by James Parkinson in 1817 (Lees, 2007), PD has become the second most common neurodegenerative disorder (Dawson and Dawson, 2003). The disease is characterized by the loss of dopaminergic neurons in the substantia nigra, and the pathological hallmark is the accumulation of α-synuclein protein aggregates called Lewy bodies (LBs). It is believed that the number and size of α-synuclein aggregates affect the progression of PD. However, the exact molecular mechanisms that contribute to dopaminergic neuron loss remain to be clarified.

To explore the molecular mechanisms of PD, we focused on sirtuins, a family of class III nicotinamide adenine dinucleotide-dependent deacetylases that deacetylate histone and nonhistone proteins. SIRT2 is one of seven members of the sirtuin family, and it plays diverse roles in cellular metabolism and aging. SIRT2 is highly expressed in the central nervous system (Maxwell et al., 2011; Zhu et al., 2012) and is located in the cytoplasm (North et al., 2003), the nucleus (Dryden et al., 2003; North et al., 2003) and mitochondria (Liu et al., 2017). It has been reported that SIRT2 plays essential roles in PD, and SIRT2 inhibitors rescue α-synuclein-mediated toxicity (Outeiro et al., 2007; Chen et al., 2015). One SIRT2 inhibitor, AK7, even protects against MPTP neurotoxicity in mice (Chen et al., 2015). The protective effects of SIRT2 inhibition are mediated through a number of pathways. First, SIRT2 can directly deacetylate α-synuclein to exacerbate α-synuclein toxicity *in vivo* (de Oliveira et al., 2017). Second, SIRT2 inhibition achieves neuroprotection by reducing sterol levels *via* the decreased nuclear trafficking of SREBP-2 (Luthi-Carter et al., 2010). Third, SIRT2 inhibition may be neuroprotective in PD by modulating a redox network (Wang et al., 2015; Guan et al., 2016). Although SIRT2 plays a key role in the development of PD, we still do not know how SIRT2 itself is regulated during the development of this disease. It has been reported that SIRT2 is a phosphorylation substrate of CDK5, which modulates the activity of SIRT2 (Pandithage et al., 2008). However, there have been no reports that CDK5 can regulate the activity of SIRT2 in PD. To obtain further insight into the mechanism by which SIRT2 is regulated, we sought to identify novel upstream kinases of SIRT2. GSK3β and CDK5 are two kinases at the center of research on Alzheimer's disease, and they share the same substrate (Wen et al., 2008). Therefore, we hypothesized that SIRT2 may be a substrate of GSK3β.

GSK3β is a serine/threonine protein kinase that is activated by neurotoxins (Hongo et al., 2012; Hernandez-Baltazar et al., 2013; Zhao et al., 2016) and PD-associated gene mutations (Wang et al., 2013; Kawakami et al., 2014). Additionally, in the postmortem PD brain, GSK3β is localized in LBs, as is phosphorylated GSK3β (Ser9; Nagao and Hayashi, 2009). Furthermore, in a study of a group of 251 Spanish patients with PD, Infante et al. (2010) found that a GSK3β (rs6438552) TT genotype, which has been shown to produce a more active isoform (Kwok et al., 2005), is associated with an elevated risk of PD. Thus, GSK3β is important in the development of PD. In accordance with these reports, GSK3β downregulation partially abrogates 6-OHDA-induced SH-SY5Y apoptotic cell death (Li et al., 2011) and MPP (+)-induced neuronal death (Petit-Paitel et al., 2009). These results indicate that GSK3β is a critical mediator of 6-OHDA/MPP (+)-induced neurotoxicity.

Based on the above information, we propose that SIRT2 may be phosphorylated by GSK3β during the development of PD. Here, we provide detailed insight into the mechanism through which GSK3β modulates SIRT2 activity and suggest that the phosphorylation of S327, S331 and S335 may be useful as a target for therapeutic intervention in PD.

MATERIALS AND METHODS

Materials

An MTT assay kit was purchased from Roche. A site-directed mutagenesis kit was purchased from Stratagene. 6-Hydroxydopamine hydrobromide (6-OHDA), DMSO, SB216763 (S3442, an inhibitor of GSK3β) and AGK2 (A8231, an inhibitor of SIRT2) were obtained from Sigma-Aldrich. Antibodies against pGSK3β (Ser9) and GSK3β were purchased from Cell Signaling (Danvers, MA, USA). Antibodies against SIRT2, ace-tubulin, α-tubulin, HA and Flag were purchased from Sigma-Aldrich. Secondary antibodies conjugated to Alexa 488 or Alexa 594 were purchased from Invitrogen. Hoechst 33258 (94403) was purchased from Sigma-Aldrich. Protein A/G-coated Sepharose beads were obtained from Santa Cruz Biotechnology (Dallas, TX, USA). An anti-phosphoserine/threonine/tyrosine antibody was obtained from Abcam (ab15556). Protein kinase CDK5/p25 (cat. 14—516) and GSK3β (cat. 14—306) were purchased from Millipore. Cells were transfected using Lipofectamine 2000 Transfection Reagent (Invitrogen, Thermo Fisher Scientific, Waltham, MA, USA). Other chemicals and reagents were of the highest analytical grade and were purchased from local commercial sources.

Cell Culture

The human neuroblastoma cell line SH-SY5Y was obtained from the American Type Culture Collection. The cells were grown in Dulbecco's modified Eagle's medium (DMEM)/Ham's F12 (1:1 mixture; HyClone) supplemented with 10% fetal bovine serum (GIBCO) in a 5% CO_2 incubator at 37°C. Human embryonic kidney cells (HEK293) were grown in DMEM (HyClone) supplemented with 10% FBS.

Pharmacological Treatments

6-OHDA was dissolved in phosphate-buffered saline (PBS) and used at a final concentration of 100 μM (Ikeda et al., 2008), which was the dose shown to induce 50% cell death within 24 h after 4 h of exposure. SB216763 and AGK2 were dissolved in DMSO. Before adding 6-OHDA, the SH-SY5Y cells were treated with SB216763 (Acevedo et al., 2014) or AGK2 (Outeiro et al., 2007) at a final concentration of 10 μM for 0.5 h (the DMSO content never exceeded 0.1%).

MTT Tests for Cell Viability

Cell viability was measured by a colorimetric MTT [3-(4,5-dimethylthiazol-2-yl)-2,5-diphenyltetrazolium bromide] assay. Briefly, the cells were seeded in a 96-well plate at a density of 5×10^4 cells/well. The cells were then pretreated with SB216763 for 0.5 h. After pretreatment, 6-OHDA was added to the culture medium to reach a final concentration of 100 μM. The control cells were not treated with SB216763 or 6-OHDA. The culture medium was changed after incubation for 4 h. Then, 16 h later, the MTT reagent was added to each well, and the cells were incubated for an additional 4 h. The absorbance of each reaction product was measured with a microplate reader at a wavelength of 595 nm. The results are expressed as a percentage of the MTT absorbance of the control cells, which was set to 100%.

Western Blot Analysis

Whole-cell lysates were prepared by incubating cells in RIPA buffer supplemented with a protease inhibitor cocktail (Selleck) according to the manufacturer's instructions. Briefly, the cells were harvested by centrifugation at 900 rpm for 5 min and washed in PBS (pH 7.2). The pellets were solubilized in the same volume of lysis buffer, kept on ice, vortexed for 5 min, and centrifuged at 13,000× *g* for 20 min at 4°C. Equal amounts of total lysate protein were loaded and separated on a 10% sodium dodecyl sulfate-polyacrylamide gel electrophoresis (SDS-PAGE) gel. The proteins were electrophoretically transferred to a PVDF membrane, and the membrane was blocked in 5% skim milk in Tris-buffered saline containing 0.1% Tween-20 (TBST) for 1 h. Then, the membranes were incubated at 4°C overnight in the presence of a primary antibody against one of the following proteins: HA, Flag, SIRT2, ace-tubulin, α-tubulin (Sigma), GSK3β or pGSK3β (Ser9). Next, the membranes were washed three times with TBST every 5 min and probed with a corresponding horseradish peroxidase (HRP)-conjugated secondary antibody at room temperature for 1 h. Probe detection was conducted using enhanced ECL Advance Western Blotting Detection Reagents (Perkin Elmer, Waltham, MA, USA) and a ChemiDoc XRS+ system (Bio-Rad, Hercules, CA, USA).

Immunofluorescence Staining

Cultured cells were fixed with PBS containing 4% paraformaldehyde for 15 min, which was followed by washing and permeabilization in PBS with 0.1% Triton X-100 for 5 min. The samples were blocked in PBS with 5% BSA and incubated with primary antibodies overnight at 4°C. The following primary antibodies were used: rabbit anti-SIRT2 (1:100) and mouse anti-acetylated α-tubulin (1:50). Secondary antibodies conjugated to Alexa 488 or Alexa 594 (1:500) were applied for 1 h at room temperature. After washing with PBS and staining with DAPI for 5 min, coverslips were mounted with Mowiol. Images of the cells were acquired at room temperature on a confocal microscope (A1+; Nikon) using either a 40× or a 60× lens. Photoshop CS (Adobe) was used to adjust the contrast and brightness.

Coimmunoprecipitation

Cells were collected and lysed in buffer containing 50 mM Tris-HCl at pH 7.4, 150 mM NaCl, and 1% NP-40. All buffers were supplemented with protease and phosphatase inhibitors. The extracted proteins were precleared by incubating the lysates with Protein A/G-coated Sepharose beads for 1 h at 4°C, and then the supernatants (500 μg, 1 μg/μl) were incubated overnight with an HA or Flag antibody at 4°C. Precipitation of the immune complexes was performed with Protein A/G-coated Sepharose beads for 2 h at 4°C. After immunoprecipitation, the beads were washed five times with lysis buffer at 4°C and suspended in 40 μl of 2× loading buffer. All samples were loaded onto a gel, processed by SDS–PAGE and analyzed by Western blot. To detect SIRT2 phosphorylation, we used an anti-phosphoserine/threonine/tyrosine antibody.

Plasmids and Transfection

GSK3β-HA and SIRT2-flag were obtained from Addgene. PCMV-HA and PCMV-Tag4A are blank plasmids that contain an HA tag and a Flag tag, respectively. A subsequent LR-recombination reaction with PGEX4T3 and phMGFP plasmids resulted in GST-tagged and GFP-tagged expression constructs. Site-directed mutagenesis was performed using a Quick change protocol to generate the S327A, S331A, S335A, S327&331&335A and S327&331&335D mutants. All constructs were verified by DNA sequencing. SIRT2-targeting shRNAs using previously identified sequences (Si et al., 2013) were cloned into a pGPU6/GFP/Neo vector from Genepharma. For transient transfection, cells were transfected using Lipofectamine 2000 Transfection Reagent according to the manufacturer's instructions.

Determining the Survival Rate of Transfected Cells

SH-SY5Y cells were transfected with plasmids (GFP, GFP-SIRT2, GFP-SIRT2SA or GFP-SIRT2SD) for 24 or 48 h to induce the expression of GFP. Chromatin condensation was detected by nuclear staining with Hoechst 33258. Briefly, the cells were fixed with 4% paraformaldehyde for 15 min, stained with PBS/0.1% TritonX-100/10 μM Hoechst 33258 for 5 min, and then visualized by fluorescence microscopy. Apoptotic cells were stained bright blue because of their chromatin condensation. Images were captured from different fields of each well for different groups of cells at 20× magnification using an Olympus fluorescence microscope. The numbers of total and live transfected cells were counted from multiple fields to obtain the percentage of live transfected cells (Dutta et al., 2018).

GST Fusion Protein Purification

The GST-SIRT2 expression plasmid was transformed into competent *Escherichia coli* BL21 cells. A single colony was inoculated in LB medium at 37°C in an orbital shaker incubator until the mid-log phase. IPTG (100 μM) was added to the culture and incubated at 20°C for 8 h. Following the incubation, the culture was centrifuged at 2,500× *g* for 10 min at 4°C, and the resulting pellet was resuspended in binding buffer [50 mM Tris-Cl, pH 8.0, 150 mM NaCl and 1× protease inhibitor cocktail (Biotool)]. The cells were lysed by sonication and centrifuged at 12,000× *g* for 30 min at 4°C. After centrifugation, the supernatant was collected, incubated with GST agarose beads (Novagen) and maintained under agitation overnight at 4°C. After overnight binding, the beads were washed with wash buffer (150 mM NaCl, 50 mM Tris-Cl, pH 7.5 and 1% Triton X-100), and the bead-bound proteins were eluted and stored in 30% glycerol-containing buffer. Other GST fusion proteins were obtained in the same way.

In vitro Kinase Assays

The phosphorylation of GST-SIRT2 was performed in a final volume of 25 μl consisting of 5 mM MOPS, pH 7.2, 0.05 mM DTT, 4 mM $MgCl_2$, 80 μm ATP, 10 μCi of [γ-32P]ATP, 0.4 mM EDTA, 1 mM EGTA, and 2.5 mM β-glycerophosphate for 30 min at 30°C in the presence or absence of CDK5/p25 or GSK3β. The reaction was terminated by the addition of 25 μl of 2× sodium dodecyl sulfate (SDS) loading buffer (187 mm Tris-HCl, pH 6.8, 30% (w/v) glycerol, 6% SDS and 15% β-mercaptoethanol). The samples were then heated at 100°C for 5 min, centrifuged in a microcentrifuge, and loaded on a gel for SDS-PAGE. Following electrophoresis, the proteins were exposed to a Kodak X-ray film for autoradiography at −80°C for 2 or 3 days.

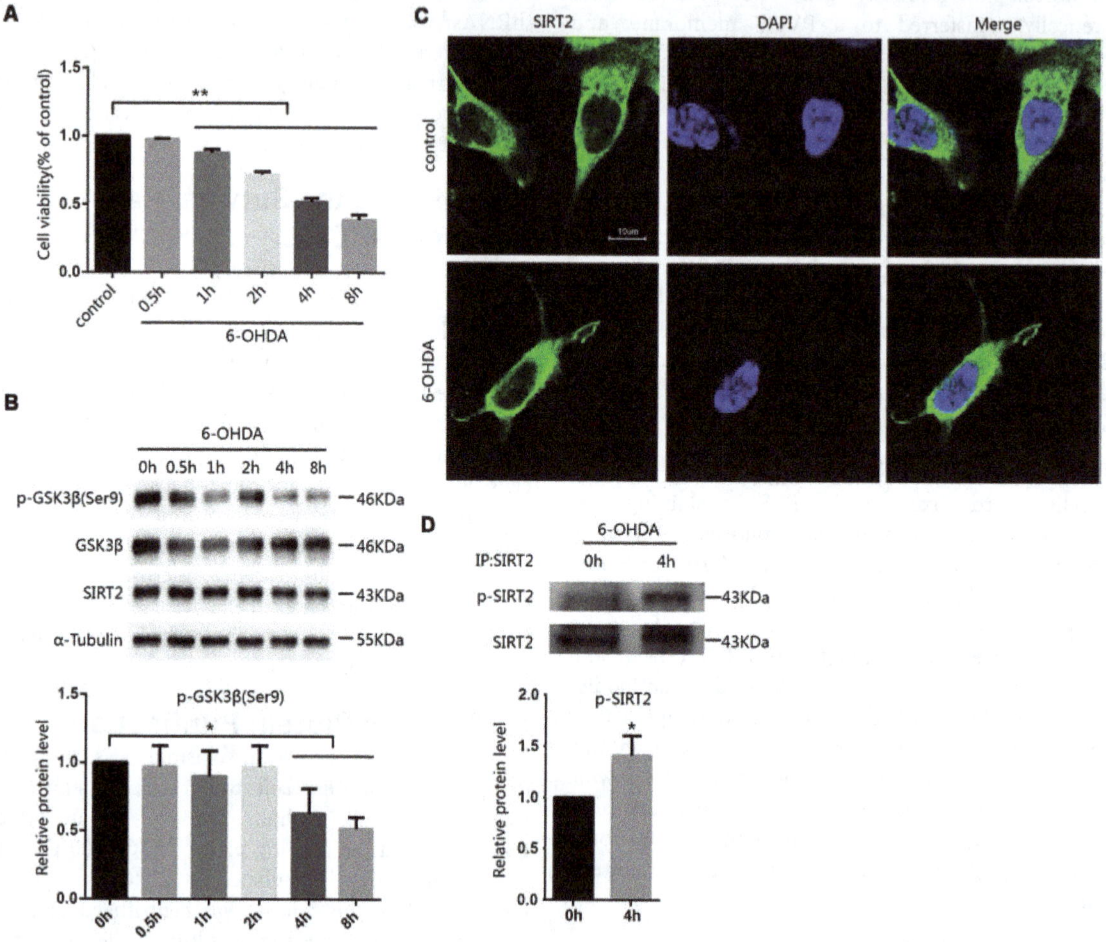

FIGURE 1 | Phosphorylation of SIRT2 increased after treatment with 6-OHDA. **(A)** SH-SY5Y cells were treated with 100 μM 6-OHDA for the indicated time. After 24 h, cell viability was measured by the MTT assay [$^{**}p < 0.01$, one-way analysis of variance (ANOVA) followed by Tukey's *post hoc* test]. **(B)** Western blot analysis showing the phosphorylation of GSK3β at Ser9 and total GSK3β, SIRT2 and α-tubulin levels in SH-SY5Y cells treated with 100 μM 6-OHDA for the indicated time. GSK3β activity was measured by detecting the phosphorylation of GSK3β at Ser9 by Western blot ($^{*}p < 0.05$, one-way ANOVA followed by Tukey's *post hoc* test; **C**). Fluorescence images representing SIRT2 immunofluorescence in phosphate-buffered saline (PBS)/6-OHDA-treated SH-SY5Y cells. Scale bar: 10 μm. **(D)** Western blot analysis showing SIRT2 phosphorylation in cells. Endogenous SIRT2 was immunoprecipitated from SH-SY5Y cells treated with or without 100 μM 6-OHDA for 4 h and probed with an anti-phosphoserine/threonine/tyrosine antibody to detect phosphorylation levels ($^{*}p < 0.05$, $^{**}p < 0.01$, two-tailed Student's *t*-test). The values are expressed as the mean ± SD, $n \geq 3$ for each group.

Phosphopeptide Identification by Mass Spectrometry (MS)

After *in vitro* phosphorylation, GST-SIRT2 was separated *via* SDS-PAGE. The gel was cut out after Coomassie blue staining, and the samples were sent to the Beijing Proteome Research Center (BPRC, China).

Statistics and Reproducibility

Statistical analysis was performed using Student's two-tailed unpaired *t*-tests for two-group comparisons and one-way analysis of variance (ANOVA) or two-way ANOVA for multigroup comparisons. *P* values < 0.05 were considered statistically significant and are indicated with asterisks ($^{*}P < 0.05$; $^{**}P < 0.01$; $^{***}P < 0.001$; $^{****}P < 0.0001$) in the figure legends. All of the data collected met the normal distribution assumptions of the tests. The data are represented as the mean ± SD. Each experiment was performed at least three times and in duplicate or more.

RESULTS

6-OHDA Elevates the Phosphorylation of SIRT2 in SH-SY5Y Cells

To investigate how toxins regulate SIRT2 function, we first established a cellular model of PD by applying 100 μM 6-OHDA to SH-SY5Y cells at the indicated times and concentrations and then assessed cell viability by the MTT assay. Cell viability decreased in a time-dependent manner following 6-OHDA exposure (**Figure 1A**). Further, we evaluated the expression of SIRT2 in SH-SY5Y cells after treatment with 6-OHDA, and SIRT2 levels showed a slight but not noticeable decrease. Furthermore, the active status of GSK3β was increased

(**Figure 1B**). Because SIRT2 can be distributed in the cytoplasm or nucleus under different conditions (Dryden et al., 2003; North et al., 2003; Liu et al., 2017), we wanted to know where SIRT2 is located under 6-OHDA treatment. We next treated SH-SY5Y cells with PBS as a control or 100 μM 6-OHDA for 4 h; later, the location of endogenous SIRT2 was assessed by immunofluorescence. We observed that SIRT2 resided in the cytoplasm for the duration of the experiment (**Figure 1C**). We next purified endogenous SIRT2 from SH-SY5Y cells treated with or without 6-OHDA and detected SIRT2 phosphorylation using an anti-phosphoserine/threonine/tyrosine antibody. We found that phosphorylated SIRT2 levels were significantly increased after treatment with 6-OHDA (**Figure 1D**).

The Protective Effect of GSK3β Inhibition Occurs Through a Blockade of SIRT2 Phosphorylation

Given that the activity of GSK3β was increased in SH-SY5Y cells treated with 6-OHDA, we blocked the activity of GSK3β in SH-SY5Y cells with SB216763 to determine whether this could protect the cells from 6-OHDA. We pretreated SH-SY5Y cells with different concentrations of SB216763 for 30 min and then applied 100 μM 6-OHDA for 4 h. After that, we measured cell viability and found that SB216763 rescued the SH-SY5Y cells from 6-OHDA (**Figure 2A**). We further analyzed the phosphorylation of endogenous SIRT2 among the control, 6-OHDA and 6-OHDA plus SB216763 groups and found that the phosphorylation of SIRT2 was increased in the 6-OHDA-treated cells, while SB216763 blocked the increase in SIRT2 phosphorylation (**Figure 2B**). These results indicate that GSK3β activation may be responsible for the increased phosphorylation of SIRT2.

SIRT2 is a tubulin deacetylase, and SB216763 increases the acetylation of tubulin (**Figure 2C**), which indicates that the decrease in SIRT2 phosphorylation mediated by SB216763 may reduce SIRT2 deacetylase activity. To further confirm this, we pretreated SH-SY5Y cells with DMSO, SB216763 or AGK2 and monitored the change in acetylated tubulin under 6-OHDA treatment. Acetylated tubulin levels decreased under 6-OHDA treatment, and both SB216763 and AGK2 reversed the decrease in acetylated tubulin levels (**Figure 2D**). To confirm that GSK3β participates in the regulation of SIRT2 deacetylase activity, we overexpressed PCMV-HA or GSK3β-HA in HEK293 cells and treated them with DMSO, SB216763 or AGK2 24 h later. The overexpression of GSK3β resulted in a decrease in acetylated tubulin levels, while SB216763 and AGK2 reversed the decrease in acetylated tubulin levels induced by the overexpression of GSK3β (**Figure 2E**). GSK3β further reduced acetylated tubulin levels relative to SIRT2 overexpression (the acetylated tubulin levels decreased by 23.73% and 40.65% in the absence or presence of GSK3β, respectively; **Figure 2F**). To further confirm that SIRT2 is the downstream target of GSK3β, we used shRNA to knock down endogenous SIRT2 (**Figure 2G**). We found that downregulated SIRT2 could reduce the toxicity of 6-OHDA, while SB216763 could not further improve cell viability after SIRT2 knockdown (**Figure 2H**). These data suggest that SIRT2 is the downstream target of GSK3β under 6-OHDA treatment. Taken together, our data demonstrate that 6-OHDA or the overexpression of GSK3β induces a decrease in acetylated tubulin levels and that inhibiting GSK3β with SB216763 counteracts this effect.

GSK3β Can Phosphorylate SIRT2 at Three Particular Sites

Given that inhibiting GSK3β blocked an increase in SIRT2 activity, we next tested whether SIRT2 interacts with GSK3β by coimmunoprecipitation (**Figures 3A,B**). Our results indicate that GSK3β and SIRT2 may interact in cells.

To test whether GSK3β directly phosphorylates SIRT2, we carried out an *in vitro* kinase assay. We purified GST-SIRT2 from *E. coli* BL21. Because it has been reported that SIRT2 is a phosphorylation substrate for CDK5, we used CDK5/p25 (p25 continues to activate CDK5) as a positive control. We found that GSK3β could phosphorylate SIRT2 (**Figure 3C**). To determine which sites are phosphorylated by GSK3β, we carried out an *in vitro* kinase assay followed by SDS-PAGE and Coomassie blue staining to detect phosphorylated SIRT2, which was later evaluated by MS (**Supplementary Figure S1**). Finally, we identified three sites that could be phosphorylated by GSK3β (**Figure 3D**). To validate the MS results, we mutated these three sites to alanine residues to mimic dephosphorylation. The mutants were purified from *E. coli* and subjected to the kinase assay. We found that each mutant decreased the phosphorylation of SIRT2 by GSK3β (**Figure 3E**). To further test whether the interaction between GSK3β and SIRT2 changes under 6-OHDA stress, we performed a coimmunoprecipitation assay. It was shown that the interaction between GSK3β and SIRT2 was increased under 6-OHDA treatment (**Figure 3F**). In conclusion, we identified S327, S331 and S335 as SIRT2 phosphorylation sites targeted by GSK3β.

SIRT2 Phosphorylation-Resistant Mutants Can Alleviate SIRT2 Toxicity in SH-SY5Y Cells

To further prove that the phosphorylation of SIRT2 by GSK3β does participate in 6-OHDA-induced SH-SY5Y cell death and that overactivated SIRT2 aggravates PD (Outeiro et al., 2007), we constructed two mutants, GFP-SIRT2SA and GFP-SIRT2-SD, to mimic dephosphorylation and phosphorylation, respectively (**Figure 4A**). Given that ace-tubulin is the substrate of SIRT2 (North et al., 2003), we measured the fluorescence intensity of ace-tubulin after the individual overexpression of GFP, GFP-SIRT2, GFP-SIRT2SA or GFP-SIRT2SD, and we found that the mutant that mimicked phosphorylation further decreased the acetylation of α-tubulin, while the mutant that mimicked dephosphorylation did not (**Figures 4B,C**). This result indicates that the phosphorylation-resistant mutant (GFP-SIRT2SA) blocks SIRT2 deacetylation activity. As we showed that GSK3β regulates the phosphorylation of SIRT2 and that the protective effect of blocking GSK3β in the PD cell model occurs through decreased SIRT2 phosphorylation,

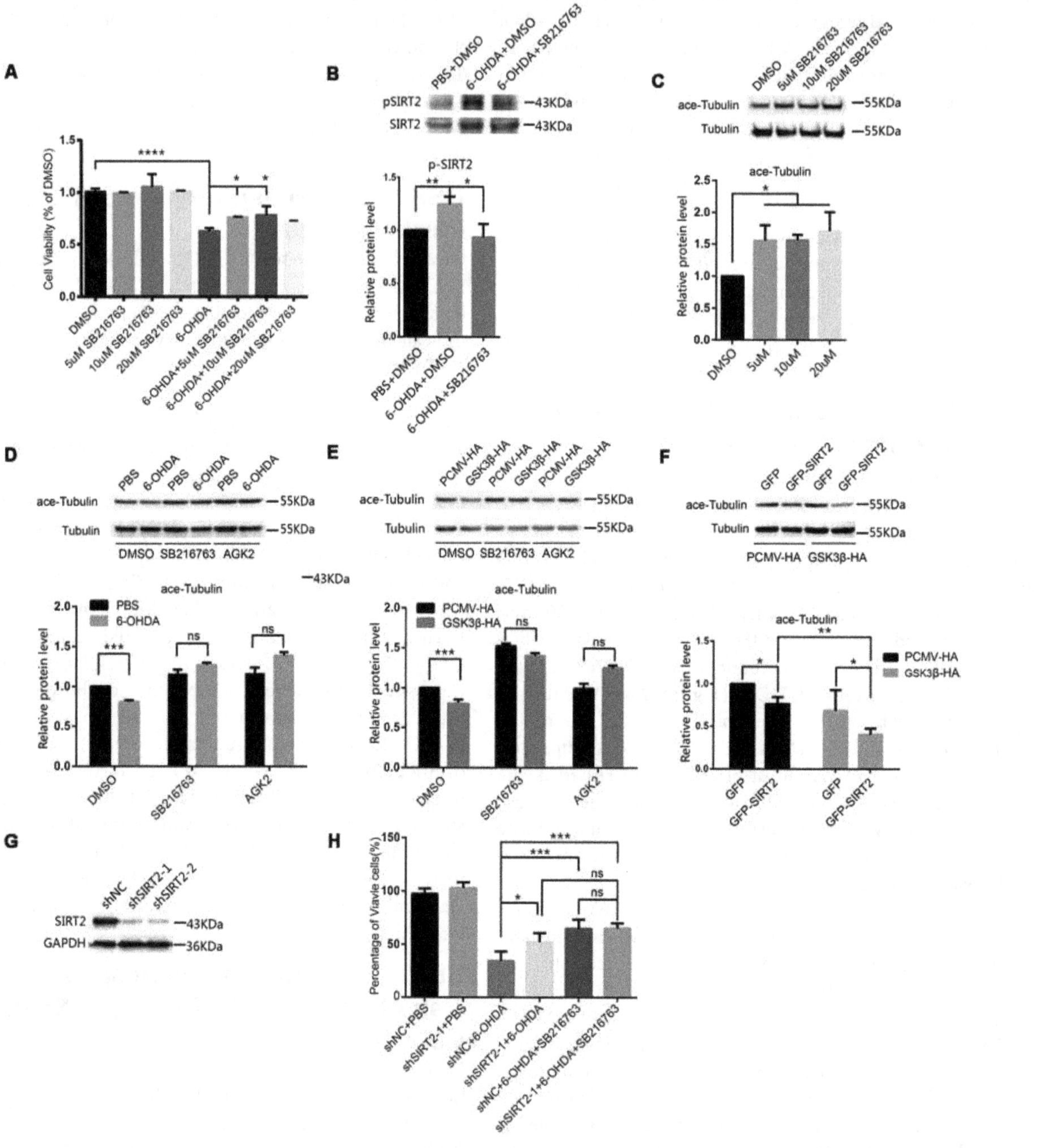

FIGURE 2 | Inhibition of GSK3β protected SH-SY5Y cells from 6-OHDA by decreasing SIRT2 phosphorylation. **(A)** SH-SY5Y cells were pretreated with different concentrations of SB216763 for 30 min and then treated with or without 100 μM 6-OHDA for 4 h. Cell viability was measured by the MTT assay (**p* < 0.05, *****p* < 0.0001, one-way ANOVA followed by Dunnett's *post hoc* test). **(B)** Endogenous SIRT2 was immunoprecipitated from whole-cell lysates, and p-SIRT2 was detected by an anti-phosphoserine/threonine/tyrosine antibody (**p* < 0.05, ***p* < 0.01, one-way ANOVA followed by Tukey's *post hoc* test). **(C)** Western blot analysis showing the acetylation of α-tubulin (ace-tubulin) and total α-tubulin levels in SH-SY5Y cells treated with DMSO or SB216763 at the indicated concentrations (**p* < 0.05, one-way ANOVA followed by Dunnett's *post hoc* test). **(D)** SH-SY5Y cells were pretreated with DMSO, 10 μM SB216763 or 10 μM AGK2 for 30 min and then treated with or without 100 μM 6-OHDA for 4 h. Ace-tubulin and α-tubulin were detected by Western blotting (****p* < 0.001, two-way ANOVA followed by Bonferroni's *post hoc* test). **(E)** HEK293 cells were treated with DMSO, 10 μM SB216763 or 10 μM AGK2 for 30 min after transfection with PCMV-HA as a control or GSK3β-HA for 24 h. Ace-tubulin and α-tubulin were detected by Western blotting (****p* < 0.001, two-way ANOVA followed by Bonferroni's *post hoc* test). **(F)** HEK293 cells were cotransfected with GFP (or GFP-SIRT2) and PCMV-HA (or GSK3β-HA) for 24 h. Ace-tubulin and α-tubulin were detected by Western blotting (**p* < 0.05, ***p* < 0.01, two-way ANOVA followed by Tukey's *post hoc* test). **(G)** The level of the SIRT2 protein was downregulated in SH-SY5Y cells transfected with SIRT2 shRNA (shSIRT2-1 or shSIRT2-2) compared to cells transfected with the control (shNC). SIRT2 and GAPDH were detected by Western blotting. **(H)** A histogram representing the percentage of viable cells. Cells were transfected with shRNA for 48 h and then treated with 6-OHDA for 4 h. The percentage of viable cells was calculated after 24 h (**p* < 0.05, ***p* < 0.01, ns, not statistically significant; one-way ANOVA followed by Tukey's *post hoc* test). The values are expressed as the mean ± SD, *n* ≥ 3 for each group.

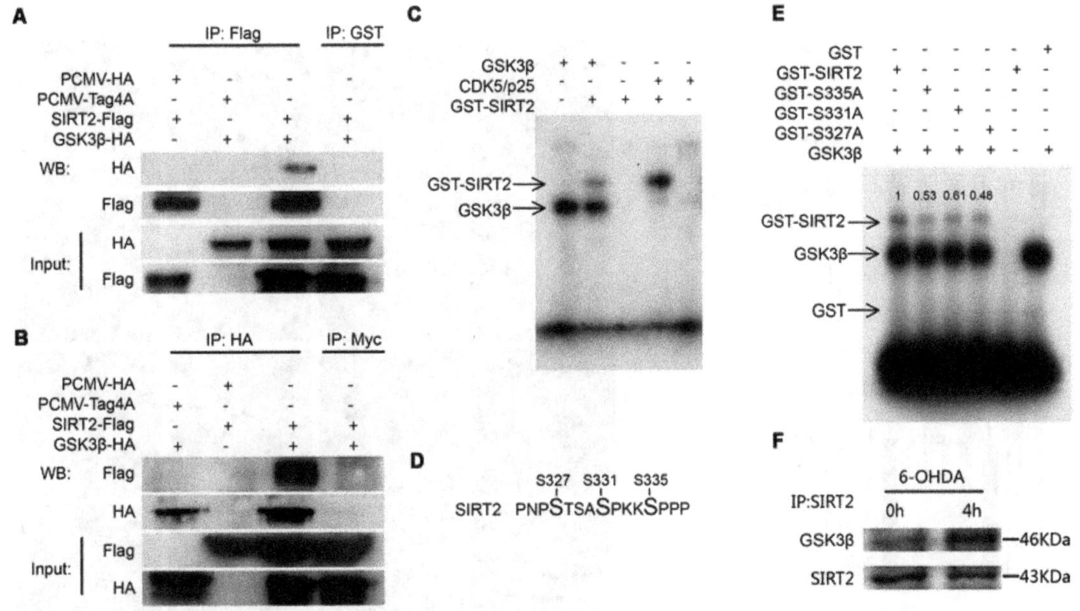

FIGURE 3 | SIRT2 could be phosphorylated by GSK3β *in vitro*. Panels **(A,B)** show the immunoprecipitation and immunoblot analyses of the interaction between SIRT2 and GSK3β in HEK293 cells expressing Flag-tagged SIRT2 or HA-tagged GSK3β. Anti-GST and anti-Myc antibodies were used as the IgG controls. **(C)** GST-SIRT2 was purified from BL21 *E. coli*, and an *in vitro* kinase assay was performed with or without GSK3β or CDK5/p25. GST-SIRT2 phosphorylation was confirmed by autoradiography. Because GSK3β is able to autophosphorylate, GSK3β bands are visible. **(D)** An *in vitro* kinase assay was performed with or without GSK3β. The samples were subjected to mass spectrometry (MS) to detect the phosphorylation of SIRT2. The S327, S331 and S335 sites were phosphorylated. **(E)** Serine was genetically mutated to alanine to mimic the dephosphorylation of the S327, S331 and S335 sites; then, the *in vitro* phosphorylation of these mutants by GSK3β was detected with autoradiography. **(F)** Endogenous SIRT2 was immunoprecipitated from SH-SY5Y cells treated with or without 100 μM 6-OHDA for 4 h. Western blotting analysis showing that the interaction between SIRT2 and GSK3β increased after treatment with 6-OHDA.

we next transfected SH-SY5Y cells with the GFP, GFP-SIRT2, GFP-SIRT2SA, or GFP-SIRT2SD plasmids for 24 h or 48 h. Cell viability was measured by live cell counting, and the data showed a notable increase in the viability of the cells overexpressing GFP-SIRT2SA (the GFP-SIRT2-overexpressing cells relative to the GFP-SIRT2SA-overexpressing cells, $^{*}P < 0.05$, $^{**}P < 0.01$), whereas there was no increase or decrease in the viability of the cells overexpressing GFP-SIRT2SD (the GFP-SIRT2-overexpressing cells relative to the GFP-SIRT2SD-overexpressing cells, $^{*}P < 0.05$, $^{***}P < 0.001$; **Figure 4D**). To assess whether AGK2 is able to block phospho-SIRT2 toxicity, we overexpressed the indicated plasmids and found that AGK2 was able to block GFP-SIRT2 toxicity but not GFP-SIRT2SD toxicity (**Figure 4E**).

These data indicate that the phosphorylation of SIRT2 by GSK3β at S327, S331 and S335 accelerates cell death. All of the data suggest that the dephosphorylation of S327, S331, and S335 decreases the activity of SIRT2, which could slow the cell death induced by SIRT2 (GFP-SIRT2) overexpression in SH-SY5Y cells.

DISCUSSION

SIRT2 appears to play a detrimental role in neurological disorders such as PD (Outeiro et al., 2007; Chen et al., 2015), Huntington's disease (Luthi-Carter et al., 2010) and ischemic stroke (Krey et al., 2015; Xie et al., 2017; She et al., 2018; Wu et al., 2018), and it is important to understand how SIRT2 is regulated since we know little about it. In the present study, we found that SIRT2 phosphorylation was increased in a cellular model of PD and that this change was mediated by the activation of GSK3β. We further identified three phosphorylation sites in SIRT2 that are targeted by GSK3β and found that a genetic mutant that mimics the dephosphorylation of SIRT2 can alleviate cell death induced by SIRT2 overexpression. Several types of evidence support this finding: (i) using Western blot analysis, we found that the phosphorylation of endogenous SIRT2 in SH-SY5Y cells is increased after treatment with 6-OHDA; (ii) SB216763, an inhibitor of GSK3β, reduced the phosphorylation of endogenous SIRT2; (iii) an *in vitro* kinase assay showed that SIRT2 is phosphorylated by GSK3β. Phosphoproteomic analysis of SIRT2 revealed that three particular sites are responsible for this phosphorylation; and (iv) genetic mutants that mimic the phosphorylation or phosphorylation resistance of the three phosphorylation sites aggravates or alleviates SIRT2-induced cell death in SH-SY5Y cells, respectively.

In this study, we first determined the subcellular location of SIRT2 under 6-OHDA treatment and found that it remains in the cytoplasm. SIRT2 regularly localizes to the cytoplasm (North et al., 2003), and it has also been reported to localize to the nucleus during the G2/M phase (Dryden et al., 2003; North et al., 2003). This prompted us to search for an upstream regulator of SIRT2 in the cytoplasm. A previous study showed that the acetylation of GSK3β increases in pathological

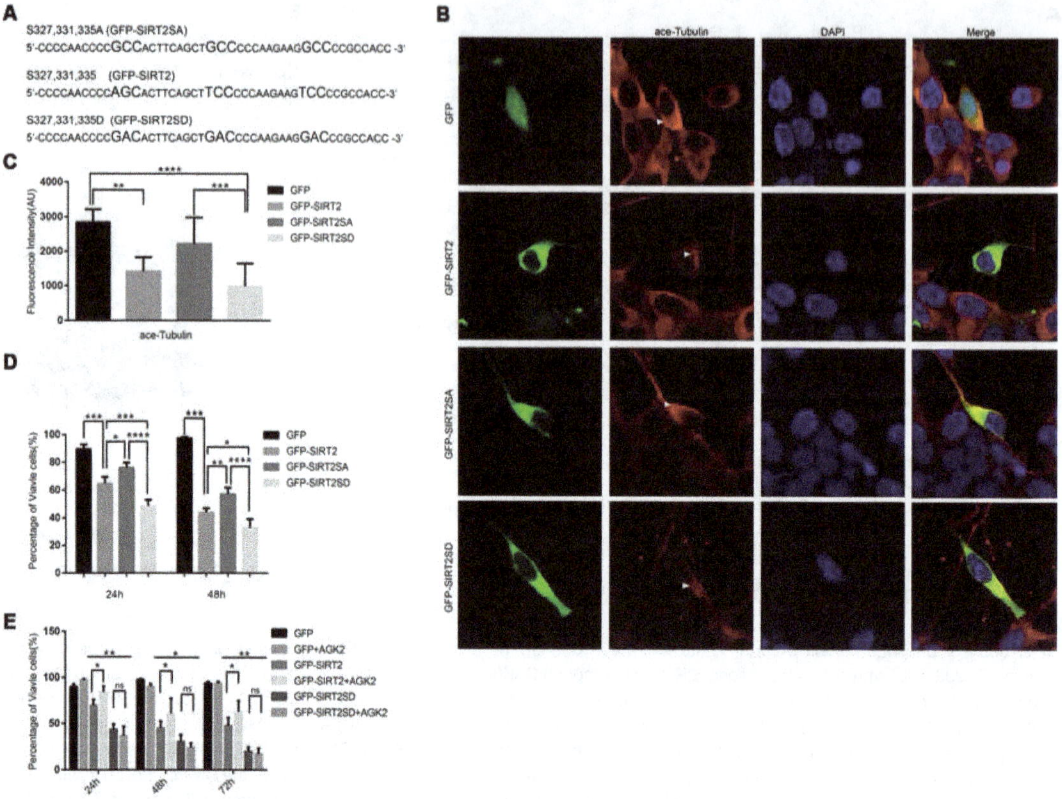

FIGURE 4 | A SIRT2 phosphorylation mimic enhanced SIRT2 cytotoxicity. **(A)** GFP-SIRT2 is the wild-type plasmid DNA sequence, GFP-SIRT2SA is the dephosphorylation mimic sequence, and GFP-SIRT2SD is the phosphorylation mimic sequence. **(B)** Fluorescence images showing ace-tubulin expression in cells transfected with GFP, GFP-SIRT2, GFP-SIRT2SA or GFP-SIRT2SD; the fluorescence intensity of ace-tubulin is shown in red (arrowheads). **(C)** A histogram representing the fluorescence intensity of ace-tubulin immunofluorescence in cells transfected with GFP, GFP-SIRT2, GFP-SIRT2SA or GFP-SIRT2SD ($^{**}p < 0.01$, $^{***}p < 0.001$, $^{****}p < 0.0001$, one-way ANOVA followed by Tukey's *post hoc* test). **(D)** A histogram representing the percentage of viable cells. The percentage of viable cells in GFP-, GFP-SIRT2-, GFP-SIRT2SA- or GFP-SIRT2SD-transfected cells was calculated after 24 and 48 h ($^{**}p < 0.01$, $^{***}p < 0.001$, $^{****}p < 0.0001$, two-way ANOVA followed by Tukey's *post hoc* test). **(E)** A histogram representing the percentage of viable cells. AGK2 was added after the cells were transfected for 24 h. The percentage of viable cells was calculated 24 h, 48 h and 72 h after the addition of AGK2 ($^{*}p < 0.05$, $^{**}p < 0.01$, two-way ANOVA followed by Tukey's *post hoc* test). The values are expressed as the mean ± SD, $n \geq 3$ for each group ($^{*}p < 0.05$, $^{**}p < 0.01$, $^{***}p < 0.005$, ns, not statistically significant; two-tailed Student's *t*-test).

cardiac hypertrophy and that SIRT2 binds to, deacetylates and activates GSK3β (Sarikhani et al., 2018). SIRT2 may also act as an upstream regulator of GSK3β to modulate the differentiation of dopaminergic neurons (Szegö et al., 2017). Here, we proposed that the increase in SIRT2 phosphorylation mediated by GSK3β affects SIRT2 catalytic activity as well. To obtain the data presented here, we used a mutant that mimics the dephosphorylation of SIRT2 (GFP-SIRT2SA) and found that it does not decrease α-tubulin acetylation, which is the opposite of what is observed with the mutant that mimics the phosphorylation of SIRT2 (GFP-SIRT2SD). Compared to GFP-SIRT2, GFP-SIRT2SA significantly increased the survival of SH-SY5Y cells. This result coincides with that of a previous study (Outeiro et al., 2007). We showed that SIRT2 phosphorylation increases after exposure to 6-OHDA, and we speculated that SIRT2 phosphorylation accelerates cell death. As expected, cell death worsened in the GFP-SIRT2SD group. Thus, the mutant that mimics the dephosphorylation of SIRT2 (GFP-SIRT2SA) can lessen the cell death induced by SIRT2 overexpression by decreasing SIRT2 deacetylase activity. All of these data suggest that there are complex regulatory relationships between SIRT2 and GSK3β.

We found that AGK2 could not inhibit GFP-SIRT2SD toxicity. This suggests that the phosphorylation sites we found here may be important for the ligand docking of AGK2. In previous studies, decreased enzymatic activity was observed in several C-terminal alanine substitution mutations, such as mutations at S327 or S331 and S335 (Nahhas et al., 2007). Interestingly, S331A and S335A individually did not affect SIRT2 enzymatic activity, but double substitutions elicited a 44% reduction in activity (Nahhas et al., 2007). These reports are consistent with our finding that GFP-SIRT2SA reduces SIRT2 deacetylation activity. In contrast, the phosphorylation of S331 or a phospho-mimicking mutant of this site also inhibits the catalytic activity of SIRT2 (Pandithage et al., 2008). This report differs from our finding that GFP-SIRT2SD does not reduce SIRT2 deacetylation activity. This may be due to the simultaneous substitution of three serine residues in SIRT2.

A preferred site for ligand binding of AGK2 is the "C-pocket" with a hydrogen-bonding pattern that mimics the action of nicotinamide, a known inhibitor of sirtuins (Outeiro et al., 2007). Since S327, S331 and S335 are located outside of the "C-pocket," these serine residues may affect the SIRT2 enzymatic activity by altering the conformation of the protein. In fact, nicotinamide blocks the activity of the phospho-mimicking mutant GST-SIRT-S331D (Pandithage et al., 2008), suggesting that AGK2 also inhibits the activity of GST-SIRT2-S331D. Similarly, we observed that AGK2 does not inhibit GFP-SIRT2SD toxicity, which may be because three simultaneous substitutions alter the conformation of the "C pocket," resulting in the failure of AGK2 docking. Our results indicate that S327, S331 and S335 can be simultaneously phosphorylated by GSK3β *in vitro*, and we are not sure whether this modification occurs *in vivo*. More experiments are needed to study this phenomenon.

Interestingly, it has been reported that CDK5 phosphorylates SIRT2 at S331 (Pandithage et al., 2008), S331 and S335 (Zhang et al., 2018), and we found that S327, S331 and S335 are phosphorylated by GSK3β. Furthermore, the phosphorylation of SIRT2 was found to be stronger after the coapplication of CDK5 and GSK3β (data not shown). These results indicate that there may be crosstalk between the GSK3β and CDK5 pathways. The data we present here suggest that phosphorylation-resistant mutants inhibit the catalytic activity of SIRT2. Nevertheless, phosphorylation by CDK5 inhibits the catalytic activity of SIRT2 (Pandithage et al., 2008). S331 is a common phosphorylation site, and the opposite effect may rely on other phosphorylation sites. Thus, targeting CDK5 and GSK3β at the same time may be a potential direction for the development of therapeutic strategies for PD. One possible approach is to block CDK5 and GSK3β simultaneously with one or two inhibitors. Using this strategy, we can obtain inactivated SIRT2 that is unphosphorylated at S327, S331 and S335. This may be the most effective strategy to suppress SIRT2 expression (Nahhas et al., 2007). There are many inhibitors currently in clinical trials that can block CDK5 and GSK3β simultaneously, such as AZD5438 and brain permeable AZD1080. Roscovitine and CHIR-99021, which are inhibitors of CDK5 and GSK3β, respectively, can also be used together. However, it is worth noting that the activities of CDK5 and GSK3β are related and that crosstalk depends on age (Engmann and Giese, 2009). In young mice, an increase in p25-induced CDK5 activity inhibits GSK3β activity by enhancing inhibitory phosphorylation at Ser-9 of GSK3β (Plattner et al., 2006). However, in older mice, GSK3β activity is enhanced in p25 transgenic mice (Plattner et al., 2006; Wen et al., 2008). Thus, the reaction of young and aged mice to the simultaneous targeting of CDK5 and GSK3β may be different.

As aging is considered a major risk factor for the development of PD, the pathways involved in aging may provide targets for therapeutic interventions for PD. SIRT2 is a member of the sirtuin family of proteins, which participate in a variety of cellular functions and play a role in aging (Maxwell et al., 2011). Outeiro et al. (2007) found that the inhibition of SIRT2 rescues α-synuclein toxicity and modifies inclusion morphology in a cellular model of PD (Dillin and Kelly, 2007; Garske et al., 2007). Later, de Oliveira et al. (2017) showed that α-synuclein is deacetylated by SIRT2 and that α-synuclein acetylation is a key regulatory mechanism governing α-synuclein aggregation and toxicity. Here, we further characterized SIRT2, showing that its activity is activated by its phosphorylation by GSK3β in a cellular model of PD. Based on the above conclusions, we elucidated a complete GSK3β-SIRT2-α-synuclein signaling cascade that participates in the development of PD. Because of the importance of α-synuclein in PD, we believe this cascade may play a vital role in PD. We may find treatments that inhibit the progression of PD by targeting this cascade.

Taken together, the data presented here highlight a previously unexplored cellular pathway that might underlie the impairment of dopaminergic neurons in PD, further underscoring the potential of the GSK3β-SIRT2-α-synuclein signaling cascade as a viable target pathway for neuroprotective therapies.

AUTHOR CONTRIBUTIONS

XW designed the experiments. SL and ZZ performed the enzyme activity assays and the biochemical analysis of the SH-SY5Y cells. LZ, SM and SLi analyzed the data. SL and ZZ wrote the manuscript with help from XW. All authors read and approved the final manuscript.

FUNDING

This work was supported by the Natural Science Foundation of Guangdong (2016A030311009), the National Natural Science Foundation of China (31371184), and the Program for Changjiang Scholars and the Innovative Research Team in University (IRT_16R37).

SUPPLEMENTARY MATERIAL

FIGURE S1 | Phosphopeptide identification by mass spectrometry (MS). **(A)** GST-SIRT2 was purified from BL21 *E. coli*, and an *in vitro* kinase assay was performed with or without GSK3β. The samples were separated *via* SDS-PAGE, and then the gel was visualized with Coomassie blue staining. The band in the red rectangle was subjected to MS. **(B)** The serine residues in red are the predicted phosphorylated sites.

REFERENCES

Acevedo, K. M., Opazo, C. M., Norrish, D., Challis, L. M., Li, Q. X., White, A. R., et al. (2014). Phosphorylation of amyloid precursor protein at threonine 668 is essential for its copper-responsive trafficking in SH-SY5Y neuroblastoma cells. *J. Biol. Chem.* 289, 11007–11019. doi: 10.1074/jbc.m113.538710

Chen, X., Wales, P., Quinti, L., Zuo, F., Moniot, S., Herisson, F., et al. (2015). The sirtuin-2 inhibitor AK7 is neuroprotective in models of Parkinson's disease but not amyotrophic lateral sclerosis and cerebral ischemia. *PLoS One* 10:e0116919. doi: 10.1371/journal.pone.0116919

Dawson, T. M., and Dawson, V. L. (2003). Molecular pathways of neurodegeneration in Parkinson's disease. *Science* 302, 819–822. doi: 10.1126/science.1087753

de Oliveira, R. M., Vicente Miranda, H., Francelle, L., Pinho, R., Szegö, E. M., Martinho, R., et al. (2017). The mechanism of sirtuin 2-mediated exacerbation of α-synuclein toxicity in models of Parkinson disease. *PLoS Biol.* 15:e2000374. doi: 10.1371/journal.pbio.2000374

Dillin, A., and Kelly, J. W. (2007). Medicine. The yin-yang of sirtuins. *Science* 317, 461–462. doi: 10.1126/science.1146585

Dryden, S. C., Nahhas, F. A., Nowak, J. E., Goustin, A. S., and Tainsky, M. A. (2003). Role for human SIRT2 NAD-dependent deacetylase activity in control of mitotic exit in the cell cycle. *Mol. Cell. Biol.* 23, 3173–3185. doi: 10.1128/mcb.23.9.3173-3185.2003

Dutta, D., Ali, N., Banerjee, E., Singh, R., Naskar, A., Paidi, R. K., et al. (2018). Low levels of prohibitin in substantia nigra makes dopaminergic neurons vulnerable in Parkinson's disease. *Mol. Neurobiol.* 55, 804–821. doi: 10.1007/s12035-016-0328-y

Engmann, O., and Giese, K. P. (2009). Crosstalk between Cdk5 and GSK3β: implications for Alzheimer's disease. *Front. Mol. Neurosci.* 2:2. doi: 10.3389/neuro.02.002.2009

Garske, A. L., Smith, B. C., and Denu, J. M. (2007). Linking SIRT2 to Parkinson's disease. *ACS Chem. Biol.* 2, 529–532. doi: 10.1021/cb700160d

Guan, Q., Wang, M., Chen, H., Yang, L., Yan, Z., and Wang, X. (2016). Aging-related 1-methyl-4-phenyl-1,2,3,6-tetrahydropyridine-induced neurochemial and behavioral deficits and redox dysfunction: improvement by AK-7. *Exp. Gerontol.* 82, 19–29. doi: 10.1016/j.exger.2016.05.011

Hernandez-Baltazar, D., Mendoza-Garrido, M. E., and Martinez-Fong, D. (2013). Activation of GSK-3β and caspase-3 occurs in Nigral dopamine neurons during the development of apoptosis activated by a striatal injection of 6-hydroxydopamine. *PLoS One* 8:e70951. doi: 10.1371/journal.pone.0070951

Hongo, H., Kihara, T., Kume, T., Izumi, Y., Niidome, T., Sugimoto, H., et al. (2012). Glycogen synthase kinase-3β activation mediates rotenone-induced cytotoxicity with the involvement of microtubule destabilization. *Biochem. Biophys. Res. Commun.* 426, 94–99. doi: 10.1016/j.bbrc.2012.08.042

Ikeda, Y., Tsuji, S., Satoh, A., Ishikura, M., Shirasawa, T., and Shimizu, T. (2008). Protective effects of astaxanthin on 6-hydroxydopamine-induced apoptosis in human neuroblastoma SH-SY5Y cells. *J. Neurochem.* 107, 1730–1740. doi: 10.1111/j.1471-4159.2008.05743.x

Infante, J., García-Gorostiaga, I., Sánchez-Juan, P., Sierra, M., Martín-Gurpegui, J. L., Terrazas, J., et al. (2010). Synergistic effect of two oxidative stress-related genes (heme oxygenase-1 and GSK3β) on the risk of Parkinson's disease. *Eur. J. Neurol.* 17, 760–762. doi: 10.1111/j.1468-1331.2009.02908.x

Kawakami, F., Shimada, N., Ohta, E., Kagiya, G., Kawashima, R., Maekawa, T., et al. (2014). Leucine-rich repeat kinase 2 regulates tau phosphorylation through direct activation of glycogen synthase kinase-3β. *FEBS J.* 281, 3–13. doi: 10.1111/febs.12579

Krey, L., Lühder, F., Kusch, K., Czech-Zechmeister, B., Könnecke, B., Fleming Outeiro, T., et al. (2015). Knockout of silent information regulator 2 (SIRT2) preserves neurological function after experimental stroke in mice. *J. Cereb. Blood Flow Metab.* 35, 2080–2088. doi: 10.1038/jcbfm.2015.178

Kwok, J. B., Hallupp, M., Loy, C. T., Chan, D. K., Woo, J., Mellick, G. D., et al. (2005). GSK3B polymorphisms alter transcription and splicing in Parkinson's disease. *Ann. Neurol.* 58, 829–839. doi: 10.1002/ana.20691

Lees, A. J. (2007). Unresolved issues relating to the shaking palsy on the celebration of James Parkinson's 250th birthday. *Mov. Disord.* 22, S327–334. doi: 10.1002/mds.21684

Li, Y., Luo, F., Wei, L., Liu, Z., and Xu, P. (2011). Knockdown of glycogen synthase kinase 3 β attenuates 6-hydroxydopamine-induced apoptosis in SH-SY5Y cells. *Neurosci. Lett.* 487, 41–46. doi: 10.1016/j.neulet.2010.09.070

Liu, G., Park, S. H., Imbesi, M., Nathan, W. J., Zou, X., Zhu, Y., et al. (2017). Loss of NAD-dependent protein deacetylase sirtuin-2 alters mitochondrial protein acetylation and dysregulates mitophagy. *Antioxid. Redox Signal.* 26, 849–863. doi: 10.1089/ars.2016.6662

Luthi-Carter, R., Taylor, D. M., Pallos, J., Lambert, E., Amore, A., Parker, A., et al. (2010). SIRT2 inhibition achieves neuroprotection by decreasing sterol biosynthesis. *Proc. Natl. Acad. Sci. U S A* 107, 7927–7932. doi: 10.1073/pnas.1002924107

Maxwell, M. M., Tomkinson, E. M., Nobles, J., Wizeman, J. W., Amore, A. M., Quinti, L., et al. (2011). The Sirtuin 2 microtubule deacetylase is an abundant neuronal protein that accumulates in the aging CNS. *Hum. Mol. Genet.* 20, 3986–3996. doi: 10.1093/hmg/ddr326

Nagao, M., and Hayashi, H. (2009). Glycogen synthase kinase-3β is associated with Parkinson's disease. *Neurosci. Lett.* 449, 103–107. doi: 10.1016/j.neulet.2008.10.104

Nahhas, F., Dryden, S. C., Abrams, J., and Tainsky, M. A. (2007). Mutations in SIRT2 deacetylase which regulate enzymatic activity but not its interaction with HDAC6 and tubulin. *Mol. Cell. Biochem.* 303, 221–230. doi: 10.1007/s11010-007-9478-6

North, B. J., Marshall, B. L., Borra, M. T., Denu, J. M., and Verdin, E. (2003). The human Sir2 ortholog, SIRT2, is an NAD+-dependent tubulin deacetylase. *Mol. Cell* 11, 437–444. doi: 10.1016/s1097-2765(03)00038-8

Outeiro, T. F., Kontopoulos, E., Altmann, S. M., Kufareva, I., Strathearn, K. E., Amore, A. M., et al. (2007). Sirtuin 2 inhibitors rescue α-synuclein-mediated toxicity in models of Parkinson's disease. *Science* 317, 516–519. doi: 10.1126/science.1143780

Pandithage, R., Lilischkis, R., Harting, K., Wolf, A., Jedamzik, B., Lüscher-Firzlaff, J., et al. (2008). The regulation of SIRT2 function by cyclin-dependent kinases affects cell motility. *J. Cell Biol.* 180, 915–929. doi: 10.1083/jcb.200707126

Petit-Paitel, A., Brau, F., Cazareth, J., and Chabry, J. (2009). Involvment of cytosolic and mitochondrial GSK-3β in mitochondrial dysfunction and neuronal cell death of MPTP/MPP-treated neurons. *PLoS One* 4:e5491. doi: 10.1371/journal.pone.0005491

Plattner, F., Angelo, M., and Giese, K. P. (2006). The roles of cyclin-dependent kinase 5 and glycogen synthase kinase 3 in tau hyperphosphorylation. *J. Biol. Chem.* 281, 25457–25465. doi: 10.1074/jbc.M603469200

Sarikhani, M., Mishra, S., Maity, S., Kotyada, C., Wolfgeher, D., Gupta, M. P., et al. (2018). SIRT2 deacetylase regulates the activity of GSK3 isoforms independent of inhibitory phosphorylation. *Elife* 7:e32952. doi: 10.7554/elife.32952

She, D. T., Wong, L. J., Baik, S. H., and Arumugam, T. V. (2018). SIRT2 inhibition confers neuroprotection by downregulation of FOXO3a and MAPK signaling pathways in ischemic stroke. *Mol. Neurobiol.* 55, 9188–9203. doi: 10.1007/s12035-018-1058-0

Si, X., Chen, W., Guo, X., Chen, L., Wang, G., Xu, Y., et al. (2013). Activation of GSK3β by Sirt2 is required for early lineage commitment of mouse embryonic stem cell. *PLoS One* 8:e76699. doi: 10.1371/journal.pone.0076699

Szegö, É. M., Gerhardt, E., and Outeiro, T. F. (2017). Sirtuin 2 enhances dopaminergic differentiation via the AKT/GSK-3β/β-catenin pathway. *Neurobiol. Aging* 56, 7–16. doi: 10.1016/j.neurobiolaging.2017.04.001

Wang, X., Guan, Q., Wang, M., Yang, L., Bai, J., Yan, Z., et al. (2015). Aging-related rotenone-induced neurochemical and behavioral deficits: role of SIRT2 and redox imbalance and neuroprotection by AK-7. *Drug Des. Devel. Ther.* 9, 2553–2563. doi: 10.2147/dddt.s81539

Wang, Y., Liu, W., He, X., and Zhou, F. (2013). Parkinson's disease-associated DJ-1 mutations increase abnormal phosphorylation of tau protein through Akt/GSK-3β pathways. *J. Mol. Neurosci.* 51, 911–918. doi: 10.1007/s12031-013-0099-0

Wen, Y., Planel, E., Herman, M., Figueroa, H. Y., Wang, L., Liu, L., et al. (2008). Interplay between cyclin-dependent kinase 5 and glycogen synthase kinase 3 β mediated by neuregulin signaling leads to differential effects on tau phosphorylation and amyloid precursor protein processing. *J. Neurosci.* 28, 2624–2632. doi: 10.1523/JNEUROSCI.5245-07.2008

Wu, D., Lu, W., Wei, Z., Xu, M., and Liu, X. (2018). Neuroprotective effect of Sirt2-specific inhibitor AK-7 against acute cerebral ischemia is P38 activation-dependent in mice. *Neuroscience* 374, 61–69. doi: 10.1016/j.neuroscience.2018.01.040

Xie, X. Q., Zhang, P., Tian, B., and Chen, X. Q. (2017). Downregulation of NAD-dependent deacetylase SIRT2 protects mouse brain against ischemic stroke. *Mol. Neurobiol.* 54, 7251–7261. doi: 10.1007/s12035-016-0173-z

Zhang, Z., Zhang, P., Qi, G. J., Jiao, F. J., Wang, Q. Z., Yan, J. G., et al. (2018). CDK5-mediated phosphorylation of Sirt2 contributes to depressive-like behavior induced by social defeat stress. *Biochim. Biophys. Acta Mol. Basis Dis.* 1864, 533–541. doi: 10.1016/j.bbadis.2017.11.012

Zhao, Q., Ye, J., Wei, N., Fong, C., and Dong, X. (2016). Protection against MPP^+-induced neurotoxicity in SH-SY5Y cells by tormentic acid via the activation of PI3-K/Akt/GSK3β pathway. *Neurochem. Int.* 97, 117–123. doi: 10.1016/j.neuint.2016.03.010

Zhu, H., Zhao, L., Wang, E., Dimova, N., Liu, G., Feng, Y., et al. (2012). The QKI-PLP pathway controls SIRT2 abundance in CNS myelin. *Glia* 60, 69–82. doi: 10.1002/glia.21248

10

Normal and Pathological Tau Uptake Mediated by M1/M3 Muscarinic Receptors Promotes Opposite Neuronal Changes

Viktoriya Morozova[1,2]*, Leah S. Cohen*[1]*, Ali El-Hadi Makki*[1]*, Alison Shur*[1,2]*, Guillermo Pilar*[3]*, Abdeslem El Idrissi*[1,2] *and Alejandra D. Alonso*[1,2]*

[1] *Department of Biology and Center for Developmental Neuroscience, College of Staten Island, The City University of New York, Staten Island, NY, United States,* [2] *Biology Program, The Graduate Center, The City University of New York, New York, NY, United States,* [3] *Department of Neurosciences, Case Western Reserve University, Cleveland, OH, United States*

***Correspondence:**
Alejandra D. Alonso
Alejandra.Alonso@csi.cuny.edu

The microtubule associated protein tau is mainly found in the cell's cytosol but recently it was also shown in the extracellular space. In neurodegenerative diseases, like Alzheimer's disease (AD), pathological tau spreads from neuron to neuron enhancing neurodegeneration. Here, we show that HEK293 cells and neurons in culture uptake extracellular normal and pathological Tau. Muscarinic receptor antagonists atropine and pirenzepine block 80% this uptake. CHO cells do not express these receptors therefore cannot uptake tau, unless transfected with M1 and/or M3 receptor. These results strongly suggest that muscarinic receptors mediate this process. Uptake of normal tau in neurons enhances neuronal process formation but a pseudophosphorylated form of tau (pathological human tau, PH-Tau) disrupts them and accumulates in the somatodendritic compartment. AD hyperphosphorylated tau (AD P-Tau) has similar effects as PH-Tau on cultured neurons. Addition of either PH-Tau or AD P-tau to neuronal cultures induced microglial activation. In conclusion, uptake of extracellular tau is mediated by muscarinic receptors with opposite effects: normal tau stabilizes neurites; whereas pathological tau disrupts this process leading to neurodegeneration.

Keywords: tau, muscarinic receptors, uptake, neurodegeneration, Alzheimer's disease

INTRODUCTION

Tau is a neuronal cytosolic microtubule associated phospho-protein whose function can be influenced by post-translational modifications. Abnormally phosphorylated tau is a common denominator in several types of dementia, including Alzheimer's disease (AD) and other tauopathies (Goedert et al., 2010; Beharry et al., 2014).

Unlike normal tau, soluble hyperphosphorylated tau taken from AD patients (AD P-tau) does not promote microtubule assembly. Instead, AD P-tau binds normal tau, sequestering it from interactions with tubulin and producing bundles of filaments observed by electron microscopy (Alonso et al., 1996). This suggests that differences in tau phosphorylation states could affect its conformation and subsequently alter protein-protein interactions and tau biological function. Seeding activity into self-assembled aggregates can lead to the development of neurofibrillary tangles. We have shown previously that pseudophosphorylation at Ser199, Thr212, Thr231, and Ser262 with inclusion of the FTDP-17 R406W mutation (Pathological Human Tau, PH-Tau) results in a protein that mimics the effect of AD P-tau in culture (Alonso et al., 2010). This protein has been studied in mammalian cell culture, Drosophila, and mouse models. The expression of PH-Tau induced microtubule disruption in all systems, and resulted in cognitive and behavior impairment in Drosophila and mice (Alonso et al., 2010; Beharry et al., 2013; Di et al., 2016).

In AD, the initial neurodegenerative lesions are in the transentorhinal cortex spreading slowly to the hippocampus and neocortex (Hyman et al., 1984; Braak and Braak, 1991; Goedert et al., 2010), leading to cognitive decline. It was proposed that pathological tau is spread from cell to cell in a prion-like fashion (Holmes and Diamond, 2014; Mudher et al., 2017). The seeding and propagation of filamentous structures by hyperpshosphorylated tau has been a central point in AD research (Alonso et al., 2016; Hu et al., 2016; Iqbal et al., 2016; Mudher et al., 2017; Shafiei et al., 2017). Cells in culture take up tau aggregates ranging in size from oligomers and short filaments (neuronal cells) to fibrils (non-neuronal cells) through endocytosis (Frost et al., 2009; Nonaka et al., 2010; Guo and Lee, 2011; Wu et al., 2013; Sanders et al., 2014; Wu et al., 2016). Recently, it has been shown that monomeric tau can enter neurons (Evans et al., 2018) and based on the kinetics of tau uptake, it was suggested that this might be a receptor-mediated process (Evans et al., 2018). Furthermore, intracerebral injections of abnormal tau showed that tau pathology propagates away from the injection site, to neighboring brain regions indicating that tau can be transferred from cell to cell (Bolmont et al., 2007; Clavaguera et al., 2009; Lasagna-Reeves et al., 2012; Clavaguera et al., 2013; Iba et al., 2013; Wu et al., 2013; Ahmed et al., 2014; Clavaguera et al., 2014). Taken together, these results have led to the tau propagation hypothesis in which tau is released from one neuron into the intra-neuronal space, and taken up by other neurons transferring tau toxicity in a similar fashion as prion proteins (as reviewed in Takeda, 2019).

In this study we demonstrate that addition of recombinant tau protein to the culture media of Human Embryonic Kidney cells (HEK293) and primary cerebellar neuronal culture results in the uptake of tau and PH-Tau. Chinese Hamster Ovary (CHO) cells are unable to uptake tau unless they are transfected with M1- and M3-type muscarinic receptors. Furthermore, uptake into both HEK293 cells and cerebellar neurons is blocked by atropine, a muscarinic receptor antagonist, and uptake in cerebellar neurons is blocked by pirenzepine, an M1 antagonist, but not AF-DX116, an M2 antagonist, or pertussis toxin (PTX), an M2/M4 antagonist. Neuronal cultures incubated with wild-type tau for 7 days show an abundant and well-organized neuritic arbor. Similar cultures exposed to PH-Tau and AD P-tau show accumulation of tau in the somatodendritic neuronal compartment and disruption of neuronal processes. Our experimental results suggest that both tau and pathogenic tau are taken up in mammalian cells and neurons in a muscarinic receptor-mediated uptake mechanism that facilitates long-term neuronal changes.

MATERIALS AND METHODS

Antibodies

The primary antibodies used in this work are as follows: tau-13 (mouse, 1:1,000,000 for Western blot, 1:1000 for immunohistochemistry), CHRM1 (rabbit, 1:1000, Invitrogen, Cat#711098), βactin (1:2500, Santa Cruz, Cat#SC4778), β-III tubulin (chicken, 1:1000, Abcam, Cat#AB107216), GFAP (rabbit, 1:1000, Invitrogen Cat#PA3-16-727), IbaI (rabbit, 1:1000, Wako Cat#019-19741). The secondary antibodies used in this work are as follows: anti-mouse IgG-HRP (1:2000, Santa Cruz, Cat#SC-516102), anti-mouse Alexa 488 (1:1000, Invitrogen, Cat#A21202), anti-chicken Alexa 555 (1:1000, Invitrogen, Cat#A21437), anti-rabbit Alexa 594 (1:1000, Invitrogen, Cat#A21203). Tau-13 antibodies were a gift from Dr. Nicholas Kanaan at Michigan State University (originally created by Dr. Lester Binder at Northwestern University).

Recombinant Protein Expression and Purification

GST-tagged proteins were transformed into BL21(DE3)pLysS cells and purified using glutathione-sepharose beads (GE Healthcare) as described (Cevher et al., 2010).

Protein Quantitation, PAGE, and Western Blot Analysis

Quantitation of protein samples was performed by either the Bradford assay or by UV quantitation. The Bradford assay was performed on recombinant proteins and cell and neuronal lysates as described by the BioRad manual. Recombinant protein was also determined by UV spectroscopy at 280 nm using the extinction coefficients of 50685 $M^{-1}cm^{-1}$ for GST-tau, 56185 $M^{-1}cm^{-1}$ for GST-PH-Tau, and 43110 $M^{-1}cm^{-1}$ for GST. Recombinant proteins (10 µg per lane), cell and neuronal lysates (7 µg per lane) were analyzed by SDS-PAGE and Western blot as described with some modifications (Grundke-Iqbal et al., 1984).

Cell Culture and Transfection

HEK293 cells were grown in DMEM cell media supplemented with 10% Fetal Bovine Serum (FBS), sodium pyruvate, Glutamax, and Antibiotic-Antimitotic. CHO cells were grown in FK12 media with 10% FBS, sodium pyruvate, Glutamax and Antibiotic-Antimitotic. Media components were from Gibco or Thermo Fisher Scientific.

Chinese Hamster Ovary cells were plated on glass coverslips overnight. Transfections were performed using LipofectamineTM 2000 (Invitrogen, Carlsbad, CA, United States), according to the manufacturer's instructions. Briefly, transfections were performed in serum-free media OptiMEM using 3 µg of total DNA and 3 µl of Lipofectamine^{TM} 2000 per 35 mm dish. Cells were incubated in transfection media for 4 h and then replaced with fresh cell media.

Preparation of Mixed Cerebellar Neuronal Culture

Cerebellar granule cells were prepared from PN7 CD1 mice. The cerebellum was removed and single cell suspension was prepared by trypsinization and trituration in 1% trypsin in Ca^{2+}, Mg^{2+} free isotonic phosphate buffer (CMF-PBS). Cells were washed in CMF-PBS and resuspended in minimum essential culture medium supplemented with 0.25% glucose, 2 mM GlutaMax, 10% Horse Serum, 5% FBS, and 25 U/ml both penicillin and streptomycin. Cells were seeded into PDL-coated dishes and incubated at 37°C, 5% CO_2. Twenty-four hours after neuronal isolation, culture media was changed to media containing 15% of N2 supplement (R&S system) and 10 μM KCl. This media was changed every 2 days. Media components were from Gibco, Sigma, or Corning.

Protein Addition to Cultures

GST, GST-tau, and GST-PH-Tau (0.4 μg/ml final concentration) were added to the cell media of HEK293 cells, CHO cells and primary neuronal cultures. HEK293 and CHO cells were incubated with proteins for 2–4 h and washed with PBS. After additional incubation for 48 h, cells were fixed, processed for immunocytochemistry and viewed by confocal microscopy. M1/M3 transfected CHO cells were incubated for 48 h, then tau or PH-tau was added to the cells as described, incubated for 4 h, then media was changed and cells were grown for another 24 h and then processed for western blot.

Neuronal cultures were incubated for 24 h in the presence of tau or PH-Tau and were either fixed and processed for immunochemistry (DIV8) or incubated for longer time periods. For longer incubation times, half of the media was removed after 24 h and replaced with fresh media. The cultures were fixed and processed at DIV10, DIV12, or DIV14.

Blocking of Muscarinic Receptors

HEK293 cells and neuronal cultures were treated with 100 μM Atropine sulfate salt monohydrate (Sigma), 10 μM Pirenzepine Dichloride (Alfa Aesar), 40 ng/ml Pertussis toxin (Enzo), or 10 μM AF-DX116 (Toriks Biochemicals) in the culture media for 10 min prior to protein addition. After pre-treatment, half of the media was removed, replaced with fresh media and tau, PH-Tau or AD P-tau were added immediately to the cultures and incubated as described above.

Immunocytochemistry of Cell and Neuronal Cultures

HEK293 and CHO cells were fixed with cold methanol at −20°C for 5 min. Fixed cells were washed with PBS three times for 5 min and then blocked with 5% Donkey serum in PBS for 1 h at room temperature. Tau-13 was added to blocking buffer and cells were incubated overnight at 4°C with agitation. Cells were washed three times for 5 min each and incubated with anti-mouse Alexa 488 in blocking buffer (1:1000 dilution) for 2 h. Finally, cells were washed three times with PBS and the coverslips were mounted on the slides using Vectashield mounting media containing DAPI (Vector Laboratories, Inc.) and viewed by confocal microscopy.

Neuronal cultures were fixed with warm 4% paraformaldehyde for 10 min at room temperature, washed with PBS three times for 5 min and permeabilized with 100% methanol at −20°C for 10 min. Permeabilized cells were washed again with PBS three times for 5 min and blocked with 5% BSA, 1% Donkey serum, 0.2% TritonX-100 in PBS for 1 h at room temperature. Tau-13, β-III tubulin, GFAP, or IbaI were added to blocking buffer and cultures were incubated overnight at 4°C. Cultures were washed with 0.2% TritonX-100 in PBS (PBS-T) three times 5 min each and incubated with anti-mouse Alexa 488, anti-chicken Alexa 555, or anti-rabbit Alexa 594 in blocking buffer for 2 h at room temperature. Cultures were washed with PBS-T and then with PBS. Coverslips were mounted as described above.

LIVE/DEAD Imaging

Neuronal cultures (DIV 14) cultured in 24-well plates were treated with reagents from the LIVE/DEAD Cell Imaging Kit (488/570) (Invitrogen) as described by the manufacturer's protocol. Analysis was performed using a Zeiss-Axio Observer Z1 Live Imager.

Stereotaxic Injections

Five-month-old CD-1 mice were anesthetized with 100 mg/kg ketamine and mounted onto a stereotaxic apparatus, and kept anesthetized under isofluorane throughout the procedure. A midsagittal incision was made and a hole was drilled using a Circuit Medic Micro Drill System into the cranium according to the following coordinates set from bregma: AP: + 2.18 mm, ML: + 2.85 mm, DV: −2.5 mm. The mice were injected with 2 μL of 2 μg/mL of either aCSF, tau, or PH-Tau with the use of a Hamilton syringe at a rate of 0.5 μL/min for 4 min of total injection time with a KD Scientific Syringe Infusion Pump. The incision was treated with garamycin and closed with surgical staples, and the mice were placed onto a heating pad while they recovered from the procedure. The mice were sacrificed after 45 days.

Cryosectioning and H&E Staining

Mice were anesthetized with 0.3 mL urethane (1 g/mL) and transcardially perfused with 0.1 M phosphate buffered saline (PBS) and 4% paraformaldehyde (PFA) in 0.1 M PBS then stored in PFA followed by 30% sucrose at 4°C. Brains were cryosectioned in sagittal vibratome sections (50 μm) and mounted onto microscope slides. Tissue sections were then incubated in the following order: PBS for 5 min, dH_2O for 1 min, hematoxylin for 4 min, running tap water for 3–5 min, dH_2O for 1 min, eosin for 2 min, 70% alcohol for 2 min, 95% alcohol for 2 min, 100% alcohol for 2 min, and xylene for 2 min. The tissue sections were covered in a Permount/xylene solution and coverslipped. The staining was observed with an EVOS PLc light microscope at 20×.

Confocal Image Acquisition, Measurements, and Statistical Analysis

Images for each set of analysis were observed under a LEICA TGS SP5 confocal laser scaning microscope (Leica Microsystems CMSGmbH, Mannheim, Germany) and obtained using the same gain, laser intensity and pinhole size. Confocal images were analyzed using ImageJ software. Images were split onto blue (DAPI), green and red channels. The same threshold was assigned to all pictures for each channel. Mean gray value was calculated from each channel and divided by the number of the nuclei. The results were graphed and compared using Excel 2010.

All experiments were performed at least three times and at least 10 images from each experiment were analyzed. Statistics were performed using Microsoft Excel 2010. Two-Sample *t*-Test assuming equal variances was used to compare samples. The data reported as mean values. An alpha level of 0.05 was used for all statistical tests. The significance was determined based on two-tailed *P* values.

RESULTS

Tau Uptake Into Cells Is Receptor Mediated

Propagation of abnormal tau in AD and other tauopathies has been proposed to occur through cell-to-cell transfer (as reviewed in Takeda, 2019). To better understand the mechanism of uptake, culture media spiked with recombinant proteins GST-tau, or GST-PH-Tau, 400 ng/mL (**Supplementary Figure S1**) was added to HEK293 or CHO cells and incubated for 4 h. After replacing the culture media, the cells were incubated in normal media for 2 days. Cells were washed to remove all extracellular tau, fixed and labeled with an anti-human tau antibody, counterstained with DAPI to observe the nuclei, and analyzed by confocal microscopy. Tau and PH-Tau were taken up into the HEK293 cells, but no uptake was observed in CHO cells (**Figure 1A**). GST alone was not detected in both cell lines (data not shown). These results indicate that tau, independent of phosphorylation state, can be uptaken in a cell-specific manner.

To determine if similar uptake can be observed in neuronal cells, primary mixed cerebellar neuronal cultures were prepared at Day 7 after birth (DIV1). Tau and PH-Tau, each at 400 ng/mL, were added to the media at DIV7 and incubated for 24 h. After incubation, the cultures were washed as above, fixed, processed for immunochemistry and double-labeled with anti-human tau and β-III tubulin (**Figure 1B**). DAPI was used as a counterstain to observe the nuclei. Both Tau and PH-Tau were taken up by neurons and accumulated at similar levels around the cell nucleus (**Figure 1B**, ROI). Uptake was observed without changes in neuritic morphology or neuronal numbers when comparing to control. Similar experiments were performed with human tau without a GST-tag and uptake was observed indicating that the uptake was due to tau and not the GST-tag (**Supplementary Figure S2**).

The different responses between HEK293 and CHO might be because HEK cells were generated from human embryonic kidney having properties similar to immature neurons and CHO cells are an epithelial cell line derived from ovaries of Chinese hamster (Shaw et al., 2002; Shafer and Williams, 2004; Lin et al., 2014). Similar to neurons, HEK293 cells express muscarinic receptors, while CHO cells do not. Neuronal muscarinic receptors have been shown to interact with tau (Gomez-Ramos et al., 2008; Gomez-Ramos et al., 2009; Avila et al., 2015). Western blot analysis of these cell lines shows that both HEK293 cells express about eight-fold higher M1 receptors (CHRM1) while primary cerebellar neuronal cultures express more than 20-fold higher M1 muscarinic receptors when compared to CHO cells (**Figure 1D**, left). Pre-treatment of cells with the muscarinic receptor antagonist atropine resulted in reduced uptake of both recombinant tau proteins in HEK293 cells and neuronal cultures (**Figure 1A**, bottom, **Figure 1B**, last column). Quantitative analysis shows that tau uptake in the neuronal cultures was reduced up to 80% of that without atropine (**Figure 1C**). Taken together these results implicate the involvement of muscarinic receptors in the uptake of tau into HEK293 cells and neurons.

Muscarinic Receptor Subtypes M1 and M3 Are Involved in the Uptake of Tau

Given that tau is uptaken by HEK293 cells and neurons but not CHO cells, and uptake is blocked by atropine, we wanted to further analyze which of the five main subtypes of muscarinic receptors were involved. Primary cerebellar cultures were treated with pirenzepine, an M1 antagonist, AF-DX116, a selective M2 antagonist, and pertussis toxin (PTX), which blocks downstream processes of G_i G protein-coupled receptors (including M2/M4) (**Figure 1C**). Pirenzepine blocked the uptake of tau and PH-Tau about 80% which is similar to atropine. Conversely, both AF-DX116 and PTX did not block the uptake of either tau protein significantly. These results further implicate the M1 muscarinic receptor but not M2/M4 in the uptake of tau into the cells.

To further examine the role of muscarinic receptor subtypes in uptake into cells, CHO cells were transiently transfected with M1-HA, M3-HA, or both. The transfected cells were cultured for 48 h and then media containing the recombinant proteins was added as described above. The cells were collected after 24 h, washed, lysed and analyzed by immunoblot using anti-human tau. In CHO cells transfected with M1 or M3 there is ~19-fold increase tau uptake (**Figure 1D**, right) compared to non-transfected CHO cells. When the cells were transfected with both M1 and M3 at the same time, the level of tau uptake increased by 31.5-fold. CHO cells transfected with either M1 or M3 appear to uptake tau at similar levels as HEK293 cells. When both receptors are present the uptake increases significantly. These results imply that both M1 and M3 are involved in the uptake of tau into cells.

Consequences of Tau Exposure in Neuronal Processes

To observe changes in neurons due to the uptake of tau or PH-Tau we performed the experiments as described above, where the neurons were exposed to tau for 24 h and cultures were allowed to grow and differentiate for up to seven more

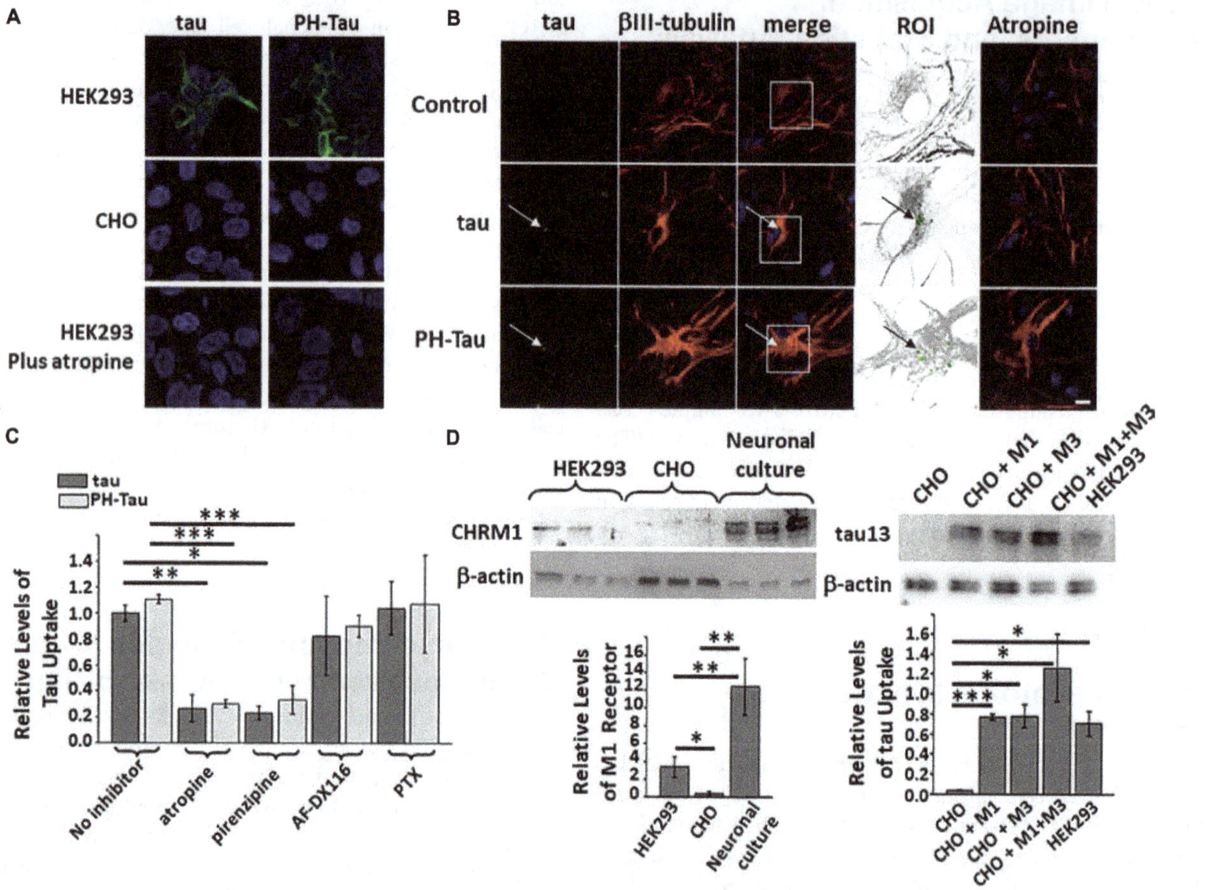

FIGURE 1 | Uptake of tau is cell-type specific. Recombinant tau and PH-Tau (400 ng/mL) were added to HEK293 and CHO cells **(A)** and to primary neuronal cultures **(B)**. Confocal analysis indicated that uptake occurred in HEK293 and neuronal cultures (white arrows) but not CHO cells and was blocked by pre-treatment with atropine. In the neuronal images, the boxed areas were zoomed 2.5× and converted (βIII-tubulin, gray; tau, green). **(C)** Quantitation of tau uptake into neuronal cultures indicates that both tau (dark bars) and PH-Tau (light bars) are uptaken at similar levels. Pre-treatment with antagonists atropine and pirenzepine block the uptake of both proteins by about 80%. Conversely, AF-DX116 and PTX do not block uptake. **(D)** Left: Western blot analysis of cultured cells and neurons to analyze the presence of the M1 muscarinic receptor. Quantitation indicated that both HEK293 and neuronal cultures have a large amount of M1 muscarinic receptors compared to CHO cells. Right: Western blot analysis of HEK293 cells transfected with M1, M3, or M1/M3 muscarinic receptors to determine tau uptake. The introduction of the muscarinic receptors resulted in the significant uptake of tau into CHO cells. Scale bar: 20 μm. All experiments were performed three times with 10 images analyzed per experiment. (*$p < 0.05$, **$p < 0.01$, ***$p < 0.001$).

days *in vitro* (**Figure 2A**). βIII-tubulin intensity at DIV10 appears to be higher in all cultures to which tau was added when compared to the control cultures. After this point, the cultures treated with PH-Tau, showed decreasing intensity of βIII-tubulin. DIV12 neurons treated with PH-Tau began to lose neurites, a feature indicative of neurodegeneration. Interestingly, the few neurons in cultures treated with pathogenic tau, which are still present at DIV14, appear more similar to neuronal processes treated with wild-type tau than those in the control. Conversely, there was an increase in βIII-tubulin intensity in cultures treated with normal tau. DIV14 neurons treated with tau appear to bundle together and to be straighter than neurons in the control samples. Levels of βIII-tubulin in culture were quantitated at DIV14 based on the confocal acquired fluorescence (**Figure 2A**, graph). The quantitative analysis confirms that by DIV14, βIII-tubulin levels increased upon addition of tau and decreased when PH-Tau was added. Based on the observed changes in βIII-tubulin for each sample, it appears that the uptake of tau reinforces neuritic growth, while the uptake of PH-Tau triggers the loss of neurites and result in neurodegeneration similar to that observed in AD pathology.

As seen in **Figure 1**, the initial uptake of tau was blocked by atropine and when these cultures were allowed to incubate for 7 days, the neurons appeared similar to cultures without tau addition (**Figure 2A**, bottom images). Quantitative analysis of cultures at DIV14 of the exposed to tau with and without atropine pre-treatment show a significant decrease in βIII-tubulin intensity when atropine was present. The neudegeneration that was induced by exposure to PH-Tau was significantly inhibited by pre-treatment with atropine (**Figure 2A**, graph). These results indicate that muscarinic receptors play a role in the uptake of tau and that blocking them can control the uptake and therefore the overall condition of the neurons.

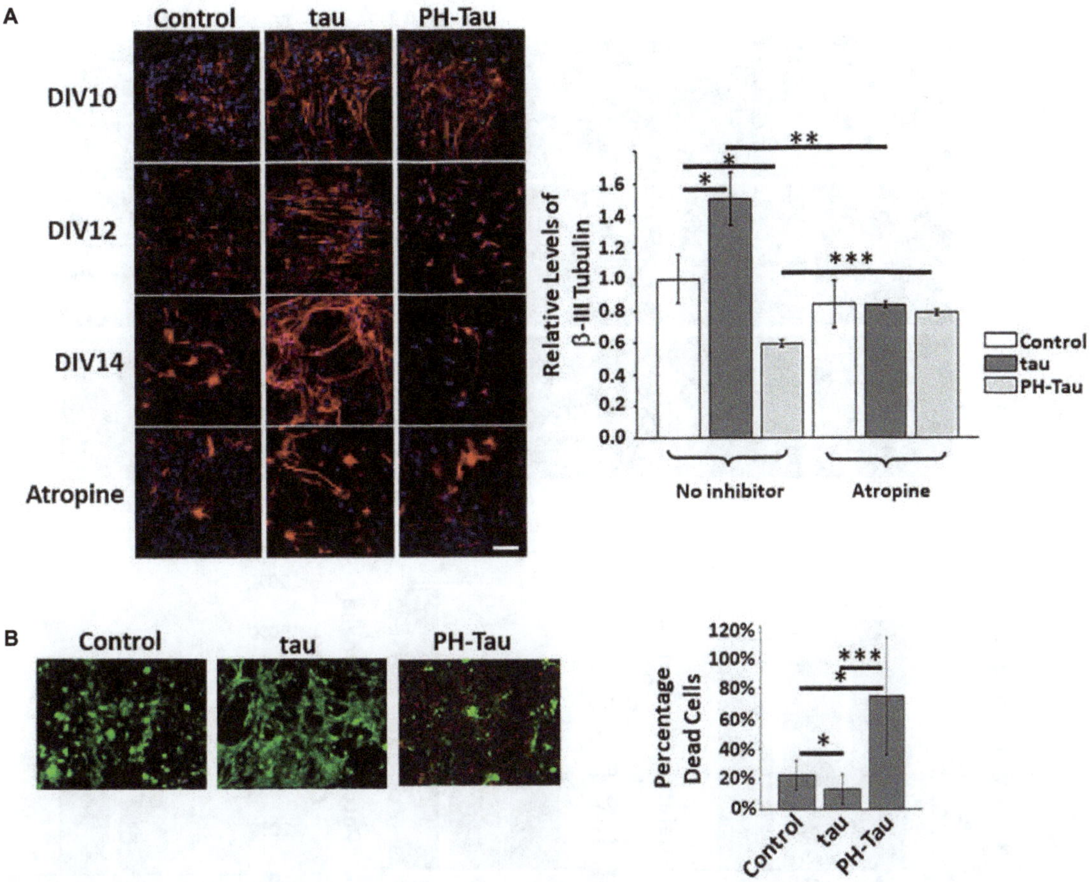

FIGURE 2 | Uptake of tau affects the neuritic morphology of neurons in culture. **(A)** Proteins were added to the neuronal culture media as described. Over a period of 7 days, the neurons were fixed and studied by confocal microscopy. The addition of WT tau appears to stabilize and organize the neuronal processes whereas PH-Tau triggers a loss if neurites over time. Pre-treatment with atropine appears to block the uptake of tau and reduces changes in neuritic morphology. Graph: Quantitation of β-III tubulin indicates that tau (dark bars) increases protein levels whereas PH-Tau (light bars) decreases the levels indicating a loss of neuritic morphology. **(B)** LIVE/DEAD Imaging of neuronal cultures after treatment with tau or PH-Tau. The number of dead cells increases significantly in cultures treated with PH-Tau. Scale bar: 20 μm. All experiments were performed three times with 10 images analyzed per experiment. (*$p < 0.05$, **$p < 0.01$, ***$p < 0.001$).

Addition of PH-Tau Results in Increased Cell Death in Neuronal Cultures

To determine if this neuronal loss was due to cell death, neuronal cultures were prepared as described and were analyzed using the LIVE/DEAD Cell Imaging Invitrogen kit (**Figure 2B**). Live neurons stain green whereas cell death is indicated by red staining. There is a significant increase in the number of red cells in the neuronal cultures treated with PH-Tau when compared to the tau-treated and control cultures. Additionally, the cells (red or green) look mostly rounded, due to a loss of neuritic projections which is consistent with the results seen above when analyzing βIII-tubulin in treated cells. The percentage of dead cells in the neuronal cultures treated with wild-type tau is decreased 50% compared to control mixed primary neuronal cultures. This may be correlated to the increase in βIII-tubulin observed above. These results indicate that the addition of wild-type tau may play a role in strengthening the health of the neurons. Conversely, addition of PH-tau results in loss of neuritic projections and induction of cellular death which is similar to phenotypes seen in neurons of AD patients.

Microglial Activation Is Triggered by the Presence of PH-Tau

An important component of inflammation seen in brains of patients with AD other tauopathies is microglia activation. Therefore we investigated if in our experiments there was a microglia modification. The neuronal cultures analyzed contain a mixture of cells including neurons, microglia, and astrocytes (**Supplementary Table S1**). Primary cerebellar neuronal cultures were treated as described above and then washed and fixed at DIV14. Immunohistochemistry was performed with antibodies against GFAP, an astrocyte marker, and Ibal, a marker for activated microglia. It is important to note that other subpopulations of microglia may stain for Iba-1 (Ito et al., 1998), however, we are looking at relative changes upon addition of tau. No significant changes were found in the levels of astrocytes as judged by the levels of GFAP

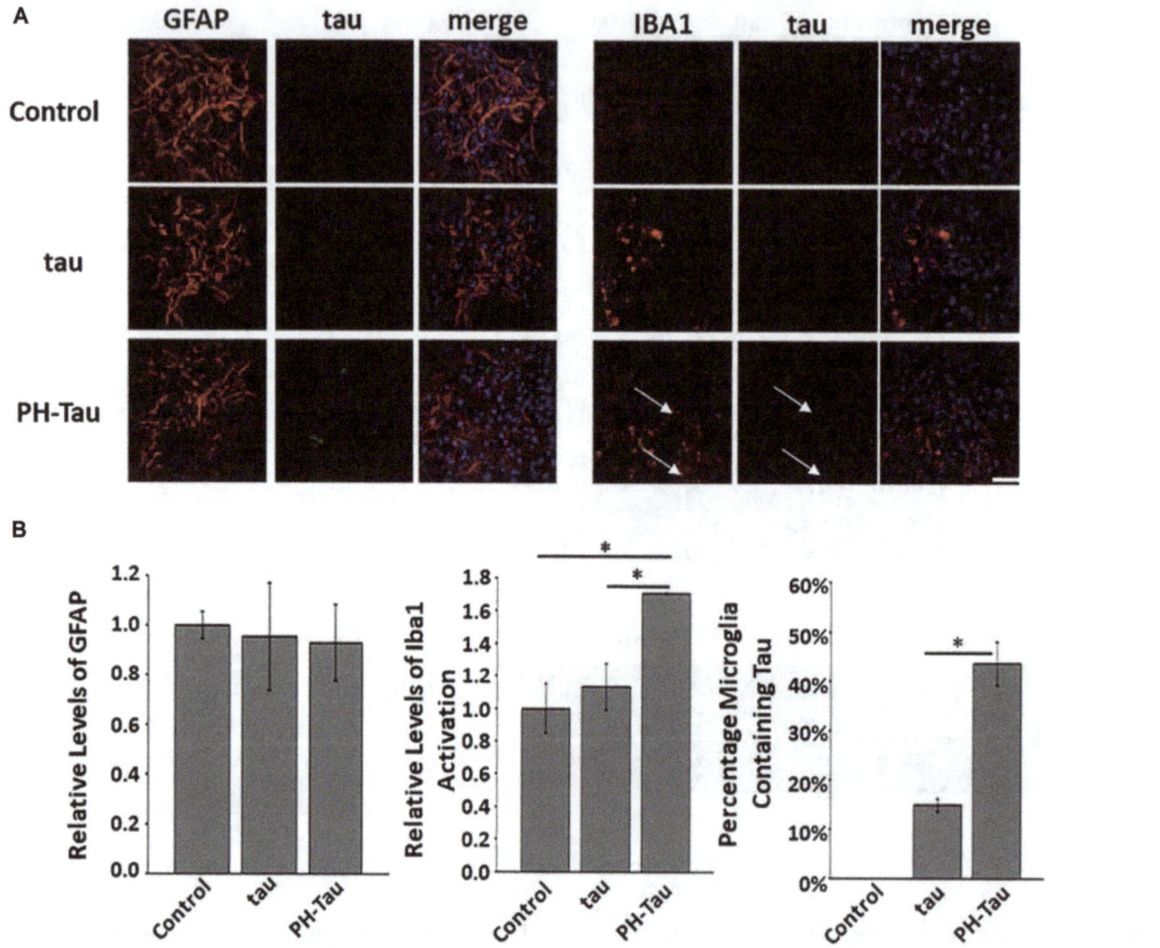

FIGURE 3 | Uptake of tau affects the microglia but not astrocytes in neuronal culture. **(A)** Proteins were added to the neuronal culture media and analyzed after 7 days. There is no significant change in the amount of GFAP fluorescence in cultures challenged with either tau or PH-Tau when compared to control. The addition of the PH-Tau but not tau appears to activate the microglia which is correlated with the uptake of tau into the cells (white arrows). Scale Bar: 20 μm. **(B)** Left: Quantitation of the GFAP levels indicates that there is no change after addition of tau to cultures. Middle: Iba1 activation indicates that PH-Tau significantly activates the microglial response. Right: This activation correlates with the amount of tau uptaken by the microglia in culture. All experiments were performed three times with 10 images analyzed per experiment. (*$p < 0.05$).

in the cultured neurons (**Figure 3A**, top). However, there was a significant increase in the activation of microglia in the cultures treated with PH-Tau when compared to control and tau-treated cultures (**Figure 3A** bottom, and **Figure 3B** left graph).

Further analysis of these cultures indicated that tau uptake into the microglia was dependent on the conformation of tau as PH-Tau was taken up to a much higher extent than the wild-type form (**Figure 3B**, right graph). The increase in microglial activation was directly correlated to the amount of tau uptake in the Iba1 active cells (**Figure 3B**, compare left and right graphs). In cultures treated with PH-Tau, 43% of activated microglia were also positive for human tau. Cultures treated with tau had significantly lower proportion of tau containing microglia which correlates to an insignificant level of Iba1 activation (**Figure 3B**, graphs). An increased microglial response could be indicative of conditions that may lead to inflammation, similar to that found in patients with AD.

PH-Tau Effectively Mimics AD P-Tau Taken From Human Brain Tissue

Alzheimer's disease P-tau, soluble, hyperphosphorylated tau extracted from the brains of human patients was used in similar experiments to those described above. The uptake of AD P-tau was shown to be similar to tau and PH-Tau and is also blocked by atropine (**Figure 4A** top and top graph). Cultures treated with PH-Tau followed a similar pattern of neurodegeneration compared to the addition of AD P-tau, showing increased βIII-tubulin at DIV10 followed by a decrease compared to control (**Figure 4A** bottom and bottom graph). Furthermore, pre-treatment with atropine resulted in very little loss of βIII-tubulin compared to control. Finally, in cultures treated with AD P-tau,

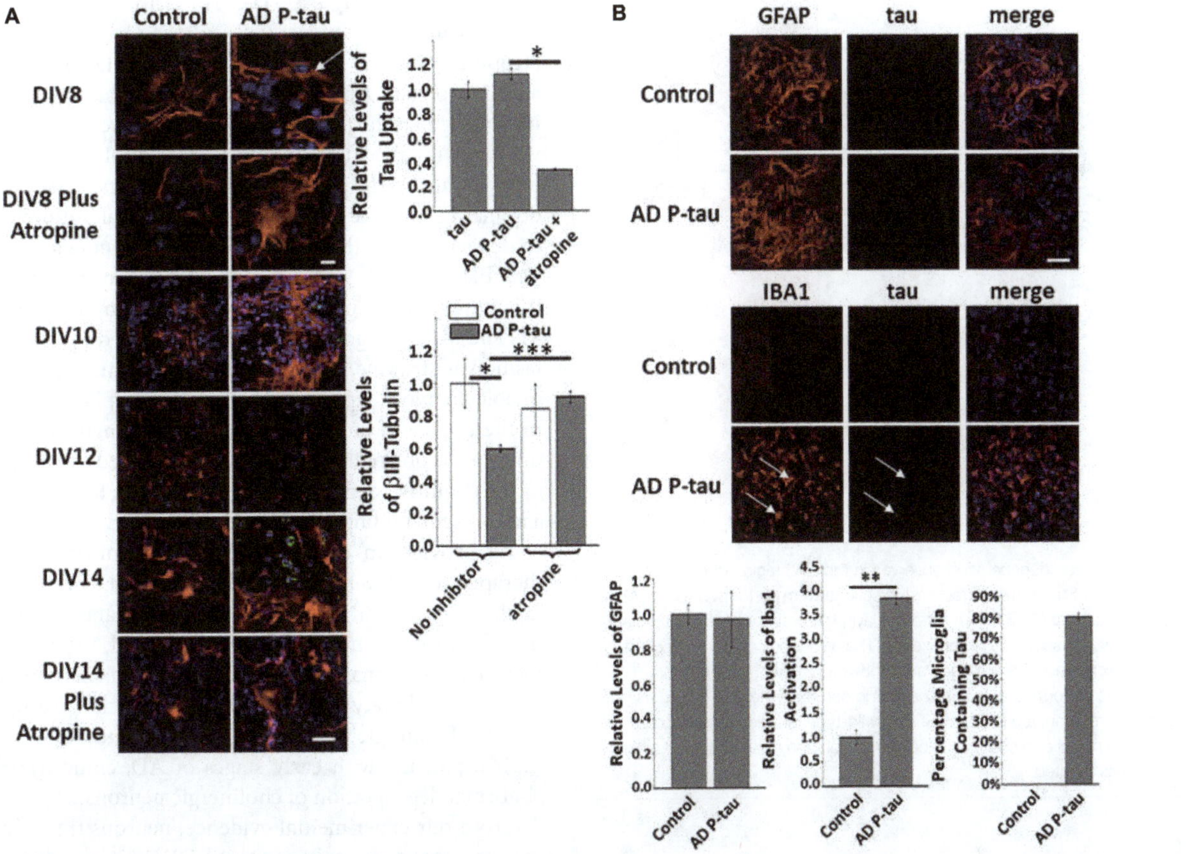

FIGURE 4 | AD P-tau addition to neuronal cultures has similar effects as PH-Tau. **(A)** AD P-tau is uptaken after incubation of 24 h and atropine blocks this uptake. The white arrow indicates where tau (green) is localized near the nucleus. No tau is observed in neurons pre-treated with atropine. Quantitation of uptake is observed in the top graph on the right. At DIV10, β-III tubulin appears to increase compared to control followed by a sharp decrease over time, see DIV12 and DIV14. The pre-treatment with atropine blocks the decrease in β-III tubulin levels. These changes are observed by confocal microscopy (images) and by quantitation of tau uptake (bar graph, top right) or β-III tubulin fluorescence (bar graph, bottom right). **(B)** Activation of microglia is observed upon addition of AD P-tau and this activation is correlated with the uptake of protein (indicated by the white arrows). GFAP levels are observed in the top row and activation of microglia is observed by an increase in fluorescence of Iba1. Bar graphs show levels of GFAP fluorescence (left), quantiation of Iba1 activation (middle) and AD P-tau uptake (right) Scale bar: 20 μm. All experiments were performed three times with 10 images analyzed per experiment. (*$p < 0.05$, **$p < 0.01$, ***$p < 0.001$).

no change was observed in GFAP staining, but microglia were activated almost four-fold more than control cells and almost 80% of these activated microglia were also positive for human tau. Taken together, these results confirm the validity of PH-Tau as a good mimic for AD P-tau and can be used as a surrogate in future studies.

Histological Evaluation of Neurodegeneration in CA3 Region of the Hippocampus

Mice received a stereotaxic intracranial injection of pure artificial cerebral spinal fluid (aCSF) or either tau or PH-Tau dissolved in aCSF. Forty-five days post injection, mice were perfused with 4% paraformaldehyde and brains were dissected and post fixed for 2 h. Coronal cryosections were stained with Haemotoxylin and Eosin (H&E). These images are representative of the (A) aCSF-injected, (B) tau-injected, and (C) PH-Tau-injected mice (**Figure 5**). The arrow indicates the injection site and the box represents the imaged area shown on the right panels. The aCSF and wild-type tau injected mice show relatively healthy neurons as demonstrated by the light appearance of neurons and their morphological integrity. Whereas the PH-Tau injected mice show relatively unhealthy neurons as evident from nuclear condensation based on intense staining and the irregular shape of the cell body.

DISCUSSION

In this study, we have observed that recombinant tau and pathological tau can be taken up from the culture media into cell lines, microglia, and neurons and that this uptake activity involves muscarinic receptors. The addition of normal tau to neurons promotes neuritic extension, while PH-Tau leads to the disruption of neuritic processes and accumulation in the somatodendritic compartment. These findings suggest a novel mechanism for the pathogenesis of hyperphosphorylated tau

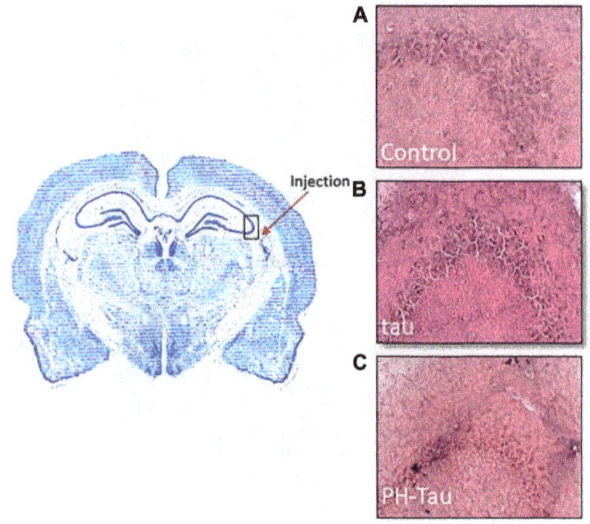

FIGURE 5 | Neurodegeneration observed in the CA3 region of the hippocampus. Stereotaxic intracranial injections were performed using **(A)** aCSF, **(B)** tau, and **(C)** PH-Tau. After 45 days, the brains were harvested and prepared by cryosectioning after fixation. The arrow indicates the injection site and the box represent the imaged area shown on the right panel. H&E staining was performed to follow changes in nerons in the CA3 region. Healthy neurons were observed in the aCSF and wild-type tau injections whereas condensed nuclei and changes in cellular morphology was observed when PH-Tau was injected.

and demonstrate additional functions for normal tau. We have further confirmed our previous study which showed that PH-Tau mimics AD P-Tau in cultured neurons. Both forms of tau caused the disruption of neuritic processes and accumulation of tau aggregates in the somatodendritic compartment.

The addition of tau to cell and neuronal cultures has been previously studied (Frost et al., 2009; Nonaka et al., 2010; Guo and Lee, 2011; Wu et al., 2013; Sanders et al., 2014; Wu et al., 2016; Evans et al., 2018). Research has indicated that the minimal unit for uptake is trimeric tau (Mirbaha et al., 2015). These tau trimers also appear to be the minimal tau toxic unit in both AD and PSP (Shafiei et al., 2017). Native gel electrophoresis indicates that the tau and PH-Tau that we are using are both mixtures of oligomeric states but that PH-Tau appears to be composed of a greater number of higher order complexes (**Supplementary Figure S3**). Furthermore, when seeded with AD P-tau the number of higher oligomeric complexes increases indicating the seeding ability of pathological tau. Our experiments show that normal tau is taken up similarly to PH-Tau. However, only PH-Tau exhibited a toxic effect indicating that it may not be the size of the aggregate that is toxic, but the phosphorylation state of tau.

To determine the importance of muscarinic receptors in intracellular uptake of tau, we added normal tau or PH-Tau to the culture media of HEK293 cells or CHO cells. Uptake of tau was only observed in HEK293 cells. Unlike HEK293 cells, CHO cells do not naturally express muscarinic receptors. Transfection of CHO cells with either M1, M3, or M1/M3 muscarinic receptors indicated that the presence of these receptors was necessary for tau uptake (**Figure 1D**). To further investigate the role of muscarinic receptors, cell cultures were pre-treated with atropine, a known muscarinic receptor antagonist, prior to the addition of tau. Atropine blocked tau uptake in HEK293 cells, indicating that the presence of muscarinic receptors is correlated with tau uptake. It is known that cortical neurons, including hippocampal cells have M1 and M3 muscarinic receptors and so do glial cells (Levey et al., 1994). Neuronal cultures were used to determine if both forms of tau could be uptaken in the brain. Tau, PH-Tau, and AD P-tau were all uptaken at similar levels and this uptake was blocked up to 80% by atropine (**Figures 1B,C, 4**). The M1 anatagonist pirenzepine blocked uptake in a similar fashion as atropine, but AF-DX116 and pertussis toxin, were both unable to block uptake. These results implicate M1 receptors in the uptake of tau (**Figure 1C**). Interestingly, a cholinesterase inhibitor is one of the medications prescribed to ameliorate some of the cognitive deficits of AD (Birks, 2006; Soukup et al., 2017). The present findings that atropine blocked the PH-Tau uptake could provide an explanation for the limited efficacy of this therapeutic intervention. Acetylcholine is one of the transmitters in the cortical and hippocampal circuits, and because PH-Tau transfer to other neurons may be blocked, other, non-effected neurons, could maintain the synaptic transmission prolonging persistence of acetylcholine in the synaptic cleft. Complementary to this cholinergic mechanism was the study of Schmitz et al. (2016), patients with early stages of AD, clinically silent, have abnormal degeneration of cholinergic neurons.

From our experimental evidence, neurons treated with wild-type tau that were cultured until DIV14 were more organized and had many more aligned neuritic processes compared to the untreated neurons (**Figure 2**). These findings suggest that extra-neuronal tau might be a physiological signal. Although the presence of tau in the extracellular space is described, there is no consensus about physiological function for this localization of tau (Chai et al., 2012; Magnoni et al., 2012; Karch et al., 2013; Bright et al., 2015; Kanmert et al., 2015). Tau increases the electrical activity of iPSC-derived or primary cortical neurons, in line with the finding that tau leads to intracellular calcium increase (Gomez-Ramos et al., 2008; Bright et al., 2015). As such, extracellular tau may play an important neuromodulatory role for cognition. In agreement with our results, Biundo et al. (2018) have shown that tau depletion in a mouse model led to age-dependent deficits in memory and synaptic plasticity, correlating with levels of normal tau expression. Considering the potential beneficial role of normal tau with respect to the electrophysiological functioning and morphology of neurons, our study further explored the effects of pathological tau. Addition of PH-Tau or AD P-tau to the culture medium induced a retraction of the neuritic processes (**Figures 2, 4**). This retraction by PH-Tau is noticeable 5 days (DIV12) after exposure (**Figure 2**). Similarly, at 45 days post injection of mice injected with PH-Tau, the neuronal nuclei began to condense and the cell bodies did not appear rounded (**Figure 5**). Though uptake of wild-type tau and PH-Tau both appear to be mediated via similar muscarinic receptors, the effects on neurons and microglia are opposite in nature. The downstream effects of each of these proteins should be further investigated.

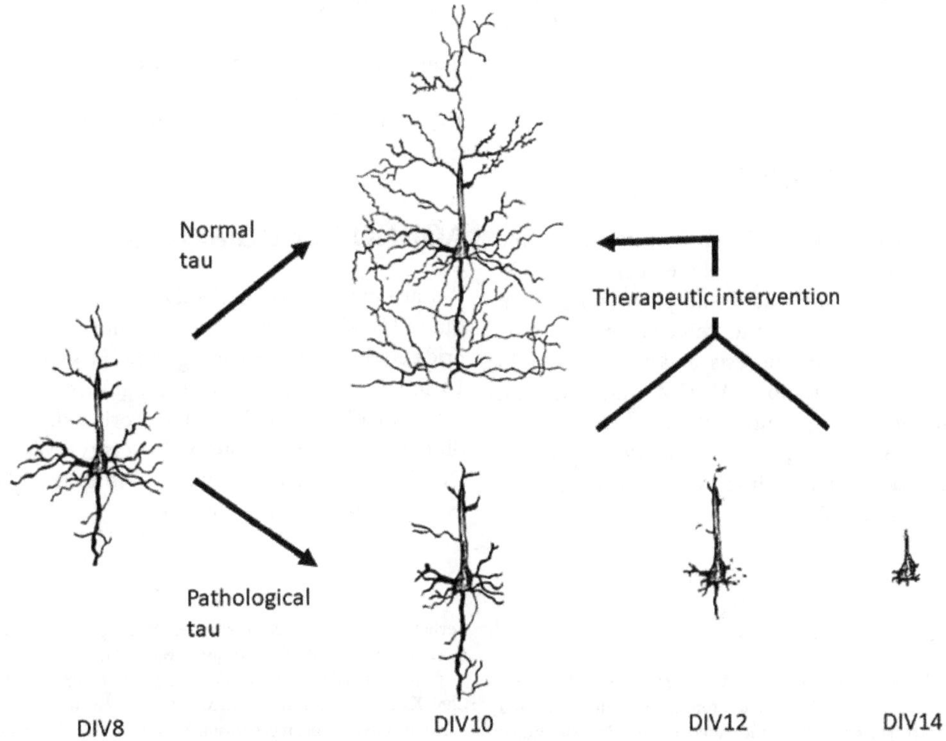

FIGURE 6 | Neuronal culture model system for the development of therapeutic interventions. We have shown that the neuronal culture system that we use can mimic neurodegeneration within 2 weeks of preparation. At DIV7, tau proteins are added to the culture medium for 24 h before exchanging the media to tau free media. Uptake of the proteins can be observed at DIV8. By DIV10, no tau is observed in the normal tau cultures, but the levels of βIII-tubulin increase. Cultures treated with pathogenic tau began to degenerate by DIV10 with significant loss of βIII-tubulin by DIV14. This system can be used to try out novel therapeutics to either halt degeneration and/or return the neurons to their original form.

Microglia activation, as indicated by an increase in Iba1 staining in cultures, after treatment with PH-Tau and ADP-Tau, while astrocytes were left unchanged (**Figures 3, 4**). This may indicate a response to the presence of pathological tau. Microglia are capable of taking up extracellular tau and have the ability to degrade the protein to remove it from the matrix (Bolós et al., 2016). Murine microglial cells from young mice have been used to clear tau from brain slices of P301S mice and from AD patients (Luo et al., 2015). Other studies have shown that microglia cluster in tau-rich regions indicating that they may play a role in the clearance of pathogenic tau (Bolós et al., 2016; Davies et al., 2017). Interestingly, there is a report of an increase in microglia that express muscarinic receptors, in particular M3, in AD mouse models (Pannell et al., 2016). Tau has been shown to bind to M1 and M3 mucarinic receptors (Gomez-Ramos et al., 2008). Therefore, activation of microglial cells that express M1 and M3 muscarinic receptors in the presence of extracellular tau for clearance further supports our findings that these specific receptor subtypes are important for tau uptake.

In this report, novel function and pathophysiology of tau in the extracellular space were investigated and neurons treated with pathological tau mimic the neurodegeneration observed in AD (**Figure 6**). This versatile model allows for the potential development of high throughput screening of novel therapeutics against tau-induced neurodegeneration. We showed that the uptake of tau is correlated with microtubule stabilization, and that the uptake of wild-type tau can increase stabilization and organization of microtubules whereas uptake of PH-Tau causes destabilization leading to neurite retraction. With these neuronal cultures therapeutic interventions can be tried at varying points of neurodegeneration with the hope of allowing the neurites to regenerate over time. Further analysis is necessary to understand the mechanisms of tau propagation, nucleation of oligomerization and induction of neurodegeneration.

With the present findings we hypothesize that under normal physiological conditions, tau is released in the extracellular space, uptaken by other neuronal cells in a muscarinic-receptor mediated pathway, and the connectivity of the neurons is reinforced. Early onset of AD progression begins with the appearance of pathological tau in a subset of neurons that can be secreted in the microenvironment, spreading its toxicity to the neighboring cells. Tau can be released as a naked pathological tau aggregates or in vesicles or exosomes. Pathological tau uptake by microglial cells induces activation, initiating an inflammatory response. Pathological tau exhibits a prion-like behavior inducing conformational changes in normal tau, disrupting microtubules or through other pathways, causing neurodegeneration. This sequence of events suggests a mechanism of propagation that exacerbates pathological conditions and that it could be a target for therapeutic intervention.

AUTHOR CONTRIBUTIONS

All authors contributed in the critical discussion of the experimental designs, results, and writing of the manuscript. VM performed the protein purifications, cell and primary neuronal culture, and immunocytochemistry and confocal imaging. LC performed the native gel electrophoresis and participated in the recombinant protein purification. AE-HM, AS, and AEL participated in the *in vivo* recombinant tau and PH-Tau stereotactic injection. GP participated in the design of the pharmacological inhibition of muscarinic receptors experiments. AA supervised the research project.

FUNDING

This study was supported at least in part by the private donation by Jeff Lin, as well as grants from the NIH (1R15AG058197-01 to AA) and PSC CUNY (60290-00 48 to AA).

ACKNOWLEDGMENTS

We are grateful to Drs. Robert Marraccino, Fred Naider, and Marta Hallak for their critical editing of the manuscript and Dr. Frida Kleiman for providing the GST expression plasmids. Tau 12 and Tau 13 antibodies were a gift from Dr. Nicholas Kanaan at the Michigan State University (originally created by Dr. Lester Binder at the Northwestern University). We are also grateful to Dr. Khalid Iqbal for providing the isolated AD P-tau and his expert opinion on drug discovery.

REFERENCES

Ahmed, Z., Cooper, J., Murray, T. K., Garn, K., McNaughton, E., Clarke, H., et al. (2014). A novel in vivo model of tau propagation with rapid and progressive neurofibrillary tangle pathology: the pattern of spread is determined by connectivity, not proximity. *Acta Neuropathol.* 127, 667–683. doi: 10.1007/s00401-014-1254-6

Alonso, A. D., Beharry, C., Corbo, C. P., and Cohen, L. S. (2016). Molecular mechanism of prion-like tau-induced neurodegeneration. *Alzheimers Dement.* 12, 1090–1097. doi: 10.1016/j.jalz.2015.12.014

Alonso, A. D., Di Clerico, J., Li, B., Corbo, C. P., Alaniz, M. E., Grundke-Iqbal, I., et al. (2010). Phosphorylation of tau at Thr212. *J. Biol. Chem.* 285, 30851–30860. doi: 10.1074/jbc.M110.110957

Alonso, A. D., Grundke-Iqbal, I., and Iqbal, K. (1996). Alzheimer's disease hyperphosphorylated tau sequesters normal tau into tangles of filaments and disassembles microtubules. *Nat. Med.* 2, 783–787. doi: 10.1038/nm0796-783

Avila, J., Gomez-Ramos, A., and Bolos, M. (2015). AD genetic risk factors and tau spreading. *Front. Aging Neurosci.* 7:99. doi: 10.3389/fnagi.2015.00099

Beharry, C., Alaniz, M. E., and Alonso, A. D. (2013). Expression of Alzheimer-like pathological human tau induces a behavioral motor and olfactory learning deficit in Drosophila melanogaster. *J. Alzheimers. Dis.* 37, 539–550. doi: 10.3233/JAD-130617

Beharry, C., Cohen, L. S., Di, J., Ibrahim, K., Briffa-Mirabella, S., and Alonso, A. D. (2014). Tau-induced neurodegeneration: mechanisms and targets. *Neurosci. Bull.* 30, 346–358. doi: 10.1007/s12264-013-1414-z

Birks, J. (2006). Cholinesterase inhibitors for Alzheimer's disease. *Cochrane Database Syst. Rev.* 25:CD005593.

Biundo, F., Del Prete, D., Zhang, H., Arancio, O., and D'Adamio, L. (2018). A role for tau in learning, memory and synaptic plasticity. *Sci. Rep.* 8:184. doi: 10.1038/s41598-018-21596-3

Bolmont, T., Clavaguera, F., Meyer-Luehmann, M., Herzig, M. C., Radde, R., Staufenbiel, M., et al. (2007). Induction of tau pathology by intracerebral infusion of amyloid-beta -containing brain extract and by amyloid-beta deposition in APP x Tau transgenic mice. *Am. J. Pathol.* 171, 2012–2020. doi: 10.2353/ajpath.2007.070403

Bolós, M., Llorens-Martín, M., Jurado-Arjona, J., Hernández, F., Rábano, A., and Avila, J. (2016). Direct evidence of internalization of tau by microglia in vitro and in vivo. *J. Alzheimers Dis.* 50, 77–87. doi: 10.3233/JAD-150704

Braak, H., and Braak, E. (1991). Neuropathological stageing of Alzheimer-related changes. *Acta Neuropathol.* 82, 239–259. doi: 10.1007/bf00308809

Bright, J., Hussain, S., Dang, V., Wright, S., Cooper, B., Byun, T., et al. (2015). Human secreted tau increases amyloid-beta production. *Neurobiol. Aging* 36, 693–709. doi: 10.1016/j.neurobiolaging.2014.09.007

Cevher, M. A., Zhang, X., Fernandez, S., Kim, S., Baquero, J., Nilsson, P., et al. (2010). Nuclear deadenylation/polyadenylation factors regulate 3' processing in response to DNA damage. *EMBO J.* 29, 1674–1687. doi: 10.1038/emboj.2010.59

Chai, X., Dage, J. L., and Citron, M. (2012). Constitutive secretion of tau protein by an unconventional mechanism. *Neurobiol. Dis.* 48, 356–366. doi: 10.1016/j.nbd.2012.05.021

Clavaguera, F., Akatsu, H., Fraser, G., Crowther, R. A., Frank, S., Hench, J., et al. (2013). Brain homogenates from human tauopathies induce tau inclusions in mouse brain. *Proc. Natl. Acad. Sci. U.S.A.* 110, 9535–9540. doi: 10.1073/pnas.1301175110

Clavaguera, F., Bolmont, T., Crowther, R. A., Abramowski, D., Frank, S., Probst, A., et al. (2009). Transmission and spreading of tauopathy in transgenic mouse brain. *Nat. Cell Biol.* 11, 909–913. doi: 10.1038/ncb1901

Clavaguera, F., Grueninger, F., and Tolnay, M. (2014). Intercellular transfer of tau aggregates and spreading of tau pathology: implications for therapeutic strategies. *Neuropharmacology* 76(Pt A), 9–15. doi: 10.1016/j.neuropharm.2013.08.037

Davies, D. S., Ma, J., Jegathees, T., and Goldsbury, C. (2017). Microglia show altered morphology and reduced arborization in human brain during aging and Alzheimer's disease. *Brain Pathol.* 27, 795–808. doi: 10.1111/bpa.12456

Di, J., Cohen, L. S., Corbo, C. P., Phillips, G. R., El Idrissi, A., and Alonso, A. D. (2016). Abnormal tau induces cognitive impairment through two different mechanisms: synaptic dysfunction and neuronal loss. *Sci. Rep.* 6:20833. doi: 10.1038/srep20833

Evans, L. D., Wassmer, T., Fraser, G., Smith, J., Perkinton, M., Billinton, A., et al. (2018). Extracellular monomeric and aggregated tau efficiently enter human neurons through overlapping but distinct pathways. *Cell Rep.* 22, 3612–3624. doi: 10.1016/j.celrep.2018.03.021

Frost, B., Jacks, R. L., and Diamond, M. I. (2009). Propagation of tau misfolding from the outside to the inside of a cell. *J. Biol. Chem.* 284, 12845–12852. doi: 10.1074/jbc.M808759200

Goedert, M., Clavaguera, F., and Tolnay, M. (2010). The propagation of prion-like protein inclusions in neurodegenerative diseases. *Trends Neurosci.* 33, 317–325. doi: 10.1016/j.tins.2010.04.003

Gomez-Ramos, A., Diaz-Hernandez, M., Rubio, A., Diaz-Hernandez, J. I, and Miras-Portugal, M. (2009). Characteristics and consequences of muscarinic receptor activation by tau protein. *Eur. Neuropsychopharmacol.* 19, 708–717. doi: 10.1016/j.euroneuro.2009.04.006

Gomez-Ramos, A., Diaz-Hernandez, M., Rubio, A., Miras-Portugal, M. T., and Avila, J. (2008). Extracellular tau promotes intracellular calcium increase through M1 and M3 muscarinic receptors in neuronal cells. *Mol. Cell. Neurosci.* 37, 673–681. doi: 10.1016/j.mcn.2007.12.010

Grundke-Iqbal, I., Iqbal, K., Tung, Y. C., and Wisniewski, H. M. (1984). Alzheimer paired helical filaments: immunochemical identification of polypeptides. *Acta Neuropathol.* 62, 259–267. doi: 10.1007/bf00687607

Guo, J. L., and Lee, V. M. (2011). Seeding of normal Tau by pathological Tau conformers drives pathogenesis of Alzheimer-like tangles. *J. Biol. Chem.* 286, 15317–15331. doi: 10.1074/jbc.M110.209296

Holmes, B. B., and Diamond, M. I. (2014). Prion-like properties of Tau protein: the importance of extracellular Tau as a therapeutic target. *J. Biol. Chem.* 289, 19855–19861. doi: 10.1074/jbc.R114.549295

Hu, W., Zhang, X., Xie, S., Chen, Y. H., Liu, F., and Iqbal, K. (2016). Hyperphosphorylation determines both the spread and the morphology of tau pathology. *Alzheimer's Dement.* 12, 1066–1077. doi: 10.1016/j.jalz.2016.01.014

Hyman, B. T., Van Hoesen, G. W., Damasio, A. R., and Barnes, C. L. (1984). Alzheimer's disease: cell-specific pathology isolates the hippocampal formation. *Science* 225, 1168–1170. doi: 10.1126/science.6474172

Iba, M., Guo, J. L., McBride, J. D., Zhang, B., Trojanowski, J. Q., and Lee, V. M. (2013). Synthetic tau fibrils mediate transmission of neurofibrillary tangles in a transgenic mouse model of Alzheimer's-like tauopathy. *J. Neurosci.* 33, 1024–1037. doi: 10.1523/jneurosci.2642-12.2013

Iqbal, K., Liu, F., and Gong, C. X. (2016). Tau and neurodegenerative disease: the story so far. *Nat. Rev. Neurol.* 12, 15–27. doi: 10.1038/nrneurol.2015.225

Ito, D., Imai, Y., Ohsawa, K., Nakajima, K., Fukuuchi, Y., and Kohsaka, S. (1998). Microglia-specific localisation of a novel calcium binding protein. Iba1. *Brain Res. Mol. Brain Res.* 57, 1–9. doi: 10.1016/s0169-328x(98)00040-0

Kanmert, D., Cantlon, A., Muratore, C. R., Jin, M., O'Malley, T. T., Lee, G., et al. (2015). C-terminally truncated forms of tau, but not full-length tau or its c-terminal fragments, are released from neurons independently of cell death. *J. Neurosci.* 35, 10851–10865. doi: 10.1523/JNEUROSCI.0387-15.2015

Karch, C. M., Jeng, A. T., and Goate, A. M. (2013). Calcium phosphatase calcineurin influences tau metabolism. *Neurobiol. Aging* 34, 374–386. doi: 10.1016/j.neurobiolaging.2012.05.003

Lasagna-Reeves, C. A., Castillo-Carranza, D. L., Sengupta, U., Sarmiento, J., Troncoso, J., Jackson, G. R., et al. (2012). Identification of oligomers at early stages of tau aggregation in Alzheimer's disease. *FASEB J.* 26, 1946–1959. doi: 10.1096/fj.11-199851

Levey, A. I., Edmunds, S. M., Heilman, C. J., Desmond, T. J., and Frey, K. A. (1994). Localization of muscarinic m3 receptor protein and M3 receptor binding in rat brain. *Neuroscience* 63, 207–221. doi: 10.1016/0306-4522(94)90017-5

Lin, Y. C., Boone, M., Meuris, L., Lemmens, I., Van Roy, N., Soete, A., et al. (2014). Genome dynamics of the human embryonic kidney 293 lineage in response to cell biology manipulations. *Nat. Commun.* 5:4767. doi: 10.1038/ncomms5767

Luo, W., Liu, W., Hu, X., Hanna, M., Caravaca, A., and Paul, S. M. (2015). Microglial internalization and degradation of pathological tau is enhanced by an anti-tau monoclonal antibody. *Sci. Rep.* 5:11161. doi: 10.1038/srep11161

Magnoni, S., Esparza, T. J., Conte, V., Carbonara, M., Carrabba, G., Holtzman, D. M., et al. (2012). Tau elevations in the brain extracellular space correlate with reduced amyloid-beta levels and predict adverse clinical outcomes after severe traumatic brain injury. *Brain* 135(Pt 4), 1268–1280. doi: 10.1093/brain/awr286

Mirbaha, H., Holmes, B. B., Sanders, D. W., Bieschke, J., and Diamond, M. I. (2015). Tau Trimers are the minimal propagation unit spontaneously internalized to seed intracellular aggregation. *J. Biol. Chem.* 290, 14893–14903. doi: 10.1074/jbc.M115.652693

Mudher, A., Colin, M., Dujardin, S., Medina, M., Dewachter, I., Alavi Naini, S. M., et al. (2017). What is the evidence that tau pathology spreads through prion-like propagation? *Acta Neuropathol. Commun.* 5:99. doi: 10.1186/s40478-017-0488-7

Nonaka, T., Watanabe, S. T., Iwatsubo, T., and Hasegawa, M. (2010). Seeded aggregation and toxicity of {alpha}-synuclein and tau: cellular models of neurodegenerative diseases. *J. Biol. Chem.* 285, 34885–34898. doi: 10.1074/jbc.m110.148460

Pannell, M., Meier, M. A., Szulzewsky, F., Matyash, V., Endres, M., Kronenberg, G., et al. (2016). The subpopulation of microglia expressing functional muscarinic acetylcholine receptors expands in stroke and Alzheimer's disease. *Brain Struct. Funct.* 221, 1157–1172. doi: 10.1007/s00429-014-0962-y

Sanders, D. W., Kaufman, S. K., DeVos, S. L., Sharma, A. M., Mirbaha, H., Li, A., et al. (2014). Distinct tau prion strains propagate in cells and mice and define different tauopathies. *Neuron* 82, 1271–1288. doi: 10.1016/j.neuron.2014.04.047

Schmitz, T. W., Nathan Spreng, R., and Alzheimer's Disease Neuroimaging, I. (2016). Basal forebrain degeneration precedes and predicts the cortical spread of Alzheimer's pathology. *Nat. Commun.* 7:13249. doi: 10.1038/ncomms13249

Shafer, S. H., and Williams, C. L. (2004). Elevated Rac1 activity changes the M3 muscarinic acetylcholine receptor-mediated inhibition of proliferation to induction of cell death. *Mol. Pharmacol.* 65, 1080–1091. doi: 10.1124/mol.65.5.1080

Shafiei, S. S., Guerrero-Munoz, M. J., and Castillo-Carranza, D. L. (2017). Tau oligomers: cytotoxicity, propagation, and mitochondrial damage. *Front Aging Neurosci.* 9:83. doi: 10.3389/fnagi.2017.00083

Shaw, G., Morse, S., Ararat, M., and Graham, F. L. (2002). Preferential transformation of human neuronal cells by human adenoviruses and the origin of HEK 293 cells. *FASEB J.* 16, 869–871. doi: 10.1096/fj.01-0995fje

Soukup, O., Winder, M., Killi, U. K., Wsol, V., Jun, D., Kuca, K., et al. (2017). Acetylcholinesterase inhibitors and drugs acting on muscarinic receptors- potential crosstalk of cholinergic mechanisms during pharmacological treatment. *Curr. Neuropharmacol.* 15, 637–653. doi: 10.2174/1570159X14666160607212615

Takeda, S. (2019). Progression of Alzheimer's disease, tau propagation, and its modifiable risk factors. *Neurosci. Res.* 141, 36–42. doi: 10.1016/j.neures.2018.08.005

Wu, J. W., Herman, M., Liu, L., Simoes, S., Acker, C. M., Figueroa, H., et al. (2013). Small misfolded Tau species are internalized via bulk endocytosis and anterogradely and retrogradely transported in neurons. *J. Biol. Chem.* 288, 1856–1870. doi: 10.1074/jbc.M112.394528

Wu, J. W., Hussaini, S. A., Bastille, I. M., Rodriguez, G. A., Mrejeru, A., Rilett, K., et al. (2016). Neuronal activity enhances tau propagation and tau pathology in vivo. *Nat. Neurosci.* 19, 1085–1092. doi: 10.1038/nn.4328

Alzheimer's Disease as a Membrane Disorder: Spatial Cross-Talk Among Beta-Amyloid Peptides, Nicotinic Acetylcholine Receptors and Lipid Rafts

Camila Fabiani[1,2] *and Silvia S. Antollini*[1,2*]

[1] *Instituto de Investigaciones Bioquímicas de Bahía Blanca CONICET-UNS, Bahía Blanca, Argentina,* [2] *Departamento de Biología, Bioquímica y Farmacia, Universidad Nacional del Sur, Bahía Blanca, Argentina*

Correspondence:
Silvia S. Antollini
silviant@criba.edu.ar

Biological membranes show lateral and transverse asymmetric lipid distribution. Cholesterol (Chol) localizes in both hemilayers, but in the external one it is mostly condensed in lipid-ordered microdomains (raft domains), together with saturated phosphatidyl lipids and sphingolipids (including sphingomyelin and glycosphingolipids). Membrane asymmetries induce special membrane biophysical properties and behave as signals for several physiological and/or pathological processes. Alzheimer's disease (AD) is associated with a perturbation in different membrane properties. Amyloid-β (Aβ) plaques and neurofibrillary tangles of tau protein together with neuroinflammation and neurodegeneration are the most characteristic cellular changes observed in this disease. The extracellular presence of Aβ peptides forming senile plaques, together with soluble oligomeric species of Aβ, are considered the major cause of the synaptic dysfunction of AD. The association between Aβ peptide and membrane lipids has been extensively studied. It has been postulated that Chol content and Chol distribution condition Aβ production and posterior accumulation in membranes and, hence, cell dysfunction. Several lines of evidence suggest that Aβ partitions in the cell membrane accumulate mostly in raft domains, the site where the cleavage of the precursor AβPP by β- and γ- secretase is also thought to occur. The main consequence of the pathogenesis of AD is the disruption of the cholinergic pathways in the cerebral cortex and in the basal forebrain. In parallel, the nicotinic acetylcholine receptor has been extensively linked to membrane properties. Since its transmembrane domain exhibits extensive contacts with the surrounding lipids, the acetylcholine receptor function is conditioned by its lipid microenvironment. The nicotinic acetylcholine receptor is present in high-density clusters in the cell membrane where it localizes mainly in lipid-ordered domains. Perturbations of sphingomyelin or cholesterol composition alter acetylcholine receptor location. Therefore, Aβ processing, Aβ partitioning, and acetylcholine receptor location and function can be manipulated by changes in membrane lipid biophysics. Understanding these mechanisms should provide insights into new therapeutic strategies for prevention and/or treatment of AD. Here, we discuss the implications of lipid-protein interactions at the cell membrane level in AD.

Keywords: Alzheimer's disease, Aβ peptide, nicotinic acetylcholine receptor, acetylcholinesterase, cell membranes, lipid rafts, cholesterol

INTRODUCTION

Biological membranes were, are, and will be complex, dynamic and controversial. Several different theories/models were postulated until the fluid-mosaic model was proposed by Singer and Nicolson (1972). This description of a biological membrane was very well accepted and gave light about membrane structure and membrane function. Although a lot of new information appeared in the following 40 years, the model was able to survive by absorbing some modifications, as it was emphasized by Nicolson (2014). **Table 1** details and compares the most important features of the original fluid-mosaic model membrane (Singer and Nicolson, 1972) and the current vision of a membrane (Engelman, 2005; Bagatolli, 2010; Goñi, 2014; Nicolson, 2014).

Nowadays, a membrane is thought of as an increasingly complex crowded structure of a great variety of *lipid* and *protein* arrangements with lateral and transverse *asymmetry*, variable *patchiness*, variable *thickness*, and higher *protein* occupancy (Engelman, 2005; Nicolson, 2014). It is universally accepted that biological membranes behave as barriers separating two fluid media and avoiding contact with each other. But being a physical barrier is not its only or main function. Many of the biochemical reactions essential for cell life (metabolic and signaling reactions involving G-protein coupled receptors as the rhodopsin or muscarinic receptor and ion channels as nicotinic, histamine, GABA or glutamate receptors among others transmembrane proteins) occur in the cell membranes, making them a truly important agent in almost all cellular physiological and pathological processes. These reactions imply molecular communication, which involves protein–protein and also protein–lipid interactions. Lipid membranes are not just a "sea" where proteins are embedded, as it was initially postulated by Singer and Nicolson. Lipids (including fatty acids, cholesterol, endocannabinoids, arachidonic acid metabolites as prostaglandins, leukotrienes, and epoxyeicosatrienoic acids, etc.) are active molecules with important implications. Lipids such as chol, cardiolipin, PIP2 and glycolipids condition the function of several transmembrane proteins, a fact reflected in the thousands of research papers that report the effect of these lipids on protein functions (Lee, 2003; Barenholz, 2004; Barrera et al., 2013). Here, we will discuss the implications of lipid-protein interactions at the cell membrane level in AD.

Abbreviations: Aβ, amyloid β protein; ACE, acetylcholinesterase; AD, Alzheimer's disease; APP, amyloid precursor protein; BACE 1, β-site APP-cleaving transmembrane aspartic protease 1; CARC, inversed CRAC; Chol, cholesterol; CRAC, Chol recognition amino acid consensus; DPPC, dipalmitoylphosphatidylcholine; l_d, liquid-disorder domain; LDM, low density membrane domain; l_o, liquid-ordered domain; M1 to M4, nAChR transmembrane segments; MuSK, muscle specific receptor tyrosine kinase; nAChR, nicotinic acetylcholine receptor; NMJ, neuromuscular junction; PA, phosphatidic acid; PC, phosphatidylcholine; PE, phosphatidylethanolamine; PRiMA, proline-rich membrane anchor; PS1, presenilin 1; PUFA, polyunsaturated fatty acid; SM, sphingomyelin.

CROSSTALK OF ALZHEIMER'S DISEASE PATHOGENESIS AND LIPID MEMBRANE

Alzheimer's disease is the most prevalent neurodegenerative disorder in the elderly, and is characterized by progressive cognitive decline. The main pathophysiological characteristics include extracellular accumulation of β-amyloid senile plaques and intracellular accumulation of neurofibrillary tangles (hyperphosphorylated microtubule-associated tau protein) (Feng and Wang, 2012; Kumar et al., 2015). A disruption of the cholinergic pathways that contribute to the cognitive impairment of AD patients is described in the cerebral cortex and in the basal forebrain. AD implicates the formation of extracellular insoluble peptides derived from the action of two transmembrane enzymes, a β-secretase (β-site APP-cleaving transmembrane aspartic protease, BACE 1) and a γ-secretase (an imprecise multimeric protein complex), on the membrane-bound APP. Aβ peptides of different lengths, containing 39–42 amino acid residues, are produced. 1–40 Aβ is produced more frequently while 1–42 Aβ is the predominant species in senile plaques (Iwatsubo et al., 1994). They are amphiphilic peptides with residues 1–28 constituting a hydrophilic domain and residues 29 up to 42 (which correspond to part of the transmembrane domain of APP), a hydrophobic one (Ji et al., 2002). Whereas low concentrations of 1–40 Aβ are related to neurotrophic properties (Yankner et al., 1990; Zou et al., 2002, 2003), 1–42 Aβ, produced in low amounts under physiological conditions, has a much higher tendency to form oligomers, protofibrils and fibrils, which are the ones that constitute AD brain plaques (Jarrett et al., 1993; Gu and Guo, 2013). The structural-activity relation between these assemblies and the differences between 1–40 Aβ and 1–42 Aβ are under continuous investigation and exceed the aim of this review. Alternatively, APP can be cleaved by another membrane enzyme (α-secretase) between amino acids 16 and 17 of the Aβ region, avoiding Aβ peptides generation and producing a neurotrophic and neuroprotective soluble AβPP (sAβPPα) through a non-amyloidogenic pathway (Thornton et al., 2006; Wang et al., 2016). In neurons, amyloidogenic and non-amyloidogenic pathways compete with each other, jumping between neuroprotection and neurodegeneration (Vetrivel and Thinakaran, 2006; Tan and Gleeson, 2019). Furthermore, in normal brains, 1–42 Aβ is produced in low picomolar concentrations and, as it will be explained later, these low, non-toxic concentrations have physiological implications in synaptic plasticity and memory, among others (Plant et al., 2003; Puzzo et al., 2008, 2011, 2015). In fact, physiological 1–42 Aβ binds to several target molecules as apoE, the receptor for advanced glycosylation end products (RAGE), serpin–enzyme complex receptor (SEC-R) and nicotinic acetylcholine (nACh) receptors (Turner et al., 2003). Thus, although during a person's lifetime there is a continuous formation of all these peptides, the deregulation of the enzymatic equilibrium with the consequent accumulation of insoluble peptides is characteristic of AD. 1–42 Aβ is the most hydrophobic peptide that forms soluble oligomeric intermediates before aggregating as insoluble plaques with cytotoxic properties in the AD brains. It induces iron and cooper reduction in the brain triggering oxidative stress and damage, it causes calcium homeostasis deregulation probably through lipid perturbation at the cell membrane, and it causes oxy-radicals formation and finally neurodegeneration (Butterfield et al., 2013; Fonseca et al., 2015; Cheignon et al., 2018). Amyloidogenic and non-amyloidogenic pathways are thought to occur in different cellular compartments depending

TABLE 1 | Comparison of the main membrane characteristics proposed by the Singer and Nicolson (1972) model and the current cell membrane vision (based on Engelman (2005), Bagatolli (2010), Goñi (2014), Nicolson (2014), and references there in).

Singer and Nicolson (1972)	Today (2019)
The membrane consists of a double layer of lipids (*bilayer*) in a *lamellar liquid-crystalline phase.* (A preliminary deviation of this concept was included in the original model: *"It is therefore not excluded that some significant fraction of the phospholipid (perhaps as much as 30 percent) is physically in a different state from the rest of the lipid."*)	In certain membranes, other phases like *liquid-ordered phases* or *non-lamellar phases* as rhombohedral, tetragonal, inverted hexagonal and cubic phases fulfill physiologically important functions. These phenomena involve membrane phase changes that are possible because of the intrinsic deformability of the membrane. Examples of transient *non-lamellar phases* can be seen during membrane fusion where from two independent bilayers originates only one which involves the coalesce of two bilayers (Chernomordik and Zimmerberg, 1995; Tenchov et al., 2006) or during pore formation by proteins as Bax/colicin family proteins and actinoporins which involves the formation of non-lamellar (semi-toroidal or toroidal) lipidic structures (Gilbert et al., 2014; Gilbert, 2016).
The membrane is considered *flat.*	Membranes are usually *curved*, dynamically modulated by the geometry of both lipids and proteins, and require *asymmetry* between both hemilayers in order to support this membrane curvature (Mouritsen and Bloom, 1984; Epand et al., 1996; Zimmerberg and Gawrisch, 2006; Bagatolli, 2010).
The protein:lipid ratio is 1.5–4, and thus proteins play an important role in the membrane structure. However, lipids and proteins do not interact strongly. They are almost independent entities, without significant perturbation of the bilayer. (A preliminary deviation of this concept was proposed in the original model: *"if it is proposed that, while the largest portion of the phospholipid is in bilayer form and not strongly coupled to proteins in the membrane a small fraction of the lipid is more tightly coupled to protein. With any membrane protein, the tightly coupled lipid might be specific; that is, the interaction might require that the phospholipid contain specific fatty acid chains or particular polar head groups. There is at present, however, no satisfactory direct evidence for such a distinctive lipid fraction".*)	The membrane is full of proteins, leaving no membrane fraction unaffected by their presence. Protein–protein interactions have functional important signaling implications. There are lipids in direct contact with the protein (boundary lipids) that provide a special lipid environment for the proteins. Some of these lipids have a fast exchange with bulk lipids (annular lipids), whereas others (non-annular lipids) are tightly bound to certain membrane proteins stabilizing their conformation and/or function.
Proteins interact with the bilayer in two different forms: as *peripheral or extrinsic proteins* (associated to the lipid bilayer polar headgroups) and as *integral or intrinsic proteins* (associated to the hydrophobic matrix).	There are also other proteins that are only part of the time docked to a membrane (*membrane associated proteins*). They are not involved in the microstructure of the membrane; however, they have important membrane functions and dynamics. For example, protein kinases C and annexins (Bazzi and Nelsestuen, 1996).
The membranes are *fluid*. Lipids and proteins have two of three different modes of motion: *rotational* around an axis perpendicular to the plane of the membrane, and freely *translational* along the plane of the membrane. *Transbilayer* diffusion is forbidden because of the energy barrier presented by the hydrophobic matrix to the polar groups of the lipids and proteins.	The high amount of transmembrane proteins plus peripheral proteins plus protein-protein interactions restricts dramatically the lateral diffusion of proteins. The membranes are seen as "more *mosaic* than *fluid.*"[1] Membrane lipids can also undergo fast transbilayer diffusion (*flip-flop* movements), which can be a protein-helped event or a spontaneous event. Scrambling of lipids contributes to the dynamic transbilayer asymmetry of the membrane; or, contrary to this, to losing the asymmetric condition by triggering a signaling process (i.e., phosphatidylserine flip-flop from the inner to the outer hemilayer and apoptosis).
The two surfaces of membranes are not identical in composition, structure, and distribution of oligosaccharides. This *asymmetry* is based on the forbidden transbilayer diffusion.	Membranes are *asymmetric*. Lipids and proteins are different in each hemilayer, this being a condition that involves lipid transporters or spontaneous lipid movements (Quinn, 2002; Daleke, 2003; van Meer, 2011). Integral proteins are naturally asymmetrical in the membrane after their initial biosynthesis. Asymmetry is essential for cells and its disruption is associated with cell activation or pathological conditions.

(Continued)

TABLE 1 | Continued

Singer and Nicolson (1972)	Today (2019)
The membrane is mainly *homogeneous.* The original model suggested that: *"Such short-range order is probably mediated by specific protein (and perhaps protein-lipid) interactions leading to the formation of stoichiometrically defined aggregates within the membrane. However, in a mosaic membrane with a lipid matrix, the long-range distribution of such aggregates would be expected to be random over the entire surface of the membrane".*	The bilayer is full of uneven *heterogeneous* patches or domains enriched in certain lipids and proteins, which confer irregular thickness in the membrane. This is the result of certain preference of protein-lipid contacts, mismatch between the length of the hydrophobic transmembrane segments of the proteins and the length of the lipid acyl chains, protein–protein contacts, the anchoring of integral proteins to cytoskeletal proteins, the poor miscibility of certain lipids, etc. These domains have very important functional implications. *Membrane rafts* (Simons and Ikonen, 1997) are one type of membrane domains. They are small (10–200 nm), transient and dynamic (short life, ~200 ms). These domains, which induce lateral order and heterogeneous organization of membranes, are a consequence of the immiscibility of certain lipids of biological membranes, leading to the coexistence of patches with different physical properties and lipid compositions. They also compartmentalize or segregate certain proteins making more efficient a variety of cellular processes. Rafts domains in eukaryotic cell membranes are liquid-ordered domains rich in cholesterol and sphingomyelin. In model membranes, a mixture of lipids that induce a segregation of liquid-ordered (lo) and liquid-disordered phases (ld) is used to study those domains. A *lo phase* is a phase with higher lateral mobility in the bilayer than in a gel phase but with the lipid acyl chains extended and ordered, whereas a *ld phase* is a fluid phase with the acyl chains of the lipids highly disordered and mobile (Simons and van Meer, 1988; Simons and Ikonen, 1997; Brown and London, 2000; London, 2005; Sonnino and Prinetti, 2013).
The membrane is an *isolated system* with no exchange of matter or energy with the environment.	All kind of signals occur in the membrane contacting with the extracellular and intracellular environment, for example molecules reaching and leaving the membrane in response to stimulus (Watson, 2015; Wen et al., 2018).

[1] *Nicolson (2014) said: "I have re-termed the model as the 'Fluid—Mosaic Membrane Model' to highlight the important role of mosaic, aggregate and domain structures in membranes and the restraints on lateral mobility of many if not most membrane protein components."*

on secretases localization. γ-secretase complex is present in multiple compartments: near 6% in the plasma membrane and the rest in intracellular organelles such as endoplasmic reticulum, late Golgi/*trans*-Golgi network and endosomes (Vetrivel et al., 2004; Chyung et al., 2005). However, α- and β-secretases are more compartmentalized. α-cleavage occurs at the cell surface (Parvathy et al., 1999; Haass et al., 2012; Sun and Roy, 2018). APP is released to the plasma membrane through the secretory pathway and stays there for a short time. Therefore, during this short time, APP is proteolytically processed by α-secretase. Anyway, near 70% of APP is internalized by endocytosis. A fraction of this APP is recycled to the cell surface and another one is degraded in lysosomes. BACE 1 is localized late in the Golgi/*trans*-Golgi network and endosomes and cleaves APP during the endocytic/recycling cycle (Koo and Squazzo, 1994); thus, β-cleavage depends on endocytosis (Koo and Squazzo, 1994; Perez et al., 1999; Huse et al., 2000; Daugherty and Green, 2001; Kamal et al., 2001; Ehehalt et al., 2003) and Aβ is produced mainly in the *trans*-Golgi network during the recycling pathway (Vetrivel and Thinakaran, 2006). Additionally, it was suggested that 1–42 Aβ is produced mainly in the endoplasmatic reticulum whereas 1–40 Aβ is produced in the *trans*-Golgi network (Annaert et al., 1999; Greenfield et al., 1999).

APP cleavage by secretases always happens in a membrane, independently of the subcellular compartment. To understand the importance of this fact, it is recommended to read the general commentary by Lukiw (2013) in *Frontiers in Physiology* titled "Alzheimer's disease (AD) as a disorder of the plasma membrane," whereas the author pointed out the implication that the membrane has in the physiopathology of this disease. Several studies postulated that membrane components condition the APP enzymatic processing. Particularly, Chol is a key element in the membrane and it has been related to AD in several ways. Lahdo and De La Fournière-Bessueille (2004) studied the minimum lipid requirements of a monolayer for the insertion of APP. They concluded that APP insertion depends on the Chol content, the Chol/PC and the Chol/SM ratios, and the monolayer membrane order. They identified a critical inflection point at near 30% Chol: at a lower ratio APP localizes in the membrane surface mainly in a β-sheet conformation, whereas as this Chol percentage increases, APP can insert spontaneously into the membrane changing its conformation (Ji et al., 2002; Lahdo and De La Fournière-Bessueille, 2004). Consequently, once APP is confined to the interior of the membrane it can perturb the biophysical properties of this membrane and the activity of several transmembrane or associated-membrane proteins. The Chol concentration and Chol location in brain plasma membranes change throughout a person's life. At early ages, about 87% of the Chol is localized mainly in the inner layer of the brain plasma membrane, but during aging, the percentage of Chol increases in the outer layer losing the initial transmembrane asymmetry and reaching at least 30 mol%, the critical value with respect to APP membrane insertion (Igbavboa et al., 1996; Wood et al., 2002). In another work, it was suggested that modifications of Chol compartmentation and the equilibrium free cholesterol/cholesteryl esters through acyl-coenzyme A:Chol acyltransferase (ACAT) activation, instead of variations of total membrane Chol, are the determinant of Aβ accumulation and cell dysfunction (Puglielli et al., 2001).

The importance of the amount of Chol for APP insertion leads us to think that APP would probably prefer raft domains (Cordy et al., 2006; Reid et al., 2007). Initial studies in the brain showed that both APP and Aβ reside in detergent-insoluble glycolipid-enriched membrane domains (DIG) (Lee et al., 1998), suggesting that those domains are the place in the membrane where the APP processing occurs. The non-amyloidogenic pathway through α-secretase is thought to occur in non-raft domains (Kojro et al., 2001; Reid et al., 2007). On the other hand, although there is no consensus about the localization of APP and BACE 1, there is agreement that APP cleavage by β- and γ-secretase occurs in raft domains (see **Table 1** for a detailed explanation of raft domains). Experiments in culture cells showed that overexpressed APP and both secretases enzymes localize in Chol-rich domains (Burns and Duff, 2002; Ehehalt et al., 2003), and that Chol depletion by Chol synthesis inhibition or Chol membrane extraction resulted in a reduction of Aβ production (Simons et al., 1998; Fassbender et al., 2001; Ehehalt et al., 2003). Several studies suggest that APP is present in two cellular pools: one in raft domains and another in non-raft domains. Ehehalt et al. (2003) concluded that this APP membrane compartmentation explains how the same protein could be processed in two different ways (generating Aβ in raft domains and being cleaved by α-secretase in non-raft domains). Furthermore, they said that although BACE 1 is present in both raft and non-raft domains it needs to be in raft domains to be functional, outside these domains the enzyme is inactive (**Figure 1a**). That is the reason why, when Chol diminishes, Aβ production also diminishes but increases αCTF (C-terminal fragment) or C83, which is a direct product of α-secretase. Thus, Chol regulates the access of α or β secretase to APP (Ehehalt et al., 2003). On the other hand, immediately after this study, a study in human hippocampal membranes showed that the vast majority of APP is located in non-raft domains, while β-secretase BACE 1 is found in two cellular pools: one in raft domains and another in non-raft domains (Abad-Rodriguez et al., 2004). These authors gave an explanation opposite to the previous one: when Chol diminishes, which is what happens in the membrane from AD patients (Mason et al., 1992; Roth et al., 1995), BACE 1 increases in non-raft domains and then an enhancement of amyloid peptide production occurs. They concluded that BACE 1 in raft domains corresponds to an inactive pool that needs to relocate to non-raft domains to perform its activity, and that it is the Chol which directly conditions APP processing by "allowing" BACE 1 to exit or not from neighboring domains (**Figure 1b**). However, they distinguished between a mild membrane Chol reduction (less than 25%), which results in an increase of APP processing, and a drastic membrane Chol reduction (more than 35%), where an overall disruption of membrane integrity occurs concomitantly with a lower Aβ production. Working with primary cultures of rat hippocampal neurons infected with recombinant Semliki Forest virus (SFV) carrying APP, Simons et al. (1998) arrived to a different conclusion. They showed that depletion of Chol up to 60–70% did not affect the amount of APPsec (the main processed form of APP in neurons obtained by direct α-cleavage), but drastically decreased the amount of Aβ. Therefore, Chol depletion appears to redirect the APP processing from amyloidogenic processing to non-amyloidogenic cleavage. One possible explanation for this is that the small raft-resident pool of APP and BACE 1 is the active one and that it generates C99 to be processed by γ-secretase (Rushworth and Hooper, 2011). Another explanation considers that the amount of both proteins in rafts is so small that the APP processing by BACE 1 is effective once a clustering of raft domains occurs during endocytosis, meanwhile, in the plasma membrane, APP will be mainly cleaved by α-secretase through a non-amyloidogenesis pathway (Ehehalt et al., 2003). Thus, it is possible that APP processing can be altered by membrane lipid composition perturbations. Eckert et al. (2003) showed that Chol depletion decreases the amount of APP in raft domains and, consequently, the production of Aβ. On the other side, Chol increment as in Niemann Pick type C model cells, causes an APP augmentation in raft domains.

A controversial point is where are secretases located, especially β-secretase, and where they function in the membrane. With respect to γ-secretase, however, there is broad consensus. It is postulated that this enzyme is localized in raft domains confirming that the last step in the generation of Aβ occurs in those domains (Vetrivel et al., 2005). These authors postulated that once APP is cleaved by β-secretase, the CTFs (or C99) produced are recruited or sequestered into raft domains where cleavage by γ-secretase takes place. They indicated that ~20% of BACE 1, less than 5% of APP and more than 70% of CTFs reside in raft domains; and, based on previous work, they assume that all cleavage occurs in these rigid domains (Vetrivel et al., 2005).

By magnetic nuclear resonance of C99, Beel et al. (2010) identified a short sequence of 5 amino acids (VGSNK) between the extracellular segment and the transmembrane domain that interacts with Chol, probably through hydrogen bonds. These authors recognize that although C99 is in raft domains, APP, which has the same loop, localizes mainly in non-raft domains, concluding that one possibility is that APP and C99 have different affinities for Chol. This Chol interaction site is also present in Aβ peptides, thus explaining the reported Chol-Aβ peptides interactions that trigger oligomerization, fibrillization, etc. (Beel et al., 2010) which will be discussed below.

Chol is not only crucial for APP processing in the membrane by compartmentalizing the location of both APP and secretases, but also for modulating the secretases activity. Briefly, Chol positively modulates BACE 1 and γ-secretase activities, and negatively modulates α-secretase (Bodovitz and Klein, 1996; Simons et al., 1998; Frears et al., 1999; Kojro et al., 2001; Wahrle et al., 2002; Ghribi et al., 2006). In lysates from human brain and in cultured cells, a certain amount of Chol stimulated β and γ-secretase activities, but at 20 μM Chol γ-secretase activity was inhibited. It is probable that high Chol can directly stabilize the activities of the enzymes to the maximum level in the correct lipid domain or can reduce enzymes degradation increasing Aβ production (Xiong et al., 2008). Furthermore, APP processing can be modulated by Chol conditioning membrane biophysical properties (Kojro et al., 2001; Fukaya et al., 2007; Kogel et al., 2008; Peters et al., 2009; Yang et al., 2010; Askarova et al., 2011). For example, substitution of Chol by lanosterol or polyunsaturated free fatty acids (PUFAs) induced an increment of membrane fluidity, which was related to an enhancement of α-secretase activity (Kojro et al., 2001; Yang et al., 2010; Askarova et al., 2011).

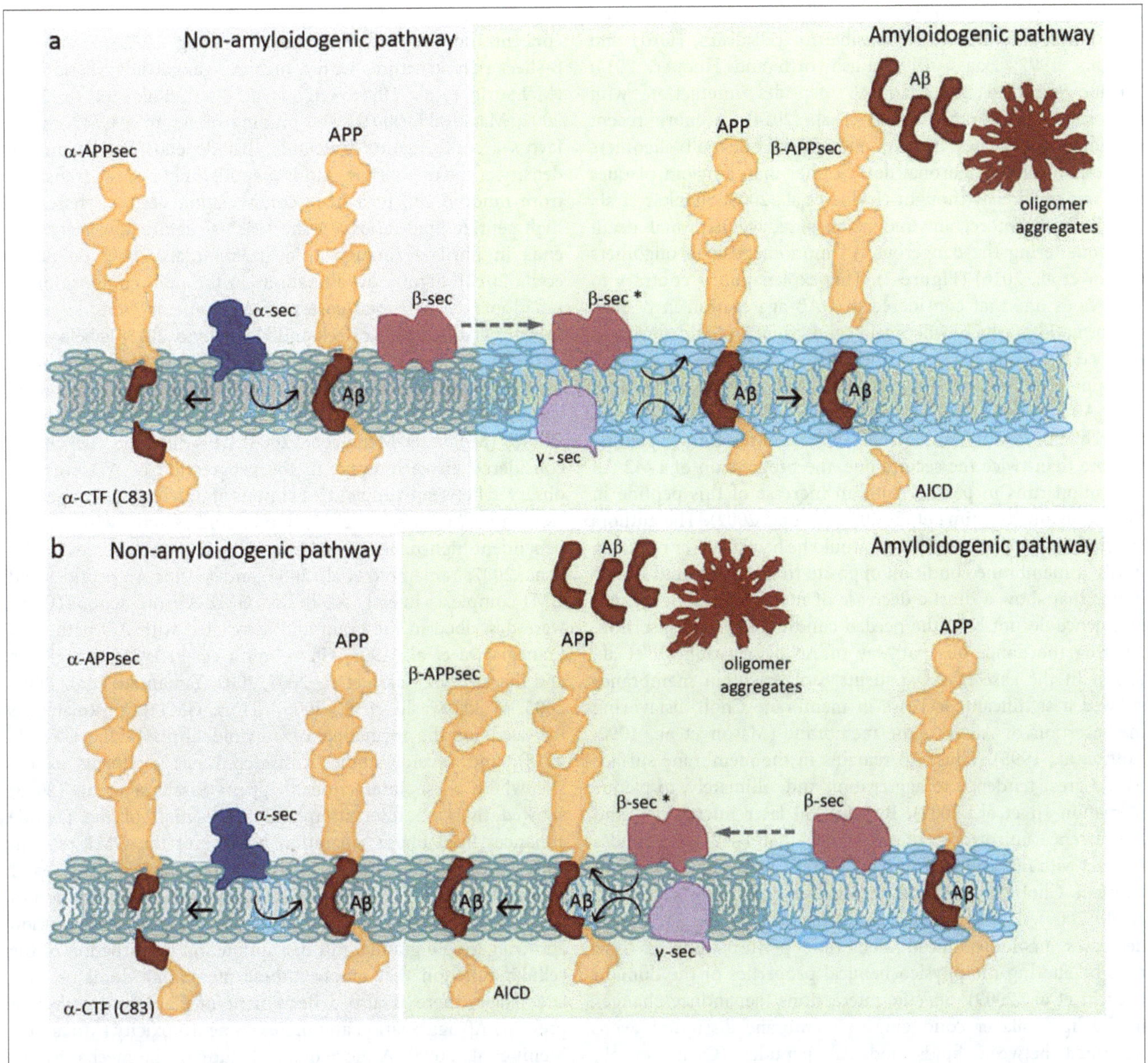

FIGURE 1 | Schematic diagram showing two distinct hypotheses of APP processing, which differ in the membrane location of the whole process. Two different colors are used to represent a raft domain and a liquid-disordered domain (light blue and gray, respectively). **(a)** Hypothesis where β sec is present in both raft and non-raft domains but needs to be in raft domains to be functional (represented as β sec*) (Ehehalt et al., 2003). **(b)** Hypothesis where β sec in raft domains corresponds to an inactive pool that needs to relocate to non-raft domains to be functional (Abad-Rodriguez et al., 2004). APP, amyloid precursor protein; α-CTF, C-terminal fragment obtained by α-secretase; α-APPsec, soluble N-terminal APP fragment obtained by α-secretase; Aβ, amyloid β peptide; β-APPsec, soluble N-terminal APP fragment obtained by β-secretase; AICD, APP intracellular domain obtained by the action of γ-secretase on β-CTF or C99 (intermediate peptide that is not shown and corresponds to Aβ plus AICD, obtained in the first step by the action of β-secretase); α-sec, α-secretase; β-sec, β-secretase; and γ-sec, γ-secretase.

Aβ RELATIONSHIP WITH AND IMPLICATIONS ON CELL MEMBRANE

Chol is also important for Aβ peptide action/effect (Eckert et al., 2003; Wood et al., 2014). Aβ peptide can adopt different conformations: a random-coil conformation in aqueous solution, an antiparallel β-sheet in the core of the amyloid plaques, and an α-helix in membranes containing Chol (Ji et al., 2002). It can exist as monomers, oligomers or as amyloid fibrils (Klein et al., 2004; Reid et al., 2007). Several studies indicate that Chol directly binds to APP as was described above (Beel et al., 2010), and also to C99 and monomeric Aβ peptides (Barrett et al., 2012), to oligomers (Ashley et al., 2006), to aggregates (Avdulov et al., 1997), and to fibrils (Harris, 2008). Considering that the mechanism by which Aβ produces brain dysfunction in AD patients is still unknown, these evidences turned the view of Aβ peptides pathogenesis from extracellular plaques (the *"amyloid theory"*: extracellular amyloid plaques are the responsible for cell death; Hardy and Higgins, 1992; Haass, 1996; Rushworth and Hooper, 2011; Serrano-Pozo et al., 2011) to Aβ peptides interaction with the plasma membrane (Relini et al., 2014). A more recent explanation indicates that Aβ monomers or small oligomers are responsible of neuronal death rather than amyloid plaques as it was previously thought (Irvine et al., 2008; Shankar et al., 2008). Furthermore, amyloid plaques reduce neuronal death by sequestering the dangerous Aβ monomers/small oligomers (Arbor et al., 2016) (**Figure 2**). This explanation is contrary to a previous one that considered that Aβ aggregation in β-sheet conformation, which will finally end as neurotoxic fibrils, is reduced by Aβ insertion as α-helix after interaction with Chol-containing membranes (Ji et al., 2002). They showed that both 1–40 Aβ and 1–42 Aβ peptides prefer Chol enriched LDM and that while in healthy humans the amount of the former peptide is more than twice the second one, the progression of 1–42 Aβ deposition runs in parallel with an increase of this peptide in LDM domains (Oshima et al., 2001; Ji et al., 2002). The authors concluded that Chol enrichment would be beneficial for reducing fibrils, a membrane condition opposite to the one found in AD brains that show a drastic decrease of membrane Chol content and hence do not have the needed conditions for Aβ insertion, favoring the dangerous pathway of Aβ aggregation (Ji et al., 2002). In the case of AD patients, isolated brain membranes showed a significant decrease in membrane Chol, disfavoring the insertion of Aβ into the membrane (Mason et al., 1992; Roth et al., 1995). Thus, Aβ remains in the membrane surface with a great tendency to aggregation and, ultimately, to plaque formation (Ji et al., 2002). By confocal laser microscopy and fluorescence anisotropy, it was shown that 1–42 Aβ peptides interact with raft domains and that there is an inverse correlation between Chol content and membrane perturbation (Cecchi et al., 2009). It was further indicated that a Chol increment decreases amyloid-induced membrane perturbations at lipid rafts by altering the physicochemical properties of the domain (Cecchi et al., 2009). Specific interactions that induce changes in the lipid bilayer conducing to membrane disruption were described between lipids and Aβ peptides (Qiang et al., 2014). Different kinds of interactions were proposed in the last few years. Vestergaard et al. (2010) performed studies of Aβ interactions with model biomimetic membranes and showed that immediately after peptide addition, membrane fluctuations/morphological changes occur. They suggested that both Chol levels and lipid composition affect how Aβ oligomers interact with the membrane. X-ray diffraction studies of the interaction between a 25–35 Aβ peptide and anionic membranes enabled the identification of immiscible Chol plaques when more than 30 mol% Chol was added. The peptide interacts with the bilayers sequestering more Chol molecules into the plaques and, hence, decreasing the amount of Chol in the membrane (Dies et al., 2014).

Chol is not the only important lipid in the Aβ-membrane interactions, there is also GM1, which is a resident lipid of raft domains (Lin et al., 2008). High Chol levels facilitate gangliosides clustering, which is postulated to modulate Aβ oligomerization. These clusters interact with Aβ peptides in a concentration dependent manner inducing Aβ aggregation in β-sheet rich structures with a high Aβ/ganglioside relationship (McLaurin et al., 1998; Ariga et al., 2001; Kakio et al., 2001, 2002; Matsuzaki, 2007). The binding of Aβ to a GM1 cluster favors a conformation transition that depends on the protein density of the membrane. At low peptide/lipid ratios a transition from random coil to α-helix conformation occurs, whereas at high peptide/lipid ratios a β-sheet rich structure appears, which ends in fibrils formation (Matsuzaki et al., 2010; Fukunaga et al., 2012). Significant alterations in the lipid composition of raft domains in frontal cortex of AD patients were described (Martín et al., 2010; Kosicek and Hecimovic, 2013; Fabelo et al., 2014). A detailed study of the lipid composition of DRM from temporal and frontal cortex of AD brains indicated that there was an increment of GM1 and GM2 in both areas of the brain studied (Molander-Melin et al., 2005). This difference, which was considered an early event in the progression of AD, was not observed between samples from brains of different ages or gender (Molander-Melin et al., 2005). Other studies agree with an age-dependent high-density GM1 clustering in synaptosomes (Gylys et al., 2007; Yamamoto et al., 2008) and specific Aβ peptides and GM1 complexes in early AD brains. GM1-Aβ interactions (GAβ) were described in the brain and associated with AD pathology (Yanagisawa et al., 1995; Choo-Smith et al., 1997; Yanagisawa and Ihara, 1998; Kakio et al., 2001, 2002; Yamamoto et al., 2004, 2005; Wakabayashi et al., 2005). Thus, GM1 is postulated as the seed for the formation of amyloid fibrils (Staneva et al., 2018), and several studies considered raft platforms as the site where these interactions happen. Sasahara et al. (2013) showed that the interaction and aggregation of the peptide enhances lipid phase separation because of the GM1 relation with Aβ aggregates. A two-step phase was postulated to occur in membranes of AD patients: at early stages the proportion of GM1 in raft domains increases accelerating Aβ plaques formation and triggering a gradual raft disruption and perturbation of the cellular function that involves these membrane domains; at a later stage, there is also a decrement in Chol content which prevents Aβ aggregation and increases neurotoxicity (Molander-Melin et al., 2005). A more detailed study of the mechanism of Aβ interaction with GM1 indicates that Aβ oligomers, which have increased hydrophobicity compared to Aβ monomers, primarily bind to GM1 initiating progressive alterations such as membrane biophysical and ion permeability perturbations that end in the well-known synaptotoxic effects of Aβ (Hong et al., 2014).

Although all data points to a direct implication of gangliosides on Aβ oligomerization, a ganglioside-independent Aβ oligomerization mechanism was also observed, suggesting that other lipid components or carbohydrates in raft domains would be also implicated (Kim et al., 2006).

One important consequence of these raft domains/Aβ peptide interaction is the occurrence of Aβ peptide aggregation and Ca^{+2} channels formation in raft domains (Lin et al., 2001). In hippocampal cell membranes this process was related to neurotoxicity (Sepúlveda et al., 2014). Di Scala et al. (2013) identified a Chol binding domain in a 20–35 fragment of 1–42 Aβ, which is also present in other peptides with high

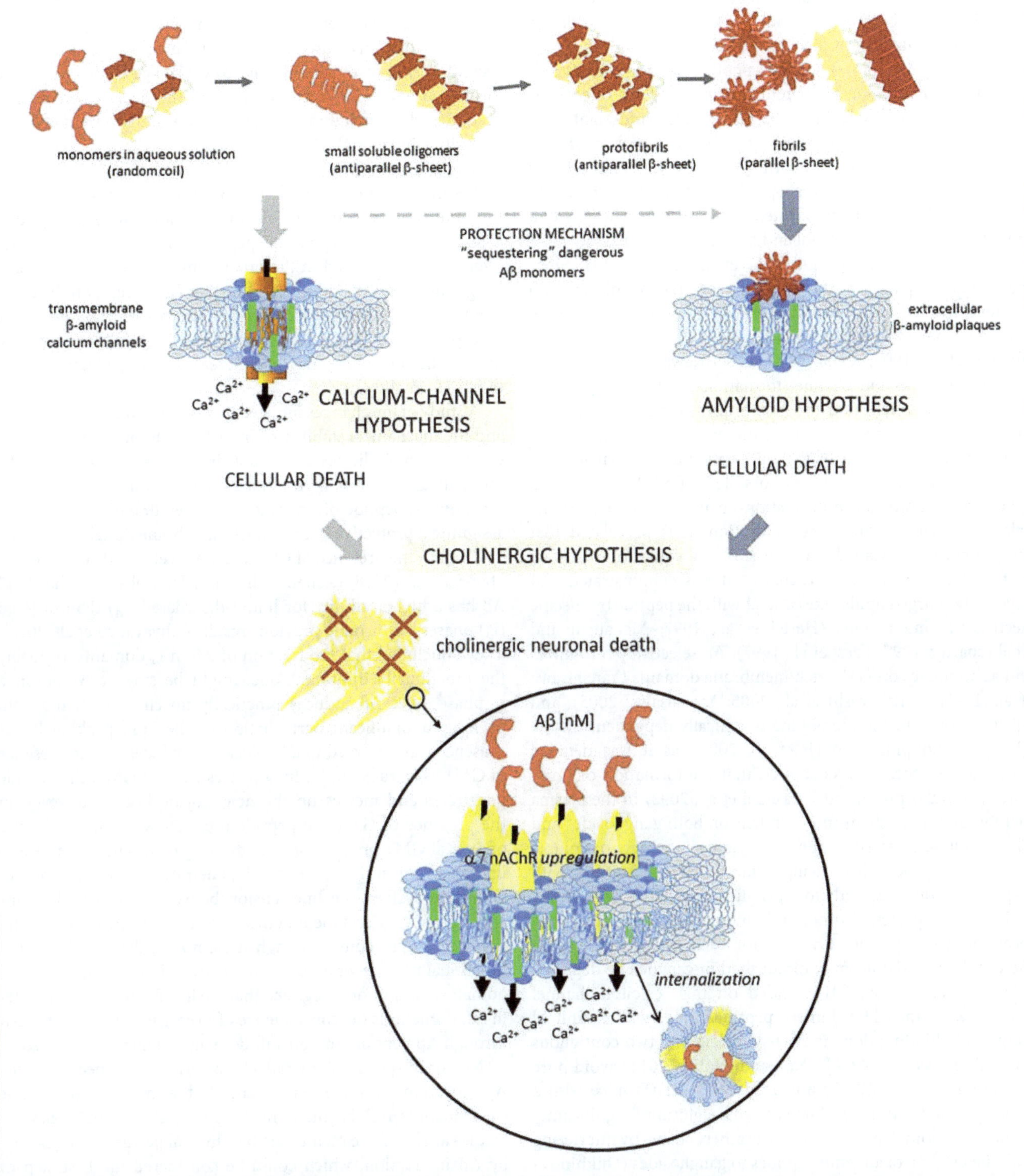

FIGURE 2 | Schematic diagram showing three different hypotheses of AD, which are closely related. Two different colors are used to represent a raft domain and a liquid-disordered domain (light blue and gray, respectively), and also within raft domains, two central lipids are identified for these hypotheses with different colors: chol and GM1 (green and blue, respectively). Aβ, amyloid β peptide; α7 nAChR, α7 nicotinic acetylcholine receptor.

Chol affinity. Interestingly, although both APP and 1–42 Aβ interact with Chol, they have distinct binding domains [17–40 Aβ for APP (Barrett et al., 2012) and 20–35 Aβ for 1–42 Aβ (Di Scala et al., 2013; Fantini et al., 2014)]. By physicochemical and *in silico* experiments, it was demonstrated that this 20–35 Aβ domain forms oligomeric Ca^{2+} channels in the plasma membrane in a Chol dependent manner (Di Scala et al., 2014). The high interaction with Chol of this 20–35 Aβ domain triggers the helix to an adequate tilted orientation inside the membrane, which allows accurate peptide-peptide interactions and the formation of the circular channel. This oligomeric channel is formed by eight 20–35 Aβ subunits and eight Chol molecules, with a pore size and an external diameter of 1.46 and 4.4 nm, respectively. The formation of these channels could help explain the neurotoxic properties of 1–42 Aβ (**Figure 2**). Similar *in silico* studies performed with 1–40 Aβ showed that the interactions between Chol and peptide are different to those observed with 1–42 Aβ (Di Scala et al., 2013, 2014). Since the initial proposal of the existence of transmembrane ion channels formed by Aβ peptides (Arispe et al., 1993a,b), lots of studies deepened in the "*β-amyloid calcium channel hypothesis*" (Pollard et al., 1995; Kagan et al., 2002; Kawahara, 2010). The first step for this ion channel formation must be the contact between the peptides and the membrane. It was demonstrated that both the lipid composition of the outer membrane and the structural conformation of the Aβ peptide are crucial for this interaction. In solution, it was possible to find Aβ as β-sheet, α-helix or random coil conformations, being the conformational balance dependent on its concentration. It is postulated that the presence of certain lipids can shift the equilibrium to one preferred conformation. Particularly, it was demonstrated that negatively charged lipids take contact with the peptide by specific electrostatic interactions (Hertel et al., 1997; McLaurin and Chakrabartty, 1997; Terzi et al., 1997). Aβ selectively recognizes and accumulates on GM1-rich membrane domains (Yanagisawa et al., 1995; Wakabayashi et al., 2005; Yanagisawa, 2005), and Aβ insertion into the membrane is critically dependent on the Chol/phospholipids ratio (Ji et al., 2002), as it was detailed above. More recent works showed that the formation of Ca^{2+} pores ("annular protofibrils," Lashuel et al., 2002) in the plasma membrane is a mechanism dependent on both gangliosides and Chol. As it was described above, amyloid monomers or soluble oligomers interact with a ganglioside at the cell surface, with a specificity that responds to a ganglioside-binding domain for each amyloid protein (common amino acid residues at specific locations, with specific variations for each ganglioside), being the Ca^{2+} pores significantly diminished in ganglioside deprived cells (Di Scala et al., 2016). Based on this "calcium-channel hypothesis" of the AD, a chimeric peptide formed with a minimal ganglioside-binding domain of α-synuclein and two contiguous His residues as in 1–42 Aβ (Yahi and Fantini, 2014) avoid pore formation by 1–42 Aβ. Treatment of WT 5XFAD mice with a sialic-specific lectin (LFA, Limax flavus agglutinin) significantly reduced amyloid depositions in the brain, probably by interfering with the binding of amyloid peptides to gangliosides (Dukhinova et al., 2019). Furthermore, Cascella et al. (2017) showed that different oligomer conformations can perturb Ca^{2+} cell-permeation by both a channel-independent mechanism as annular protofibrils, or by a channel-dependent one (through NMDA-R and AMPA-R).

Aβ peptides that stay in the membrane surface are in a β-sheet conformation, and once inside the membrane they turn their conformation to an α-helix (Yu and Zheng, 2012). Other studies suggested that 1–40 Aβ interacts with the membrane in two sequential steps. The first one involves the formation of a pore-like structure and membrane permeation, and the second one involves subsequent growth of aggregates with fibril formation and lipid clustering around the fiber which implies lipid extraction, membrane fragmentation, and loss of membrane integrity (Engel et al., 2008; Stefani, 2010; Milanesi et al., 2012; Sciacca et al., 2012; Relini et al., 2013; Kotler et al., 2014).

Recently, Rondelli et al. (2016) described more in detail the interactions between cell membranes and Aβ peptides. Those interactions depend on peptide conformation: structural oligomers are imbibed in the outer hemilayer of the membrane triggering more Aβ addition and further elongation; on the other hand, early labile oligomers in equilibrium with monomers are incorporated as monomers deeply in the membrane coming up to the inner hemilayer, whereas Aβ organization leads to pore formation.

A study of the changes induced by 1–42 Aβ on the morphology and the mechanical stability of model membranes with different Chol content indicates that Chol drives 1–42 Aβ toward rafts domains and that at high Chol concentration the presence of the amyloid peptide did not alter any membrane property, thus assigning a protective effect against membrane destabilization by 1–42 Aβ to the presence of Chol (Seghezza et al., 2014). Recently, Staneva et al. (2018) deepened this idea. They observed that 1–42 Aβ has a higher affinity for liquid-disordered (l_d) than ordered (l_o) phases, confirming previous results (Ahyayauch et al., 2012). They concluded that the fraction of Aβ in l_o domains, probably the functionally important one, might be smaller. While in a l_o phase 1–42 Aβ induces practically no changes in the lipid packing, a significant perturbation of the lipid packing by its presence was observed in a l_d phase. They focus on the presence of GM1 as a crucial lipid. In l_d phases without GM1, the peptide penetrates and messes up the neighboring lipids. However, in the presence of GM1 the peptide interacts with the headgroup of several GM1 promoting a condensing effect and an increased lipid packing and decreases Aβ penetration. The presence of GM1 could affect the line tension between l_o and l_d domains which in turn affects the kinetics of domains formation, growth, shape and size. Thus, although it cannot be discarded that the functional peptide, or at least a minority of it, binds directly to l_o domains, the authors suggested that the fibrillation of Aβ peptides in raft domains is the consequence of a reorganization modulated through Aβ peptides in non-raft domains (Staneva et al., 2018).

Not only specific lipid raft characteristics are necessary for Aβ insertion into the membrane, but also its insertion has consequences on the membrane (Chang et al., 2017). Several studies analyzed the membrane biophysical perturbations caused by Aβ interaction, which could be considered the first step of its biological effect (Kanfer et al., 1999; Chochina et al., 2001; Eckert et al., 2003). A decrease in the fluidity of mouse brain membranes, human lymphocyte membranes and membranes from rat cortex, hippocampus and striatum was observed in the presence of 25–35 Aβ and 1–40 Aβ, and in all cases the effect was dependent on peptide concentration (Müller et al., 1995). Low concentrations of Aβ significantly perturb membrane fluidity by specifically altering the acyl-chain mobility of brain membranes, an effect dependent on peptide length, with almost no effect at the polar head groups (Müller et al., 2001). Lately, it was observed that monomeric 1–40 Aβ has no effect on membrane fluidity, while oligomeric forms do (Peters et al., 2009). Contrary to these results, by exposition of hippocampal neurons to nanomolar concentrations of Aβ oligomers for 24 h we could not observe changes in membrane fluidity tested with three different fluorescence probes (Uranga et al., 2017). Peters et al. (2009) showed that membrane perturbation by Aβ is a consequence of Aβ complexing with GM1; thus, it is possible that in our experiments the cell membrane did not have the correct GM1/Chol relationship. A previous study of the interaction of 1–42 Aβ with planar bilayers had already demonstrated that the Chol content is directly correlated with Aβ assembly on the membrane surface, that during this process membrane changes occur, and that all this process is governed by lipid bilayer composition (Yip et al., 2002). Thus, membrane lipid environment modulates Aβ production and at the same time Aβ causes a membrane perturbation that positively feedbacks its own production (Peters et al., 2009). Moreover, Aβ insertion into the membrane not only potentiates Aβ production but also unspecifically activates a variety of membrane processes which could eventually end in neuronal cell death (Kanfer et al., 1999). 25–35 Aβ peptide interacts with phospholipids through electrostatic interactions favoring peptide aggregation which causes perturbations at the lipid-water interphase of the membrane (Martínez-Senac et al., 1999). Mass spectroscopy studies showed that Aβ inserts into model membranes containing Chol, but not in the absence of Chol (Ji et al., 2002). This study also indicated that the membrane insertion is initiated by the C-terminus of the Aβ peptide which has the hydrophobic domain.

Brain membranes from middle aged mice were more susceptible to Aβ perturbations than membranes from aged mice; and *in vitro* studies showed that a decrease in membrane Chol content enhanced Aβ effect, while an increase in membrane Chol strongly decreased the perturbation effect (Kirsch et al., 2002), suggesting that Chol protects neuronal membranes from Aβ perturbations and neurotoxicity (Eckert et al., 2003). However, they also observed *in vivo* that a reduction of Chol levels by approx. 30% by treatment with lovastatin (HMG-CoA-reductase inhibitor) resulted in moderated membrane alterations without acyl chain flexibility perturbations and reduced Aβ bulk fluidity perturbation (Kirsch et al., 2002). A possible explanation is that Chol membrane modification involves different membrane Chol pools with different sensitivity for Aβ perturbations whether it is *in vitro* or *in vivo*, with the one at the membrane acyl-chain being the most receptive (Kirsch et al., 2003).

Another important consequence of an enhanced Aβ production linked to lipid membrane is oxidative stress with an excess of lipid peroxidation and increased lipid susceptibility to oxidative damage, which exacerbates Aβ toxicity in the membrane (Behl et al., 1994; Opazo et al., 2002; Cutler et al., 2004; Boyd-Kimball et al., 2005; Wu and Luo, 2005). It is reported that Aβ prefers to interact with membranes with high oxidatively damaged phospholipids (Zampagni et al., 2010), particularly in raft domains, and that these membranes promote misfolding and aggregations of Aβ peptides into fibrils (Shringarpure et al., 2000; Magni et al., 2002; Zhang et al., 2004; Bieschke et al., 2005; Lee et al., 2006; Murray et al., 2007), whereas the misfolded peptides promote more oxidative damage in the membrane, conducing to a positive feedback (Murray et al., 2007). Aβ increases 4-hydroxy-2-nonenal (HNE) production which promotes oxidative damage and also induces Aβ to form β-structure and amyloid fibrils (Mark et al., 1997; Lauderback et al., 2001; Murray et al., 2005, 2007).

Even though it is not a topic of interest for this review, it is important to remember that just as Chol is a crucial lipid molecule for Aβ processing and Aβ membrane effects, the round trip is also valid since Aβ has an impact on Chol homeostasis (Koudinova et al., 2000; Michikawa et al., 2001; Gong et al., 2002; Michikawa, 2003; Koudinov and Koudinova, 2004; Grimm et al., 2005, 2007). This ultimate effect suggests that Aβ down-regulates Chol content and also raft content (Beel et al., 2010). Thus, the peptide behaves as a Chol sensor: when there is high Chol content in a membrane, the amyloidogenic pathway is favored and, thus, an enhancement takes place in Aβ processing, which in turn reduces both Chol uptake and biosynthesis, following up a negative feedback mechanism (Beel et al., 2010).

CROSSTALK BETWEEN AMYLOID HYPOTHESIS AND CHOLINERGIC HYPOTHESIS

The basis of AD pathogenesis is still controversial today, even though several hypotheses try to explain it, such as the Aβ amyloid cascade (Hardy and Allsop, 1991; Hardy and Higgins, 1992), the hyperphosphorylated microtubule-associated tau (Götz et al., 2004), abnormalities of the cholinergic system (Bartus et al., 1982), oxidative stress (Butterfield and Boyd-Kimball, 2005), etc. Even though the amyloid hypothesis is the most popular explanation for the mechanism of AD, it fails to explain several aspects of this multifactorial etiopathology (Herrup, 2015). In addition, until now, the majority of clinical trials conducted to diminish the amount of Aβ did not give good results (Puzzo et al., 2015; Maia and Sousa, 2019). Although these failures are not enough to discard the amyloid hypothesis (see for example Rosenblum, 2014), attention is now focused on the cholinergic hypothesis since it became the main therapeutic strategy for this disease (**Figure 2**). As we will work out in the following paragraphs, these two hypotheses are highly linked.

The cholinergic system involves two families of receptors, nAChR and muscarinic acetylcholine receptors (mAChR). Although both types of receptors are related with cognitive processes (Ghoneim and Mewaldt, 1977; Petersen, 1977; Sarter and Paolone, 2011) and are affected in AD, only the relation between nAChR and AD has been largely studied (Lombardo and Maskos, 2014).

The nAChR is an integral membrane protein that belongs to the Cys-loop superfamily of ligand-gated ion channels (Karlin and Akabas, 1995; Le Novère and Changeux, 1995; Changeux and Edelstein, 1998; Paterson and Nordberg, 2000). The binding of its natural agonist acetylcholine triggers a conformational change that ends in the opening of a channel and the flux of positive ions across the membrane, causing membrane depolarization and a subsequence intracellular cascade of events (Lindstrom, 2003; Brown, 2006; McKay et al., 2007; Pohanka, 2012). The nAChR presents a pentameric arrangement, with each subunit having a large N-terminal extracellular domain, four transmembrane segments (M1–M4), a small cytoplasmic domain between M3 and M4, and a short C-terminal extracellular domain. To this day, 16 different nAChR subunits (including: α1-7, α9-10, β1-4, γ, δ, and ε) that form homologous and heterologous receptors with distinct structures, functions and locations are known (Champtiaux et al., 2003; Dajas-Bailador and Wonnacott, 2004; Fucile, 2004; Giniatullin et al., 2005; Gotti et al., 2006a, 2007, 2009; Albuquerque et al., 2009; Shen and Yakel, 2009). The muscle-type nAChR of the electric organ of *Torpedo*, first receptor described and still the prototype of the family, is formed by $\alpha 1_2\beta 1\delta\gamma$ (similar to embryonic muscle nAChR of vertebrates, which change to $\alpha 1_2\beta 1\varepsilon\gamma$ in adult). Two receptor subtypes are highly expressed in the central nervous system: the heteropentamer α4β2 nAChR and the homopentamer α7 nAChR (Schmidt and Freeman, 1980; Sargent et al., 1991; Clarke, 1992; Sargent and Garrett, 1995; Cooper et al., 1999; Nashmi et al., 2003; Scholze et al., 2011). The latter is particularly important in AD (Ma and Qian, 2019). It is present in high density in the striatum, thalamus, neocortex, and limbic system suggesting a central role in normal cognition and, hence, in age-related cognitive decline (Bigl et al., 1982; Mesulam et al., 1983; Muir et al., 1993; Sarter and Bruno, 1997; Wenk, 1997; Woolf, 1998; Guillem et al., 2011). It was shown that α7 nAChR is important for growth, development and aging, regulating the plasticity of the neural circuit, neuronal differentiation, proliferation, apoptosis and clearance of aged neurons (Nees, 2015). The levels of this receptor change during development and adult stage, and in AD patients, they decrease significantly (Bowen et al., 1976; Perry et al., 1981, 1985, 1987, 1988; Whitehouse et al., 1981, 1982, 1986; Coyle et al., 1983; Shimohama et al., 1986; Nordberg et al., 1995; Paterson and Nordberg, 2000; Auld et al., 2002; Gotti et al., 2006b; Kim et al., 2013; Ma and Qian, 2019).

Activation of the α7 nAChR opens a high permeability Ca^{++} channel that consequently activates voltage-dependent Ca^{++} channels (Perry et al., 1992; Sharma and Vijayaraghavan, 2001) and triggers an intracellular signaling cascade through activation of a protein kinase. In the case of activation of presynaptic α7 nAChR, the final event is the fusion of vesicles loaded with neurotransmitters (glutamic acid, norepinephrine, acetylcholine, dopamine and GABA) to the presynaptic membrane and the massive release of these neurotransmitters to the synaptic cleft (Wonnacott et al., 2006; Ma and Qian, 2019). Postsynaptic α7 nAChR depolarize the postsynaptic membrane and participate in signal transduction (Messi et al., 1997; Morley and Happe, 2000; Berg and Conroy, 2002). ACE metabolizes acetylcholine after its release to the synaptic cleft ending the cholinergic stimulus (Bowen et al., 1976; Davies and Maloney, 1976; Coyle et al., 1983; Auld et al., 2002).

The cholinergic hypothesis of AD focuses on the fact that in brains of AD patients there is a decrease in the total amount of nAChRs (Whitehouse et al., 1982; Banerjee et al., 2000), which is an outcome of progressive death of forebrain cholinergic neurons with an extended cholinergic presynaptic denervation (Bartus et al., 1982; Court et al., 2000; Graham et al., 2002; Contestabile, 2011; Hampel et al., 2018). This is considered a consequence of enhanced Aβ production (Liu and Wu, 2006). Banerjee et al. (2000) observed that in the remaining cholinergic neurons there was a higher amount of nAChR, which suggests a possible compensatory mechanism. Many efforts were performed to ameliorate this loss. However, current approved pharmacological agents, such as physostigmine, tacrine, donepezil, rivastigmine and galantamine (Martorana et al., 2010), are targeted to inhibit ACE function increasing the amount of acetylcholine at the synapse cleft and ameliorating the clinical symptoms of AD without halting the progress of the disease.

The affinity of α7 nAChR for 1–42 Aβ is in the low picomolar concentration, a range estimated to occur in healthy brains, while the affinity of α4β2 nAChR for 1–42 Aβ is between 100 to 5000 times lower (Wang et al., 2000a); thus, it is expected that both α7 nAChR and 1–42 Aβ could associate under physiological conditions. Puzzo et al. (2015) hypothesized that under physiological conditions a positive feedback mechanism occurs: synaptic activity induces Aβ release that acts as an endogenous ligand and modulates α7 nAChR, which in turn induces release of neurotransmitters and enhances synaptic plasticity and memory. Under pathological conditions, abnormal accumulation of Aβ (nanomolar concentration, Näslund et al., 1994, 2000; Tapiola et al., 2000; Andreasen et al., 2003) induces a negative feedback mechanism which implies inhibition and internalization of α7 nAChR, leading to synaptic dysfunction and memory loss. The Aβ-α7 complex influences tau hyperphosphorylation (Wang et al., 2003) and its internalization leads to plaque formation (Nagele et al., 2003, 2004; Dineley, 2007).

It is thought that the soluble form of Aβ interacts with α7 nAChR with apparently high affinity (Wang et al., 2000a) regulating its function (Dineley et al., 2001; Liu et al., 2001; Pettit et al., 2001). However, there is no consensus about the nature and consequences of this interaction (Farhat and Ahmed, 2017). While several studies propose an agonist-like effect for presynaptic nicotinic receptors (Dineley et al., 2002; Dougherty et al., 2003; Wu et al., 2007; Puzzo et al., 2008; Mehta et al., 2009; Lilja et al., 2011; Arora et al., 2013), others propose an inhibitory action (Dineley et al., 2001; Liu et al., 2001; Pettit et al., 2001; Tozaki et al., 2002; Lee and Wang, 2003; Wu et al., 2004; Wang et al., 2009; Parri et al., 2011), and others a concentration-dependent relationship with a stimulatory effect at picomolar Aβ concentration and an inhibitory effect at high nanomolar Aβ concentration (Puzzo et al., 2008). The variability between all the performed studies is so large in terms of *in vitro* and *in vivo* models, Aβ concentrations and Aβ preparations/conformations, and other conditions, that it is difficult to find a rule for the data obtained. Khan et al. (2010) gave a possible explanation for these inconsistency centered in a different Aβ effect on pre or postsynaptic receptors. Aβ induces a rapid stabilization of an inactive/desensitized state of postsynaptic receptors, resulting in an antagonist effect, and a slower desensitization of presynaptic receptors resulting in an agonist-like effect. The authors pointed to differences in the lipid microenvironment of the pre and postsynaptic α7 nAChR for these different desensitization rates. Presynaptic terminals have abundance of raft domains, and experimental disruption of these domains dramatically attenuates Aβ evoked α7 nAChR currents (Khan et al., 2010). With respect to the concentration-dependent effect, it is important to take into consideration that in a normal central nervous system 1–42 Aβ is found, although at low picomolar concentrations. Under this condition, it is postulated that Aβ exerts a positive effect on synaptic plasticity and memory formation (Phinney et al., 2003; Plant et al., 2003; Puzzo et al., 2008, 2011, 2015; Puzzo and Arancio, 2013). However, in a pathological condition, Aβ cannot exert its physiological function and hence a feedback mechanism induces more Aβ production, leading to an enhancement of the peptide with the subsequent reduction of α7 nAChR with Aβ removal and synaptic alteration and memory loss (Phinney et al., 2003; Puzzo et al., 2015).

Interaction of Aβ with α7 nAChR increases Aβ internalization (Nagele et al., 2002; D'Andrea and Nagele, 2006) and accumulation in lysosomes causing an excessive intraneuronal 1-42 Aβ accumulation. The majority of the amyloid plaques proceed from the lysis of degenerated, Aβ-overburdened neurons (Wang et al., 2000b; Gyure et al., 2001; Langui et al., 2004; Nunomura et al., 2010; Palop and Mucke, 2010; Li et al., 2011; Deutsch et al., 2014, 2016). Additionally, the formation of the Aβ-α7 nAChR complex may influence the membrane lipid and membrane protein organization (Deutsch et al., 2014, 2016; Ma and Qian, 2019). At the same time, the internalization of the Aβ-α7 nAChR complex triggers an upregulation of the α7 nAChR and magnifies the toxicity of the pathology (Molinari et al., 1998; Xiu et al., 2005; Yu et al., 2005; Liu et al., 2013, 2015; Shen and Wu, 2015) (**Figure 2**). In AD patients and preclinical AD models, a high expression of α7 nAChR was described (Hellström-Lindahl et al., 1999, 2004a,b; Dineley et al., 2002; Jones et al., 2006; Counts et al., 2007; Ikonomovic et al., 2009). Chronic exposure to Aβ enhances the expression of α7 nAChR in neuron and glia cells (Yu et al., 2005; Liu et al., 2013). Also, an age-dependent increase of cell surface α7 nAChR was observed in 5xFAD mice, a model that rapidly develops amyloid pathology (Jin et al., 2015). Several studies contributed to this hypothesis. Treatment of PC12 cells with 1–42 Aβ increased cell surface α7 nAChR, suggesting that the peptide induces translocation of the receptor toward the plasma membrane (Jin et al., 2015). They observed that the agonist nicotine prevented Aβ induced cell death, whereas the competitive antagonist α-bungarotoxin potentiates the peptide effect, indicating that α7 nAChR plays a role in protecting neuronal cells from Aβ 1–42 peptide (Dziewczapolski et al., 2009; Wang et al., 2009; Jin et al., 2015). Contrary to this, Liu et al. (2015) concluded that upregulation of α7 nAChR induced by Aβ is necessary to mediate peptide neurotoxicity, both in hippocampal neurons and differentiated cholinergic SH-SY5Ycells. α7 nAChR function, which is exacerbated by its upregulation, may be necessary for the toxicity of Aβ aggregates; this effect was prevented by α7 nAChR inhibition or deletion. Previous studies showed that the blockade of α7 nAChR significantly ameliorated attentional deficits (Levin et al., 2013; Burke et al., 2014). Likewise, the deletion of α7 nAChR gene was correlated with an improvement in synaptic plasticity and a reduction in cognitive deficiency (Dziewczapolski et al., 2009). Two possible cytotoxic α7 nAChR-mediated mechanisms were proposed: one considers that the α7 nAChR increment in the membrane conduces to a high calcium permeability, which could be the ultimate responsible for cell toxicity, and the other that the high Aβ-α7 nAChR complex internalization and intracellular accumulation leads to neurotoxicity (Liu et al., 2015). Thus, while several studies point to α7 nAChR activation as a beneficial treatment, others suggest that a function inhibition for a beneficial effect is necessary.

A different hypothesis about Aβ and α7 nAChR relationship was postulated by Small et al. (2007). They concluded that Aβ does not bind directly to α7 nAChR but to the lipids of the plasma membrane, and that the perturbation of the structure or fluidity of the lipid microenvironment of the receptor could be the responsible for toxicity through an alteration of the receptor function. Their conclusion is supported by previous evidence that showed that Aβ binds strongly to lipids (Subasinghe et al., 2003; Hou et al., 2005). We will return to this issue later.

We here described the most relevant information about the interaction between Aβ and α7 nAChR, and its final consequences, focusing on the events that occur through the membrane. However, not only the interactions between Aβ and α7 nAChR are important. Other proteins that interact with α7 nAChR including Lynx proteins, NMDA-receptors and the Wnt/β-catenin pathway are important as well. All those interactions that modulate receptor function are specifically altered in AD and can lead to differences in the clinical effect of nAChR ligands in AD (Thomsen et al., 2016). It is also important to take into account that there is an internal cascade of signaling downstream α7 nAChR activation that involves several other active molecules, such as glycogen synthase kinase-3β (GSK-3β), phosphoinosite 3-kinase (PI3K)-Akt, Wnt and the mitogen-activated protein kinase (MAPK) signaling pathway, which are also altered in AD (see Ma and Qian, 2019 for a further explanation).

The last step in cholinergic signaling is the degradation of acetylcholine by the enzyme ACE to end the synaptic transmission. ACE is a globular non-transmembrane protein that can exist in different molecular forms, depending on the splicing of the ACE gene (Henderson et al., 2010). Although all ACE molecular forms and variants have similar catalytic activity, they also have other non-catalytic, non-classical functions, which depend on the multiple molecular forms of this enzyme and on cell types and cellular compartments (Small et al., 1996; Grisaru et al., 1999; Massoulié, 2002; Hicks et al., 2011). In non-neuronal tissues, ACE regulates cell proliferation, differentiation, apoptosis and cell–cell interaction, which is important to take into consideration when ACE inhibitors for AD are designed (Lazarevic-Pasti et al., 2017). ACE_T is the predominant form in central nervous system, which has a C-terminal α-helix peptide of 40 amino acids named T peptide. Through disulphure bondings between these peptides they can be found as homodimers and homotetramers of ACE_T. Also, the T peptide binds to hydrophobic proline-rich domains of membrane anchoring-proteins (like collagen-like Q subunit in NMJ and proline-rich membrane anchor, PRiMA, in the central nervous system; Massoulié et al., 2005). In the central nervous system, the majority of ACE is found as tetrameric ACE_T (G4) bound to PRiMA (Navaratnam et al., 2000; Perrier et al., 2002; Massoulié et al., 2005), which constitute the functional units at cholinergic synapse (Perrier et al., 2002; Dvir et al., 2010; Henderson et al., 2010; Hicks et al., 2011). PRiMA could bring the membrane-bound ACE together with other proteins in specialized membrane areas, such as raft domains, specifically with α7 nAChR at basal forebrains cholinergic neurons (Henderson et al., 2005; Hicks et al., 2012). A significant proportion of ACE_T is effectively located in raft domains through a Chol-binding domain of 13 amino acids of PRiMA (a CRAC, Chol recognition amino acid consensus, sequence), and Chol depletion or mutations at this domain reduced the lipid raft-PRiMA association (Xie et al., 2010a,b). A diminution of ACE activity in the cerebral cortex and other areas in AD patients was described, being the G4-PRiMA complex the ACE form markedly altered, whereas the ACE monomeric form was almost preserved (Atack et al., 1983; Fishman et al., 1986; Sáez-Valero et al., 1999). Interactions of PRiMA subunit with presenilin 1 (PS1, the catalytic subunit of γ-secretase), which is an aspartyl protease that cleaves substrates inside membrane, were described to occur in raft domains (García-Ayllón et al., 2014). This interaction could explain, in part, the cellular release of ACE through a shedding mechanism that was postulated to involve a metalloprotease (Hicks et al., 2013a). Furthermore, a direct relationship between PS1 and ACE was observed, with an overexpression of ACE related to higher levels of PS1, ACE knockdown leaded to decreased PS1 and a mutated PS1 was related with decreased ACE in the brain (Silveyra et al., 2008, 2012). At the same time, it was also observed that ACE inhibits AβPP processing through γ-secretase (Niu et al., 2012), perhaps, acting as an inhibitor of the secretase by interacting with PS1 (Campanari et al., 2014). In AD, ACE activity is diminished and hence impedes its potentiality to modulate γ-secretase (Campanari et al., 2014).

Interactions of ACE with Aβ are important in AD (Inestrosa et al., 1996; Wang et al., 2000b; Small et al., 2007), as the peptide alters several ACE properties such as its pH optimum and inhibitor sensitivity (Geula and Mesulam, 1989), making Aβ even more neurotoxic (Inestrosa et al., 1996; Alvarez et al., 1998). Moreover, ACE was detected in amyloid plaques evidencing the high affinity between both molecules and suggesting that ACE could promote Aβ aggregation (Morán et al., 1993; Inestrosa et al., 1996). Even more, in some cerebral areas of AD patients almost all ACE is in these complexes. The binding between Aβ and ACE occurs at the ACE peripheral anionic site (PAS); ACE inhibitors that bind to the anionic site (i.e., propidium), as well as antibodies against it, significantly reduce fibril formation (Reyes et al., 1997; Bartolini et al., 2003). Although the ACE catalytic domain does not participate of this interaction (Inestrosa et al., 1996), new compounds with a dual action (blocking PAS and catalytic site) are being designed, looking for the prevention of fibril aggregation with the aim of reversing the progression of the disease and, at the same time, inhibiting acetylcholine degradation to ameliorate the symptomatology (Alptüzün et al., 2010).

Furthermore, a negative relationship between APP and ACE was observed, as an overexpression of APP repressed ACE transcription with reductions of both ACE levels and ACE activity (Hicks et al., 2013b). A similar negative regulation was observed between APP and PRiMA; however, it is not clear if there is a direct downregulation by APP or if this diminution is a consequence of decreased ACE levels (Hicks et al., 2013b; Nalivaeva and Turner, 2016). The authors proposed that this ACE downregulation could be a novel neuroprotective function of APP.

nAChR AND MEMBRANE LIPIDS

As we said in the previous section, there are several nAChR subtypes depending on the individual pentameric arrangement. Summing up, all nAChR have two well defined structural domains: the neurotransmitter-binding site extracellular domain and the transmembrane domain containing the ion pore. Whereas the extracellular domain is the site where the agonists or different activators/inhibitors bind, the transmembrane region, besides having the ion pore, exhibits extensive contacts with the surrounding lipids through structural motifs remarkably conserved along phylogenic evolution (Antollini et al., 2005; Unwin, 2005; Jha et al., 2007; Baenziger and Corringer, 2011; Baenziger and daCosta, 2013; Barrantes, 2015). It is well known that a correct allosteric coupling between both domains is crucial for nAChR function, strongly dependent on its surrounding lipid, which modulates the relative proportion of nAChR in its resting or desensitized states (daCosta et al., 2002; Baenziger et al., 2000, 2008, 2015; daCosta and Baenziger, 2009; Barrantes, 2010; Barrantes et al., 2010; Hénault et al., 2015). The most studied nicotinic receptor is the muscle nAChR, which is not only the paradigm of all other nAChR but also of the entire cys-loop superfamily. In the following paragraphs we will discuss the relationship between distinct lipids or raft domains and the muscle nAChR, knowledge that can be extended to other members of the family, in particular to α7 nAChR.

Several years ago, Marsh and Barrantes (1978) described a layer of immobilized lipids that encircle the muscle nAChR with characteristics different from those of bulk lipids. Subsequent studies assigned an important role to these bounded lipids on muscle nAChR (Criado et al., 1982; Ellena et al., 1983; Ochoa et al., 1983; Sunshine and McNamee, 1992, 1994; Narayanaswami et al., 1993; Fernández-Ballester et al., 1994; Dreger et al., 1997; Barrantes, 2002, 2007; Quesada et al., 2016). The presence of both Chol and negatively charged lipids in the nAChR-lipid microenvironment is necessary to stabilize the nAChR in a functional conformation (Criado et al., 1984; Fong and McNamee, 1986; Butler and McNamee, 1993; Méthot et al., 1995; Antollini et al., 1996). However, there is no consensus about if it is the entity/identity of the lipid itself or the fluidity that each lipid confers to the membrane the responsible of this role. In spite of this controversy, the importance of a proper lipid microenvironment for muscle nAChR becomes clear when highly hydrophobic molecules, such as free fatty acids or steroids, perturb nAChR function through the membrane localizing at the lipid-nAChR interphase (Andreasen and McNamee, 1980; Villar et al., 1988; Bouzat et al., 1993; Bouzat and Barrantes, 1996; Nurowska and Ruzzier, 1996, 2002; Minota and Watanabe, 1997; Blanton et al., 1999; Garbus et al., 2001, 2002; Antollini and Barrantes, 2002, 2016; Fernández Nievas et al., 2007, 2008). Working with reconstituted *Torpedo* nAChR, Jones and McNamee (1988) distinguished two different populations of lipids in the nAChR-lipid microenvironment region: annular and non-annular lipids. Annular lipids interact with the protein in a relatively less specific manner with a fast rate of exchange with bulk lipids. Contrarily, non-annular lipids are in close contact with the protein, probably in between α-helix transmembrane segments or subunits, and can be associated to lipid binding sites with a slow exchange rate with bulk lipids (Lee, 2003). We identified the same two types of lipids in native *Torpedo* membranes (Antollini and Barrantes, 1998). The entity/identity of non-annular lipids are considered crucial for nAChR function; in the case of annular lipids the biophysical characteristics are more relevant. This is in concordance with other studies that assigned several roles to the lipids in a membrane, two of the main ones being: a collective one, in which they form a viscoelastic lipid "solvent" with the above-mentioned heterogeneities; and an individual one as signaling molecules (Piomelli et al., 2007).

Two annular lipids that are of particular interest are negative lipids and SM. With respect to the requirement of negative lipids, PA is particularly of interest. The segregation of PA domains containing nAChR and the stabilization of a functional conformation of the receptor by PA were described (daCosta et al., 2002, 2004; Poveda et al., 2002, 2008; Wenz and Barrantes, 2005; Dickey and Faller, 2008). SM showed moderated affinity for the nAChR (Bonini et al., 2002) but it is important for proper nAChR stability in the membrane. Its deficit affects the efficiency of the nAChR assembly process and the nAChR targeting to the membrane and increases the rate of turnover (Roccamo et al., 1999; Baier and Barrantes, 2007). Moreover, SM is important for membrane biophysical properties as it is asymmetrically distributed between both membrane hemilayers and it is one of the main actors of lipid raft domains, being both aspects that impact on nAChR (Perillo et al., 2016).

A separate paragraph is for Chol, a key lipid for nAChR (Middlemas and Raftery, 1987). This lipid molecule can be found in every region of a membrane: as a bulk, annular or non-annular lipid. In the first two cases, it probably plays an important function conditioning the physical properties of the environment, mainly because of its participation in raft domain formation and in the maintenance of the asymmetrical membrane condition. As a non-annular lipid, the occurrence of allosteric binding sites is postulated (Addona et al., 1998). It was suggested that the binding domain for Chol is at the nAChR lipid-protein interface, taking contact with the transmembrane subunits αM4, αM1, and γM4 (Corbin et al., 1998); other studies identified interactions of Chol with the transmembrane segments M1, M3, and M4 of each subunit (Hamouda et al., 2006). By fluorescence quenching and energy-transfer measurements of *T. californica* reconstituted membranes, sites accessible to Chol but not to phospholipids were identified (Narayanaswami and McNamee, 1993). Using Molecular Dynamics simulations of the nAChR structure, Brannigan et al. (2008) identified 15 Chol binding sites, large hydrophobic intersubunit and intrasubunit gaps. The location of Chol molecules at these sites improved nAChR stability; and in the case of intrasubunit sites, occupation of these sites by Chol precludes the nAChR from collapsing. A recent study using coarse-grained molecular dynamics simulations suggested that while long n-3 chains (in this case, docosahexaenoic acid, 22:6) have a high propensity for annular and non-annular sites, displacing Chol and occupying sites even deeper within the bundle, shorter n-6 chains do not displace Chol from non-annular sites as efficiently as long n-3 chains (Sharp et al., 2019).

Considering the intimate and close relationship between Chol and the muscle nAChR, studies looking for a consensus about specific Chol domains in the nAChR subunits were performed. A CRAC sequence in a region immediately adjacent to the M1 transmembrane domain of all the subunits of the muscle nAChR was identified (Baier et al., 2011). These sequences are located exiting the membrane bilayer, which suggests that they are probably not good partners for Chol in the hydrophobic membrane environment. However, a novel Chol recognizing domain was identified by *in silico* studies, a sequence opposite to a CRAC one (inverted CRAC or "CARC" sequence) at M1, M3, and M4, which is located inside the membrane and is highly preserved in the evolutionary scale, from prokaryotes to humans (Baier et al., 2011; Di Scala et al., 2017). These *in silico* results were also experimentally confirmed (Fantini et al., 2016). Furthermore, the authors concluded that a CARC sequence generally exhibits more affinity for Chol than a CRAC one (Fantini and Barrantes, 2013), and that it is of high affinity, lipid specific, and saturable (Fantini et al., 2016).

Chol not only conditions nAChR function but also its stability in the plasma membrane. There are some controversies about how the nAChR is organized in the membrane. At the NMJ, supramolecular aggregations of nAChRs (micron-sized two-dimensional clusters) are postulated to occur in Chol-rich lipid microdomains, together with several postsynaptic proteins including rapsyn, MuSK and Src-family kinases. Chol would stabilize NMJ and promote its maturation (Willmann et al., 2006). Depletion of cell-surface Chol produced a marked alteration of the organization of the nAChR (Kellner et al., 2007). One hypothesis for this situation is that after an agrin (extracellular heparan sulfate proteoglycan that aggregates nAChRs on cultured myotubes) stimulus, nAChR and MuSK translocate into raft domains where nAChR clustering occurs, as raft domains concentrate the agrin/MuSK signaling, nAChR and rapsyn. Disruption of these microdomains by Chol depletion inhibits agrin stimulation and formation and maintenance of nAChR clusters (Zhu et al., 2006). A contemporary study suggested that agrin causes the translocation of nAChR into raft domains, which is in agreement with the mentioned hypothesis (Campagna and Fallon, 2006). A slightly different hypothesis indicates that agrin does not reclute nAChRs into raft domains, as they are already in those domains independently of agrin activation, but it triggers the coalescence of raft domains conducing to nAChR clustering and it is also responsible for its maintenance, as Chol is necessary for all this process (Stetzkowski-Marden et al., 2006a,b; Cartaud et al., 2011). A previous study supports this hypothesis where the authors observed that nAChR subunits and rapsyn are cotargeted in the exocytic pathway to the cell surface inserted in Chol-rich microdomains (Marchand et al., 2002). Furthermore, Chol depletion affects the maintenance of the nAChR in the plasma membrane by several mechanisms. Treatments of cells with methyl-β-cyclodextrin, which extracts Chol from the membrane, enhanced nAChR internalization by endocytosis with a marked decrease of the number of nAChR domains, concomitantly with a gain-of-function of the remaining nAChR (Borroni et al., 2007; Borroni and Barrantes, 2011; Kamerbeek et al., 2013). Furthermore, chronic treatments with mevinolin, an inhibitor of 3-hydroxy-3-methyl-glutaryl-CoA reductase and hence of Chol synthesis, inhibited the trafficking of the receptor toward the membrane surface, which caused low nAChR cell-surface expression, and increased the intracellular nAChR pools (Pediconi et al., 2004). Moreover, Chol conditions muscle nAChR cell-surface diffusion (Baier et al., 2010; Mosqueira et al., 2018) and nAChR stability in confined raft domains (Mosqueira et al., 2018).

Different results of the interaction between muscle nAChR and lipid domains were obtained in model systems. We observed that reconstituted *Torpedo* nAChR in symmetric model membranes with coexistence of liquid-ordered (l_o) and liquid-disordered (l_d) domains was distributed homogeneously, without preference for any domain (Bermúdez et al., 2010). However, similar experiments with a synthetic peptide corresponding to the γM4 peptide showed a marked preference of this peptide for l_o domains (de Almeida et al., 2004; Bermúdez et al., 2010). Thus, although this transmembrane segment could give the nAChR the potentiality to localize in raft domains, it is not sufficient and other conditions must occur which influence nAChR partition profile. One of these mentioned conditions is membrane asymmetry. By increasing SM in the outer hemilayer, we observed an increment of the *Torpedo* nAChR in l_o domains, and the same was observed when specific SM species instead of brain SM were used in symmetric models (Perillo et al., 2016). Recently, by using coarse-grained molecular dynamics simulations of nAChR inserted in a ternary system of DPPC:Chol:PE or PC with PUFA, the authors concluded that nAChR partitioned in l_d domains poor in Chol (Sharp et al., 2019). The simulated membrane, despite having l_o and l_d domains, (a) did not have SM of any species, which is a critical lipid for raft domains in biological membranes, (b) used PUFA which are known to behave as nAChR inhibitors probably by competition with Chol for non-annular sites, as the authors observed in the study, and (c) was symmetric, a condition different to the natural asymmetry of biological membranes. Thus, this work emphasizes that it is not just the presence of an l_o domain, but also its physicochemical characteristics and specific lipid components which condition nAChRs agglomeration.

With respect to neuronal nAChR, it was observed that α7 nAChR is associated with Chol-rich microdomains at somatic spine-rich regions of ciliary neurons and that the

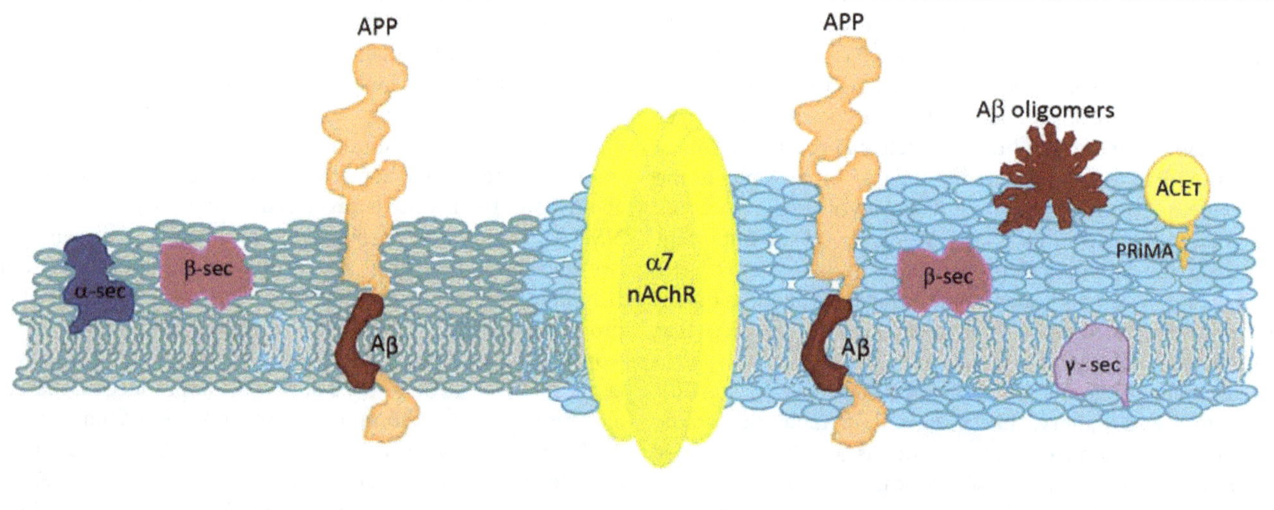

FIGURE 3 | Schematic diagram of a plasma membrane, depicting the spatial relationship between the molecules involved in Aβ synthesis and the cholinergic system. Two different colors are used to represent a raft domain and a liquid-disordered domain (light blue and gray, respectively). APP, amyloid precursor protein; Aβ, amyloid β peptide; α7 nAChR, α7 nicotinic acetylcholine receptor; ACE_T, tetrameric acetylcholinesterase; α-sec, α-secretase; β-sec, β-secretase; γ-sec, γ-secretase; and PRiMA, proline-rich membrane anchor.

maintenance of these receptors within these domains is Chol-dependent (Brusés et al., 2001). Furthermore, in PC-12 cells, a rat pheochromocytoma cell line, α7 nAChR location in raft domains is necessary to regulate cAMP signal through the nicotinic activation, signaling that was altered by Chol depletion (Oshikawa et al., 2003). A similar relation between α7 nAChR location at raft domains and efficiently signaling, with a direct Chol influence, was also observed in CG neurons (Liu et al., 2008). Disruption of raft domains in the same CG neurons increased the mobility of α7 nAChRs in the synaptic space (Fernandes et al., 2010). Disruption of raft domains by removal of Chol and/or SM in rat primary hippocampal neurons slowed the kinetics of α7 nAChR desensitization through increasing the rate of recovery from desensitization and increased the agonist affinity and single-channel conductance (Colón-Sáez and Yakel, 2011). The authors observed the effects of raft domains disruption also on α3β2 nAChRs functionality. These results confirm that, as with muscle nAChR, neuronal nAChR functionality is modulated by its lipid microenvironment with the raft domains integrity a critical factor. On the contrary, α7 nAChR at non-neural tissues, in rat arterial endothelial (RAEC) and human venous endothelial (HUVEC), was found to occur in non-raft subcellular membrane fractions (Peña et al., 2011).

CONCLUSION

Alzheimer's disease is a progressive neurodegenerative condition, the etiopathogenic mechanisms of which are not totally understood. Due to its multifactorial character, the development of new drugs and effective treatments is still a challenge (Dineley, 2007). Here, we intended to focus only in the processes related to this disease that occur in the cell membrane, which allows to observe the multiple crosslinking between specific lipids and the membrane proteins involved in the amyloid process. In a dry human brain, half of its weight corresponds to lipids, molecules with great chemical diversity and complex dynamical heterogeneities (Piomelli et al., 2007). Thus, it is not surprising that through the years more and more biological functions are being related to them. Raft domains are implicated in several of the events involved in AD. Chol is a very important lipid at synaptic membranes (Barrantes, 2007) and it is also a principal author in AD, together with other lipids such as GM1, SM or PA. It is not surprising that APP, Aβ, nAChR and G4-PRiMA all have Chol-recognition amino acid sequences. Although there are still some controversies, there is no doubt that APP processing, Aβ production and Aβ action are intimately related to raft domains, and that the cholinergic system function is highly conditioned by both raft domains and Aβ. A continuous crosstalk between amyloid processing and cholinergic signaling occurs at physiological and pathological conditions, and shifting from one condition to the other is triggered by an imbalance in Aβ synthesis, being Chol homeostasis intimately implicated (**Figure 3**). Currently, the only available treatment for AD is a group of drugs that inhibit ACE. A better understanding of Aβ-α7 nAChR interactions and of the implication of Chol in particular, and membrane heterogeneities in general, could allow for a deepening of the understanding of this neurodegenerative pathology and could help define new therapeutic strategies and potential novel molecular targets.

The World Health Organization (WHO) declared dementia as a public health priority (in *Priority Medicines for Europe and the World "A Public Health Approach to Innovation"* by Saloni Tanna). The number of people worldwide with this condition is in continuous growth: whereas in 2010 this number was estimated to be 35.6 million, it is expected to be near 115.4 million in 2050, in line with the view that this number nearly doubles every 20 years. AD is the most common form of dementia and, hence, it has become a major public health problem because of the continuous increase in the age of the population (in fact, in 2050 it is expected that 22% of the world population will be aged 60 and over). Thus, it is imperative to count with specific biomarkers for early stages of the disease, to improve detection and evaluation and, of course, with effective therapies. At present, the only treatment available is symptomatic: ACE inhibitors, like physostigmine, tacrine, donepezil, rivastigmine, and galantamine. Although new knowledge is continuously emerging, until now and as suggested in this work, there is no consensus among the different coexisting hypotheses around this subject, several of which are antagonistic. This fact clearly contributes to the current situation: there is not a single specific AD treatment commercially available. A great variety of molecular targets were proposed for AD treatment, a few of which were explained here (like β and γ-secretases, α7 nAChR and ACE), and plenty of studies have been conducted on them. Much effort has been invested in this area, but more is still required. Science is facing a huge challenge. Further studies that contribute to the description and explanation of the AD etiopathology will be crucial for a final consensus on AD. Multitarget-drug design is an interesting strategy as AD involves a large number of different molecules. And finally, it should not be forgotten that membrane lipids are not just a "sea" where proteins function but, as explained in detail above, they are necessary for the proper function of these proteins. Chol, GM1, SM, among others, are important lipids for AChR function, conformation and membrane stabilization, and also for Aβ processing and Aβ-membrane insertion. Thus, lipid membrane perturbation, and hence, raft domains alteration and membrane signal perturbation, directly impact in several hot points of AD etiopathology and, for this reason, they can also be considered as interesting molecular targets for AD.

AUTHOR CONTRIBUTIONS

CF and SA contributed to the design, analysis, interpretation, and writing of the manuscript.

FUNDING

This work was supported by grants from the Universidad Nacional del Sur (UNS) and Consejo Nacional de Investigaciones Científicas y Técnicas (CONICET) to SA.

REFERENCES

Abad-Rodriguez, J., Ledesma, M. D., Craessaerts, K., Perga, S., Medina, M., Delacourte, A., et al. (2004). Neuronal membrane cholesterol loss enhances amyloid peptide generation. *J. Cell. Biol.* 167, 953–960. doi: 10.1083/jcb.200404149

Addona, G. H., Sandermann, H., and Kloczewiak, M. A. (1998). Where does cholesterol act during activation of the nicotinic acetylcholine receptor? *Biochim. Biophys. Acta* 1370, 299–309. doi: 10.1016/s0005-2736(97)00280-0

Ahyayauch, H., Raab, M., Busto, J. V., Andraka, N., Arrondo, J. L., Masserini, M., et al. (2012). Binding of β-amyloid (1-42) peptide to negatively charged phospholipid membranes in the liquid-ordered state: modeling and experimental studies. *Biophys. J.* 103, 453–463. doi: 10.1016/j.bpj.2012.06.043

Albuquerque, E. X., Pereira, E. F. R., Alkondon, M., and Rogers, S. W. (2009). Mammalian nicotinic acetylcholine receptors: from structure to function. *Physiol. Rev.* 89, 73–120. doi: 10.1152/physrev.00015.2008

Alptüzün, V., Prinz, M., Hörr, V., Scheiber, J., Radacki, K., Fallarero, A., et al. (2010). Interaction of (benzylidene-hydrazono)-1,4-dihydropyridines with beta-amyloid, acetylcholine, and butyrylcholine esterases. *Bioorg. Med. Chem.* 218, 2049–2059. doi: 10.1016/j.bmc.2010.01.002

Alvarez, A., Alarcón, R., Opazo, C., Campos, E. O., Muñoz, F. J., Calderón, F. H., et al. (1998). Stable complexes involving acetylcholinesterase and amyloid-beta peptide change the biochemical properties of the enzyme and increase the neurotoxicity of Alzheimer's fibrils. *J. Neurosci.* 18, 3213–3223. doi: 10.1523/jneurosci.18-09-03213.1998

Andreasen, N., Sjögren, M., and Blennow, K. (2003). CSF markers for Alzheimer's disease: total tau, phospho-tau and Abeta42. *World J. Biol. Psychiatry* 4, 147–155. doi: 10.1080/15622970310029912

Andreasen, T. J., and McNamee, M. G. (1980). Inhibition of ion permeability control properties of acetylcholine receptor from Torpedo californica by long-chain fatty acids. *Biochemistry* 19, 4719–4726. doi: 10.1021/bi00561a027

Annaert, W. G., Levesque, L., Craessaerts, K., Dierinck, I., Snellings, G., Westaway, D., et al. (1999). Presenilin 1 controls gamma-secretase processing of amyloid precursor protein in pre-golgi compartments of hippocampal neurons. *J. Cell. Biol.* 147, 277–294. doi: 10.1083/jcb.147.2.277

Antollini, S. S., and Barrantes, F. J. (1998). Disclosure of discrete sites for phospholipid and sterols at the protein-lipid interface in native acetylcholine receptor-rich membrane. *Biochemistry* 37, 16653–16662. doi: 10.1021/bi9808215

Antollini, S. S., and Barrantes, F. J. (2002). Unique effects of different fatty acid species on the physical properties of the torpedo acetylcholine receptor membrane. *J. Biol. Chem.* 277, 1249–1254. doi: 10.1074/jbc.M106618200

Antollini, S. S., and Barrantes, F. J. (2016). Fatty Acid Regulation of Voltage- and Ligand-Gated Ion Channel Function. *Front. Physiol.* 28:573. doi: 10.3389/fphys.2016.00573

Antollini, S. S., Soto, M. A., Bonini de Romanelli, I., Gutiérrez-Merino, C., Sotomayor, P., and Barrantes, F. J. (1996). Physical state of bulk and protein-associated lipid in nicotinic acetylcholine receptor-rich membrane studied by laurdan generalized polarization and fluorescence energy transfer. *Biophys. J.* 70, 1275–1284. doi: 10.1016/s0006-3495(96)79684-4

Antollini, S. S., Xu, Y., Jiang, H., and Barrantes, F. J. (2005). Fluorescence and molecular dynamics studies of the acetylcholine receptor gammaM4 transmembrane peptide in reconstituted systems. *Mol. Membr. Biol.* 22, 471–483. doi: 10.1080/09687860500367915

Arbor, S. C., Lafontaine, M., and Cumbay, M. (2016). Amyloid-beta Alzheimer targets -protein processing, lipid rafts, and amyloid-beta pores. *Yale J. Biol. Med.* 89, 5–21.

Ariga, T., Kobayashi, K., Hasegawa, A., Kiso, M., Ishida, H., and Miyatake, T. (2001). Characterization of high-affinity binding between gangliosides and amyloid beta-protein. *Arch. Biochem. Biophys.* 388, 225–230. doi: 10.1006/abbi.2001.2304

Arispe, N., Pollard, H. B., and Rojas, E. (1993a). Giant multilevel cation channels formed by Alzheimer disease amyloid beta-protein [A beta P-(1-40)] in bilayer membranes. *Proc. Natl. Acad. Sci. U.S.A.* 90, 10573–10577. doi: 10.1073/pnas.90.22.10573

Arispe, N., Rojas, E., and Pollard, H. B. (1993b). Alzheimer disease amyloid beta protein forms calcium channels in bilayer membranes: blockade by tromethamine and aluminum. *Proc. Natl. Acad. Sci. U.S.A.* 90, 567–571. doi: 10.1073/pnas.90.2.567

Arora, K., Alfulaij, N., Higa, J. K., Panee, J., and Nichols, R. A. (2013). Impact of sustained exposure to β-amyloid on calcium homeostasis and neuronal integrity in model nerve cell system expressing α4β2 nicotinic acetylcholine receptors. *J. Biol. Chem.* 288, 11175–11190. doi: 10.1074/jbc.M113.453746

Ashley, R. H., Harroun, T. A., Hauss, T., Breen, K. C., and Bradshaw, J. P. (2006). Autoinsertion of soluble oligomers of Alzheimer's Abeta(1-42) peptide into cholesterol-containing membranes is accompanied by relocation of the sterol towards the bilayer surface. *BMC. Struct. Biol.* 6:21. doi: 10.1186/1472-6807-6-21

Askarova, S., Yang, X., and Lee, J. C. (2011). Impacts of membrane biophysics in Alzheimer's Disease: from amyloid precursor protein processing to Aβ peptide-induced membrane changes. *Int. J. Alzheimers Dis.* 2011:134971. doi: 10.4061/2011/134971

Atack, J. R., Perry, E. K., Bonham, J. R., Perry, R. H., Tomlinson, B. E., Blessed, G., et al. (1983). Molecular forms of acetylcholinesterase in senile dementia of Alzheimer type: selective loss of the intermediate (10S) form. *Neurosci. Lett.* 40, 199–204. doi: 10.1016/0304-3940(83)90302-6

Auld, D. S., Kornecook, T. J., Bastianetto, S., and Quirion, R. (2002). Alzheimer's disease and the basal forebrain cholinergic system: relations to beta-amyloid peptides, cognition, and treatment strategies. *Prog. Neurobiol.* 68, 209–245. doi: 10.1016/s0301-0082(02)00079-5

Avdulov, N. A., Chochina, S. V., Igbavboa, U., Warden, C. S., Vassiliev, A. V., and Wood, W. G. (1997). Lipid binding to amyloid beta-peptide aggregates: preferential binding of cholesterol as compared with phosphatidylcholine and fatty acids. *J. Neurochem.* 69, 1746–1752. doi: 10.1046/j.1471-4159.1997.69041746.x

Baenziger, J. E., and Corringer, P. J. (2011). 3D structure and allosteric modulation of the transmembrane domain of pentameric ligand-gated ion channels. *Neuropharmacology* 60, 116–125. doi: 10.1016/j.neuropharm.2010.08.007

Baenziger, J. E., and daCosta, C. J. B. (2013). Molecular mechanisms of acetylcholine receptor-lipid interactions: from model membranes to human biology. *Biophys. Rev.* 5, 1–9. doi: 10.1007/s12551-012-0078-77

Baenziger, J. E., Hénault, C. M., Therien, J. P. D., and Sun, J. (2015). Nicotinic acetylcholine receptor-lipid interactions: mechanistic insight and biological function. *Biochim. Biophys. Acta Biomembr.* 1848, 1806–1817. doi: 10.1016/j.bbamem.2015.03.010

Baenziger, J. E., Morris, M., Darsaut, T. E., and Ryan, S. E. (2000). Effect of membrane lipid composition on the conformational equilibria of the Nicotinic acetylcholine receptor. *J. Biol. Chem.* 275, 777–784. doi: 10.1074/jbc.275.2.777

Baenziger, J. E., Ryan, S. E., Goodreid, M. M., Vuong, N. Q., Sturgeon, R. M., and Corrie, J. B. (2008). Lipid composition alters drug action at the Nicotinic acetylcholine receptor. *Mol. Pharmacol.* 73, 880–890. doi: 10.1124/mol.107.039008

Bagatolli, L. A. (2010). Microscopy imaging of membrane domains. *Biochim. Biophys. Acta* 1798:1285. doi: 10.1016/j.bbamem.2010.05.023

Baier, C. J., and Barrantes, F. J. (2007). Sphingolipids are necessary for nicotinic acetylcholine receptor export in the early secretory pathway. *J. Neurochem.* 101, 1072–1084. doi: 10.1111/j.1471-4159.2007.04561.x

Baier, C. J., Fantini, J., and Barrantes, F. J. (2011). Disclosure of cholesterol recognition motifs in transmembrane domains of the human nicotinic acetylcholine receptor. *Sci. Rep.* 1:69. doi: 10.1038/srep00069

Baier, C. J., Gallegos, C. E., Levi, V., and Barrantes, F. J. (2010). Cholesterol modulation of nicotinic acetylcholine receptor surface mobility. *Eur. Biophys* 39, 213–227. doi: 10.1007/s00249-009-0521-522

Banerjee, C., Nyengaard, J. R., Wevers, A., de Vos, R. A., Jansen Steur, E. N., Lindstrom, J., et al. (2000). Cellular expression of alpha7 Nicotinic Acetylcholine receptor protein in the temporal cortex in Alzheimer's and Parkinson's disease - A stereological approach. *Neurobiol. Dis.* 7, 666–672. doi: 10.1006/nbdi.2000.0317

Barenholz, Y. (2004). Sphingomyelin and cholesterol: from membrane biophysics and rafts to potential medical applications. *Subcell. Biochem.* 37, 167–215. doi: 10.1007/978-1-4757-5806-1_5

Barrantes, F. J. (2002). Lipid matters: nicotinic acetylcholine receptor-lipid interactions. *Mol. Membr. Biol.* 219, 277–284. doi: 10.1080/09687680210166226

Barrantes, F. J. (2007). Cholesterol effects on nicotinic acetylcholine receptor. *Neurochem.* 103, 72–80. doi: 10.1111/j.1471-4159.2007.04719.x

Barrantes, F. J. (2010). Cholesterol effects on nicotinic acetylcholine receptor: cellular aspects. *Subcell. Biochem.* 51, 467–487. doi: 10.1007/978-90-481-8622-8_17

Barrantes, F. J. (2015). Phylogenetic conservation of protein-lipid motifs in pentameric ligand-gated ion channels. *Biochim. Biophys. Acta* 1848, 1796–1805. doi: 10.1016/j.bbamem.2015.03.028

Barrantes, F. J., Borroni, V., and Vallés, S. (2010). Neuronal nicotinic acetylcholine receptor – cholesterol crosstalk in Alzheimer's disease. *FEBS Lett.* 584, 1856–1863. doi: 10.1016/j.febslet.2009.11.036

Barrera, N. P., Zhou, M., and Robinson, C. V. (2013). The role of lipids in defining membrane protein interactions: insights from mass spectrometry. *Trends. Cell. Biol.* 23, 1–8. doi: 10.1016/j.tcb.2012.08.007

Barrett, P. J., Song, Y., Horn, W. D., Van Hustedt, E. J., Johanna, M., Hadziselimovic, A., et al. (2012). The amyloid precursor protein has a flexible transmembrane domain and binds cholesterol. *Science.* 336, 1168–1171. doi: 10.1126/science.1219988

Bartolini, M., Bertucci, C., Cavrini, V., and Andrisano, V. (2003). Beta-Amyloid aggregation induced by human acetylcholinesterase: inhibition studies. *Biochem. Pharmacol.* 65, 407–416. doi: 10.1016/s0006-2952(02)01514-9

Bartus, R. T., Dean, R. L., Beer, B., and Lippa, A. S. (1982). The cholinergic hypothesis of geriatric memory dysfunction. *Science* 1217, 408–414. doi: 10.1126/science.7046051

Bazzi, M. D., and Nelsestuen, G. L. (1996). Extensive segregation of acidic phospholipids in membranes induced by protein kinase C and related proteins. *Biochemistry* 32, 7961–7969. doi: 10.1021/bi00246a013

Beel, A. J., Sakakura, M., Barrett, P. J., and Sanders, C. R. (2010). Direct binding of cholesterol to the amyloid precursor protein: an important interaction in lipid-Alzheimer's disease relationships? *Biochim. Biophys. Acta* 1801, 975–982. doi: 10.1016/j.bbalip.2010.03.008

Behl, C., Davis, J. B., Lesley, R., and Schubert, D. (1994). Hydrogen peroxide mediates amyloid beta protein toxicity. *Cell* 77, 817–827. doi: 10.1016/0092-8674(94)90131-7

Berg, D. K., and Conroy, W. G. (2002). Nicotinic alpha 7 receptors: synaptic options and downstream signaling in neurons. *J. Neurobiol.* 53, 512–523. doi: 10.1002/neu.10116

Bermúdez, V., Antollini, S. S., Nievas, G. A. F., Aveldaño, M. I., and Barrantes, F. J. (2010). Partition profile of the nicotinic acetylcholine receptor in lipid domains upon reconstitution. *J. Lipid Res.* 51, 2629–2641. doi: 10.1194/jlr.M005132

Bieschke, J., Zhang, Q., Powers, E. T., Lerner, R. A., and Kelly, J. W. (2005). Oxidative metabolites accelerate Alzheimer's amyloidogenesis by a two-step mechanism, eliminating the requirement for nucleation. *Biochemistry* 44, 4977–4983. doi: 10.1021/bi0501030

Bigl, V., Woolf, N. J., and Butcher, L. L. (1982). Cholinergic projections from the basal forebrain to frontal, parietal, temporal, occipital, and cingulate cortices: a combined fluorescent tracer and acetylcholinesterase analysis. *Brain Res. Bull.* 8, 727–749. doi: 10.1016/0361-9230(82)90101-0

Blanton, M. P., Xie, Y., Dangott, L. J., and Cohen, J. B. (1999). The steroid promegestone is a noncompetitive antagonist of the Torpedo nicotinic acetylcholine receptor that interacts with the lipid-protein interface. *Mol. Pharmacol.* 55, 269–278. doi: 10.1124/mol.55.2.269

Bodovitz, S., and Klein, W. L. (1996). Cholesterol Modulates alpha-Secretase Cleavage of Amyloid Precursor Protein. *J. Biol. Chem.* 271, 4436–4440. doi: 10.1074/jbc.271.8.4436

Bonini, I. C., Antollini, S. S., Gutiérrez-Merino, C., and Barrantes, F. J. (2002). Sphingomyelin composition and physical asymmetries in native acetylcholine receptor-rich membranes. *Eur. Biophys. J.* 31, 417–427. doi: 10.1007/s00249-002-0230-236

Borroni, V., Baier, C. J., Lang, T., Bonini, I., White, M. M., Garbus, I., et al. (2007). Cholesterol depletion activates rapid internalization of submicron-sized acetylcholine receptor domains at the cell membrane. *Mol. Membr. Biol.* 24, 1–15. doi: 10.1080/09687860600903387

Borroni, V., and Barrantes, F. J. (2011). Cholesterol Modulates the Rate and Mechanism of Acetylcholine Receptor Internalization. *J Biol Chem.* 286, 17122–17132. doi: 10.1074/jbc.M110.211870

Bouzat, C., and Barrantes, F. J. (1996). Modulation of muscle nicotinic acetylcholine receptors by the glucocorticoid hydrocortisone. Possible allosteric mechanism of channel blockade. *J. Biol. Chem.* 271, 25835–25841. doi: 10.1074/jbc.271.42.25835

Bouzat, C. B., Lacorazza, H. D., de Jiménez Bonino, M. B., and Barrantes, F. J. (1993). Effect of chemical modification of extracellular histidyl residues on the channel properties of the nicotinic acetylcholine receptor. *Pflugers. Arch.* 423, 365–371. doi: 10.1007/bf00374929

Bowen, D. M., Smith, C. B., White, P., and Davison, A. N. (1976). Neurotransmitter-related enzymes and indices of hypoxia in senile dementia and other abiotrophies. *Brain* 99, 459–496. doi: 10.1093/brain/99.3.459

Boyd-Kimball, D., Castegna, A., Sultana, R., Poon, H. F., Petroze, R., Lynn, B. C., et al. (2005). Proteomic identification of proteins oxidized by Abeta(1-42) in synaptosomes: implications for Alzheimer's disease. *Brain Res.* 1044, 206–215. doi: 10.1016/j.brainres.2005.02.086

Brannigan, G., Hénin, J., Law, R., Eckenhoff, R., and Klein, M. L. (2008). Embedded cholesterol in the nicotinic acetylcholine receptor. *Proc. Natl. Acad. Sci. U.S.A.* 105, 14418–14423. doi: 10.1073/pnas.0803029105

Brown, D. A. (2006). Acetylcholine. *Br. J. Pharmacol.* 147(Suppl. 1), S120–S126. doi: 10.1038/sj.bjp.0706474

Brown, D. A., and London, E. (2000). Structure and function of sphingolipid- and cholesterol-rich membrane rafts. *J. Biol. Chem.* 275, 17221–17224. doi: 10.1074/jbc.r000005200

Brusés, J. L., Chauvet, N., and Rutishauser, U. (2001). Membrane lipid rafts are necessary for the maintenance of the (alpha)7 nicotinic acetylcholine receptor in somatic spines of ciliary neurons. *J. Neurosci.* 21, 504–512. doi: 10.1523/jneurosci.21-02-00504.2001

Burke, D. A., Heshmati, P., Kholdebarin, E., and Levin, E. D. (2014). Decreasing nicotinic receptor activity and the spatial learning impairment caused by the NMDA glutamate antagonist dizocilpine in rats. *Eur. J. Pharmacol.* 741, 132–139. doi: 10.1016/j.ejphar.2014.07.030

Burns, M., and Duff, K. (2002). Cholesterol in Alzheimer's disease and tauopathy. *Ann. N. Y. Acad. Sci.* 977, 367–375. doi: 10.1111/j.1749-6632.2002.tb04839.x

Butler, D. H., and McNamee, M. G. (1993). FTIR analysis of nicotinic acetylcholine receptor secondary structure in reconstituted membranes. *Biochim. Biophys. Acta* 11150, 17–24. doi: 10.1016/0005-2736(93)90116-h

Butterfield, D. A., and Boyd-Kimball, D. (2005). The critical role of methionine 35 in Alzheimer's amyloid beta-peptide (1-42)-induced oxidative stress and neurotoxicity. *Biochim. Biophys. Acta* 1703, 149–156. doi: 10.1016/j.bbapap.2004.10.014

Butterfield, D. A., Swomley, A. M., and Sultana, R. (2013). Amyloid β-Peptide (1–42)-induced oxidative stress in Alzheimer disease: importance in disease Pathogenesis and Progression. *Antioxid. Redox. Signal.* 19, 823–835. doi: 10.1089/ars.2012.5027

Campagna, J. A., and Fallon, J. (2006). Lipid rafts are involved in C95 (4,8) agrin fragment-induced acetylcholine receptor clustering. *Neuroscience* 138, 123–132. doi: 10.1016/j.neuroscience.2005.11.019

Campanari, M. L., García-Ayllón, M. S., Belbin, O., Galcerán, J., Lleó, A., and Sáez-Valero, J. (2014). Acetylcholinesterase modulates presenilin-1 levels and γ-secretase activity. *J. Alzheimers Dis.* 41, 911–924. doi: 10.3233/JAD-140426

Cartaud, A., Stetzkowski-Marden, F., Maoui, A., and Cartaud, J. (2011). Agrin triggers the clustering of raft-associated acetylcholine receptors through actin cytoskeleton reorganization. *Biol. Cell.* 103, 287–301. doi: 10.1042/BC20110018

Cascella, R., Evangelisti, E., Bigi, A., Becatti, M., Fiorillo, C., Stefani, M., et al. (2017). Soluble oligomers require a ganglioside to trigger neuronal calcium overload. *J. Alzheimers. Dis.* 60, 923–938. doi: 10.3233/JAD-170340

Cecchi, C., Nichino, D., Zampagni, M., Bernacchioni, C., Evangelisti, E., Pensal, A., et al. (2009). A protective role for lipid raft cholesterol against amyloid-induced membrane damage in human neuroblastoma cells. *Biochim. Biophys. Acta* 1788, 2204–2216. doi: 10.1016/j.bbamem.2009.07.019

Champtiaux, N., Gotti, C., Cordero-Erausquin, M., David, D. J., Przybylski, C., Léna, C., et al. (2003). Subunit composition of functional nicotinic receptors in dopaminergic neurons investigated with knock-out mice. *J. Neurosci.* 23, 7820–7829. doi: 10.1523/jneurosci.23-21-07820.2003

Chang, T., Yamauchi, Y., Hasan, M. T., and Chang, C. (2017). Cellular cholesterol homeostasis and Alzheimer's disease. *J. Lipid. Res.* 58, 2239–2254. doi: 10.1194/jlr.R075630

Changeux, J. P., and Edelstein, S. J. (1998). Allosteric receptors after 30 years. *Neuron* 21, 959–980. doi: 10.1016/s0896-6273(00)80616-9

Cheignon, C., Tomas, M., Bonnefont-Rousselot, D., Faller, P., Hureau, C., and Collin, F. (2018). Oxidative stress and the amyloid beta peptide in Alzheimer's disease. *Redox Biol.* 14, 450–464. doi: 10.1016/j.redox.2017.10.014

Chernomordik, L. V., and Zimmerberg, J. (1995). Bending membranes to the task: structural intermediates in bilayer fusion. *Curr. Opin. Struct. Biol.* 5, 541–547. doi: 10.1016/0959-440x(95)80041-7

Chochina, S. V., Avdulov, N. A., Igbavboa, U., Cleary, J. P., O'Hare, E. O., and Wood, W. G. (2001). Amyloid beta-peptide1-40 increases neuronal membrane fluidity: role of cholesterol and brain region. *J. Lipid Res.* 42, 1292–1297.

Choo-Smith, L. P., Garzon-Rodriguez, W., Glabe, C. G., and Surewicz, W. K. (1997). Acceleration of amyloid fibril formation by specific binding of Abeta-(1-40) peptide to ganglioside-containing membrane vesicles. *J. Biol. Chem.* 272, 22987–22990. doi: 10.1074/jbc.272.37.22987

Chyung, J. H., Raper, D. M., and Selkoe, D. J. (2005). Gamma-secretase exists on the plasma membrane as an intact complex that accepts substrates and effects intramembrane cleavage. *J. Biol. Chem.* 280, 4383–4392. doi: 10.1074/jbc.M409272200

Clarke, P. B. (1992). The fall and rise of neuronal alpha-bungarotoxin binding proteins. *Trends Pharmacol. Sci.* 113, 407–413. doi: 10.1016/0165-6147(92)90125-p

Colón-Sáez, J. O., and Yakel, J. L. (2011). The α7 nicotinic acetylcholine receptor function in hippocampal neurons is regulated by the lipid composition of the plasma membrane. *J. Physiol.* 589, 3163–3174. doi: 10.1113/jphysiol.2011.209494

Contestabile, A. (2011). The history of the cholinergic hypothesis. *Behav. Brain Res.* 221, 334–340. doi: 10.1016/j.bbr.2009.12.044

Cooper, S. T., Harkness, P. C., Baker, E. R., and Millar, N. S. (1999). Up-regulation of cell-surface alpha4beta2 neuronal Nicotinic receptors by lower temperature and expression of chimeric subunits. *J. Biol. Chem.* 274, 27145–27152. doi: 10.1074/jbc.274.38.27145

Corbin, J., Wang, H. H., and Blanton, M. P. (1998). Identifying the cholesterol binding domain in the nicotinic acetylcholine receptor with [125I] azido-cholesterol. *Biochim. Biophys. Acta* 1414, 65–74. doi: 10.1016/s0005-2736(98)00153-9

Cordy, J. M., Hooper, N. M., and Turner, A. J. (2006). The involvement of lipid rafts in Alzheimer's disease. *Mol. Membr. Biol.* 23, 111–122. doi: 10.1080/09687860500496417

Counts, S. E., He, B., Che, S., Ikonomovic, M. D., DeKosky, S. T., Ginsberg, S. D., et al. (2007). Alpha7 nicotinic receptor up-regulation in cholinergic basal forebrain neurons in Alzheimer disease. *Arch. Neurol.* 64, 1771–1776. doi: 10.1001/archneur.64.12.1771

Court, J. A., Piggott, M. A., Lloyd, S., Cookson, N., Ballard, C. G., McKeith, I. G., et al. (2000). Nicotine binding in human striatum: elevation in schizophrenia and reductions in dementia with Lewy bodies, Parkinson's disease and Alzheimer's disease and in relation to neuroleptic medication. *Neuroscience* 98, 79–87. doi: 10.1016/s0306-4522(00)00071-3

Coyle, J. T., Price, D. L., and DeLong, M. R. (1983). Alzheimer's disease: a disorder of cortical cholinergic innervation. *Science* 219, 1184–1190. doi: 10.1126/science.6338589

Criado, M., Eibl, H., and Barrantes, F. J. (1984). Functional properties of the acetylcholine receptor incorporated in model lipid membranes. Differential effects of chain length and head group of phospholipids on receptor affinity states and receptor-mediated ion translocation. *J. Biol. Chem.* 259, 9188–9198.

Criado, M., Vaz, W. L., Barrantes, F. J., and Jovin, T. M. (1982). Translational diffusion of acetylcholine receptor (monomeric and dimeric forms) of Torpedo marmorata reconstituted into phospholipid bilayers studied by fluorescence recovery after photobleaching. *Biochemistry* 21, 5750–5755. doi: 10.1021/bi00266a004

Cutler, R. G., Kelly, J., Storie, K., Pedersen, W. A., Tammara, A., Hatanpaa, K., et al. (2004). Involvement of oxidative stress-induced abnormalities in ceramide and cholesterol metabolism in brain aging and Alzheimer's disease. *Proc. Natl. Acad. Sci. U.S.A.* 101, 2070–2075. doi: 10.1073/pnas.0305799101

daCosta, C. J., Ogrel, A. A., McCardy, E. A., Blanton, M. P., and Baenziger, J. E. (2002). Lipid-protein interactions at the nicotinic acetylcholine receptor. A functional coupling between Nicotinic receptors and Phosphatidic acid-containing lipid bilayers. *J. Biol. Chem.* 277, 201–208. doi: 10.1074/jbc.M108341200

daCosta, C. J., Wagg, I. D., McKay, M. E., and Baenziger, J. E. (2004). Phosphatidic acid and phosphatidylserine have distinct structural and functional interactions with the nicotinic acetylcholine receptor. *J. Biol. Chem.* 279, 14967–14974. doi: 10.1074/jbc.M310037200

daCosta, C. J. B., and Baenziger, J. E. (2009). A lipid-dependent uncoupled conformation of the acetylcholine receptor. *J. Biol. Chem.* 284, 17819–17825. doi: 10.1074/jbc.M900030200

Dajas-Bailador, F., and Wonnacott, S. (2004). Nicotinic acetylcholine receptors and the regulation of neuronal signalling. *Trends. Pharmacol. Sci.* 25, 317–324. doi: 10.1016/s0165-6147(04)00118-x

Daleke, D. L. (2003). Regulation of transbilayer plasma membrane phospholipid asymmetry. *J. Lipid Res.* 44, 233–242. doi: 10.1194/jlr.r200019-jlr200

D'Andrea, M. R., and Nagele, R. G. (2006). Targeting the alpha 7 nicotinic acetylcholine receptor to reduce amyloid accumulation in Alzheimer's disease pyramidal neurons. *Curr. Pharm. Des.* 12, 677–684. doi: 10.2174/138161206775474224

Daugherty, B. L., and Green, S. A. (2001). Endosomal sorting of amyloid precursor protein-P-selectin chimeras influences secretase processing. *Traffic* 2, 908–916. doi: 10.1034/j.1600-0854.2001.21206.x

Davies, P., and Maloney, A. J. (1976). Selective loss of central cholinergic neurons in Alzheimer's disease. *Lancet* 2:1403. doi: 10.1016/s0140-6736(76)91936-x

de Almeida, R. F., Loura, L. M., Prieto, M., Watts, A., Fedorov, A., and Barrantes, F. J. (2004). Cholesterol modulates the organization of the gammaM4 transmembrane domain of the muscle nicotinic acetylcholine receptor. *Biophys. J.* 86, 2261–2272. doi: 10.1016/S0006-3495(04)74284-74288

Deutsch, S. I., Burket, J. A., and Benson, A. D. (2014). Targeting the α7 nicotinic acetylcholine receptor to prevent progressive dementia and improve cognition in adults with Down's syndrome. *Prog. Neuropsychopharmacol. Biol. Psychiatry* 254, 131–139. doi: 10.1016/j.pnpbp.2014.05.011

Deutsch, S. I., Burket, J. A., Benson, A. D., and Urbano, M. R. (2016). The 15q13.3 deletion syndrome: Deficient α(7)-containing nicotinic acetylcholine receptor-mediated neurotransmission in the pathogenesis of neurodevelopmental disorders. *Prog. Neuropsychopharmacol. Biol Psychiatry* 64, 09–17. doi: 10.1016/j.pnpbp.2015.08.001

Di Scala, C., Baier, C. J., Evans, L. S., Williamson, P. T. F., Fantini, J., and Barrantes, F. J. (2017). Relevance of CARC and CRAC Cholesterol-Recognition Motifs in the Nicotinic Acetylcholine Receptor and Other Membrane-Bound Receptors. *Curr. Top. Membr.* 80, 3–23. doi: 10.1016/bs.ctm.2017.05.001

Di Scala, C., Chahinian, H., Yahi, N., Garmy, N., and Fantini, J. (2014). Interaction of Alzheimer's β-amyloid peptides with cholesterol: mechanistic insights into amyloid pore formation. *Biochemistry* 53, 4489–4502. doi: 10.1021/bi500373k

Di Scala, C., Yahi, N., Boutemeur, S., Flores, A., Rodriguez, L., Chahinian, H., et al. (2016). Common molecular mechanism of amyloid pore formation by Alzheimer's β-amyloid peptide and α-synuclein. *Sci. Rep.* 29:28781. doi: 10.1038/srep28781

Di Scala, C., Yahi, N., Lelièvre, C., Garmy, N., Chahinian, H., and Fantini, J. (2013). Biochemical identification of a linear cholesterol-binding domain within Alzheimer's β amyloid peptide. *ACS Chem. Neurosci.* 4, 509–517. doi: 10.1021/cn300203a

Dickey, A. N., and Faller, R. (2008). Behavioral differences between Phosphatidic acid and Phosphatidylcholine in the Presence of the Nicotinic Acetylcholine receptor. *Biophys. J.* 95, 5637–5647. doi: 10.1529/biophysj.108.136895

Dies, H., Toppozini, L., and Rheinstädter, M. C. (2014). The interaction between amyloid-β peptides and anionic lipid membranes containing cholesterol and melatonin. *PLoS One* 9:e99124. doi: 10.1371/journal.pone.0099124

Dineley, K. T. (2007). Beta-amyloid peptide–nicotinic acetylcholine receptor interaction: the two faces of health and disease. *Front. Biosci.* 12:5030–5038.

Dineley, K. T., Bell, K. A., Bui, D., and Sweatt, J. D. (2002). Beta -Amyloid peptide activates alpha 7 nicotinic acetylcholine receptors expressed in Xenopus oocytes. *J. Biol. Chem.* 277, 25056–25061. doi: 10.1074/jbc.M200066200

Dineley, K. T., Westerman, M., Bui, D., Bell, K., Ashe, K. H., and Sweatt, J. D. (2001). Beta-amyloid activates the mitogen-activated protein kinase cascade via hippocampal alpha7 nicotinic acetylcholine receptors: in vitro and in vivo mechanisms related to Alzheimer's disease. *J. Neurosci.* 21, 4125–4133. doi: 10.1523/jneurosci.21-12-04125.2001

Dougherty, J. J., Wu, J., and Nichols, R. A. (2003). Beta-amyloid regulation of presynaptic nicotinic receptors in rat hippocampus and neocortex. *J. Neurosci.* 23, 6740–6747. doi: 10.1523/jneurosci.23-17-06740.2003

Dreger, M., Krauss, M., Herrmann, A., and Hucho, F. (1997). Interactions of the Nicotinic acetylcholine receptor Transmembrane segments with the Lipid Bilayer in Native receptor-rich membranes. *Biochemistry* 36, 839–847. doi: 10.1021/bi960666z

Dukhinova, M., Veremeyko, T., Yung, A. W. Y., Kuznetsova, I. S., Lau, T. Y. B., Kopeikina, E., et al. (2019). Fresh evidence for major brain gangliosides as a target for the treatment of Alzheimer's disease. *Neurobiol. Aging* 77, 128–143. doi: 10.1016/j.neurobiolaging.2019.01.020

Dvir, H., Silman, I., Harel, M., Rosenberry, T. L., and Sussman, J. L. (2010). Acetylcholinesterase: from 3D structure to function. *Chem. Biol. Interact.* 187, 10–22. doi: 10.1016/j.cbi.2010.01.042

Dziewczapolski, G., Glogowski, C. M., Masliah, E., and Heinemann, S. F. (2009). Deletion of the alpha 7 nicotinic acetylcholine receptor gene improves cognitive deficits and synaptic pathology in a mouse model of Alzheimer's disease. *J. Neurosci.* 29, 8805–8815. doi: 10.1523/JNEUROSCI.6159-08.2009

Eckert, G. P., Kirsch, C., Leutz, S., Wood, W. G., and Müller, W. E. (2003). Cholesterol Modulates Amyloid Beta-peptide's Membrane Interactions. *Pharmacopsychiatry* 36(Suppl. 2), S136–S143. doi: 10.1055/s-2003-43059

Ehehalt, R., Keller, P., Haass, C., Thiele, C., and Simons, K. (2003). Amyloidogenic processing of the Alzheimer beta-amyloid precursor protein depends on lipid rafts. *J. Cell. Biol.* 160, 113–123. doi: 10.1083/jcb.200207113

Ellena, J. F., Blazing, M. A., and McNamee, M. G. (1983). Lipid-protein interactions in reconstituted membranes containing Acetylcholine receptor. *Biochemistry* 22, 5523–5535. doi: 10.1021/bi00293a012

Engel, M. F., Khemtémourian, L., Kleijer, C. C., Meeldijk, H. J., Jacobs, J., Verkleij, A. J., et al. (2008). Membrane damage by human islet amyloid polypeptide through fibril growth at the membrane. *Proc. Natl. Acad. Sci. U.S.A.* 105, 6033–6038. doi: 10.1073/pnas.0708354105

Engelman, D. M. (2005). Membranes are more mosaic than fluid. *Nature* 438, 578–580. doi: 10.1038/nature04394

Epand, R. F., Kraayenhof, R., Sterk, G. J., Wong Fong Sang, H. W., and Epand, R. M. (1996). Fluorescent probes of membrane surface properties. *Biochim Biophys Acta* 1284, 191–195.

Fabelo, N., Martín, V., Marín, R., Moreno, D., Ferrer, I., and Díaz, M. (2014). Altered lipid composition in cortical lipid rafts occurs at early stages of sporadic Alzheimer's disease and facilitates APP/BACE1 interactions. *Neurobiol. Aging* 35, 1801–1812. doi: 10.1016/j.neurobiolaging.2014.02.005

Fantini, J., and Barrantes, F. J. (2013). How cholesterol interacts with membrane proteins: an exploration of cholesterol-binding sites including CRAC, CARC, and tilted domains. *Front. Physiol.* 4:31. doi: 10.3389/fphys.2013.00031

Fantini, J., Di Scala, C., Evans, L. S., Williamson, P. T. F., and Barrantes, F. J. (2016). Open a mirror code for protein- cholesterol interactions in the two leaflets of biological membranes. *Sci. Rep.* 26:21907. doi: 10.1038/srep21907

Fantini, J., Di Scala, C., Yahi, N., Troadec, J. D., Sadelli, K., and Chahinian, H. (2014). Bxarotene blocks calcium-permeable ion channels formed by neurotoxic Alzheimer's β-amyloid peptides. *ACS Chem. Neurosci.* 5, 216–224. doi: 10.1021/cn400183w

Farhat, S. M., and Ahmed, T. (2017). Neuroprotective and Neurotoxic implications of α7 Nicotinic Acetylcholine receptor and Aβ Interaction: Therapeutic options in Alzheimer's Disease. *Curr. Drug. Targets* 18, 1537–1544. doi: 10.2174/1389450117666161005145143

Fassbender, K., Masters, C., and Beyreuther, K. (2001). Alzheimer's disease: molecular concepts and therapeutic targets. *Naturwissenschaften* 88, 261–267. doi: 10.1007/s001140100237

Feng, Y., and Wang, X. (2012). Antioxidant therapies for Alzheimer's disease. *Oxid. Med. Cell. Longev.* 2012:472932. doi: 10.1155/2012/472932

Fernandes, C. C., Berg, D. K., and Gómez-Varela, D. (2010). Lateral mobility of nicotinic acetylcholine receptors on neurons is determined by receptor composition, local domain, and cell type. *J. Neurosci.* 30, 8841–8851. doi: 10.1523/JNEUROSCI.6236-09.2010

Fernández Nievas, G. A., Barrantes, F. J., and Antollini, S. S. (2007). Conformation-sensitive steroid and fatty acid sites in the transmembrane domain of the nicotinic acetylcholine receptor. *Biochemistry* 46, 3503–3512. doi: 10.1021/bi061388z

Fernández Nievas, G. A., Barrantes, F. J., and Antollini, S. S. (2008). Modulation of nicotinic acetylcholine receptor conformational state by free fatty acids and steroids. *J. Biol. Chem.* 283, 21478–21486. doi: 10.1074/jbc.M800345200

Fernández-Ballester, G., Castresana, J., Fernandez, A. M., Arrondo, J. L., Ferragut, J. A., and Gonzalez-Ros, J. M. (1994). Role of cholesterol as a structural and functional effector of the nicotinic acetylcholine receptor. *Biochem. Soc. Trans.* 122, 776–780. doi: 10.1042/bst0220776

Fishman, E. B., Siek, G. C., MacCallum, R. D., Bird, E. D., Volicer, L., and Marquis, J. K. (1986). Distribution of the molecular forms of acetylcholinesterase in human brain: alterations in dementia of the Alzheimer type. *Ann. Neurol.* 119, 246–252. doi: 10.1002/ana.410190305

Fong, T. M., and McNamee, M. G. (1986). Correlation between acetylcholine receptor function and structural properties of membranes. *Biochemistry* 25, 830–840. doi: 10.1021/bi00352a015

Fonseca, A. C., Moreira, P. I., Oliveira, C. R., Cardoso, S. M., Pinton, P., and Pereira, C. F. (2015). Amyloid-Beta disrupts calcium and redox homeostasis in brain endothelial cells. *Mol. Neurobiol* 51, 610–622. doi: 10.1007/s12035-014-8740-8747

Frears, E. R., Stephens, D. J., Walters, C. E., Davies, H., and Austen, B. M. (1999). The role of cholesterol in the biosynthesis of beta-amyloid. *Neuroreport* 10, 1699–1705. doi: 10.1097/00001756-199906030-00014

Fucile, S. (2004). Ca^{2+} permeability of nicotinic acetylcholine receptors. *Cell. Calcium* 35, 1–8. doi: 10.1016/j.ceca.2003.08.006

Fukaya, T., Gondaira, T., Kashiyae, Y., Kotani, S., Ishikura, Y., Fujikawa, S., et al. (2007). Arachidonic acid preserves hippocampal neuron membrane fluidity in senescent rats. *Neurobiol. Aging* 28, 1179–1186. doi: 10.1016/j.neurobiolaging.2006.05.023

Fukunaga, S., Ueno, H., Yamaguchi, T., Yano, Y., Hoshino, M., and Matsuzaki, K. (2012). GM1 cluster mediates formation of toxic Aβ fibrils by providing hydrophobic environments. *Biochemistry* 51, 8125–8131. doi: 10.1021/bi300839u

Garbus, I., Bouzat, C., and Barrantes, F. J. (2001). Steroids differentially inhibit the nicotinic acetylcholine receptor. *Neuroreport* 12, 227–231. doi: 10.1097/00001756-200102120-00010

Garbus, I., Roccamo, A. M., and Barrantes, F. J. (2002). Identification of threonine 422 in transmembrane domain alpha M4 of the nicotinic acetylcholine receptor as a possible site of interaction with hydrocortisone. *Neuropharmacology* 43, 65–73. doi: 10.1016/s0028-3908(02)00068-0

García-Ayllón, M., Campanari, M., Montenegro, M., Cuchillo-ibáñez, I., Belbin, O., Lleó, A., et al. (2014). Neurobiology of aging Presenilin-1 influences processing of the acetylcholinesterase membrane anchor PRiMA. *Neurobiol. Aging* 35, 1526–1536. doi: 10.1016/j.neurobiolaging.2014.01.147

Geula, C., and Mesulam, M. (1989). Special properties of cholinesterases in the cerebral cortex of Alzheimer's disease. *Brain Res.* 498, 185–189. doi: 10.1016/0006-8993(89)90419-8

Ghoneim, M. M., and Mewaldt, S. P. (1977). Studies on human memory: the interactions of diazepam, scopolamine, and physostigmine. *Psychopharmacology* 52, 1–6. doi: 10.1007/bf00426592

Ghribi, O., Larsen, B., Schrag, M., and Herman, M. M. (2006). High cholesterol content in neurons increases BACE, β -amyloid, and phosphorylated tau levels in rabbit hippocampus. *Exp. Neurol.* 200, 460–467. doi: 10.1016/j.expneurol.2006.03.019

Gilbert, R. J. (2016). Protein-lipid interactions and non-lamellar lipidic structures in membrane pore formation and membrane fusion. *Biochim. Biophys. Acta* 1858, 487–499. doi: 10.1016/j.bbamem.2015.11.026

Gilbert, R. J., Dalla Serra, M., Froelich, C. J., Wallace, M. I., and Anderluh, G. (2014). Membrane pore formation at protein-lipid interfaces. *Trends Biochem. Sci.* 39, 510–516. doi: 10.1016/j.tibs.2014.09.002

Giniatullin, R., Nistri, A., and Yakel, J. L. (2005). Desensitization of nicotinic ACh receptors: shaping cholinergic signaling. *Trends. Neurosci.* 28, 371–378. doi: 10.1016/j.tins.2005.04.009

Gong, J. S., Sawamura, N., Zou, K., Sakai, J., Yanagisawa, K., and Michikawa, M. (2002). Amyloid beta-protein affects cholesterol metabolism in cultured neurons: implications for pivotal role of cholesterol in the amyloid cascade. *Neurosci. Res.* 70, 438–446. doi: 10.1002/jnr.10347

Goñi, F. M. (2014). The basic structure and dynamics of cell membranes?: an update of the Singer - Nicolson model. *Biochim. Biophys. Acta* 1838, 1467–1476. doi: 10.1016/j.bbamem.2014.01.006

Gotti, C., Clementi, F., Fornari, A., Gaimarri, A., Guiducci, S., Manfredi, I., et al. (2009). Structural and functional diversity of native brain neuronal nicotinic receptors. *Biochem. Pharmacol.* 78, 703–711. doi: 10.1016/j.bcp.2009.05.024

Gotti, C., Moretti, M., Gaimarri, A., Zanardi, A., Clementi, F., and Zoli, M. (2007). Heterogeneity and complexity of native brain nicotinic receptors. *Biochem. Pharmacol.* 74, 1102–1111. doi: 10.1016/j.bcp.2007.05.023

Gotti, C., Riganti, L., Vailati, S., and Clementi, F. (2006b). Brain neuronal nicotinic receptors as new targets for drug discovery. *Curr. Pharm. Des.* 12, 407–428. doi: 10.2174/138161206775474486

Gotti, C., Zoli, M., and Clementi, F. (2006a). Brain nicotinic acetylcholine receptors: native subtypes and their relevance. *Trends Pharmacol. Sci.* 27, 482–491. doi: 10.1016/j.tips.2006.07.004

Götz, J., Schild, A., Hoerndli, F., and Pennanen, L. (2004). Amyloid-induced neurofibrillary tangle formation in Alzheimer's disease: insight from transgenic mouse and tissue-culture models. *Int. J. Dev. Neurosci.* 22, 453–465. doi: 10. 1016/j.ijdevneu.2004.07.013

Graham, A. J., Martin-Ruiz, C. M., Teaktong, T., Ray, M. A., and Court, J. A. (2002). Human brain nicotinic receptors, their distribution and participation in neuropsychiatric disorders. *Curr. Drug. Targets CNS Neurol. Disord.* 4, 387–397. doi: 10.2174/1568007023339283

Greenfield, J. P., Tsai, J., Gouras, G. K., Hai, B., Thinakaran, G., Checler, F., et al. (1999). Endoplasmic reticulum and trans-Golgi network generate distinct populations of Alzheimer beta-amyloid peptides. *Proc. Natl. Acad. Sci. U.S.A.* 96, 742–747. doi: 10.1073/pnas.96.2.742

Grimm, M. O., Grimm, H. S., and Hartmann, T. (2007). Amyloid beta as a regulator of lipid homeostasis. *Trends. Mol. Med.* 13, 337–344. doi: 10.1016/j.molmed. 2007.06.004

Grimm, M. O., Grimm, H. S., Pätzold, A. J., Zinser, E. G., Halonen, R., Duering, M., et al. (2005). Regulation of cholesterol and sphingomyelin metabolism by amyloid- β and presenilin. *Nat. Cell. Biol.* 7, 1118–1123. doi: 10.1038/ ncb1313

Grisaru, D., Sternfeld, M., Eldor, A., Glick, D., and Soreq, H. (1999). Structural roles of acetylcholinesterase variants in biology and pathology. *Eur. J. Biochem.* 264, 672–686. doi: 10.1046/j.1432-1327.1999.00693.x

Gu, L., and Guo, Z. (2013). Alzheimer's Aβ42 and Aβ40 peptides form interlaced amyloid fibrils. *J. Neurochem.* 126, 305–311. doi: 10.1111/jnc.12202

Guillem, K., Bloem, B., Poorthuis, R. B., Loos, M., Smit, A. B., Maskos, U., et al. (2011). Nicotinic acetylcholine receptor β2 subunits in the medial prefrontal cortex control attention. *Science* 333, 888–891. doi: 10.1126/science.1207079

Gylys, K. H., Fein, J. A., Yang, F., Miller, C. A., and Cole, G. M. (2007). Increased cholesterol in Abeta-positive nerve terminals from Alzheimer's disease cortex. *Neurobiol. Aging* 28, 8–17. doi: 10.1016/j.neurobiolaging.2005.10.018

Gyure, K. A., Durham, R., Stewart, W. F., Smialek, J. E., and Troncoso, J. C. (2001). Intraneuronal abeta-amyloid precedes development of amyloid plaques in Down syndrome. *Arch. Pathol. Lab. Med.* 125, 489–492.

Haass, C. (1996). The molecular significance of amyloid beta-peptide for Alzheimer's disease. *Eur. Arch. Psychiatry. Clin. Neurosci.* 246, 118–123.

Haass, C., Kaether, C., Thinakaran, G., and Sisodia, S. (2012). Trafficking and Proteolytic Processing of APP. *Cold. Spring. Harb. Perspect. Med.* 2, 1–25. doi: 10.1101/cshperspect.a006270

Hamouda, A. K., Chiara, D. C., Sauls, D., Cohen, J. B., and Blanton, M. P. (2006). Cholesterol interacts with transmembrane alpha-helices M1, M3, and M4 of the Torpedo nicotinic acetylcholine receptor: photolabeling studies using [3H]Azicholesterol. *Biochemistry* 45, 976–986. doi: 10.1021/bi051978h

Hampel, H., Mesulam, M. M., Cuello, A. C., Farlow, M. R., Giacobini, E., and Grossberg, G. T. (2018). The cholinergic system in the pathophysiology and treatment of Alzheimer's disease. *Brain* 141, 1917–1933. doi: 10.1093/brain/ awy132

Hardy, J. A., and Allsop, D. (1991). Amyloid deposition as the central event in the aetiology of Alzheimer's disease. *Trends. Pharmacol.* 12, 383–388. doi: 10.1016/0165-6147(91)90609-v

Hardy, J. A., and Higgins, G. A. (1992). Alzheimer's Disease?: the amyloid cascade hypothesis. *Science* 256, 184–185.

Harris, J. R. (2008). Cholesterol binding to amyloid-b fibrils: a TEM study. *Micron* 39, 1192–1196. doi: 10.1016/j.micron.2008.05.001

Hellström-Lindahl, E., Court, J., Keverne, J., Svedberg, M., Lee, M., Marutle, A., et al. (2004a). Nicotine reduces A beta in the brain and cerebral vessels of APPsw mice. *Eur. J. Neurosci.* 19, 2703–2710. doi: 10.1111/j.0953-816X.2004.03377.x

Hellström-Lindahl, E., Mousavi, M., Ravid, R., and Nordberg, A. (2004b). Reduced levels of Abeta 40 and Abeta 42 in brains of smoking controls and Alzheimer's patients. *Neurobiol. Dis.* 15, 351–360. doi: 10.1016/j.nbd.2003.11.024

Hellström-Lindahl, E., Mousavi, M., Zhang, X., Ravid, R., and Nordberg, A. (1999). Regional distribution of nicotinic receptor subunit mRNAs in human brain: comparison between Alzheimer and normal brain. *Brain Res. Mol. Brain. Res.* 661, 94–103. doi: 10.1016/s0169-328x(99)00030-3

Hénault, C. M., Sun, J., Therien, J. P., daCosta, C. J., Carswell, C. L., Labriola, J. M., et al. (2015). The role of the M4 lipid-sensor in the folding, trafficking, and allosteric modulation of nicotinic acetylcholine receptors. *Neuropharmacology* 296, 157–168. doi: 10.1016/j.neuropharm.2014.11.011

Henderson, Z., Boros, A., Janzso, G., Westwood, A. J., Monyer, H., and Halasy, K. (2005). Somato-dendritic nicotinic receptor responses recorded *in vitro* from the medial septal diagonal band complex of the rodent. *J. Physiol. Lond.* 562, 165–182. doi: 10.1113/jphysiol.2004.070300

Henderson, Z., Matto, N., John, D., Nalivaeva, N. N., and Turner, A. J. (2010). Co-localization of PRiMA with acetylcholinesterase in cholinergic neurons of rat brain: an immunocytochemical study. *Brain Res.* 1344, 34–42. doi: 10.1016/j. brainres.2010.05.022

Herrup, K. (2015). The case for rejecting the amyloid cascade hypothesis. *Nat. Neurosci.* 18, 794–799. doi: 10.1038/nn.4017

Hertel, C., Terzi, E., Hauser, N., Jakob-Rotne, R., Seelig, J., and Kemp, J. A. (1997). Inhibition of the electrostatic interaction between beta-amyloid peptide and membranes prevents beta-amyloid-induced toxicity. *Proc. Natl. Acad. Sci. U.S.A.* 94, 9412–9416. doi: 10.1073/pnas.94.17.9412

Hicks, D. A., John, D., Makova, N. Z., Henderson, Z., Nalivaeva, N. N., and Turner, A. J. (2011). Membrane targeting, shedding and protein interactions of brain acetylcholinesterase. *J. Neurochem.* 116, 742–746. doi: 10.1111/j.1471-4159.2010.07032.x

Hicks, D. A., Makova, N. Z., Gough, M., Parkin, E. T., Nalivaeva, N. N., and Turner, A. J. (2013b). The amyloid precursor protein represses expression of acetylcholinesterase in neuronal cell lines. *J. Biol. Chem.* 288, 26039–26051. doi: 10.1074/jbc.M113.461269

Hicks, D. A., Makova, N. Z., Nalivaeva, N. N., and Turner, A. J. (2013a). Chemico-Biological Interactions Characterisation of acetylcholinesterase release from neuronal cells. *Chem. Biol. Interact.* 203, 302–308. doi: 10.1016/j.cbi.2012. 09.019

Hicks, D. A., Nalivaeva, N. N., and Turner, A. J. (2012). Lipid rafts and Alzheimer's disease?: protein-lipid interactions and perturbation of signaling. *Front. Physiol.* 3:189. doi: 10.3389/fphys.2012.00189

Hong, S., Ostaszewski, B. L., Yang, T., Malley, T. T. O., Jin, M., Yanagisawa, K., et al. (2014). Soluble Aβ oligomers are rapidly sequestered from brain ISF in vivo and bind GM1 ganglioside on cellular membranes. *Neuron.* 82, 308–319. doi: 10.1016/j.neuron.2014.02.027

Hou, X., Richardson, S. J., Aguilar, M. I., and Small, D. H. (2005). Binding of amyloidogenic transthyretin to the plasma membrane alters membrane fluidity and induces neurotoxicity. *Biochemistry* 44, 11618–11627. doi: 10.1021/ bi050700m

Huse, J. T., Pijak, D. S., Leslie, G. J., Lee, V. M., and Doms, R. W. (2000). Maturation and endosomal targeting of beta-site amyloid precursor protein-cleaving enzyme. The Alzheimer's disease beta-secretase. *J. Biol. Chem.* 275, 33729–33737. doi: 10.1074/jbc.M004175200

Igbavboa, U., Avdulov, N. A., Schroeder, F., and Wood, W. G. (1996). Increasing age alters transbilayer fluidity and cholesterol asymmetry in synaptic plasma membranes of mice. *J. Neurochem.* 66, 1717–1725. doi: 10.1046/j.1471-4159. 1996.66041717.x

Ikonomovic, M. D., Wecker, L., Abrahamson, E. E., Wuu, J., Counts, S. E., Ginsberg, S. D., et al. (2009). Cortical alpha7 nicotinic acetylcholine receptor and beta-amyloid levels in early Alzheimer disease. *Arch. Neurol.* 66, 646–651. doi: 10.1001/archneurol.2009.46

Inestrosa, N. C., Alvarez, A., and Calderón, F. (1996). Acetylcholinesterase is a senile plaque component that promotes assembly of amyloid beta-peptide into Alzheimer's filaments. *Mol. Psychiatry* 1, 359–361.

Irvine, G. B., El-agnaf, O. M., Shankar, G. M., and Walsh, D. M. (2008). Protein aggregation in the brain: the molecular basis for Alzheimer's and Parkinson' s diseases. *Mol. Med.* 14, 451–464. doi: 10.2119/2007-00100

Iwatsubo, T., Odaka, A., Suzuki, N., Mizusawa, H., Nukina, N., and Ihara, Y. (1994). Visualization of A beta 42(43) and A beta 40 in senile plaques with end-specific

A beta monoclonals: evidence that an initially deposited species is A beta 42(43). *Neuron* 13, 45–53. doi: 10.1016/0896-6273(94)90458-8

Jarrett, J. T., Berger, E. P., and Lansbury, P. T. Jr. (1993). The carboxy terminus of the beta amyloid protein is critical for the seeding of amyloid formation: implications for the pathogenesis of Alzheimer's disease. *Biochemistry* 32, 4693–4697. doi: 10.1021/bi00069a001

Jha, A., Cadugan, D. J., Purohit, P., and Auerbach, A. (2007). Acetylcholine receptor gating at extracellular transmembrane domain interface: the cys-loop and M2-M3 linker. *J. Gen. Physiol.* 130, 547–558. doi: 10.1085/jgp.200709856

Ji, S. R., Wu, Y., and Sui, S. F. (2002). Cholesterol is an important factor affecting the membrane insertion of beta-amyloid peptide (A beta 1-40), which may potentially inhibit the fibril formation. *J. Biol. Chem.* 277, 6273–6279. doi: 10.1074/jbc.M104146200

Jin, Y., Tsuchiya, A., Kanno, T., and Nishizaki, T. (2015). Biochemical and biophysical research communications Amyloid- b peptide increases cell surface localization of a7 ACh receptor to protect neurons from amyloid b -induced damage. *Biochem. Biophys. Res. Commun.* 468, 157–160. doi: 10.1016/j.bbrc.2015.10.141

Jones, I. W., Westmacott, A., Chan, E., Jones, R. W., Dineley, K., and O'Neill, M. J. (2006). Alpha7 nicotinic acetylcholine receptor expression in Alzheimer's disease: receptor densities in brain regions of the APP(SWE) mouse model and in human peripheral blood lymphocytes. *J. Mol. Neurosci.* 30, 83–84. doi: 10.1385/JMN:30:1:83

Jones, O. T., and McNamee, M. G. (1988). Annular and nonannular binding sites for cholesterol associated with the nicotinic acetylcholine receptor. *Biochemistry* 127, 2364–2374. doi: 10.1021/bi00407a018

Kagan, B. L., Hirakura, Y., Azimov, R., Azimova, R., and Lin, M. (2002). The channel hypothesis of Alzheimer's disease: current status. *Peptides* 23, 1311–1315. doi: 10.1016/s0196-9781(02)00067-0

Kakio, A., Nishimoto, S., Yanagisawa, K., Kozutsumi, Y., and Matsuzaki, K. (2002). Interactions of amyloid beta-protein with various gangliosides in raft-like membranes: importance of GM1 ganglioside-bound form as an endogenous seed for Alzheimer amyloid. *Biochemistry* 241, 7385–7390. doi: 10.1021/bi0255874

Kakio, A., Nishimoto, S. I., Yanagisawa, K., Kozutsumi, Y., and Matsuzaki, K. (2001). Cholesterol-dependent formation of GM1 ganglioside-bound amyloid beta-protein, an endogenous seed for Alzheimer amyloid. *J. Biol. Chem.* 276, 24985–24990. doi: 10.1074/jbc.M100252200

Kamal, A., Almenar-Queralt, A., LeBlanc, J. F., Roberts, E. A., and Goldstein, L. S. (2001). Kinesin-mediated axonal transport of a membrane compartment containing beta-secretase and presenilin-1 requires APP. *Nature* 414, 643–648. doi: 10.1038/414643

Kamerbeek, C. B., Borroni, V., Pediconi, M. F., Sato, S. B., Kobayashi, T., and Barrantes, F. J. (2013). Antibody-induced acetylcholine receptor clusters inhabit liquid-ordered and liquid-disordered domains. *Biophys. J.* 150, 1601–1611. doi: 10.1016/j.bpj.2013.08.03

Kanfer, J. N., Sorrentino, G., and Sitar, D. S. (1999). Amyloid beta peptide membrane perturbation is the basis for its biological effects. *Neurochem. Res.* 24, 1621–1630.

Karlin, A., and Akabas, M. H. (1995). Toward a structural basis for the function of nicotinic acetylcholine receptors and their cousins. *Neuron* 15, 1231–1244. doi: 10.1016/0896-6273(95)90004-7

Kawahara, M. (2010). Neurotoxicity of β-amyloid protein: oligomerization, channel formation, and calcium dyshomeostasis. *Curr. Pharm. Des.* 16, 2779–2789. doi: 10.2174/138161210793176545

Kellner, R. R., Baier, C. J., Willig, K. I., Hell, S. W., and Barrantes, F. J. (2007). Nanoscale organization of nicotinic acetylcholine receptors revealed by stimulated emission depletion microscopy. *Neuroscience* 144, 135–143. doi: 10.1016/j.neuroscience.2006.08.071

Khan, G. M., Tong, M., Jhun, M., Arora, K., and Nichols, R. A. (2010). Beta-Amyloid activates presynaptic alpha7 nicotinic acetylcholine receptors reconstituted into a model nerve cell system: involvement of lipid rafts. *Eur. J. Neurosci.* 231, 788–796. doi: 10.1111/j.1460-9568.2010.07116.x

Kim, H.-J., Moon, W.-J., and Han, S.-H. (2013). Differential cholinergic pathway involvement in Alzheimer's disease and subcortical ischemic vascular dementia. *J. Alzheimers Dis.* 35, 129–136. doi: 10.3233/JAD-122320

Kim, S., Yi, J., and Ko, Y. (2006). Amyloid b Oligomerization Is Induced by Brain Lipid Rafts. *J. Cell. Biochem.* 99, 878–889. doi: 10.1002/jcb.20978

Kirsch, C., Eckert, G. P., and Mueller, W. E. (2002). Cholesterol attenuates the membrane perturbing properties of beta-amyloid peptides. *Amyloid* 9, 149–159.

Kirsch, C., Eckert, G. P., and Mueller, W. E. (2003). Statin effects on cholesterol micro-domains in brain plasma membranes. *Biochem. Pharmacol.* 65, 843–856. doi: 10.1016/s0006-2952(02)01654-4

Klein, W. L., Steine, W. B. Jr., and Teplow, D. B. (2004). Small assemblies of unmodified amyloid beta-protein are the proximate neurotoxin in Alzheimer's disease. *Neurobiol. Aging* 25, 569–580. doi: 10.1016/j.neurobiolaging.2004.02.010

Kogel, D., Copanaki, E., Hartig, U., Bottner, S., Peters, I., Muller, W. E., et al. (2008). "Modulation of membrane fluidity by omega 3 fatty acids: enhanced generation of sAPPalpha is required for the neuroprotective effects of DHA," in *The 38th Annual Meeting of the Society for Neuroscience*, Washington, DC, 15–19.

Kojro, E., Gimpl, G., Lammich, S., Marz, W., and Fahrenholz, F. (2001). Low cholesterol stimulates the nonamyloidogenic pathway by its effect on the alpha -secretase ADAM 10. *Proc. Natl. Acad. Sci. U.S.A.* 98, 5815–5820. doi: 10.1073/pnas.081612998

Koo, E. H., and Squazzo, S. L. (1994). Evidence that production and release of amyloid beta-protein involves the endocytic pathway. *J. Biol. Chem.* 269, 17386–17389.

Kosicek, M., and Hecimovic, S. (2013). Phospholipids and Alzheimer's disease: alterations, mechanisms and potential biomarkers. *Int. J. Mol. Sci.* 214, 1310–1322. doi: 10.3390/ijms14011310

Kotler, S. A., Walsh, P., Brender, J. R., and Ramamoorthy, A. (2014). Differences between amyloid-β aggregation in solution and on the membrane: insights into elucidation of the mechanistic details of Alzheimer's disease. *Chem. Soc. Rev.* 19, 6692–6700. doi: 10.1039/c3cs60431d

Koudinov, A. R., and Koudinova, N. V. (2004). Cholesterol homeostasis failure as a unifying cause of synaptic degeneration. *J. Neurol. Sci.* 229-230, 233–240. doi: 10.1016/j.jns.2004.11.036

Koudinova, N. V., Koudinov, A. R., and Yavin, E. (2000). Alzheimer's Abeta1-40 peptide modulates lipid synthesis in neuronal cultures and intact rat fetal brain under normoxic and oxidative stress conditions. *Neurochem. Res.* 25, 653–660.

Kumar, A., Singh, A., and Ekavali. (2015). A review on Alzheimer's disease pathophysiology and its management: an update. *Pharmacol. Rep.* 67, 195–203. doi: 10.1016/j.pharep.2014.09.004

Lahdo, R., and De La Fournière-Bessueille, L. (2004). Insertion of the amyloid precursor protein into lipid monolayers: effects of cholesterol and apolipoprotein E. *Biochem. J.* 382, 987–994. doi: 10.1042/BJ20040777

Langui, D., Girardot, N., El, Hachimi KH, Allinquant, B., Blanchard, V., Pradier, L., et al. (2004). Subcellular topography of neuronal Abeta peptide in APPxPS1 transgenic mice. *Am. J. Pathol.* 165, 1465–1477. doi: 10.1016/s0002-9440(10)63405-0

Lashuel, H. A., Hartley, D., Petre, B. M., Walz, T., and Lansbury, P. T. Jr. (2002). Neurodegenerative disease: amyloid pores from pathogenic mutations. *Nature* 418:291. doi: 10.1038/418291a

Lauderback, C. M., Hackett, J. M., Keller, J. N., Varadarajan, S., Szweda, L., Kindy, M., et al. (2001). Vulnerability of synaptosomes from apoE knock-out mice to structural and oxidative modifications induced by A beta(1-40): implications for Alzheimer's disease. *Biochemistry* 240, 2548–2554. doi: 10.1021/bi002312k

Lazarevic-Pasti, T., Leskovac, A., Momic, T., Petrovic, S., and Vasic, V. (2017). Modulators of Acetylcholinesterase activity: from Alzheimer's disease to anti-cancer drugs. *Curr. Med. Chem.* 24, 3283–3309. doi: 10.2174/0929867324666170705123509

Le Novère, N., and Changeux, J. P. (1995). Molecular evolution of the nicotinic acetylcholine receptor: an example of multigene family in excitable cells. *J Mol. Evol.* 40, 155–172. doi: 10.1007/bf00167110

Lee, A. G. (2003). Lipid - protein interactions in biological membranes: a structural perspective. *Biochim. Biophys. Acta* 1612, 1–40. doi: 10.1016/S0005-2736(03)00056-57

Lee, D. H. S., and Wang, H.-Y. (2003). Differential physiologic responses of α7 nicotinic acetylcholine receptors to β-amyloid$_{1-40}$ and β-amyloid$_{1-42}$. *J. Neurobiol.* 55, 25–30. doi: 10.1002/neu.10203

Lee, E. B., Leng, L. Z., Zhang, B., Kwong, L., Trojanowski, J. Q., Abel, T., et al. (2006). Targeting amyloid-β peptide (Aβ) oligomers by passive immunization with a conformation-selective monoclonal antibody improves learning and memory in Aβ precursor protein (APP) transgenic mice. *J. Biol. Chem.* 281, 4292–4299. doi: 10.1074/jbc.M511018200

Lee, S. J., Liyanage, U., Bickel, P. E., Xia, W., Lansbury, P. T. Jr., and Kosik, K. S. (1998). A detergent-insoluble membrane compartment contains A beta in vivo. *Nat. Med.* 4, 730–734. doi: 10.1038/nm0698-730

Levin, E. D., Cauley, M., and Rezvani, A. H. (2013). Improvement of attentional function with antagonism of nicotinic receptors in female rats. *Eur. J. Pharmacol.* 702, 269–274. doi: 10.1016/j.ejphar.2013.01.056

Li, L., Cheung, T., Chen, J., and Herrup, K. (2011). A comparative study of five mouse models of Alzheimer's disease: cell cycle events reveal new insights into neurons at risk for death. *Int. J. Alzheimers Dis.* 2011:171464. doi: 10.4061/2011/171464

Lilja, A. M., Porras, O., Storelli, E., Nordberg, A., and Marutle, A. (2011). Functional interactions of fibrillar and oligomeric amyloid-β with alpha7 nicotinic receptors in Alzheimer's disease. *J. Alzheimers Dis.* 23, 335–347. doi: 10.3233/JAD-2010-101242

Lin, H., Bhatia, R., and Lal, R. (2001). Amyloid beta protein forms ion channels: implications for Alzheimer's diseases pathophysiology. *FASEB J.* 15, 2433–2444. doi: 10.1096/fj.01-0377com

Lin, M. S., Chen, L. Y., Wang, S. S., Chang, Y., and Chen, W. Y. (2008). Examining the levels of ganglioside and cholesterol in cell membrane on attenuation the cytotoxicity of beta-amyloid peptide. *Colloids Surf. B. Biointerfaces* 65, 172–177. doi: 10.1016/j.colsurfb.2008.03.012

Lindstrom, J. M. (2003). Nicotinic acetylcholine receptors of muscles and nerves: comparison of their structures, functional roles, and vulnerability to pathology. *Ann. N.Y. Acad. Sci.* 998, 41–52. doi: 10.1196/annals.1254.007

Liu, Q., Kawai, H., and Berg, D. K. (2001). Beta -Amyloid peptide blocks the response of alpha 7-containing nicotinic receptors on hippocampal neurons. *Proc. Natl. Acad. Sci. U.S.A.* 98, 4734–4739. doi: 10.1073/pnas.081553598

Liu, Q., and Wu, J. (2006). Neuronal nicotinic acetylcholine receptors serve as sensitive targets that mediate beta-amyloid neurotoxicity. *Acta. Pharmacol. Sin.* 27, 1277–1286. doi: 10.1111/j.1745-7254.2006.00430.x

Liu, Q., Xie, X., Emadi, S., Sierks, M. R., and Wu, J. (2015). A novel nicotinic mechanism underlies b -amyloid-induced neurotoxicity. *Neuropharmacology* 97, 457–463. doi: 10.1016/j.neuropharm.2015.04.025

Liu, Q., Xie, X., Lukas, R. J., St John, P. A., and Wu, J. (2013). A novel nicotinic mechanism underlies β-amyloid-induced neuronal hyperexcitation. *J. Neurosci.* 33, 7253–7263. doi: 10.1523/JNEUROSCI.3235-12.2013

Liu, R., Gu, R., Qi, X., Zhang, T., Zhao, Y., and He, Y. (2008). Decreased Nicotinic receptors and cognitive deficit in rats intracerebroventricularly injected with beta-amyloid peptide (1-42) and fed a high-cholesterol diet. *J. Neurosci. Res.* 86, 183–193. doi: 10.1002/jnr.21463

Lombardo, S., and Maskos, U. (2014). Neuropharmacology Role of the nicotinic acetylcholine receptor in Alzheimer's disease pathology and treatment. *Neuropharmacology* 96, 255–262. doi: 10.1016/j.neuropharm.2014.11.018

London, E. (2005). How principles of domain formation in model membranes may explain ambiguities concerning lipidraft formation in cells. *Biochim. Biophys. Acta* 30, 203–220. doi: 10.1016/j.bbamcr.2005.09.002

Lukiw, W. J. (2013). Alzheimer's disease (AD) as a disorder of the plasma membrane. *Front. Physiol.* 4:24. doi: 10.3389/fphys.2013.00024

Ma, K., and Qian, Y. (2019). Neuropeptides Alpha 7 nicotinic acetylcholine receptor and its effects on Alzheimer's disease. *Neuropeptides* 73, 96–106. doi: 10.1016/j.npep.2018.12.003

Magni, F., Galbusera, C., Tremolada, L., Ferrarese, C., and Kienle, M. G. (2002). Characterisation of adducts of the lipid peroxidation product 4-hydroxy-2-nonenal and amyloid beta-peptides by liquid chromatography/electrospray ionisation mass spectrometry. *Rapid. Commun. Mass. Spectrom.* 16, 1485–1493. doi: 10.1002/rcm.743

Maia, M. A., and Sousa, E. (2019). BACE-1 and γ-secretase as therapeutic targets for Alzheimer's disease. *Pharmaceuticals* 12:41. doi: 10.3390/ph12010041

Marchand, S., Devillers-thie, A., Pons, S., Changeux, J., and Cartaud, J. (2002). Rapsyn escorts the Nicotinic Acetylcholine receptor along the exocytic pathway via association with lipid rafts. *J. Neurosci.* 22, 8891–8901. doi: 10.1523/jneurosci.22-20-08891.2002

Mark, R., Lovell, M. A., Markesbery, W., Koiiuchida, I., and Mattson, P. (1997). A role for 4-Hydroxynonenal, an aldehydic product of lipid peroxidation, in disruption of ion homeostasis and neuronal death induced by amyloid-beta peptide. *J. Neurochem.* 68, 255–264. doi: 10.1046/j.1471-4159.1997.68010255.x

Marsh, D., and Barrantes, F. J. (1978). Immobilized lipid in acetylcholine receptor-rich membranes from Torpedo marmorata. *Proc. Natl. Acad. Sci. U.S.A.* 75, 4329–4333. doi: 10.1073/pnas.75.9.4329

Martín, V., Fabelo, N., Santpere, G., Puig, B., Marín, R., Ferrer, I., et al. (2010). Lipid alterations in lipid rafts from Alzheimer's disease human brain cortex. *J. Alzheimers. Dis.* 19, 489–502. doi: 10.3233/JAD-2010-1242

Martínez-Senac, M., Villalaín, J., and Gómez-Fernández, J. C. (1999). Structure of the Alzheimer beta-amyloid peptide (25-35) and its interaction with negatively charged phospholipid vesicles. *Eur. J. Biochem.* 265, 744–753. doi: 10.1046/j.1432-1327.1999.00775.x

Martorana, A., Esposito, Z., and Koch, G. (2010). Beyond the cholinergic hypothesis: do current drugs work in Alzheimer's disease? *CNS Neurosci. Ther.* 16, 235–245. doi: 10.1111/j.1755-5949.2010.00175.x

Mason, R. P., Shoemaker, W. J., Shajenko, L., Chambers, T. E., and Herbette, L. G. (1992). Evidence for changes in the Alzheimer's disease brain cortical membrane structure mediated by cholesterol. *Neurobiol. Aging* 13, 413–419. doi: 10.1016/0197-4580(92)90116-f

Massoulié, J. (2002). The origin of the molecular diversity and functional anchoring of cholinesterases. *Neurosignals* 11, 130–143. doi: 10.1159/000065054

Massoulié, J., Bon, S., Perrier, N., and Falasca, C. (2005). The C-terminal peptides of acetylcholinesterase: cellular trafficking, oligomerization and functional anchoring. *Chem. Biol. Interact.* 157-158, 3–14. doi: 10.1016/j.cbi.2005.10.002

Matsuzaki, K. (2007). Physicochemical interactions of amyloid β -peptide with lipid bilayers. *Biochim. Biophys. Acta* 1768, 1935–1942. doi: 10.1016/j.bbamem.2007.02.009

Matsuzaki, K., Kato, K., and Yanagisawa, K. (2010). Abeta polymerization through interaction with membrane gangliosides. *Biochim. Biophys. Acta* 1801, 868–877. doi: 10.1016/j.bbalip.2010.01.008

McKay, B. E., Placzek, A. N., and Dani, J. A. (2007). Regulation of synaptic transmission and plasticity by neuronal nicotinic acetylcholine receptors. *Biochem. Pharmacol.* 74, 1120–1133. doi: 10.1016/j.bcp.2007.07.001

McLaurin, J., and Chakrabartty, A. (1997). Characterization of the interactions of Alzheimer beta-amyloid peptides with phospholipid. *Eur. J. Biochem.* 1245, 355–363. doi: 10.1111/j.1432-1033.1997.t01-2-00355.x

McLaurin, J., Franklin, T., Fraser, P. E., and Chakrabartty, A. (1998). Structural transitions associated with the interaction of Alzheimer beta-amyloid peptides with gangliosides. *J. Biol. Chem.* 273, 4506–4515. doi: 10.1074/jbc.273.8.4506

Mehta, T. K., Dougherty, J. J., Wu, J., Choi, C. H., Khan, G. M., and Nichols, R. A. (2009). Defining pre-synaptic nicotinic receptors regulated by beta amyloid in mouse cortex and hippocampus with receptor null mutants. *J. Neurochem.* 109, 1452–1458. doi: 10.1111/j.1471-4159.2009.06070.x

Messi, M. L., Renganathan, M., Grigorenko, E., and Delbono, O. (1997). Activation of alpha7 nicotinic acetylcholine receptor promotes survival of spinal cord motoneurons. *FEBS Lett.* 411, 32–38. doi: 10.1016/s0014-5793(97)00600-5

Mesulam, M. M., Mufson, E. J., Levey, A. I., and Wainer, B. H. (1983). Cholinergic innervation of cortex by the basal forebrain: cytochemistry and cortical connections of the septal area, diagonal band nuclei, nucleus basalis (substantia innominata), and hypothalamus in the rhesus monkey. *J. Comp. Neurol.* 20, 170–197. doi: 10.1002/cne.902140206

Méthot, N., Demers, C. N., and Baenziger, J. E. (1995). Structure of both the ligand- and lipid-dependent channel-inactive states of the nicotinic acetylcholine receptor probed by FTIR spectroscopy and hydrogen exchange. *Biochemistry* 34, 15142–15149. doi: 10.1021/bi00046a021

Michikawa, M. (2003). The role of cholesterol in pathogenesis of Alzheimer's disease: dual metabolic interaction between amyloid β-protein and cholesterol. *Mol. Neurobiol.* 27, 1–12. doi: 10.1385/MN:27:1:1

Michikawa, M., Gong, J. S., Fan, Q. W., Sawamura, N., and Yanagisawa, K. (2001). A novel action of alzheimer's amyloid beta-protein (Abeta): oligomeric Abeta promotes lipid release. *J. Neurosci.* 218, 7226–7235.

Middlemas, D. S., and Raftery, M. A. (1987). Identification of Subunits of Acetylcholine Receptor That Interact with a Cholesterol Photoaffinity Probe. *Biochemistry* 126, 1219–1223. doi: 10.1021/bi00379a003

Milanesi, L., Sheynis, T., Xue, W. F., Orlova, E. V., Hellewell, A. L., Jelinek, R., et al. (2012). Direct three-dimensional visualization of membrane disruption by amyloid fibrils. *Proc. Natl. Acad. Sci. U.S.A.* 109, 20455–20460. doi: 10.1073/pnas.1206325109

Minota, S., and Watanabe, S. (1997). Inhibitory effects of arachidonic acid on nicotinic transmission in bullfrog sympathetic neurons. *J. Neurophysiol.* 178, 2396–2401. doi: 10.1152/jn.1997.78.5.2396

Molander-Melin, M., Blennow, K., Bogdanovic, N., Dellheden, B., and Fredman, P. (2005). Structural membrane alterations in Alzheimer brains found to be associated with regional disease development; increased density of gangliosides GM1 and GM2 and loss of cholesterol in detergent- resistant membrane domains. *J. Neurochem.* 92, 171–182. doi: 10.1111/j.1471-4159.2004.02849.x

Molinari, E. J., Delbono, O., Messi, M. L., Renganathan, M., Arneric, S. P., Sullivan, J. P., et al. (1998). Up-regulation of human alpha7 nicotinic receptors by chronic treatment with activator and antagonist ligands. *Eur. J. Pharmacol.* 347, 131–139. doi: 10.1016/s0014-2999(98)00084-3

Morán, M. A., Mufson, E. J., and Gómez-Ramos, P. (1993). Colocalization of cholinesterases with beta amyloid protein in aged and Alzheimer's brains. *Acta Neuropathol.* 85, 362–369. doi: 10.1007/bf00334445

Morley, B. J., and Happe, H. K. (2000). Cholinergic receptors: dual roles in transduction and plasticity. *Hear. Res.* 147, 104–112. doi: 10.1016/s0378-5955(00)00124-6

Mosqueira, A., Camino, P. A., and Barrantes, F. J. (2018). Cholesterol modulates acetylcholine receptor diffusion by tuning confinement sojourns and nanocluster stability. *Sci. Rep.* 8:11974. doi: 10.1038/s41598-018-30384

Mouritsen, O. G., and Bloom, M. (1984). Mattress model of lipid-protein interactions in membranes. *Biophys J.* 46, 141–153. doi: 10.1016/s0006-3495(84)84007-2

Muir, J. L., Page, K. J., Sirinathsinghji, D. J., Robbins, T. W., and Everitt, B. J. (1993). Excitotoxic lesions of basal forebrain cholinergic neurons: effects on learning, memory and attention. *Behav. Brain Res.* 157, 123–131. doi: 10.1016/0166-4328(93)90128-d

Müller, W. E., Kirsch, C., and Eckert, G. P. (2001). Membrane-disordering effects of beta-amyloid peptides. *Biochem. Soc. Trans.* 29, 617–623. doi: 10.1042/bst0290617

Müller, W. E., Koch, S., Eckert, A., Hartmann, H., and Scheuer, K. (1995). β-amyloid peptide decreases membrane fluidity. *Brain Res.* 674, 133–136. doi: 10.1016/0006-8993(94)01463-R

Murray, I. V. J., Liu, L., Komatsu, H., Uryu, K., Xiao, G., John, A., et al. (2007). Membrane-mediated amyloidogenesis and the promotion of oxidative lipid damage by amyloid beta proteins. *J. Biol. Chem.* 282, 9335–9345. doi: 10.1074/jbc.M608589200

Murray, J. K., Farooqi, B., Sadowsky, J. D., Scalf, M., Freund, W. A., Smith, L. M., et al. (2005). Efficient synthesis of a beta-peptide combinatorial library with microwave irradiation. *J. Am. Chem. Soc.* 127, 13271–13280. doi: 10.1021/ja052733v

Nagele, R. G., D'Andrea, M. R., Anderson, W. J., and Wang, H. Y. (2002). Intracellular accumulation of beta-amyloid(1-42) in neurons is facilitated by the alpha 7 nicotinic acetylcholine receptor in Alzheimer's disease. *Neuroscience* 110, 199–211. doi: 10.1016/s0306-4522(01)00460-2

Nagele, R. G., D'Andrea, M. R., Lee, H., Venkataraman, V., and Wang, H. Y. (2003). Astrocytes accumulate A beta 42 and give rise to astrocytic amyloid plaques in Alzheimer disease brains. *Brain Res.* 971, 197–209. doi: 10.1016/s0006-8993(03)02361-8

Nagele, R. G., Wegiel, J., Venkataraman, V., Imaki, H., Wang, K.-C., and Wegiel, J. (2004). Contribution of glial cells to the development of amyloid plaques in Alzheimer's disease. *Neurobiol. Aging* 25, 663–674. doi: 10.1016/j.neurobiolaging.2004.01.007

Nalivaeva, N. N., and Turner, A. J. (2016). Chemico-Biological Interactions AChE and the amyloid precursor protein (APP) -Cross-talk in Alzheimer's disease. *Chem. Biol. Interact.* 259, 301–306. doi: 10.1016/j.cbi.2016.04.009

Narayanaswami, V., Kim, J., and McNamee, M. G. (1993). Protein-lipid interactions and *Torpedo californica* nicotinic acetylcholine receptor function. 1. Spatial disposition of cysteine residues in the γ subunit analyzed by fluorescence-quenching and energy-transfer measurements. *Biochemistry* 32, 12413–12419. doi: 10.1021/bi00097a020

Narayanaswami, V., and McNamee, M. G. (1993). Protein-lipid interactions and Torpedo californica nicotinic acetylcholine receptor function. 2. Membrane fluidity and ligand-mediated alteration in the accessibility of gamma subunit cysteine residues to cholesterol. *Biochemistry* 123, 12420–12427. doi: 10.1021/bi00097a021

Nashmi, R., Dickinson, M. E., McKinney, S., Jareb, M., Labarca, C., Fraser, S. E., et al. (2003). Assembly of alpha4beta2 nicotinic acetylcholine receptors assessed with functional fluorescently labeled subunits: effects of localization, trafficking, and nicotine-induced upregulation in clonal mammalian cells and in cultured midbrain neurons. *J. Neurosci.* 23, 11554–11567. doi: 10.1523/jneurosci.23-37-11554.2003

Näslund, J., Haroutunian, V., Mohs, R., Davis, K. L., Davies, P., Greengard, P., et al. (2000). Correlation between elevated levels of amyloid beta-peptide in the brain and cognitive decline. *JAMA* 283, 1571–1577.

Näslund, J., Schierhorn, A., Hellman, U., Lannfelt, L., Roses, A. D., Tjernberg, L. O., et al. (1994). Relative abundance of Alzheimer A beta amyloid peptide variants in Alzheimer disease and normal aging. *Proc. Natl. Acad. Sci. U.S.A.* 91, 8378–8382. doi: 10.1073/pnas.91.18.8378

Navaratnam, D. S., Fernando, F. S., Priddle, J. D., Giles, K., Clegg, S. M., Pappin, D. J., et al. (2000). Hydrophobic protein that copurifies with human brain acetylcholinesterase: amino acid sequence, genomic organization, and chromosomal localization. *J. Neurochem.* 74, 2146–2153. doi: 10.1046/j.1471-4159.2000.0742146.x

Nees, F. (2015). The nicotinic cholinergic system function in the human brain. *Neuropharmacology* 96, 289–301. doi: 10.1016/j.neuropharm.2014.10.021

Nicolson, G. L. (2014). The fluid-mosaic model of membrane structure?: still relevant to understanding the structure, function and dynamics of biological membranes after more than 40 years. *Biochim. Biophys. Acta.* 1838, 1451–1466. doi: 10.1016/j.bbamem.2013.10.019

Niu, X., Zhang, X., Xie, J., and Zhang, X. (2012). Acetylcholinesterase blocks cleavage of APP by γ-secretase in 293 cells and mouse brain. *Mol. Neurodegener.* 7(Suppl. 1):S11. doi: 10.1186/1750-1326-7-S1-S11

Nordberg, A., Lundqvist, H., Hartvig, P., Lilja, A., and Långström, B. (1995). Kinetic analysis of regional (S)(-)11C-nicotine binding in normal and Alzheimer brains–in vivo assessment using positron emission tomography. *Alzheimer Dis. Assoc. Disord.* 9, 21–27. doi: 10.1097/00002093-199505000-00006

Nunomura, A., Tamaoki, T., Tanaka, K., Motohashi, N., Nakamura, M., and Hayashi, T. (2010). Intraneuronal amyloid beta accumulation and oxidative damage to nucleic acids in Alzheimer disease. *Neurobiol. Dis.* 37, 731–737. doi: 10.1016/j.nbd.2009.12.012

Nurowska, E., and Ruzzier, F. (1996). Corticosterone modifies the murine muscle acetylcholine receptor channel kinetics. *Neuroreport* 8, 77–80. doi: 10.1097/00001756-199612200-00016

Nurowska, E., and Ruzzier, F. (2002). Modulation of acetylcholine receptor channel kinetics by hydrocortisone. *Biochim. Biophys. Acta* 1564, 14–20. doi: 10.1016/s0005-2736(02)00356-5

Ochoa, E. L., Dalziel, A. W., and McNamee, M. G. (1983). Reconstitution of acetylcholine receptor function in lipid vesicles of defined composition. *Biochim. Biophys. Acta* 1727, 151–162. doi: 10.1016/0005-2736(83)90379-6

Opazo, C., Huang, X., Cherny, R. A., Moir, R. D., Roher, A. E., White, A. R., et al. (2002). Metalloenzyme-like activity of Alzheimer's disease beta-amyloid. Cu-dependent catalytic conversion of dopamine, cholesterol, and biological reducing agents to Neurotoxic H(2)O(2). *J. Biol. Chem.* 277, 40302–40308. doi: 10.1074/jbc.M206428200

Oshikawa, J., Toya, Y., Fujita, T., Egawa, M., Kawabe, J., Umemura, S., et al. (2003). Nicotinic acetylcholine receptor alpha 7 regulates cAMP signal within lipid rafts. *Am. J. Physiol. Cell. Physiol.* 285, C567–C574.

Oshima, N., Morishima-kawashima, M., Yamaguchi, H., Yoshimura, M., Schenk, D., and Ihara, Y. (2001). Accumulation of amyloid beta - protein in the low - density membrane domain accurately reflects the extent of beta -amyloid deposition in the Brain. *Am. J. Pathol.* 158, 2209–2218. doi: 10.1016/s0002-9440(10)64693-7

Palop, J. J., and Mucke, L. (2010). Amyloid-beta-induced neuronal dysfunction in Alzheimer's disease: from synapses toward neural networks. *Nat. Neurosci.* 13, 812–818. doi: 10.1038/nn.2583

Parri, H. R., Hernandez, C. M., and Dineley, K. T. (2011). Research update: Alpha7 nicotinic acetylcholine receptor mechanisms in Alzheimer's disease. *Biochem. Pharmacol.* 82, 931–942. doi: 10.1016/j.bcp.2011.06.039

Parvathy, S., Hussain, I., Karran, E. H., Turner, A. J., and Hooper, N. M. (1999). Cleavage of Alzheimer's amyloid precursor protein by alpha. -secretase occurs at the surface of neuronal cells. *Biochemistry* 38, 9728–9734. doi: 10.1021/bi9906827

Paterson, D., and Nordberg, A. (2000). Neuronal nicotinic receptors in the human brain. *Prog. Neurobiol.* 61, 75–111. doi: 10.1016/s0301-0082(99)00045-3

Pediconi, M. F., Gallegos, C. E., and Barrantes, F. J. (2004). Metabolic cholesterol depletion hinders cell-surface trafficking of the nicotinic acetylcholine receptor. *Neuroscience* 128, 239–249. doi: 10.1016/j.neuroscience.2004.06.007

Peña, V. B., Bonini, I. C., Antollini, S. S., Kobayashi, T., and Barrantes, F. J. (2011). A7-Type Acetylcholine Receptor Localization and Its Modulation By Nicotine and Cholesterol in Vascular Endothelial Cells. *J. Cell. Biochem.* 112, 3276–3288. doi: 10.1002/jcb.23254

Perez, R. G., Soriano, S., Hayes, J. D., Ostaszewski, B., Xia, W., Selkoe, D. J., et al. (1999). Mutagenesis identifies new signals for beta-amyloid precursor protein endocytosis, turnover, and the generation of secreted fragments, including Abeta42. *J. Biol. Chem.* 274, 18851–18856. doi: 10.1074/jbc.274.27.18851

Perillo, V. L., Peñalva, D. A., Vitale, A. J., Barrantes, F. J., and Antollini, S. S. (2016). Transbilayer asymmetry and sphingomyelin composition modulate the preferential membrane partitioning of the nicotinic acetylcholine receptor in Lo domains. *Arch. Biochem. Biophys.* 591, 76–86. doi: 10.1016/j.abb.2015.12.003

Perrier, A. L., Massoulié, J., and Krejci, E. (2002). PRiMA: the membrane anchor of acetylcholinesterase in the brain. *Neuron.* 33, 275–285.

Perry, E. K., Blessed, G., Tomlinson, B. E., Perry, R. H., Crow, T. J., Cross, A. J., et al. (1981). Neurochemical activities in human temporal lobe related to aging and Alzheimer-type changes. *Neurobiol. Aging* 2, 251–266.

Perry, E. K., Curtis, M., Dick, D. J., Candy, J. M., Atack, J. R., Bloxham, C. A., et al. (1985). Cholinergic correlates of cognitive impairment in Parkinson's disease: comparisons with Alzheimer's disease. *J. Neurol. Neurosurg. Psychiatry* 48, 413–421.

Perry, E. K., Johnson, M., Kerwin, J. M., Piggott, M. A., Court, J. A., Shaw, P. J., et al. (1992). Convergent cholinergic activities in aging and Alzheimer's disease. *Neurobiol. Aging* 13, 393–400. doi: 10.1016/0197-4580(92)90113-c

Perry, E. K., Perry, R. H., Smith, C. J., Dick, D. J., Candy, J. M., Edwardson, J. A., et al. (1987). Nicotinic receptor abnormalities in Alzheimer's and Parkinson's diseases. *J. Neurol. Neurosurg. Psychiatry* 50, 806–809.

Perry, G., Lipphardt, S., Mulvihill, P., Kancherla, M., Mijares, M., Gambetti, P., et al. (1988). Amyloid precursor protein in senile plaques of Alzheimer disease. *Lancet* 2, 746–751.

Peters, I., Igbavboa, U., Schütt, T., Haidari, S., Hartig, U., Rosello, X., et al. (2009). The interaction of beta-amyloid protein with cellular membranes stimulates its own production. *Biochim. Biophys. Acta* 1788, 964–972. doi: 10.1016/j.bbamem.2009.01.012

Petersen, R. C. (1977). Scopolamine induced learning failures in man. *Psychopharmacology* 52, 283–289. doi: 10.1007/BF00426713

Pettit, D. L., Shao, Z., and Yakel, J. L. (2001). Beta-Amyloid(1-42) peptide directly modulates nicotinic receptors in the rat hippocampal slice. *J. Neurosci.* 21:RC120.

Phinney, A. L., Horne, P., Yang, J., Janus, C., Bergeron, C., and Westaway, D. (2003). Mouse models of Alzheimer's disease: the long and filamentous road. *Neurol. Res.* 25, 590–600. doi: 10.1179/016164103101202020

Piomelli, D., Astarita, G., and Rapaka, R. (2007). A neuroscientist's guide to lipidomics. *Nat. Rev. Neurosci.* 8, 743–754. doi: 10.1038/nrn2233

Plant, L. D., Boyle, J. P., Smith, I. F., Peers, C., and Pearson, H. A. (2003). The production of amyloid beta peptide is a critical requirement for the viability of central neurons. *J. Neurosci.* 23, 5531–5535. doi: 10.1523/jneurosci.23-13-05531.2003

Pohanka, M. (2012). Alpha7 nicotinic acetylcholine receptor is a target in pharmacology and toxicology. *Int. J. Mol. Sci.* 13, 2219–2238. doi: 10.3390/ijms13022219

Pollard, H. B., Arispe, N., and Rojas, E. (1995). Ion Channel Hypothesis for Alzheimer Amyloid Peptide Neurotoxicity. *Cell. Mol. Neurobiol.* 15, 513–526. doi: 10.1007/bf02071314

Poveda, J. A., Encinar, J. A., Fernández, A. M., Mateo, C. R., Ferragut, J. A., and González-Ros, J. M. (2002). Segregation of phosphatidic acid-rich domains in reconstituted acetylcholine receptor membranes. *Biochemistry* 41, 12253–12262. doi: 10.1021/bi0200099

Poveda, J. A., Fernández, A. M., and Encinar, J. A. (2008). Protein-promoted membrane domains. *Biochim. Biophys. Acta* 1778, 1583–1590. doi: 10.1016/j.bbamem.2008.01.021

Puglielli, L., Konopka, G., Pack-Chung, E., Ingano, L. A. M., Berezovska, O., Hyman, B. T., et al. (2001). Acyl-coenzyme A: cholesterol acyltransferase modulates the generation of the amyloid β-peptide. *Nat. Cell. Biol.* 3, 905–912. doi: 10.1038/ncb1001-905

Puzzo, D., and Arancio, O. (2013). Amyloid-β peptide: Dr. Jekyll or Mr. Hyde? *J. Alzheimers Dis.* 33, S111–S120.

Puzzo, D., Gulisano, W., Arancio, O., and Palmeri, A. (2015). The keystone of Alzheimer pathogenesis might be sought in Aβ physiology. *Neuroscience* 307, 26–36. doi: 10.1016/j.neuroscience.2015.08.039

Puzzo, D., Privitera, L., Fa', M., Staniszewski, A., Hashimoto, G., Aziz, F., et al. (2011). Endogenous amyloid-β is necessary for hippocampal synaptic plasticity and memory. *Ann. Neurol.* 69, 819–830. doi: 10.1002/ana.22313

Puzzo, D., Privitera, L., Leznik, E., Fà, M., Staniszewski, A., Palmeri, A., et al. (2008). Picomolar amyloid-beta positively modulates synaptic plasticity and memory in hippocampus. *J. Neurosci.* 28, 14537–14545. doi: 10.1523/JNEUROSCI.2692-08.2008

Qiang, W., Yau, W. M., and Schulte, J. (2014). Fibrillation of β amyloid peptides in the presence of phospholipid bilayers and the consequent membrane disruption. *Biochim. Biophys. Acta* 1848, 266–276. doi: 10.1016/j.bbamem.2014.04.011

Quesada, O., González-Freire, C., Ferrer, M. C., Colón-Sáez, J. O., Fernández-García, E., Mercado, J., et al. (2016). Uncovering the lipidic basis for the preparation of functional nicotinic acetylcholine receptor detergent complexes for structural studies. *Sci. Rep.* 19:32766. doi: 10.1038/srep32766

Quinn, P. J. (2002). Plasma membrane phospholipid asymmetry. *Subcell Biochem.* 36, 39–60. doi: 10.1007/0-306-47931-1_3

Reid, P. C., Urano, Y., Kodama, T., and Hamakubo, T. (2007). Alzheimer's Disease?: cholesterol, membrane rafts, isoprenoids and statins. *J. Cell. Mol. Med.* 11, 383–392. doi: 10.1111/j.1582-4934.2007.00054.x

Relini, A., Marano, N., and Gliozzi, A. (2013). Misfolding of amyloidogenic proteins and their interactions with membranes. *Biomolecules* 27, 20–55. doi: 10.3390/biom4010020

Relini, A., Marano, N., and Gliozzi, A. (2014). Probing the interplay between amyloidogenic proteins and membranes using lipid monolayers and bilayers. *Adv. Colloid Interface Sci.* 207, 81–92. doi: 10.1016/j.cis.2013.10.015

Reyes, A. E., Perez, D. R., Alvarez, A., Garrido, J., Gentry, M. K., and Doctor, B. P. (1997). A monoclonal antibody against acetylcholinesterase inhibits the formation of amyloid fibrils induced by the enzyme. *Biochem. Biophys. Res. Commun.* 232, 652–655. doi: 10.1006/bbrc.1997.6357

Roccamo, A. M., Pediconi, M. F., Aztiria, E., Zanello, L., Wolstenholme, A., and Barrantes, F. J. (1999). Cells defective in sphingolipids biosynthesis express low amounts of muscle nicotinic acetylcholine receptor. *Eur. J. Neurosci.* 11, 1615–1623. doi: 10.1046/j.1460-9568.1999.00574.x

Rondelli, V., Brocca, P., Motta, S., Messa, M., Colombo, L., Salmona, M., et al. (2016). Amyloid - β Peptides in interaction with raft-mime model membranes: a neutron reflectivity insight. *Sci. Rep.* 16:20997. doi: 10.1038/srep20997

Rosenblum, W. I. (2014). Why Alzheimer trials fail: removing soluble oligomeric beta amyloid is essential, inconsistent, and difficult. *Neurobiol. Aging* 35, 969–974. doi: 10.1016/j.neurobiolaging.2013.10.085

Roth, G. S., Joseph, J. A., and Mason, R. P. (1995). Membrane alterations as causes of impaired signal transduction in Alzheimer's disease and aging. *Trends. Neurosci.* 18, 203–206. doi: 10.1016/0166-2236(95)93902-a

Rushworth, J. V., and Hooper, N. M. (2011). Lipid rafts: linking Alzheimer's Amyloid- β production, aggregation, and toxicity at neuronal membranes. *Int. J. Alzheimers Dis.* 2011:603052. doi: 10.4061/2011/603052

Sáez-Valero, J., Sberna, G., McLean, C. A., and Small, D. H. (1999). Molecular isoform distribution and glycosylation of acetylcholinesterase are altered in brain and cerebrospinal fluid of patients with Alzheimer's disease. *J. Neurochem.* 72, 1600–1608. doi: 10.1046/j.1471-4159.1999.721600.x

Sargent, P. B., Bryan, G. K., Streichert, L. C., and Garrett, E. N. (1991). Denervation does not alter the number of neuronal bungarotoxin binding sites on autonomic neurons in the frog cardiac ganglion. *J. Neurosci.* 11, 3610–3623. doi: 10.1523/jneurosci.11-11-03610.1991

Sargent, P. B., and Garrett, E. N. (1995). The characterization of alpha-bungarotoxin receptors on the surface of parasympathetic neurons in the frog heart. *Brain Res.* 680, 99–107. doi: 10.1016/0006-8993(95)00250-t

Sarter, M., and Bruno, J. P. (1997). Cognitive functions of cortical acetylcholine: toward a unifying hypothesis. *Brain Res.* 23, 28–46. doi: 10.1016/s0165-0173(96)00009-4

Sarter, M., and Paolone, G. (2011). Deficits in attentional control: cholinergic mechanisms and circuitry-based treatment approaches. *Behav. Neurosci.* 125, 825–835. doi: 10.1037/a0026227

Sasahara, K., Morigaki, K., and Shinya, K. (2013). Effects of membrane interaction and aggregation of amyloid β-peptide on lipid mobility and membrane domain structure. *Phys. Chem. Chem. Phys.* 15, 8929–8939. doi: 10.1039/c3cp44517h

Schmidt, J. T., and Freeman, J. A. (1980). Electrophysiologic evidence that retinotectal synaptic transmission in the goldfish is nicotinic cholinergic. *Brain Res.* 187, 129–142. doi: 10.1016/0006-8993(80)90499-0

Scholze, P., Ciuraszkiewicz, A., Groessl, F., Orr-Urtreger, A., McIntosh, J. M., and Huck, S. (2011). α4β2 nicotinic acetylcholine receptors in the early postnatal mouse superior cervical ganglion. *Dev. Neurobiol.* 71, 390–399. doi: 10.1002/dneu.20870

Sciacca, M. F., Kotler, S. A., Brender, J. R., Chen, J., Lee, D. K., and Ramamoorthy, A. (2012). Two-step mechanism of membrane disruption by Aβ through membrane fragmentation and pore formation. *Biophys. J.* 103, 702–710. doi: 10.1016/j.bpj.2012.06.045

Seghezza, S., Diaspro, A., Canale, C., and Dante, S. (2014). Cholesterol drives aβ(1-42) interaction with lipid rafts in model membranes. *Langmuir* 30, 13934–13941. doi: 10.1021/la502966m

Sepúlveda, F. J., Fierro, H., Fernandez, E., Castillo, C., Peoples, R. W., Opazo, C., et al. (2014). Nature of the neurotoxic membrane actions of amyloid-β on hippocampal neurons in Alzheimer's disease. *Neurobiol. Aging* 5, 472–481. doi: 10.1016/j.neurobiolaging.2013.08.035

Serrano-Pozo, A., Frosch, M. P., Masliah, E., and Hyman, B. T. (2011). Neuropathological alterations in Alzheimer disease. *Cold. Spring. Harb. Perspect. Med.* 1:a006189. doi: 10.1101/cshperspect.a006189

Shankar, G. M., Li, S., Mehta, T. H., Garcia-Munoz, A., Shepardson, N. E., Smith, I., et al. (2008). Amyloid-beta protein dimers isolated directly from Alzheimer's brains impair synaptic plasticity and memory. *Nat. Med.* 14, 837–842. doi: 10.1038/nm1782

Sharma, G., and Vijayaraghavan, S. (2001). Nicotinic cholinergic signaling in hippocampal astrocytes involves calcium-induced calcium release from intracellular stores. *Proc. Natl. Acad. Sci. U.S.A.* 98, 4148–4153. doi: 10.1073/pnas.071540198

Sharp, L., Salari, R., and Brannigan, G. (2019). Boundary lipids of the nicotinic acetylcholine receptor: spontaneous partitioning via coarse-grained molecular dynamics simulation. *Biochim. Biophys. Acta. Biomembr.* 1861, 887–896. doi: 10.1016/j.bbamem.2019.01.005

Shen, J., and Wu, J. (2015). Nicotinic cholinergic mechanisms in Alzheimer's disease. *Int. Rev. Neurobiol.* 124, 275–292. doi: 10.1016/bs.irn.2015.08.00

Shen, J. X., and Yakel, J. L. (2009). Nicotinic acetylcholine receptor-mediated calcium signaling in the nervous system. *Acta Pharmacol. Sin.* 30, 673–680. doi: 10.1038/aps.2009.64

Shimohama, S., Taniguchi, T., Fujiwara, M., and Kameyama, M. (1986). Changes in nicotinic and muscarinic cholinergic receptors in Alzheimer-type dementia. *J. Neurochem.* 46, 288–293. doi: 10.1111/j.1471-4159.1986.tb12960.x

Shringarpure, R., Grune, T., Sitte, N., and Davies, K. J. (2000). 4-Hydroxynonenal-modified amyloid-beta peptide inhibits the proteasome: possible importance in Alzheimer's disease. *Cell. Mol. Life Sci.* 57, 1802–1809. doi: 10.1007/pl00000660

Silveyra, M. X., Evin, G., Montenegro, M. F., Vidal, C. J., Martínez, S., and Culvenor, J. G. (2008). Presenilin 1 interacts with acetylcholinesterase and alters its enzymatic activity and glycosylation. *Mol. Cell. Biol.* 28, 2908–2919. doi: 10.1128/MCB.02065-2067

Silveyra, M. X., García-Ayllón, M. S., Serra-Basante, C., Mazzoni, V., García-Gutierrez, M. S., and Manzanares, J. (2012). Changes in acetylcholinesterase expression are associated with altered presenilin-1 levels. *Neurobiol. Aging* 33, 627–637. doi: 10.1016/j.neurobiolaging.2011.04.006

Simons, K., and Ikonen, E. (1997). Functional rafts in cell membranes. *Nature* 387, 569–572. doi: 10.1038/42408

Simons, K., and van Meer, G. (1988). Lipid sorting in epithelial cells. *Biochemistry* 23, 6197–6202. doi: 10.1021/bi00417a001

Simons, M., Keller, P., De Strooper, B., Beyreuther, K., Dotti, C. G., and Simons, K. (1998). Cholesterol depletion inhibits the generation of beta-amyloid in hippocampal neurons. *Proc. Natl. Acad. Sci. U.S.A.* 95, 6460–6464. doi: 10.1073/pnas.95.11.6460

Singer, A. S. J., and Nicolson, G. L. (1972). The Fluid Mosaic Model of the Structure of Cell Membranes. *Science* 175, 720–731. doi: 10.1126/science.175.4023.720

Small, D. H., Maksel, D., Kerr, M. L., Ng, J., Hou, X., Chu, C., et al. (2007). The b -amyloid protein of Alzheimer's disease binds to membrane lipids but does not bind to the a 7 nicotinic acetylcholine receptor. *J. Neurochem.* 101, 1527–1538. doi: 10.1111/j.1471-4159.2006.04444.x

Small, D. H., Michaelson, S., and Sberna, G. (1996). Non-classical actions of cholinesterases: role in cellular differentiation, tumorigenesis and Alzheimer's disease. *Neurochem. Int.* 28, 453–483. doi: 10.1016/0197-0186(95)00099-2

Sonnino, S., and Prinetti, A. (2013). Membrane domains and the "lipid raft" concept. *Curr Med Chem.* 20, 4–21. doi: 10.2174/0929867311320010003

Staneva, G., Puff, N., Stanimirov, S., Tochev, T., Angelova, M. I., and Seigneuret, M. (2018). The Alzheimer's disease amyloid-β peptide affects the size-dynamics of raft-mimicking Lo domains in GM1-containing lipid bilayers. *Soft. Matter.* 14, 9609–9618. doi: 10.1039/c8sm01636d

Stefani, M. (2010). Biochemical and biophysical features of both oligomer/fibril and cell membrane in amyloid cytotoxicity. *FEBS J.* 277, 4602–4613. doi: 10.1111/j.1742-4658.2010.07889.x

Stetzkowski-Marden, F., Gaus, K., Recouvreur, M., Cartaud, A., and Cartaud, J. (2006a). Agrin elicits membrane lipid condensation at sites of acetylcholine receptor clusters in C2C12 myotubes. *J. Lipid. Res.* 47, 2121–2133. doi: 10.1194/jlr.M600182-JLR200

Stetzkowski-Marden, F., Recouvreur, M., Camus, G., Cartaud, A., Marchand, S., and Cartaud, J. (2006b). Rafts are required for acetylcholine receptor clustering. *J. Mol. Neurosci.* 30, 37–38. doi: 10.1385/JMN:30:1:37

Subasinghe, S., Unabia, S., Barrow, C. J., Mok, S. S., Aguilar, M. I., and Small, D. H. (2003). Cholesterol is necessary both for the toxic effect of Abeta peptides on vascular smooth muscle cells and for Abeta binding to vascular smooth muscle cell membranes. *J. Neurochem.* 84, 471–479. doi: 10.1046/j.1471-4159.2003.01552.x

Sun, J., and Roy, S. (2018). The physical approximation of APP and BACE-1: a key event in alzheimer's disease pathogenesis. *Dev. Neurobiol.* 78, 340–347. doi: 10.1002/dneu.22556

Sunshine, C., and McNamee, M. G. (1992). Lipid modulation of nicotinic acetylcholine receptor function: the role of neutral and negatively charged lipids. *Biochim. Biophys. Acta* 1108, 240–246. doi: 10.1016/0005-2736(92)90031-g

Sunshine, C., and McNamee, M. G. (1994). Lipid modulation of nicotinic acetylcholine receptor function: the role of membrane lipid composition and fluidity. *Biochim. Biophys. Acta* 1191, 59–64. doi: 10.1016/0005-2736(94)90233-X

Tan, J. Z. A., and Gleeson, P. A. (2019). The role of membrane trafficking in the processing of amyloid precursor protein and production of amyloid peptides in Alzheimer's disease. *BBA - Biomembr.* 1861, 697–712. doi: 10.1016/j.bbamem.2018.11.013

Tapiola, T., Pirttilä, T., Mehta, P. D., Alafuzofff, I., Lehtovirta, M., and Soininen, H. (2000). Relationship between apoE genotype and CSF beta-amyloid (1-42) and tau in patients with probable and definite Alzheimer's disease. *Neurobiol. Aging* 21, 735–740. doi: 10.1016/s0197-4580(00)00164-0

Tenchov, B. G., MacDonald, R. C., and Siegel, D. P. (2006). Cubic phases in phosphatidylcholine-cholesterol mixtures: cholesterol as membrane "fusogen". *Biophys. J.* 91, 2508–2516. doi: 10.1529/biophysj.106.083766

Terzi, E., Hölzemann, G., and Seelig, J. (1997). Interaction of Alzheimer beta-amyloid peptide(1-40) with lipid membranes. *Biochemistry* 36, 14845–14852. doi: 10.1021/bi971843e

Thomsen, M. S., Andreasen, J. T., Arvaniti, M., and Kohlmeier, K. A. (2016). Nicotinic Acetylcholine receptors in the pathophysiology of Al zheimer's disease: the role of protein-protein interactions in current and future treatment. *Curr. Pharm. Des.* 22, 2015–2034. doi: 10.2174/1381612822666160127112357

Thornton, E., Vink, R., Blumbergs, P. C., and Van Den Heuvel, C. (2006). Soluble amyloid precursor protein alpha reduces neuronal injury and improves functional outcome following diffuse traumatic brain injury in rats. *Brain Res.* 1094, 38–46. doi: 10.1016/j.brainres.2006.03.107

Tozaki, H., Matsumoto, A., Kanno, T., Nagai, K., Nagata, T., Yamamoto, S., et al. (2002). The inhibitory and facilitatory actions of amyloid-beta peptides on nicotinic ACh receptors and AMPA receptors. *Biochem. Biophys. Res. Commun.* 294, 42–45. doi: 10.1016/S0006-291X(02)00429-421

Turner, P. R., O'Connor, K., Tate, W. P., and Abraham, W. C. (2003). Roles of amyloid precursor protein and its fragments in regulating neural activity, plasticity and memory. *Prog Neurobiol.* 70, 1–32. doi: 10.1016/s0301-0082(03)00089-3

Unwin, N. (2005). Refined structure of the nicotinic acetylcholine receptor at 4A resolution. *J. Mol. Biol.* 346, 967–989. doi: 10.1016/j.jmb.2004.12.031

Uranga, R. M., Alza, N. P., Conde, M. A., Antollini, S. S., and Salvador, G. A. (2017). Phosphoinositides: two-path signaling in neuronal response to Oligomeric amyloid β peptide. *Mol. Neurobiol.* 54, 3236–3252. doi: 10.1007/s12035-016-9885-9883

van Meer, G. (2011). Dynamic transbilayer lipid asymmetry. *Cold Spring Harb. Perspect. Biol.* 3:004671. doi: 10.1101/cshperspect.a004671

Vestergaard, M., Hamada, T., Morita, M., and Takagi, M. (2010). Cholesterol, Lipids, Amyloid Beta, and Alzheimer' s. *Curr. Alzheimer Res.* 7, 262–270. doi: 10.2174/156720510791050821

Vetrivel, K. S., Cheng, H., Kim, S., Chen, Y., Barnes, N. Y., Parent, A. T., et al. (2005). Spatial segregation of gamma-secretase and substrates in distinct membrane domains. *J. Biol. Chem.* 280, 25892–25900. doi: 10.1074/jbc.M503570200

Vetrivel, K. S., Cheng, H., Lin, W., Sakurai, T., Li, T., Nukina, N., et al. (2004). Association of γ-secretase with lipid rafts in post-Golgi and endosome membranes. *J. Biol. Chem.* 279, 44945–44954. doi: 10.1074/jbc.M407986200

Vetrivel, K. S., and Thinakaran, G. (2006). Amyloidogenic processing of beta-amyloid precursor protein in intracellular compartments. *Neurology* 66, 69–73. doi: 10.1212/01.wnl.0000192107.17175.39

Villar, M. T., Artigues, A., Ferragut, J. A., and Gonzalez-Ros, J. M. (1988). Phospholipase A2 hydrolysis of membrane phospholipids causes structural alteration of the nicotinic acetylcholine receptor. *Biochim. Biophys. Acta* 938, 35–43. doi: 10.1016/0005-2736(88)90119-8

Wahrle, S., Das, P., Nyborg, A. C., Mclendon, C., Shoji, M., Kawarabayashi, T., et al. (2002). Cholesterol-dependent gamma-secretase activity in buoyant cholesterol-rich membrane microdomains. *Neurobiol. Dis.* 9, 11–23. doi: 10.1006/nbdi.2001.0470

Wakabayashi, M., Okada, T., Kozutsumi, Y., and Matsuzaki, K. (2005). GM1 ganglioside-mediated accumulation of amyloid beta-protein on cell membranes. *Biochem. Biophys. Res. Commun.* 328, 1019–1023. doi: 10.1016/j.bbrc.2005.01.060

Wang, H.-Y., Lee, D. H., Davis, C. B., and Shank, R. P. (2000a). Amyloid peptide Abeta(1-42) binds selectively and with picomolar affinity to alpha7 nicotinic acetylcholine receptors. *J. Neurochem.* 75, 1155–1161. doi: 10.1046/j.1471-4159.2000.0751155.x

Wang, H.-Y., Lee, D. H. S., D'Andrea, M. R., Peterson, P. A., Shank, R. P., and Reitz, A. B. (2000b). β-amyloid$_{1-42}$ binds to α7 nicotinic acetylcholine receptor with high affinity. Implications for Alzheimer's disease pathology. *J. Biol. Chem.* 275, 5626–5632. doi: 10.1074/jbc.275.8.5626

Wang, H. Y., Li, W., Benedetti, N. J., and Lee, D. H. (2003). Alpha 7 nicotinic acetylcholine receptors mediate beta-amyloid peptide-induced tau protein phosphorylation. *J. Biol. Chem.* 278, 1547–1553. doi: 10.1074/jbc.M212532200

Wang, H. Y., Stucky, A., Liu, J., Shen, C., Trocme-Thibierge, C., and Morain, P. (2009). Dissociating beta-amyloid from alpha 7 nicotinic acetylcholine receptor by a novel therapeutic agent, S 24795, normalizes alpha 7 nicotinic acetylcholine and NMDA receptor function in Alzheimer's disease brain. *J. Neurosci.* 229, 10961–10973. doi: 10.1523/JNEUROSCI.6088-08.2009

Wang, Y., Qu, D., and Wang, K. (2016). Therapeutic approaches to Alzheimer's disease through stimulating of non-amyloidogenic processing of amyloid precursor protein. *Eur. Rev. Med. Pharmacol. Sci.* 20, 2389–2403.

Watson, H. (2015). Biological membranes. *Essays Biochem.* 59, 43–69. doi: 10.1042/bse0590043

Wen, P.-C., Mahinthichaichan, P., Trebesch, N., Jiang, T., Zhao, Z., Shinn, E., et al. (2018). Microscopic view of lipids and their diverse biological functions. *Curr. Opin. Struct. Biol.* 51, 177–186. doi: 10.1016/j.sbi.2018.07.003

Wenk, G. L. (1997). The nucleus basallis magnocellularis cholinergic system: one hundred years of progress. *Neurobiol. Learn. Mem.* 67, 85–95. doi: 10.1006/nlme.1996.3757

Wenz, J. J., and Barrantes, F. J. (2005). Nicotinic acetylcholine receptor induces lateral segregation of phosphatidic acid and phosphatidylcholine in reconstituted membranes. *Biochemistry* 44, 398–410. doi: 10.1021/bi048026g

Whitehouse, P. J., Martino, A. M., Antuono, P. G., Lowenstein, P. R., Coyle, J. T., Price, D. L., et al. (1986). Nicotinic acetylcholine binding sites in Alzheimer's disease. *Brain Res.* 371, 146–151. doi: 10.1016/0006-8993(86)90819-x

Whitehouse, P. J., Price, D. L., Clark, A. W., Coyle, J. T., and DeLong, M. R. (1981). Alzheimer disease: evidence for selective loss of cholinergic neurons in the nucleus basalis. *Ann. Neurol.* 10, 122–126. doi: 10.1002/ana.410100203

Whitehouse, P. J., Struble, R. G., Clark, A. W., and Price, D. L. (1982). Alzheimer disease: plaques, tangles, and the basal forebrain. *Ann. Neurol.* 12:494. doi: 10.1002/ana.410120517

Willmann, R., Pun, S., Sadasivam, G., Santos, A. F., Caroni, P., and Fuhrer, C. (2006). Cholesterol and lipid microdomains stabilize the postsynapse at the neuromuscular junction. *EMBO J.* 25, 4050–4060. doi: 10.1038/sj.emboj.7601288

Wonnacott, S., Barik, J., Dickinson, J., and Jones, I. W. (2006). Nicotinic receptors modulate transmitter cross talk in the CNS: Nicotinic modulation of transmitters. *J. Mol. Neurosci.* 30, 137–140. doi: 10.1385/JMN:30:1:137

Wood, W. G., Li, L., Müller, W. E., and Eckert, G. P. (2014). Cholesterol as a causative factor in Alzheimer disease: a debatable hypothesis. *J.Neurochem.* 129, 559–572. doi: 10.1111/jnc.12637

Wood, W. G., Schroeder, F., Igbavboa, U., Avdulov, N. A., and Chochina, S. V. (2002). Brain membrane cholesterol domains, aging and amyloid beta-peptides. *Neurobiol. Aging* 23, 685–694. doi: 10.1016/s0197-4580(02)00018-0

Woolf, N. J. (1998). A structural basis for memory storage in mammals. *Prog. Neurobiol.* 55, 59–77. doi: 10.1016/s0301-0082(97)00094-4

Wu, J., Khan, G. M., and Nichols, R. A. (2007). Dopamine release in prefrontal cortex in response to beta-amyloid activation of alpha7 nicotinic receptors. *Brain Res.* 1182, 82–89. doi: 10.1016/j.brainres.2007.08.079

Wu, J., Kuo, Y. P., George, A. A., Xu, L., Hu, J., and Lukas, R. J. (2004). Beta-Amyloid directly inhibits human alpha4beta2-nicotinic acetylcholine receptors heterologously expressed in human SH-EP1 cells. *J. Biol. Chem.* 279, 37842–37851. doi: 10.1074/jbc.M400335200

Wu, Y., and Luo, Y. (2005). Transgenic C. *elegans as a model in Alzheimer's research. Curr. Alzheimer. Res.* 2, 37–45. doi: 10.2174/1567205052772768

Xie, H. Q., Leung, K. W., Chen, V. P., Chan, G. K. L., Xu, S. L., Guo, A. J. Y., et al. (2010a). Chemico-Biological Interactions PRiMA directs a restricted localization of tetrameric AChE at synapses. *Chem. Biol. Interact.* 187, 78–83. doi: 10.1016/j.cbi.2010.02.018

Xie, H. Q., Liang, D., Leung, K. W., Chen, V. P., Zhu, K. Y., Chan, W. K. B., et al. (2010b). Targeting Acetylcholinesterase to Membrane Rafts a function mediated by the proline-rich membrane anchor (PRiMA) in neurons. *J. Biol. Chem.* 285, 11537–11546. doi: 10.1074/jbc.M109.038711

Xiong, H., Callaghan, D., Jones, A., Walker, D. G., Lue, L. F., and Beach, T. G. (2008). Cholesterol retention in Alzheimer's brain is responsible for high beta- and gamma-secretase activities and Abeta production. *Neurobiol. Dis.* 29, 422–437. doi: 10.1016/j.nbd.2007.10.005

Xiu, J., Nordberg, A., Zhang, J. T., and Guan, Z. Z. (2005). Expression of nicotinic receptors on primary cultures of rat astrocytes and up-regulation of the alpha7, alpha4 and beta2 subunits in response to nanomolar concentrations of the beta-amyloid peptide(1-42). *Neurochem. Int.* 47, 281–290. doi: 10.1016/j.neuint.2005.04.023

Yahi, N., and Fantini, J. (2014). Deciphering the glycolipid code of Alzheimer's and Parkinson's amyloid proteins allowed the creation of a universal ganglioside-binding peptide. *PLoS One.* 9:e104751. doi: 10.1371/journal.pone.0104751

Yamamoto, N., Hasegawa, K., Matsuzaki, K., Naiki, H., and Yanagisawa, K. (2004). Environment- and mutation-dependent aggregation behavior of Alzheimer amyloid beta-protein. *J. Neurochem.* 90, 62–69. doi: 10.1111/j.1471-4159.2004.02459.x

Yamamoto, N., Matsubara, T., Sato, T., and Yanagisawa, K. (2008). Age-dependent high-density clustering of GM1 ganglioside at presynaptic neuritic terminals promotes amyloid β -protein fi brillogenesis. *Biochim. Biophys. Acta* 1778, 2717–2726. doi: 10.1016/j.bbamem.2008.07.028

Yamamoto, N., Matsuzaki, K., and Yanagisawa, K. (2005). Cross-seeding of wild-type and hereditary variant-type amyloid beta-proteins in the presence of gangliosides. *J. Neurochem.* 95, 1167–1176. doi: 10.1111/j.1471-4159.2005.03444.x

Yanagisawa, K. (2005). GM1 ganglioside and the seeding of amyloid in Alzheimer's disease: endogenous seed for Alzheimer amyloid. *Neuroscientist* 11, 250–260. doi: 10.1177/1073858405275177

Yanagisawa, K., and Ihara, Y. (1998). GM1 ganglioside-bound amyloid beta-protein in Alzheimer's disease brain. *Neurobiol. Aging* 19(1 Suppl.), S65–S67. doi: 10.1177/1073858405275177

Yanagisawa, K., Odaka, A., Suzuki, N., and Ihara, Y. (1995). GM1 ganglioside-bound amyloid beta-protein (A beta): a possible form of preamyloid in Alzheimer's disease. *Nat. Med.* 1, 1062–1066. doi: 10.1038/nm1095-1062

Yang, X., Askarova, S., and Lee, J. C.-M. (2010). Membrane biophysics and mechanics in Alzheimer's disease. *Mol. Neurobiol.* 41, 138–148. doi: 10.1007/s12035-010-8121-9

Yankner, B. A., Duffy, L. K., and Kirschner, D. A. (1990). Neurotrophic and neurotoxic effects of amyloid beta protein: reversal by tachykinin neuropeptides. *Science* 250, 279–282. doi: 10.1126/science.2218531

Yip, C. M., Darabie, A. A., and McLaurin, J. (2002). Abeta42-peptide assembly on lipid bilayers. *J. Mol. Biol.* 318, 97–107. doi: 10.1016/s0022-2836(02)00028-1

Yu, W. F., Guan, Z. Z., Bogdanovic, N., and Nordberg, A. (2005). High selective expression of alpha7 nicotinic receptors on astrocytes in the brains of patients with sporadic Alzheimer's disease and patients carrying Swedish APP 670/671 mutation: a possible association with neuritic plaques. *Exp. Neurol.* 2192, 215–225. doi: 10.1016/j.expneurol.2004.12.015

Yu, X., and Zheng, J. (2012). Cholesterol promotes the interaction of Alzheimer β-amyloid monomer with lipid bilayer. *J. Mol. Biol.* 421, 561–571. doi: 10.1016/j.jmb.2011.11.006

Zampagni, M., Evangelisti, E., Cascella, R., Liguri, G., Becatti, M., Pensalfini, A., et al. (2010). Lipid rafts are primary mediators of amyloid oxidative attack on plasma membrane. *J. Mol. Med.* 88, 597–608. doi: 10.1007/s00109-010-0603-608

Zhang, Q., Powers, E. T., Nieva, J., Huff, M. E., Dendle, M. A., Bieschke, J., et al. (2004). Metabolite-initiated protein misfolding may trigger Alzheimer's disease. *Proc. Natl. Acad. Sci. U.S.A.* 101, 4752–4757. doi: 10.1073/pnas.040092 4101

Zhu, D., Xiong, W. C., and Mei, L. (2006). Lipid rafts serve as a signaling platform for Nicotinic Acetylcholine receptor clustering. *J. Neurosci.* 26, 4841–4851. doi: 10.1523/JNEUROSCI.2807-05.2006

Zimmerberg, J., and Gawrisch, K. (2006). The physical chemistry of biological membranes. *Nat. Chem. Biol.* 2, 564–567. doi: 10.1038/nchembio11 06-564

Zou, K., Gong, J. S., Yanagisawa, K., and Michikawa, M. (2002). A novel function of monomeric amyloid beta-protein serving as an antioxidant molecule against metal-induced oxidative damage. *J. Neurosci.* 22, 4833–4841. doi: 10.1523/jneurosci.22-12-04833.2002

Zou, K., Kim, D., Kakio, A., Byun, K., Gong, J. S., Kim, J., et al. (2003). Amyloid beta-protein (Abeta)1-40 protects neurons from damage induced by Abeta1-42 in culture and in rat brain. *J. Neurochem.* 87, 609–619. doi: 10.1046/j.1471-4159.2003.02018.x

12

Molecular Modulation of Human α7 Nicotinic Receptor by Amyloid-β Peptides

*Matías Lasala, Camila Fabiani, Jeremías Corradi, Silvia Antollini and Cecilia Bouzat**

Instituto de Investigaciones Bioquímicas de Bahía Blanca (INIBIBB), Departamento de Biología, Bioquímica y Farmacia, Universidad Nacional del Sur-Consejo Nacional de Investigaciones Científicas y Técnicas (CONICET), Bahía Blanca, Argentina

Correspondence:
Cecilia Bouzat
inbouzat@criba.edu.ar

Amyloid β peptide (Aβ) is a key player in the development of Alzheimer's disease (AD). It is the primary component of senile plaques in AD patients and is also found in soluble forms. Cholinergic activity mediated by α7 nicotinic receptors has been shown to be affected by Aβ soluble forms. To shed light into the molecular mechanism of this effect, we explored the direct actions of oligomeric $A\beta_{1-40}$ and $A\beta_{1-42}$ on human α7 by fluorescence spectroscopy and single-channel recordings. Fluorescence measurements using the conformational sensitive probe crystal violet (CrV) revealed that in the presence of Aβ α7 undergoes concentration-dependent conformational changes. Exposure of α7 to 100 pM Aβ changes CrV K_D towards that of the desensitized state. However, α7 is still reactive to high carbamylcholine (Carb) concentrations. These observations are compatible with the induction of active/desensitized states as well as of a novel conformational state in the presence of both Aβ and Carb. At 100 nM Aβ, α7 adopts a resting-state-like structure which does not respond to Carb, suggesting stabilization of α7 in a blocked state. In real time, we found that Aβ is capable of eliciting α7 channel activity either in the absence or presence of the positive allosteric modulator (PAM) PNU-120596. Activation by Aβ is favored at picomolar or low nanomolar concentrations and is not detected at micromolar concentrations. At high Aβ concentrations, the mean duration of activation episodes elicited by ACh in the presence of PNU-120596 is significantly reduced, an effect compatible with slow open-channel block. We conclude that Aβ directly affects α7 function by acting as an agonist and a negative modulator. Whereas the capability of low concentrations of Aβ to activate α7 could be beneficial, the reduced α7 activity in the presence of higher Aβ concentrations or its long exposure may contribute to the cholinergic signaling deficit and may be involved in the initiation and development of AD.

Keywords: nicotinic receptor, patch-clamp recordings, single-channel currents, Cys-loop receptor, amyloid peptide, crystal violet

Abbreviations: ACh, acetylcholine; Carb, carbamylcholine; $A\beta_{1-42}$, amyloid-β_{1-42} peptide; $A\beta_{1-40}$, amyloid-β_{1-40} peptide; nAChR, nicotinic acetylcholine receptor; CrV, crystal violet; NS-1738, N-(5-Chloro-2-hydroxyphenyl)-N′-[2-chloro-5-(trifluoromethyl) phenyl]urea; PNU-120596, [N-(5-Chloro-2,4-dimethoxyphenyl)-N′-(5-methyl-3-isoxazolyl)-urea].

INTRODUCTION

Alzheimer's disease (AD) is a progressive neurodegenerative disease characterized by loss of memory, multiple cognitive impairments and changes in personality and behavior. Memory impairment in AD is associated with neuronal degeneration as well as synaptic damage. Although AD is a multifactorial disease, accumulation of amyloid-β peptides (Aβ) is one of the major pathological factors. Accumulation phase starts with low molecular weight fractions of Aβ (monomers, dimers, or trimers) and continues with larger oligomers or insoluble amyloid fibrils (Sadigh-Eteghad et al., 2014). Although plaques remain the principal identifiers and predictors of Alzheimer's disease, a clear paradigm shift has occurred that emphasizes the primacy of Aβ oligomers in disease causation (Lacor et al., 2004; Shankar et al., 2008; Hayden and Teplow, 2013; Collins-Praino et al., 2014). Despite all research efforts, there are still many unsolved aspects regarding the molecular mechanisms underlying Aβ pathogenic actions. One of these mechanisms involves the interaction of Aβ with synaptic receptors, which consequently emerge as novel druggable sites to restore cognitive functions in AD patients (Kandimalla and Reddy, 2017).

Cholinergic neurons with a pivotal role in learning and memory are mainly involved in the pathogenesis of AD. Indeed, inhibitors of acetylcholinesterase (AChE), which by decreasing ACh breakdown enhance cholinergic neurotransmission, are to date one of the main specific therapeutic drugs, although their efficacy is limited (Kandimalla and Reddy, 2017).

The α7 nicotinic acetylcholine receptor (nAChR) has been shown to be associated with AD. α7 is highly expressed in hippocampus, cortex and several subcortical limbic regions and is involved in cognition, sensory processing information, attention, working memory, and reward pathways (Lendvai et al., 2013). Reduction of α7 in brain, particularly in the hippocampus, has been reported in AD patients (Buckingham et al., 2009; Dineley et al., 2015).

α7 is a pentameric ligand-gated ion channel that responds to ACh by opening an intrinsic channel permeable to cations that triggers rapid membrane depolarization and calcium influx (Wonnacott, 2014). However, α7 also acts as a metabotropic receptor and triggers several signal transduction pathways as well as the release of calcium from intracellular stores (Kabbani et al., 2013; Egea et al., 2015; Guan et al., 2015; Corradi and Bouzat, 2016; Bouzat et al., 2018). This metabotropic activity has been associated to synaptic plasticity and neuroprotection, including against Aβ damage (Buckingham et al., 2009; Inestrosa et al., 2013; Jin et al., 2015).

Enhancement of α7 activity is emerging as a therapeutic strategy for cognitive impairment in AD. Positive allosteric modulators (PAMs) are the most promising therapeutic compounds because they maintain the temporal and spatial characteristics of endogenous activation, are more selective than agonists, and reduce tolerance due to desensitization (Chatzidaki and Millar, 2015; Terry et al., 2015; Corradi and Bouzat, 2016; Echeverria et al., 2016; Yang et al., 2017; Bouzat et al., 2018). Based on their effects on macroscopic currents, PAMs have been classified as type I PAMs, that mainly enhance agonist-induced peak currents, and type II PAMs, that enhance agonist-elicited currents and also decrease desensitization and recover receptors from desensitized states (Bertrand and Gopalakrishnan, 2007; Grønlien et al., 2007; Andersen et al., 2016).

Both α7 agonist- and antagonist-like actions of Aβ have been described in different cells and tissues (Wu et al., 2004; Khan et al., 2010; Li et al., 2011; Parri et al., 2011; Sadigh-Eteghad et al., 2014; Liu et al., 2015; Yan et al., 2015). Studies have been focused mainly on evaluation of the effects of Aβ on α7 metabotropic activity, which includes signaling pathways, such as ERK/MAPK, PI3K/AKT, JAK-2/STAT-3 and intracellular calcium mobilization. The acute effects of Aβ on α7 electrical activity have been explored at the macroscopic current level. Despite problems of comparability and some dissimilar results, probably due to variations on the aggregation state and concentration of amyloid peptides (see Buckingham et al., 2009), the consensus indicates that low concentrations of Aβ (picomolar) activate α7 whereas higher concentrations lead to current inhibition (Liu et al., 2001; Dineley et al., 2002; Grassi et al., 2003; Pym et al., 2005; Parri et al., 2011).

To shed light into the molecular mechanism of the direct action of Aβ on α7, we expressed human α7 on mammalian cells and evaluated functional effects by fluorescence spectroscopic measurements and electrophysiological recordings. We used Aβ preparations enriched in oligomeric forms since these species were shown to be involved in cognitive impairment, inhibition of long-term potentiation, memory loss and α7 modulation (Walsh et al., 2002; Wang et al., 2002; Cleary et al., 2005; Parri et al., 2011). By taking advantage of the potential of single-channel recordings in providing information unattainable by macroscopic measurements, we deciphered the direct molecular effects of oligomeric Aβ as activator and inhibitor of α7 channels. By using a fluorescent conformational probe, we revealed that Aβ elicits different concentration-dependent conformational changes and induces novel conformational states.

MATERIALS AND METHODS

Drugs

Acetylcholine (ACh) and human amyloid-β1–42 ($A\beta_{1-42}$) were purchased from Sigma-Aldrich (St. Louis, MO, USA); NS-1738 N-(5-Chloro-2-hydroxyphenyl)-N′-[2-chloro-5-(trifluoromethyl) phenyl]urea, PNU-120596 [N-(5-Chloro-2,4-dimethoxyphenyl)-N′-(5-methyl-3-isoxazolyl)-urea] and rat amyloid-β1–40 ($A\beta_{1-40}$) were obtained from Tocris Biosciences (Bristol, UK).

Receptor Expression

BOSC-23 cells, derived from HEK 293 cells (Pear et al., 1993), were transfected by calcium phosphate procedure with human α7 cDNA subcloned in pRBG4 vector (Bouzat et al., 1994). Plasmids harboring cDNAs of the α7 chaperone proteins Ric-3 and NACHO were incorporated to favor α7 expression (Bouzat et al., 2008; Andersen et al., 2016; Nielsen et al., 2018). All transfections were carried out for about 12–18 h in Dulbecco's Modified Eagle Medium (DMEM) with 10%

fetal bovine serum and terminated by exchanging the medium. Cells were used for single-channel recordings 2–4 days after transfection. To facilitate identification of transfected cells, a separate plasmid encoding green fluorescent protein was included in all transfections.

Amyloid-β Peptide Preparations

$A\beta_{1-40}$ or $A\beta_{1-42}$ were resuspended in dimethyl sulfoxide at a concentration of 10 mg/ml (peptide stock solution) and stored in aliquots at −80°C. Aβ oligomers were prepared immediately prior to use according to previously published methods (Uranga et al., 2016; Pascual et al., 2017). Briefly, aliquots of peptide stock (10 μl) were added to 280 μl of phosphate buffered saline (PBS; pH 7.4) and stirred continuously (300 rpm) for 120 min and stored at 4°C until use.

Transmission electron microscopy (TEM) studies were carried out according to previously published methods with slight modifications (Uranga et al., 2016; Pascual et al., 2017). Briefly, 10 μl media containing the peptide was placed on a carbon-coated grid and incubated for 60 s. Ten microliters of 0.5% glutaraldehyde was added to the grid followed by incubation for an additional 60 s. The grid was then washed with drops of water and dried. Finally, the grid was stained for 2 min with 2% uranyl acetate and air dried. The grid was subsequently examined under a Jeol 100 Cx II electron microscope (Uranga et al., 2016). TEM photomicrographs showed that Aβ preparations included spheroidal structures individually or in small groups (**Supplementary Figure S1**). These ultrastructural forms were compatible with a heterogeneous array of oligomers, thus discarding the presence of fibrils (Uranga et al., 2016; Pascual et al., 2017).

Single-Channel Recordings

Single-channel recordings were obtained in the cell-attached patch configuration. The bath and pipette solutions contained 142 mM KCl, 5.4 mM NaCl, 1.8 mM $CaCl_2$, 1.7 mM $MgCl_2$ and 10 mM HEPES (pH 7.4). For potentiation, 1 μM PNU-120596 or 10 μM NS-1738 were added to the pipette solution together with ACh.

Single-channel currents were digitized at 5–10 μs intervals, low-pass filtered at a cut-off frequency of 10 kHz using an Axopatch 200B patch-clamp amplifier (Molecular Devices Corp., CA, USA). Single-channel events were idealized by the half amplitude threshold criterion using the program QuB 2.0.0.28 (Qin et al., 1996, 1997; State University of New York at Buffalo) with a digital low-pass filter at 9 kHz. A filter of 3 kHz was used in recordings with PNU-120596 to facilitate the analysis. The open and closed time histograms obtained from idealization were fitted by the maximum interval likelihood (MIL) function in QuB (Qin et al., 1996, 1997), with a dead time of 0.1 ms. This analysis was performed by sequentially adding an open and/or closed state to a starting C ↔ O model in order to properly fit the corresponding histograms (Fabiani et al., 2018; Lasala et al., 2018). Final models contained five-six closed states and three-four open states for α7 in the presence of ACh plus PNU-120596, five-six closed states and three open states for α7 in the presence of ACh plus NS-1738, or three closed states and one-two open states for α7 in the presence of ACh and absence of PAMs.

Clusters were identified as a series of closely separated openings preceded and followed by closings longer than a critical duration. Different critical closed times were calculated by MIL between each closed component. Critical times between the third and fourth closed components for α7 in the presence of PNU-120596 (∼30–60 ms) or NS-1738 (∼2–8 ms) were selected in QuB to chop the idealized data and create a sub-data set that only contained clusters to define mean cluster duration.

Fluorimetric Measurements

Fluorimetric measurements were performed in a SLM model 4800 fluorimeter (SLM Instruments, Urbana, IL, USA) using a vertically polarized light beam from an Hannovia 200-W mercury/xenon arc obtained with a Glan-Thompson polarizer (4 nm excitation and emission slits).

Crystal violet (CrV) was used as a probe to detect conformational changes (Lurtz and Pedersen, 1999; Sun et al., 2017; Fabiani et al., 2018). nAChR-rich membranes were prepared from *Torpedo californica* electric tissue as described previously (Fernández Nievas et al., 2008; Perillo et al., 2012; Fabiani et al., 2018). CrV experiments using *Torpedo* membranes or α7-expressing cells were conducted as described previously for the *Torpedo* nAChR (Fernández Nievas et al., 2008; Perillo et al., 2012; Fabiani et al., 2018). *Torpedo* membranes or BOSC-23 cells expressing α7 were resuspended on phosphate saline buffer with a protein concentration of 100 μg/ml or up to an absorbance value of ∼0.5 at 280 nM measured on a Jasco V-630 spectrophotometer (JASCO Deutschland GmbH), respectively. The suspended cells or membranes were incubated with Aβ oligomers for 20 min. For measurements conducted in the desensitized state, the membrane or cell suspensions were additionally incubated for 15 min with 1 mM or 20 mM carbamylcholine (Carb), respectively. The suspensions were subsequently titrated with increasing concentrations of CrV (in water). After each addition of CrV, the samples were incubated for 15 min before obtaining the fluorescence emission spectra. CrV was excited at 600 nm, and the fluorescence emission spectra were collected from 605 to 700 nm. Before the first addition of CrV, a background fluorescence emission spectrum was obtained for each sample. The spectrum was then subtracted from the emission spectra obtained in the presence of CrV and the maximum intensity (at 623–625 nm) was measured. To determine the CrV dissociation constant (K_D), the value of the CrV maximum fluorescence emission was plotted as a function of the logarithmic CrV concentration (M). The resulting sigmoid curve was fitted by the Boltzmann function and the K_D was calculated using the program Origin 7.0 (OriginLab Corporation).

Statistical Analysis

Intergroup comparisons were carried out using one-way analyses of variance (ANOVA), Dunnett's multiple comparisons test (Graphpad PRISM software). The values represent the average ± SD of the total number of samples indicated. Statistically significance difference was established at p-values <0.05.

RESULTS

Amyloid β Oligomers Induce Conformational Changes in α7

To examine the potential of oligomeric Aβ peptides to directly affect α7, we first used the conformational-sensitive probe CrV and measured its affinity for the receptor before and after exposure to Aβ by fluorescence spectroscopy.

CrV has been extensively used for studies in the *Torpedo* muscle nAChR where it shows low affinity for the resting state (K_D values ~400 nM, Fernández Nievas et al., 2008; Perillo et al., 2012) and high affinity for the desensitized state (K_D values ~60 nM; Fernández Nievas et al., 2008; Perillo et al., 2012; Fabiani et al., 2018; **Figure 1A**).

We first determined if CrV can be used as a conformational probe for the human α7 receptor. Suspensions of BOSC-23 cells expressing α7 were titrated with increasing concentrations of CrV. Saturable CrV binding yielded a K_D value of 492 ± 41 nM for resting α7 receptors, indicating an affinity similar to that for the muscle nAChR in the resting state. Interestingly, measurements in the desensitized state, which was induced by 20-min preincubation with Carb, yielded a K_D value of 680 ± 89 nM for CrV binding (**Figures 1A,B**). The maximal fluorescence intensities of the samples were similar at resting and desensitized conditions, thus discarding that the lower affinity for the desensitized state corresponds to reduced binding of the probe in the latter state. These results indicate that CrV saturates its binding sites at both conditions with different affinities. Thus, opposite to its binding affinity profile for the muscle nAChR, CrV shows higher affinity for resting than for desensitized states in α7.

We next determined the effects of low (0.1 nM) and high (100 nM) $A\beta_{1-40}$ concentrations on α7 conformation by measuring CrV K_D values to resting and desensitized states (**Figure 1B**).

Exposure of α7 in the resting state (in the absence of Carb) to 0.1 nM $A\beta_{1-40}$ increased the CrV K_D towards that of the desensitized state, indicating that amyloid peptides induce conformational changes in α7. Interestingly, subsequent addition of Carb induced a further displacement to higher K_D values, suggesting that the agonist can lead to further conformational changes (**Figure 1B**). K_D values for desensitized conditions were statistically significantly different in the absence and presence of Aβ (**Figure 1B**). Similar results were obtained with 0.1 nM $A\beta_{1-42}$.

On the other hand, incubation of resting α7 receptors with 1,000-fold higher $A\beta_{1-40}$ concentration (100 nM) did not induce statistically significant changes in the CrV K_D value (**Figure 1B**). Furthermore, the K_D value remained constant even after addition of 20 mM Carb, indicating that α7 was not reactive to the agonist. Similar results were obtained with high (100 nM) $A\beta_{1-42}$.

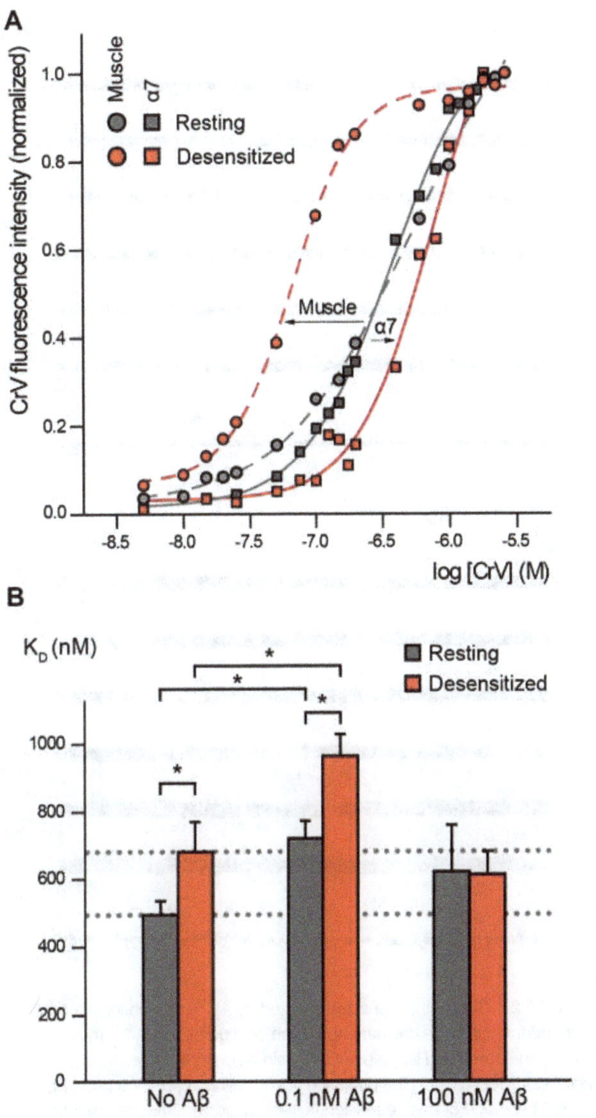

FIGURE 1 | α7 conformational changes depend on Amyloid β peptide (Aβ) concentrations. **(A)** Crystal violet (CrV) titration curves obtained with muscle nicotinic acetylcholine receptor (nAChR) from *T. californica* rich membranes (circles) and with human α7 (squares) in the absence (gray, Resting) and presence of carbamylcholine (Carb; red, desensitized). The arrows indicate the changes from resting to desensitized conditions for each nAChR type. **(B)** Changes in K_D values of CrV by the exposure to low (0.1 nM) and high (100 nM) concentrations of $A\beta_{1-40}$. K_D values of CrV were calculated from the titration curves, in the absence and presence of 20 mM Carb (gray and red columns, respectively). Each column corresponds to the average ± SD of more than four independent experiments. Statistically significant differences are shown by asterisks, *p < 0.05.

Oligomeric Amyloid-β Peptides at Low Concentrations Trigger Human α7 Channel Opening

Once established that oligomeric Aβ peptides induce conformational changes that are sensitive to concentration, we took advantage of the potential of single-channel recordings to reveal the mechanistic basis of this modulation.

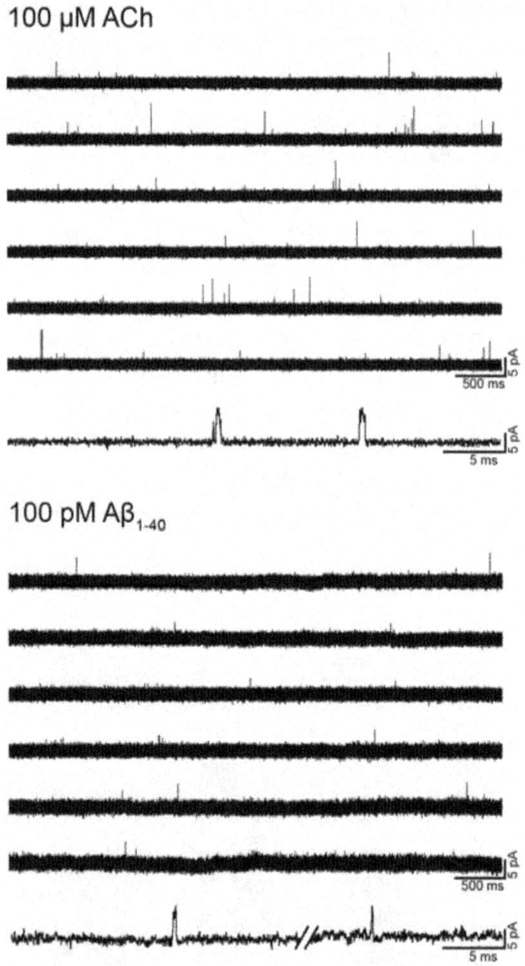

FIGURE 2 | Single-channel activity elicited by Aβ. Single-channel recordings were performed in the cell-attached patch configuration at −70 mV membrane potential. Representative α7 single-channel traces from a continuous recording in the presence of 100 μM acetylcholine (ACh) or 100 pM $A\beta_{1-40}$. For each condition, a trace at higher temporal resolution is shown (bottom traces). Channel openings are shown as upward deflections. Filter: 9 kHz.

To first determine if Aβ can activate human α7, we examined single-channel activity from BOSC-23 cells expressing the receptor (**Figure 2**). In the presence of 100 μM ACh, α7 exhibits single brief openings flanked by long closings, or less often, several openings in quick succession, which are called bursts (Bouzat et al., 2008; Andersen et al., 2016). The mean open duration was 0.36 ± 0.07 ms (n = 3) and the mean burst duration was 0.77 ± 0.21 ms (n = 3; **Figure 2**). No α7 channel activity was detected in the absence of agonist. However, 100 pM $A\beta_{1-40}$ elicited the typical α7 channel openings (**Figure 2**). The number of active patches was lower than in the presence of ACh (28% transfected cells showed channel activity). Channel activity was not detected if $A\beta_{1-40}$ was increased to 10 nM and 100 nM (n = 16 patches of different cells and transfections), indicating that activation is favored at low concentrations. These experiments were performed in parallel with recordings with ACh as the agonist to discard that the lack of channel activity was due to the lack of functional expression.

We next performed recordings in the presence of the type II PAM PNU-120596, which increases the probability of agonist-elicited channel opening and, consequently, favors the detection of infrequent opening events (daCosta et al., 2011; Andersen et al., 2016). By itself, PNU-120596 cannot elicit channel activation (Hurst et al., 2005). In the presence of 1 μM PNU-120596, α7 channel activity elicited by ACh (100 μM) appears in long activation periods of high frequency, named clusters, whose mean duration is about 1–3 s (**Figure 3**, **Table 1**; Andersen et al., 2016).

In the absence of ACh, $A\beta_{1-40}$ or $A\beta_{1-42}$ at a low concentration (100 pM) elicited clusters of PNU-120596-potentiated α7 channels (**Figure 3**). Again, the proportion of active patches was lower than in the presence of ACh. Whereas almost all patches (>90%) showed channel activity with ACh, the percentage of active patches was reduced in the presence of $A\beta_{1-40}$ or $A\beta_{1-42}$ as agonists (**Table 1**). Moreover, as Aβ concentration increased, the number of patches showing α7 activity decreased. As shown in **Table 1**, at 100 pM 43% and 78% of the patches showed clusters elicited by $A\beta_{1-40}$ or $A\beta_{1-42}$, respectively, but no channel activity was detected at 100 nM. Thus, also in the presence of a PAM, activation by Aβ is favored at picomolar or low nanomolar concentrations.

Although the frequency of clusters is usually variable among patches from different cell transfections, it was systematically lower in the presence of Aβ with respect to ACh as illustrated in typical recordings shown in **Figure 3**. For a better comparison, recordings with ACh or Aβ were performed in the same batch of transfected cells.

In the presence of ACh and PNU-120596, each cluster is composed of two or three bursts that contain long-duration openings separated by brief closings (daCosta et al., 2011; Andersen et al., 2016). Clusters elicited by Aβ in the presence of PNU-120596 showed the typical architecture observed with ACh (**Figure 3**). The analysis showed no statistically significant differences in the mean cluster duration at all tested

TABLE 1 | Activation of α7 by Amyloid β peptide (Aβ) in the presence of N-(5-Chloro-2,4-dimethoxyphenyl)-N′-(5-methyl-3-isoxazolyl)-urea (PNU)-120596.

[ACh] (μM)	Aβ	[Aβ] (nM)	% active patches (n)	Mean cluster duration (ms)
100	No	0	100 (6)	2263 ± 990
0	$A\beta_{1-40}$	0.1	42.9 (7)	762 ± 316
0		1	22.2 (18)	2016 ± 1364
0		10	30.0 (10)	5229 ± 1392*
0		100	0 (9)	Nd
0	$A\beta_{1-42}$	0.1	77.8 (9)	1401 ± 805
0		1	46.2 (13)	1208 ± 946
0		10	33.3 (9)	1751 ± 766
0		100	0 (6)	Nd

*Single-channel currents from cells expressing human α7 were recorded in the presence of 1 μM PNU-120596 plus 100 μM acetylcholine (ACh) or Aβ at the indicated concentrations. The mean cluster duration was obtained from the corresponding histograms. Nd: not detected. Statistical comparisons were performed against the corresponding control condition using analyses of variance (ANOVA; Dunnett's multiple comparisons test). *$p < 0.05$.*

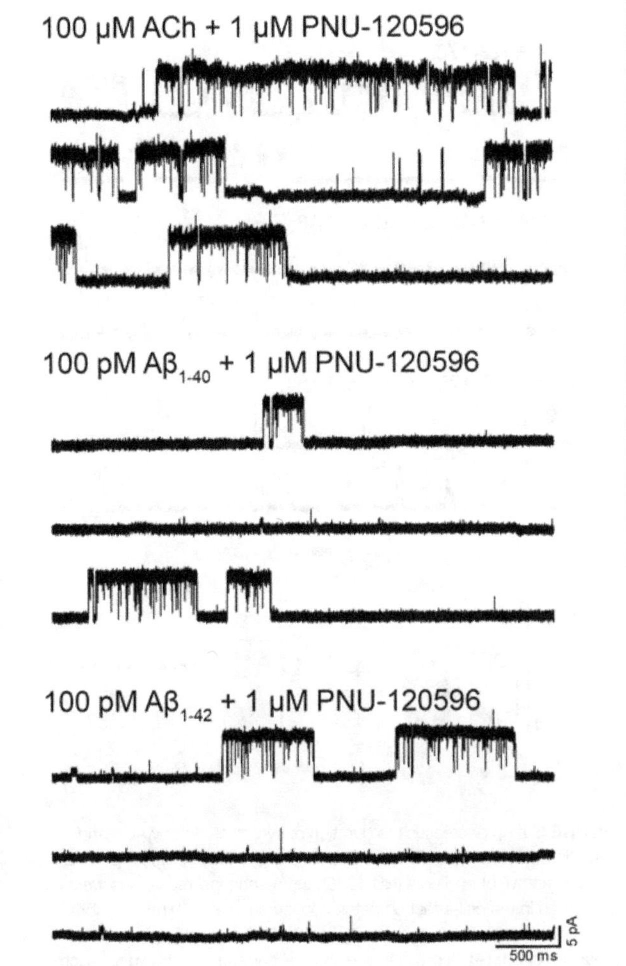

FIGURE 3 | Single-channel activity elicited by Aβ in the presence of N-(5-Chloro-2,4-dimethoxyphenyl)-N′-(5-methyl-3-isoxazolyl)-urea (PNU-120596). Single-channel recordings were performed in the cell-attached patch configuration at −70 mV membrane potential. Representative α7 single-channel traces from a continuous recording in the presence of the type II positive allosteric modulator (PAM) PNU-120596 (1 μM) together with 100 μM ACh, 100 pM $A\beta_{1-40}$ or 100 pM $A\beta_{1-42}$. Channel openings are shown as upward deflections.

concentrations, except for 10 nM $A\beta_{1-40}$ at which clusters were slightly prolonged (**Table 1**).

The results confirm that Aβ at picomolar and low nanomolar concentrations can trigger activation of α7 channels.

Amyloid-β Peptides Decrease the Duration of α7 Activation Episodes

We next explored the effect of Aβ on ACh-elicited channels. To this end, we recorded channels activated by 100 μM ACh in the presence of $A\beta_{1-42}$ (10 and 100 nM). The mean durations of openings and bursts at both Aβ concentrations were slightly briefer than the control but the differences were not statistically significant (**Table 2**). Due to the very brief durations, differences on these values may be inaccurate since they approach the resolution limit of our system. We therefore tested the effect of Aβ (10–1,000 nM) on ACh-activated channels in the presence 1 μM PNU-120596, which by increasing the duration of the activation episodes allows a better description of the molecular effects.

TABLE 2 | Effect of Aβ on ACh-elicited channel activity.

PAM	Aβ	Aβ (nM)	*n*	Mean open duration (ms)	Mean cluster/burst duration (ms)
No	No	0	3	0.36 ± 0.07	0.77 ± 0.21
	$A\beta_{1-42}$	10	3	0.26 ± 0.02	0.48 ± 0.06
		100	3	0.27 ± 0.04	0.49 ± 0.11
PNU-120596	No	0	6	159.6 ± 69.6	2263 ± 990
	$A\beta_{1-40}$	50	3	176.7 ± 22.5	2220 ± 256
		100	5	61.6 ± 33.1*	698 ± 409*
		1,000	3	23.4 ± 22.0*	931 ± 303*
	$A\beta_{1-42}$	10	5	61.1 ± 23.8*	888 ± 261*
		100	5	54.7 ± 47.8*	755 ± 560*
		1,000	6	59.6 ± 32.2*	883 ± 289*
NS-1738	No	0	12	4.2 ± 1.8	31.1 ± 8.8
	$A\beta_{1-40}$	100	10	2.7 ± 1.1*	8.4 ± 4.8****
	$A\beta_{1-42}$	100	4	2.1 ± 1.0*	10.7 ± 2.4****

*Single-channel recordings from cells expressing human α7 were recorded in the presence of 100 μM ACh, 100 μM ACh plus 1 μM PNU-120596 or 100 μM ACh plus 10 μM N-(5-Chloro-2-hydroxyphenyl)-N′-[2-chloro-5-(trifluoromethyl) phenyl]urea (NS-1738). The effects of Aβ was evaluated for all conditions. The mean open and cluster durations were obtained from the corresponding histograms. Statistical comparisons were performed against the corresponding control condition using ANOVA (Dunnett's multiple comparisons test). *$p < 0.05$, ****$p < 0.0001$.*

The presence of $A\beta_{1-40}$ or $A\beta_{1-42}$ reduced the mean duration of openings and clusters elicited by ACh and potentiated by PNU-120596 as a function of concentration (**Figure 4A**). Whereas 50 nM $A\beta_{1-40}$ did not affect open and cluster durations, 10 nM $A\beta_{1-42}$ reduced these durations. The mean open and cluster durations were statistically significantly briefer than the control at concentrations equal and higher than 100 nM for $A\beta_{1-40}$ and 10 nM for $A\beta_{1-42}$ ($p < 0.05$, **Table 2**). At these concentrations, the mean durations were reduced about 3-fold (**Figure 4B**).

To further determine if the effect of Aβ on α7 potentiation is specific for type II PAMs, we evaluated the action on channels activated by ACh and potentiated by NS-1738, which is a type I PAM (Timmermann et al., 2007; Andersen et al., 2016). In the presence of ACh, NS-1738 (10 μM) increased the mean open duration from about 0.3 ms to about 4 ms and opening events appeared grouped in bursts of about 30 ms (**Figure 5**, **Table 2**). In the presence of 100 nM $A\beta_{1-40}$ or $A\beta_{1-42}$, the mean burst duration was reduced to about 3-fold and the mean open duration was also statistically significantly briefer than in the control condition (**Figure 5**, **Table 2**).

Thus, we conclude that episodes elicited by ACh and potentiated by both types of PAMs are reduced by Aβ at high nanomolar concentrations.

DISCUSSION

Low concentrations (picomolar) of soluble Aβ peptides in the brain of healthy people have been reported to play physiological roles whereas in AD patients concentrations increase to the nanomole range and trigger the formation of insoluble plaques,

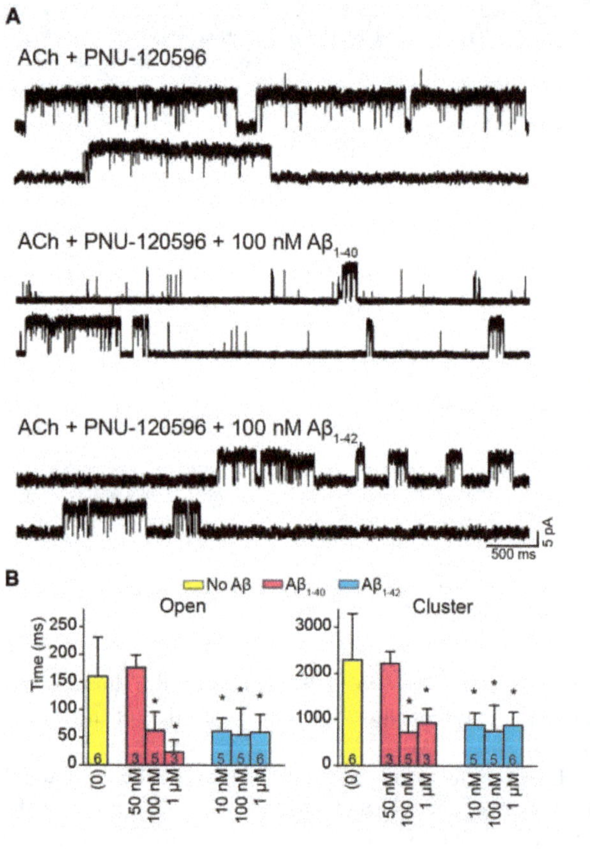

FIGURE 4 | Aβ decreases the duration of activation episodes elicited by ACh and potentiated by PNU-120596. Single-channel recordings were performed in the cell-attached patch configuration at −70 mV membrane potential with 100 μM ACh and 1 μM PNU-120596 and in the absence or presence of Aβ. **(A)** Representative clusters are shown for each condition. Channels are shown as upward deflections. **(B)** Decrease of mean open and cluster durations by Aβ. Each value corresponds to the mean ± SD of different recordings. The number of recordings for each condition is shown in the bars. The cluster and open durations for each recording were obtained from the corresponding histograms and correspond to the slowest open components $^{*}p < 0.05$.

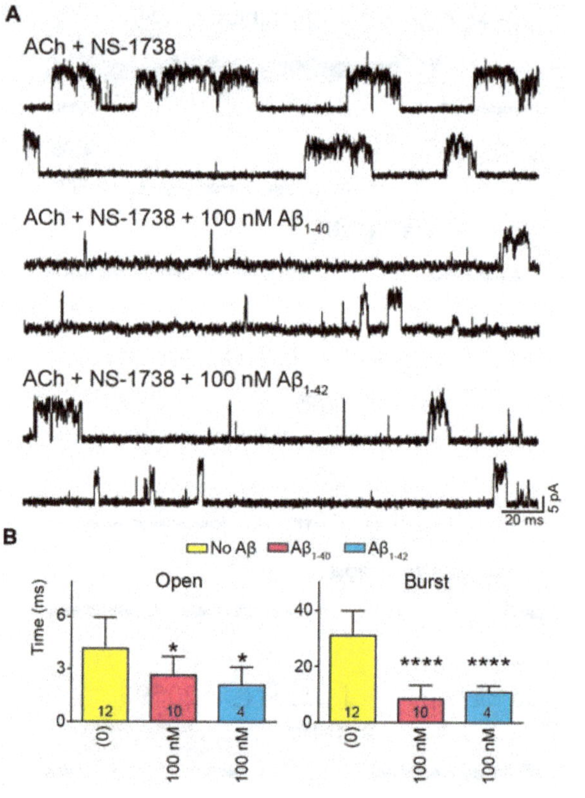

FIGURE 5 | Aβ decreases the duration of events elicited by ACh and potentiated by the type I PAM N-(5-Chloro-2-hydroxyphenyl)-N′-[2-chloro-5-(trifluoromethyl) phenyl]urea (NS-1738). Single-channel recordings were performed in the cell-attached patch configuration at −70 mV membrane potential with100 μM ACh and 10 μM NS-1738 and in the absence or presence of Aβ. **(A)** Representative channel currents are shown for each condition. **(B)** Decrease of mean open and burst durations by Aβ. Each value corresponds to the mean ± SD of *n* different recordings (shown in the bars). The open and burst durations for each recording were obtained from the corresponding histograms and correspond to the slowest open components $^{*}p < 0.05$, $^{****}p < 0.0001$.

a major neuropathologic hallmark of AD (Dineley, 2007; Parihar and Brewer, 2010; Collins-Praino et al., 2014; Puzzo et al., 2015). However, the possibility that Aβ oligomers play an important role in AD progression has gained weight (Miñano-Molina et al., 2011; Puzzo et al., 2015). Moreover, in the absence of plaques, intraneuronal accumulation of Aβ peptide has been shown to correlate with the initial steps in the tau-phosphorylation cascade, alterations in ERK2 signaling and impairment of higher CNS functions in rats (Echeverria et al., 2004a,b). Another feature of AD is the severe cholinergic deficit, which involves mainly α4β2 and α7 receptors. It has been established that α7 exhibits an exceptionally high Aβ affinity, an interaction that may influence synaptic transmission and plasticity and may also contribute to Aβ-mediated synaptic neural network dysfunction and to the severe cholinergic deficit (Wang et al., 2000; Buckingham et al., 2009; Puzzo et al., 2011; Dineley et al., 2015). Several reports have described the intracellular pathways involved in Aβ toxicity as well as crosstalk between Aβ- and α7-triggered signaling pathways (see review in Buckingham et al., 2009; Dougherty et al., 2003; Parri et al., 2011). However, the molecular mechanism by which Aβ affects α7 ionotropic activity is not well understood and has been explored mainly at the macroscopic current level. Thus, we took advantage of two different approaches to decipher the molecular basis of the direct actions of oligomeric Aβ at α7. Our spectroscopic results revealed that α7 adopts distinct stable conformations depending on the Aβ concentration range, and our single-channel recordings revealed that Aβ triggers α7 channel openings at low concentrations (picomolar to low nanomolar range) whereas at high concentrations (nanomolar to low micromolar range) it decreases the duration of ACh-elicited activation episodes. Both results fully support the idea that Aβ can act as an agonist and a negative modulator of α7 at different, physiologically attainable, concentrations.

One of the main concerns of working with Aβ is related to the standardization of the oligomeric preparations since aggregation is a dynamic and complex process, which is highly sensitive to preparation, experimental and analyzing conditions (Bitan et al., 2005; Buckingham et al., 2009; Hayden and Teplow, 2013; Watt et al., 2013). Thus, preparations are usually heterogenous since many types of soluble species co-exist. However, this scenario mimics the physiological/pathological situations where different oligomeric species and fibrils co-exist in a dynamic equilibrium (Walsh et al., 2000; Shankar et al., 2008; Noguchi et al., 2009; Santos et al., 2012; Esparza et al., 2016). Nevertheless, the results obtained with different Aβ oligomer preparations have yielded rather consistent results (Palop and Mucke, 2010). In particular, the effects exerted by our Aβ preparations, which are compatible with a heterogeneous array of oligomers and the absence of fibrils, are in general agreement with previous reported effects of oligomeric preparations on α7 (Liu et al., 2001; Dineley et al., 2002; Khan et al., 2010; Tong et al., 2011).

α7 ionotropic activity is characterized by very brief, sub-millisecond opening events and rapid desensitization (Bouzat et al., 2008; Corradi and Bouzat, 2016). We found that Aβ is capable of eliciting α7 activity either in the absence or presence of the type II PAM PNU-120596. In both conditions, activation by Aβ was favored at 100 pM or low nanomolar concentrations and was not detected at micromolar concentrations, in close agreement with macroscopic recordings of α7 expressed in oocytes (Dineley et al., 2002, 2015). Channel activity elicited by Aβ was significantly reduced with respect to that elicited by ACh in terms of the number of active patches and frequency of opening events. However, once opened, the mean open duration, cluster architecture and mean cluster duration were similar to those of ACh-elicited channel activity.

Conformational changes of α7 driven by the sole presence of Aβ at a low concentration were sensed by CrV. At 100 pM, oligomeric Aβ drove α7 conformation towards that of desensitized receptors but the subsequent addition of Carb allowed further conformational changes. Although this method senses conformations under equilibrium and cannot provide information about CrV K_D for open channels, the fact that in the presence of Aβ α7 is still responsive to Carb is compatible with the induction of both active and desensitized states. Nevertheless, the conformation of α7 in the presence of low Aβ and high Carb concentrations is different to that of the desensitized state (high Carb alone) as sensed by CrV, thus indicating the induction of a novel conformational state.

The enhancement of α7 activity as a protective role in AD and for the treatment of cognitive and memory impairment associated to neurological disorders appears to be well established (Inestrosa et al., 2013; Lendvai et al., 2013; Wallace and Bertrand, 2013; Uteshev, 2014; Dineley et al., 2015; Corradi and Bouzat, 2016; Yang et al., 2017). Also, a protective, physiological role has been proposed for soluble Aβ at low concentrations in healthy individuals (Giuffrida et al., 2009; Puzzo et al., 2015). Thus, the capability of low concentration Aβ preparations to activate α7 could be related to beneficial physiological effects. However, it would be expected that long-term exposure of an activator would lead to receptor desensitization.

Several reports have shown that high concentrations of Aβ have an inhibitory effect on the amplitude of α7-activated macroscopic currents as well as on signaling pathways (Dineley et al., 2002; Parri et al., 2011). In close agreement, we found that in the presence of PAMs the mean duration of activation episodes (clusters or bursts), which arise from a single receptor molecule, as well as the open channel lifetime are significantly reduced by high concentrations of oligomeric Aβ. There was also a trend of reduced mean durations in the absence of PAMs, but values were not statistically significantly different to the control. However, due to the very brief durations, which are close to the time-resolution limit of our system, such reduction may be underestimated. From a mechanistic point of view, the decreased duration of activation episodes and openings may be compatible with increased desensitization and/or channel block. We can discard fast open-channel blockade since brief closings corresponding to blocked openings (flickering) were not detected. However, enhanced desensitization and slow channel block processes are difficult to distinguish by electrophysiological techniques (Arias et al., 2009; Bouzat and Sine, 2018). CrV experiments showed that at high Aβ concentrations α7 adopts a conformational state which is not different to the resting state in terms of CrV K_D values and from this state α7 is not further reactive to Carb. In agreement with these observations, it was shown for the muscle nAChR that the channel blocker QX-314 does not change the CrV K_D value of the resting state and that this value remains constant even in the presence of Carb (Fabiani et al., 2018). Thus, we can infer that oligomeric Aβ at high concentrations behave as a slow channel blocker of α7. The reduced α7 activity in the presence of Aβ may contribute to the cholinergic signaling deficit and thus may be involved in the initiation and development of AD.

The combined action of PAMs and Aβ suggests that α7 potentiation by PAMs would be probably lower than expected in AD patients. By macroscopic current recordings it has been shown that $A\beta_{1-42}$ inhibits α4β2 and α2β2 receptors and this inhibition is prevented in the presence of a PAM (Pandya and Yakel, 2011). These results are not in full disagreement with ours because, though reduced, we still detected potentiation. The characterization of the influence of Aβ on α7 potentiation contributes to a better extrapolation of the molecular effects of PAMs to their potential therapeutic effects.

A collateral but still important result of our study is the demonstration of different CrV binding profiles between α7 and muscle nAChRs. In the muscle nAChR, the CrV affinity for the desensitized state is greater than for the resting state whereas in α7 it is the other way around. CrV binds to luminal non-competitive antagonist sites which are localized in the channel vestibule (Lurtz and Pedersen, 1999). Our results showed that the conformation of this region is similar for both receptors in the resting state, but it is different in the desensitized state. Thus, the structural arrangements induced by prolonged exposure to Carb are different between muscle and α7 nAChRs. Overall, the use of a conformational probe has proved to be useful for revealing receptor subtype specific structural arrangements associated with functional states and opens doors to further studies in this respect.

The binding site of Aβ remains undefined. Computer docking studies suggested that Aβ may interact with α7 at agonist binding-site interfaces (Espinoza-Fonseca, 2004) and the conserved tyrosine 188 at Loop C of the agonist binding site was proposed to be involved in α7 activation by Aβ (Tong et al., 2011). On the other hand, the transmembrane cavity, a binding site of different allosteric ligands in the Cys-loop receptor family (Gill et al., 2011; Sauguet et al., 2015; Corradi and Bouzat, 2016), was proposed to be involved in the noncompetitive block of Aβ on α4β2 (Pandya and Yakel, 2011). Our spectroscopic results demonstrating that in the presence of low Aβ concentrations α7 is still reactive to Carb suggest that Aβ does not occupy orthosteric agonist binding sites and, in consequence, activation may be mediated by allosteric sites. Allosteric activation of α7 through a transmembrane site has been shown for 4BP-TQS. However, the activity profile is strikingly different to that of ACh, which is not the case of Aβ (Gill et al., 2011; Lasala et al., 2018). Alternatively, Aβ may not occupy the five orthosteric agonist sites but may still be able to induce activation; the remaining sites, subsequently occupied by Carb, may favor activation and desensitization. This possibility is in line with our previous reports showing that occupancy of only one of the five ACh-binding sites is required for α7 activation (Andersen et al., 2013). At high concentrations, Aβ may probably inhibit α7 by acting through an allosteric site, different from that of CrV since it does not interfere with its binding. Dual actions as low-efficacy agonists and channel blockers have been described for several compounds acting at different sites of nAChRs (reviewed in Bouzat and Mukhtasimova, 2018; Bouzat and Sine, 2018).

Overall, our study provides information from a molecular perspective to understand Aβ complex actions at the higher cellular level.

AUTHOR CONTRIBUTIONS

ML, CF, JC, SA and CB contributed to study design, analysis and interpretation of data. ML and CF: acquisition of data. CB and SA contributed to writing.

FUNDING

This work was supported by grants from Universidad Nacional del Sur (UNS) to CB and SA; Agencia Nacional de Promoción Científica y Tecnológica (ANPCYT) to CB and JC; Consejo Nacional de Investigaciones Científicas y Técnicas (CONICET) Argentina to CB and SA.

ACKNOWLEDGMENTS

We are thankful to Drs. Romina Uranga, Gabriela Salvador, Ana Pascual and Susana Pasquare (INIBIBB, Argentina) for help and advice with Aβ preparations.

REFERENCES

Andersen, N., Corradi, J., Sine, S. M., and Bouzat, C. (2013). Stoichiometry for activation of neuronal α7 nicotinic receptors. *Proc. Natl. Acad. Sci. U S A* 110, 20819–20824. doi: 10.1073/pnas.1315775110

Andersen, N. D., Nielsen, B. E., Corradi, J., Tolosa, M. F., Feuerbach, D., Arias, H. R., et al. (2016). Exploring the positive allosteric modulation of human α7 nicotinic receptors from a single-channel perspective. *Neuropharmacology* 107, 189–200. doi: 10.1016/j.neuropharm.2016.02.032

Arias, H. R., Gumilar, F., Rosenberg, A., Targowska-Duda, K. M., Feuerbach, D., Jozwiak, K., et al. (2009). Interaction of bupropion with muscle-type nicotinic acetylcholine receptors in different conformational states. *Biochemistry* 48, 4506–4518. doi: 10.1021/bi802206k

Bertrand, D., and Gopalakrishnan, M. (2007). Allosteric modulation of nicotinic acetylcholine receptors. *Biochem. Pharmacol.* 74, 1155–1163. doi: 10.1016/j.bcp.2007.07.011

Bitan, G., Fradinger, E. A., Spring, S. M., and Teplow, D. B. (2005). Neurotoxic protein oligomers—what you see is not always what you get. *Amyloid* 12, 88–95. doi: 10.1080/13506120500106958

Bouzat, C., Bartos, M., Corradi, J., and Sine, S. M. (2008). The interface between extracellular and transmembrane domains of homomeric Cys-loop receptors governs open-channel lifetime and rate of desensitization. *J. Neurosci.* 28, 7808–7819. doi: 10.1523/jneurosci.0448-08.2008

Bouzat, C., Bren, N., and Sine, S. M. (1994). Structural basis of the different gating kinetics of fetal and adult acetylcholine receptors. *Neuron* 13, 1395–1402. doi: 10.1016/0896-6273(94)90424-3

Bouzat, C., Lasala, M., Nielsen, B. E., Corradi, J., and Esandi, M. D. C. (2018). Molecular function of α7 nicotinic receptors as drug targets. *J. Physiol.* 596, 1847–1861. doi: 10.1113/JP275101

Bouzat, C., and Mukhtasimova, N. (2018). The nicotinic acetylcholine receptor as a molecular machine for neuromuscular transmission. *Curr. Opin. Physiol.* 4, 40–48. doi: 10.1016/j.cophys.2018.04.008

Bouzat, C., and Sine, S. M. (2018). Nicotinic acetylcholine receptors at the single-channel level. *Br. J. Pharmacol.* 175, 1789–1804. doi: 10.1111/bph.13770

Buckingham, S. D., Jones, A. K., Brown, L. A., and Sattelle, D. B. (2009). Nicotinic acetylcholine receptor signalling: roles in Alzheimer's disease and amyloid neuroprotection. *Pharmacol. Rev.* 61, 39–61. doi: 10.1124/pr.108.000562

Chatzidaki, A., and Millar, N. S. (2015). Allosteric modulation of nicotinic acetylcholine receptors. *Biochem. Pharmacol.* 97, 408–417. doi: 10.1016/j.bcp.2015.07.028

Cleary, J. P., Walsh, D. M., Hofmeister, J. J., Shankar, G. M., Kuskowski, M. A., Selkoe, D. J., et al. (2005). Natural oligomers of the amyloid-β protein specifically disrupt cognitive function. *Nat. Neurosci.* 8, 79–84. doi: 10.1038/nn1372

Collins-Praino, L. E., Francis, Y. I., Griffith, E. Y., Wiegman, A. F., Urbach, J., Lawton, A., et al. (2014). Soluble amyloid β levels are elevated in the white matter of Alzheimer's patients, independent of cortical plaque severity. *Acta Neuropathol. Commun.* 2:83. doi: 10.1186/s40478-014-0083-0

Corradi, J., and Bouzat, C. (2016). Understanding the bases of function and modulation of 7 nicotinic receptors: implications for drug discovery. *Mol. Pharmacol.* 90, 288–299. doi: 10.1124/mol.116.104240

daCosta, C. J. B., Free, C. R., Corradi, J., Bouzat, C., and Sine, S. M. (2011). Single-channel and structural foundations of neuronal 7 acetylcholine receptor potentiation. *J. Neurosci.* 31, 13870–13879. doi: 10.1523/jneurosci.2652-11.2011

Dineley, K. T. (2007). β-amyloid peptide—nicotinic acetylcholine receptor interaction: the two faces of health and disease. *Front. Biosci.* 12, 5030–5038. doi: 10.2741/2445

Dineley, K. T., Bell, K. A., Bui, D., and Sweatt, J. D. (2002). β-Amyloid peptide activates α 7 nicotinic acetylcholine receptors expressed in *Xenopus* oocytes. *J. Biol. Chem.* 277, 25056–25061. doi: 10.1074/jbc.M200066200

Dineley, K. T., Pandya, A. A., and Yakel, J. L. (2015). Nicotinic ACh receptors as therapeutic targets in CNS disorders. *Trends Pharmacol. Sci.* 36, 96–108. doi: 10.1016/j.tips.2014.12.002

Dougherty, J. J., Wu, J. L., and Nichols, R. A. (2003). β-amyloid regulation of presynaptic nicotinic receptors in rat hippocampus and neocortex. *J. Neurosci.* 23, 6740–6747. doi: 10.1523/jneurosci.23-17-06740.2003

Echeverria, V., Ducatenzeiler, A., Alhonen, L., Janne, J., Grant, S. M., Wandosell, F., et al. (2004a). Rat transgenic models with a phenotype of intracellular Aβ accumulation in hippocampus and cortex. *J. Alzheimers Dis.* 6, 209–219. doi: 10.3233/jad-2004-6301

Echeverria, V., Ducatenzeiler, A., Dowd, E., Jänne, J., Grant, S. M., Szyf, M., et al. (2004b). Altered mitogen-activated protein kinase signaling, tau hyperphosphorylation and mild spatial learning dysfunction in transgenic rats expressing the β-amyloid peptide intracellularly in hippocampal and cortical neurons. *Neuroscience* 129, 583–592. doi: 10.1016/j.neuroscience.2004.07.036

Echeverria, V., Yarkov, A., and Aliev, G. (2016). Positive modulators of the α7 nicotinic receptor against neuroinflammation and cognitive impairment in Alzheimer's disease. *Prog. Neurobiol.* 144, 142–157. doi: 10.1016/j.pneurobio.2016.01.002

Egea, J., Buendia, I., Parada, E., Navarro, E., León, R., and Lopez, M. G. (2015). Anti-inflammatory role of microglial α7 nAChRs and its role in neuroprotection. *Biochem. Pharmacol.* 97, 463–472. doi: 10.1016/j.bcp.2015.07.032

Esparza, T. J., Wildburger, N. C., Jiang, H., Gangolli, M., Cairns, N. J., Bateman, R. J., et al. (2016). Soluble amyloid-β aggregates from human Alzheimer's disease brains. *Sci. Rep.* 6:38187. doi: 10.1038/srep38187

Espinoza-Fonseca, L. M. (2004). Base docking model of the homomeric α7 nicotinic receptor-β-amyloid(1–42) complex. *Biochem. Biophys. Res. Commun.* 320, 587–591. doi: 10.1016/j.bbrc.2004.05.207

Fabiani, C., Murray, A. P., Corradi, J., and Antollini, S. S. (2018). A novel pharmacological activity of caffeine in the cholinergic system. *Neuropharmacology* 135, 464–473. doi: 10.1016/j.neuropharm.2018.03.041

Fernández Nievas, G. A., Barrantes, F. J., and Antollini, S. S. (2008). Modulation of nicotinic acetylcholine receptor conformational state by free fatty acids and steroids. *J. Biol. Chem.* 283, 21478–21486. doi: 10.1074/jbc.M800345200

Gill, J. K., Savolainen, M., Young, G. T., Zwart, R., Sher, E., and Millar, N. S. (2011). Agonist activation of α7 nicotinic acetylcholine receptors *via* an allosteric transmembrane site. *Proc. Natl. Acad. Sci. U S A* 108, 5867–5872. doi: 10.1073/pnas.1017975108

Giuffrida, M. L., Caraci, F., Pignataro, B., Cataldo, S., De Bona, P., Bruno, V., et al. (2009). β-amyloid monomers are neuroprotective. *J. Neurosci.* 29, 10582–10587. doi: 10.1523/JNEUROSCI.1736-09.2009

Grassi, F., Palma, E., Tonini, R., Amici, M., Ballivet, M., and Eusebi, F. (2003). Amyloid β1–42peptide alters the gating of human and mouse α-bungarotoxin-sensitive nicotinic receptors. *J. Physiol.* 547, 147–157. doi: 10.1113/jphysiol.2002.035436

Grønlien, J. H., Håkerud, M., Ween, H., Thorin-hagene, K., Briggs, C. A., Gopalakrishnan, M., et al. (2007). Distinct profiles of α7 nAChR positive allosteric modulation revealed by structurally diverse chemotypes. *Mol. Pharmacol.* 72, 715–724. doi: 10.1124/mol.107.035410

Guan, Y.-Z., Jin, X.-D., Guan, L.-X., Yan, H.-C., Wang, P., Gong, Z., et al. (2015). Nicotine inhibits microglial proliferation and is neuroprotective in global ischemia rats. *Mol. Neurobiol.* 51, 1480–1488. doi: 10.1007/s12035-014-8825-3

Hayden, E. Y., and Teplow, D. B. (2013). Amyloid β-protein oligomers and Alzheimer's disease. *Alzheimers Res. Ther.* 5:60. doi: 10.1186/alzrt226

Hurst, R. S., Hajós, M., Raggenbass, M., Wall, T. M., Higdon, N. R., Lawson, J. A., et al. (2005). A novel positive allosteric modulator of the α7 neuronal nicotinic acetylcholine receptor: *in vitro* and *in vivo* characterization. *J. Neurosci.* 25, 4396–4405. doi: 10.1523/JNEUROSCI.5269-04.2005

Inestrosa, N. C., Godoy, J. A., Vargas, J. Y., Arrazola, M. S., Rios, J. A., Carvajal, F. J., et al. (2013). Nicotine prevents synaptic impairment induced by amyloid-β oligomers through α7-nicotinic acetylcholine receptor activation. *Neuromolecular Med.* 15, 549–569. doi: 10.1007/s12017-013-8242-1

Jin, Y., Tsuchiya, A., Kanno, T., and Nishizaki, T. (2015). Amyloid-β peptide increases cell surface localization of α7 ACh receptor to protect neurons from amyloid β-induced damage. *Biochem. Biophys. Res. Commun.* 468, 157–160. doi: 10.1016/j.bbrc.2015.10.141

Kabbani, N., Nordman, J. C., Corgiat, B. A., Veltri, D. P., Shehu, A., Seymour, V. A., et al. (2013). Are nicotinic acetylcholine receptors coupled to G proteins? *Bioessays* 35, 1025–1034. doi: 10.1002/bies.201300082

Kandimalla, R., and Reddy, P. H. (2017). Therapeutics of neurotransmitters in Alzheimer's disease. *J. Alzheimers Dis.* 57, 1049–1069. doi: 10.3233/JAD-161118

Khan, G. M., Tong, M., Jhun, M., Arora, K., and Nichols, R. A. (2010). β-Amyloid activates presynaptic α7 nicotinic acetylcholine receptors reconstituted into a model nerve cell system: involvement of lipid rafts. *Eur. J. Neurosci.* 31, 788–796. doi: 10.1111/j.1460-9568.2010.07116.x

Lacor, P. N., Buniel, M. C., Chang, L., Fernandez, S. J., Gong, Y., Viola, K. L., et al. (2004). Synaptic targeting by Alzheimer's-related amyloid β oligomers. *J. Neurosci.* 24, 10191–10200. doi: 10.1523/JNEUROSCI.3432-04.2004

Lasala, M., Corradi, J., Bruzzone, A., Esandi, M. D. C., and Bouzat, C. (2018). A human-specific, truncated α7 nicotinic receptor subunit assembles with full-length α7 and forms functional receptors with different stoichiometries. *J. Biol. Chem.* 293, 10707–10717. doi: 10.1074/jbc.RA117.001698

Lendvai, B., Kassai, F., Szájli, A., and Némethy, Z. (2013). α7 nicotinic acetylcholine receptors and their role in cognition. *Brain Res. Bull.* 93, 86–96. doi: 10.1016/j.brainresbull.2012.11.003

Li, S. F., Wu, M. N., Wang, X. H., Yuan, L., Yang, D., and Qi, J. S. (2011). Requirement of α7 nicotinic acetylcholine receptors for amyloid β protein-Induced depression of hippocampal long-term potentiation in CA1 region of rats *in vivo*. *Synapse* 65, 1136–1143. doi: 10.1002/syn.20951

Liu, Q., Kawai, H., and Berg, D. K. (2001). β-Amyloid peptide blocks the response of α 7-containing nicotinic receptors on hippocampal neurons. *Proc. Natl. Acad. Sci. U S A* 98, 4734–4739. doi: 10.1073/pnas.081553598

Liu, Q., Xie, X., Emadi, S., Sierks, M. R., and Wu, J. (2015). A novel nicotinic mechanism underlies β-amyloid-induced neurotoxicity. *Neuropharmacology* 97, 457–463. doi: 10.1016/j.neuropharm.2015.04.025

Lurtz, M. M., and Pedersen, S. E. (1999). Aminotriarylmethane dyes are high-affinity noncompetitive antagonists of the nicotinic acetylcholine receptor. *Mol. Pharmacol.* 55, 159–167. doi: 10.1124/mol.55.1.159

Miñano-Molina, A. J., España, J., Martín, E., Barneda-Zahonero, B., Fadó, R., Solé, M., et al. (2011). Soluble oligomers of amyloid-β peptide disrupt membrane trafficking of α-amino-3-hydroxy-5-methylisoxazole-4-propionic acid receptor contributing to early synapse dysfunction. *J. Biol. Chem.* 286, 27311–27321. doi: 10.1074/jbc.M111.227504

Nielsen, B. E., Minguez, T., Bermudez, I., and Bouzat, C. (2018). Molecular function of the novel α7β2 nicotinic receptor. *Cell. Mol. Life Sci.* 75, 2457–2471. doi: 10.1007/s00018-017-2741-4

Noguchi, A., Matsumura, S., Dezawa, M., Tada, M., Yanazawa, M., Ito, A., et al. (2009). Isolation and characterization of patient-derived, toxic, high mass amyloid β-protein (Aβ) assembly from Alzheimer disease brains. *J. Biol. Chem.* 284, 32895–32905. doi: 10.1074/jbc.M109.000208

Palop, J., and Mucke, L. (2010). Amyloid-β induced neuronal dysfunction in Alzheimer's disease: from synapses toward neural networks. *Nat. Neurosci.* 13, 812–818. doi: 10.1038/nn.2583

Pandya, A., and Yakel, J. L. (2011). Allosteric modulator desformylflustrabromine relieves the inhibition of α2β2 and α4β2 nicotinic acetylcholine receptors by β-amyloid 1–42 peptide. *J. Mol. Neurosci.* 45, 42–47. doi: 10.1007/s12031-011-9509-3

Parihar, M. S., and Brewer, G. J. (2010). Amyloid-β as a modulator of synaptic plasticity. *J. Alzheimers Dis.* 22, 741–763. doi: 10.3233/JAD-2010-101020

Parri, H. R., Hernandez, C. M., and Dineley, K. T. (2011). Research update: α7 nicotinic acetylcholine receptor mechanisms in Alzheimer's disease. *Biochem. Pharmacol.* 82, 931–942. doi: 10.1016/j.bcp.2011.06.039

Pascual, A. C., Gaveglio, V. L., Giusto, N. M., and Pasquaré, S. J. (2017). 2-Arachidonoylglycerol metabolism is differently modulated by oligomeric and fibrillar conformations of amyloid β in synaptic terminals. *Neuroscience* 362, 168–180. doi: 10.1016/j.neuroscience.2017.08.042

Perillo, V. L., Fernández-Nievas, G. A., Vallés, A. S., Barrantes, F. J., and Antollini, S. S. (2012). The position of the double bond in monounsaturated free fatty acids is essential for the inhibition of the nicotinic acetylcholine receptor. *Biochim. Biophys. Acta* 1818, 2511–2520. doi: 10.1016/j.bbamem.2012.06.001

Pear, W. S., Nolan, G. P., Scott, M. L., and Baltimore, D. (1993). Production of high-titer helper-free retroviruses by transient transfection. *Proc. Natl. Acad. Sci. U S A* 90, 8392–8396. doi: 10.1109/ICDMW.2006.113

Puzzo, D., Gulisano, W., Arancio, O., and Palmeri, A. (2015). The keystone of Alzheimer pathogenesis might be sought in Aβ physiology. *Neuroscience* 307, 26–36. doi: 10.1016/j.neuroscience.2015.08.039

Puzzo, D., Privitera, L., Fa', M., Staniszewski, A., Hashimoto, G., Aziz, F., et al. (2011). Endogenous amyloid-β is necessary for hippocampal synaptic plasticity and memory. *Ann. Neurol.* 69, 819–830. doi: 10.1002/ana.22313

Pym, L., Kemp, M., Raymond-Delpech, V., Buckingham, S., Boyd, C. A. R., and Sattelle, D. (2005). Subtype-specific actions of β-amyloid peptides on recombinant human neuronal nicotinic acetylcholine receptors (α7, α4β2, α3β4) expressed in *Xenopus laevis* oocytes. *Br. J. Pharmacol.* 146, 964–971. doi: 10.1038/sj.bjp.0706403

Qin, F., Auerbach, A., and Sachs, F. (1996). Estimating single-channel kinetic parameters from idealized patch-clamp data containing missed events. *Biophys. J.* 70, 264–280. doi: 10.1016/s0006-3495(96)79568-1

Qin, F., Auerbach, A., and Sachs, F. (1997). Maximum likelihood estimation of aggregated Markov processes. *Proc. Biol. Sci.* 264, 375–383. doi: 10.1098/rspb.1997.0054

Sadigh-Eteghad, S., Talebi, M., Farhoudi, M., Golzari, S. E. J., Sabermarouf, B., and Mahmoudi, J. (2014). β-amyloid exhibits antagonistic effects on α 7 nicotinic acetylcholine receptors in orchestrated manner. *J. Med. Hypotheses Ideas* 8, 49–52. doi: 10.1016/j.jmhi.2014.01.001

Santos, A. N., Ewers, M., Minthon, L., Simm, A., Silber, R.-E., Blennow, K., et al. (2012). Amyloid-β oligomers in cerebrospinal fluid are associated with cognitive decline in patients with Alzheimer's disease. *J. Alzheimers Dis.* 29, 171–176. doi: 10.3233/JAD-2012-111361

Sauguet, L., Shahsavar, A., and Delarue, M. (2015). Crystallographic studies of pharmacological sites in pentameric ligand-gated ion channels. *Biochim. Biophys. Acta* 1850, 511–523. doi: 10.1016/j.bbagen.2014.05.007

Shankar, G. M., Li, S., Mehta, T. H., Garcia-Munoz, A., Shepardson, N. E., Smith, I., et al. (2008). Amyloid-β protein dimers isolated directly from Alzheimer's brains impair synaptic plasticity and memory. *Nat. Med.* 14, 837–842. doi: 10.1038/nm1782

Sun, J., Comeau, J. F., and Baenziger, J. E. (2017). Probing the structure of the uncoupled nicotinic acetylcholine receptor. *Biochim. Biophys. Acta Biomembr.* 1859, 146–154. doi: 10.1016/j.bbamem.2016.11.009

Terry, A. V. Jr., Callahan, P. M., and Bertrand, D. (2015). R-(+) and S-(-) isomers of cotinine augment cholinergic responses *in vitro* and *in vivo*. *J. Pharmacol. Exp. Ther.* 352, 405–418. doi: 10.1124/jpet.114.219881

Timmermann, D. B., Grønlien, J. H., Kohlhaas, K. L., Nielsen, E. Ø., Dam, E., Jørgensen, T. D., et al. (2007). An allosteric modulator of the α7 nicotinic acetylcholine receptor possessing cognition-enhancing properties *in vivo*. *J. Pharmacol. Exp. Ther.* 323, 294–307. doi: 10.1124/jpet.107.120436

Tong, M., Arora, K., White, M. M., and Nichols, R. A. (2011). Role of key aromatic residues in the ligand-binding domain of α7 nicotinic receptors in the agonist action of β-amyloid. *J. Biol. Chem.* 286, 34373–34381. doi: 10.1074/jbc.M111.241299

Uranga, R. M., Alza, N. P., Conde, M. A., Antollini, S. S., and Salvador, G. A. (2016). Phosphoinositides: two-path signaling in neuronal response to oligomeric amyloid β peptide. *Mol. Neurobiol.* 54, 3236–3252. doi: 10.1007/s12035-016-9885-3

Uteshev, V. V. (2014). The therapeutic promise of positive allosteric modulation of nicotinic receptors. *Eur. J. Pharmacol.* 727, 181–185. doi: 10.1016/j.ejphar.2014.01.072

Wallace, T. L., and Bertrand, D. (2013). α7 neuronal nicotinic receptors as a drug target in schizophrenia. *Expert Opin. Ther. Targets* 17, 139–155. doi: 10.1517/14728222.2013.736498

Walsh, D. M., Klyubin, I., Fadeeva, J. V., Cullen, W. K., Anwyl, R., Wolfe, M. S., et al. (2002). Naturally secreted oligomers of amyloid β protein potently inhibit hippocampal long-term potentiation *in vivo*. *Nature* 416, 535–539. doi: 10.1038/416535a

Walsh, D. M., Tseng, B. P., Rydel, R. E., Podlisny, M. B., and Selkoe, D. J. (2000). The oligomerization of amyloid β-protein begins intracellularly in cells derived from human brain. *Biochemistry* 39, 10831–10839. doi: 10.1021/bi001048s

Wang, H.-Y., Lee, D. H. S., D'Andrea, M. R., Peterson, P. A., Shank, R. P., and Reitz, A. B. (2000). β-Amyloid1–42 Binds to α 7 nicotinic acetylcholine receptor with high affinity. Implications for Alzheimer's disease pathology. *J. Biol. Chem.* 275, 5626–5632. doi: 10.1074/jbc.275.8.5626

Wang, H. W., Pasternak, J. F., Kuo, H., Ristic, H., Lambert, M. P., Chromy, B., et al. (2002). Soluble oligomers of β amyloid (1–42g) inhibit long-term potentiation but not long-term depression in rat dentate gyrus. *Brain Res.* 924, 133–140. doi: 10.1016/s0006-8993(01)03058-x

Watt, A. D., Perez, K. A., Rembach, A., Sherrat, N. A., Hung, L. W., Johanssen, T., et al. (2013). Oligomers, fact or artefact? SDS-PAGE induces dimerization of β-amyloid in human brain samples. *Acta Neuropathol.* 125, 549–564. doi: 10.1007/s00401-013-1083-z

Wonnacott, S. (2014). Nicotinic ACh receptors. *Tocris Biosci. Sci. Rev. Ser. Nicotinic*, 1–31.

Wu, J., Kuo, Y.-P. P., George, A. A., Xu, L., Hu, J., Lukas, R. J., et al. (2004). β-amyloid directly inhibits human α4β2-nicotinic acetylcholine receptors heterologously expressed in human SH-EP1 cells. *J. Biol. Chem.* 279, 37842–37851. doi: 10.1074/jbc.m400335200

Yan, H., Pan, N., Xue, F., Zheng, Y., Li, C., Chang, Y., et al. (2015). The coupling interface and pore domain codetermine the single-channel activity of theα7 nicotinic receptor. *Neuropharmacology* 95, 448–458. doi: 10.1016/j.neuropharm.2015.04.010

Yang, T., Xiao, T., Sun, Q., and Wang, K. (2017). The current agonists and positive allosteric modulators of α7 nAChR for CNS indications in clinical trials. *Acta Pharm. Sin. B* 7, 611–622. doi: 10.1016/j.apsb.2017.09.001

13

Processing Bodies Oscillate in Neuro 2A Cells

*Melisa Malcolm[1,2], Lucía Saad[1,2], Laura Gabriela Penazzi[1,2] and Eduardo Garbarino-Pico[1,2]**

[1] Departamento de Química Biológica Ranwel Caputto, Facultad de Ciencias Químicas, Universidad Nacional de Córdoba (UNC), Córdoba, Argentina, [2] CONICET-UNC, Centro de Investigaciones en Química Biológica de Córdoba (CIQUIBIC), Córdoba, Argentina

***Correspondence:**
Eduardo Garbarino-Pico
egarbarino@unc.edu.ar

Circadian rhythms are biological variables that oscillate with periods close to 24 h that are generated internally by biological clocks. Depending on the tissue/cell type, about 5–20% of genes are expressed rhythmically. Unexpectedly, the correlation between the oscillations of messengers and the proteins they encode is low. We hypothesize that these discrepancies could be because in certain phases of the circadian cycle some messengers could be translationally silenced and stored. Processing bodies (PBs) are membraneless organelles formed by ribonucleoprotein aggregates located in the cytoplasm. They contain silenced messengers and factors involved in mRNA processing. A previous work showed that the number of cells containing these mRNA granules varies when comparing two time-points in U2OS cell cultures and that these differences disappear when an essential clock gene is silenced. Here we evaluate whether PBs oscillate in Neuro2A cells. We analyzed in cell cultures synchronized with dexamethasone the variations in the number, the signal intensity of the markers used (GE-1/HEDLS and DDX6), and the area of PBs between 8 and 68 h post-synchronization. All three parameters oscillated with periods compatible with a circadian regulated process. The most robust rhythm was the number of PBs. These rhythms could be generated by oscillations in proteins that have been involved in the nucleation of these foci such as LSM1, TTP, and BRF1. The described phenomenon would allow to explain the differences observed in the temporal profiles of some messengers and their proteins and to understand how circadian clocks can control post-transcriptionally cellular functions.

Keywords: processing bodies, circadian rhythms, Neuro 2A, RNA granules, GE1/Hedls, DDX6/P54/RCK, membraneless organelles

INTRODUCTION

Throughout evolution, living beings have developed mechanisms capable of measuring time and controlling numerous functions in a cyclic manner. Most of these oscillations have a period of 1 day in natural environments and close to 24 h in constant conditions. These mechanisms are called biological clocks and the functions they control circadian rhythms.

They are believed to confer adaptative advantages by predicting the cyclic changes in the environment caused by the rotation of the Earth (e.g., light/dark and temperature cycles) and temporarily organizing physiology (Schibler et al., 2015; Bass and Lazar, 2016; Takahashi, 2017). Examples of circadian rhythms are cycles of sleep/wakefulness, locomotor activity or body temperature. In neurons, rhythms have been described in firing rate, gene expression, the activity of enzymes and channels and even in synaptic plasticity, among others. The molecular clockwork consists of a group of genes that mutually regulate each other through interconnected transcription-translation negative feedback loops (TTFLs) (Takahashi, 2017). These circuits rhythmically regulate the abundance of messengers encoded by ~5–20% of genes in different tissues/organs and about 50% of mRNAs oscillate in at least some tissue (Zhang et al., 2014). Importantly, post-transcriptional regulation also plays a very important role in the generation of rhythms in protein abundance (Green, 2018). This is reflected in the poor correlation that exists between variations in the abundance of transcripts and their corresponding proteins (Reddy et al., 2006; Mauvoisin et al., 2014; Robles et al., 2014).

In the last two decades, new types of intracellular compartments characterized by not being delimited by membranes have been described in eukaryotic cells, collectively called membraneless organelles or RNA granules. They are condensed liquid-like droplets of ribonuleoprotein complexes (Courchaine et al., 2016; Sfakianos et al., 2016; Shin and Brangwynne, 2017). In cytosol, these subcompartments include processing bodies (PBs), stress granules, germ granules and neuronal granules. PBs are constitutively present, contain translationally silent mRNAs and factors involved in messengers 5′→3′ degradation, repression of translation, and RNA interference (Decker and Parker, 2012; Ivanov et al., 2018; Standart and Weil, 2018). Because of this, and other indirect evidence, it has been proposed that these foci would play a role in mRNA degradation (Sheth and Parker, 2003). However, it was also demonstrated that some messengers localizing in PBs can be translated again, consequently they would also serve as storage places (Brengues et al., 2005). Recently, it was possible to purify PBs and determine the identity of many of the proteins and mRNAs that compose them (Hubstenberger et al., 2017). From these studies it was proposed that PBs would store mRNA regulons, that is groups of transcripts coding for proteins with regulatory functions of specific pathways, while messengers with basic functions are virtually excluded (for example, transcripts coding for histone methylases but not for histones were found in PBs) (Hubstenberger et al., 2017; Standart and Weil, 2018). Thus, PBs have a role in the post-transcriptional regulation of gene expression, remarkably they would store silenced the mRNAs of groups of genes that modulate specific functions.

Since it is proposed that PBs store silenced messengers, if these structures were to oscillate, this would help to explain (at least partially) the discrepancies observed when analyzing the mRNA and protein profiles corresponding to a number of genes (Reddy et al., 2006; Mauvoisin et al., 2014; Robles et al., 2014). That is, if the messengers of a particular gene are mostly located in PBs, no matter how abundant, this will not be reflected in their protein levels or translation rate. If it is also considered that these foci contain fundamentally transcripts of regulatory factors (Hubstenberger et al., 2017; Standart and Weil, 2018), changes in their abundance and/or size would contribute to understanding the pathways by which many rhythmic cellular processes are regulated. In fact, Jang et al. (2015) have demonstrated changes in the number of cells containing PBs in cultures of U2OS cells (human osteosarcoma cell line). They decided to study this because previously, by ribosome profiling, they had found that the translation of *Lsm1* was circadian modulated into U2OS cells. LSM1 is a marker of PBs (Ingelfinger et al., 2002; Kedersha and Anderson, 2007). They also demonstrated that silencing a fundamental clock gene in the circadian clock molecular mechanism abrogates those differences (Jang et al., 2015). Given that this work analyzes only two time-points post-synchronization with dexamethasone (4 and 16 h), and that one of these is very close to the addition of this synchronizing agent that dramatically affects cellular physiology, we decided to analyze whether the number and size of PBs varies for 68 h in a neuroblastoma cell line. In this Brief Research Report we show that these two parameters oscillate cyclically in cultures of Neuro 2A cells.

MATERIALS AND METHODS

Cell Culture

Mouse Albino neuroblastoma (Neuro 2a) cells (ATCC) were cultured in Minimum Essential Medium (MEM, Gibco) supplemented with 10% fetal bovine serum (FBS, Internegocios S.A, Argentina), in a 37°C incubator with 5% CO_2 according ATCC recommendations. These cells have been used before for studying circadian rhythms in cell cultures (Chilov et al., 2001; Margadant et al., 2007; Repouskou et al., 2010; Chang and Guarente, 2013). Cells were grown on coverslips in a 24-well plate until they reached ~70% of confluence, and then maintained in serum starvation conditions (0.25%, see below) to prevent the progression of the cell cycle. This is important to ensure that changes observed over time are regulated by the circadian clock and not by the cell cycle. Initially we tried to completely eliminate serum from the medium, but cells did not survive the 68 h that the experiment required. Subsequently we tested for 96 h different serum concentrations: 0, 0.1, 0.25, and 0.5%. Cells died at serum concentration lower than 0.25% and proliferate at 0.5% FBS; thus we chose 0.25% FBS, a concentration in which the number of cells did not vary during the 96 h analyzed. To control that the cells were not proliferating, we analyzed cultures grown in the same conditions by flow cytometry with propidium iodide. Indeed, when the cultures contained only 0.25% FBS in the medium, the cells were arrested. For circadian clock synchronization (i.e., to entrain the cell population to the same circadian phase), cells were treated for 1 h with 100 nM dexamethasone (Balsalobre et al., 2000; Nagoshi et al., 2005; Repouskou et al., 2010); then culture medium was replaced with fresh 0.25% FBS-MEM.

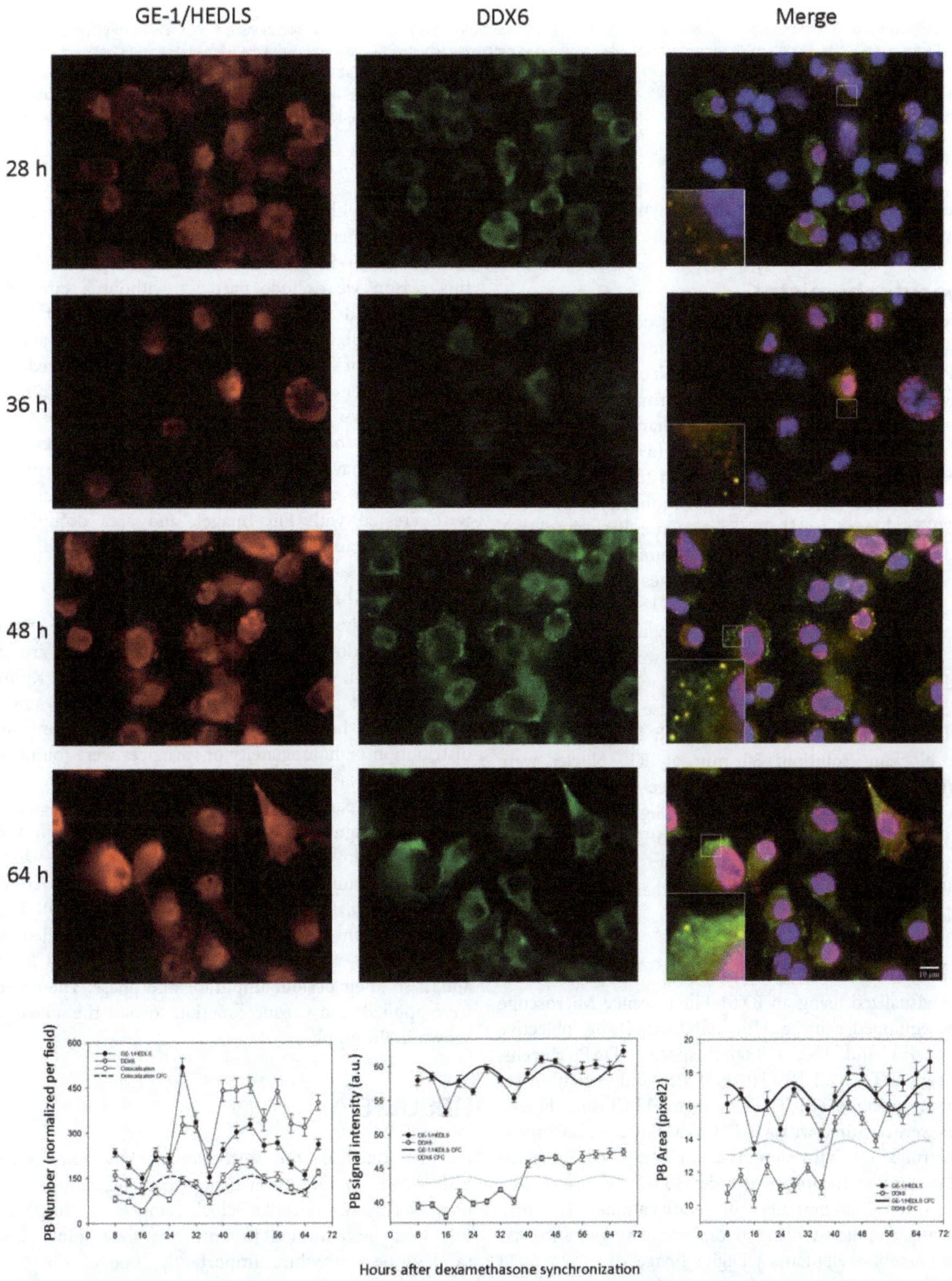

FIGURE 1 | Processing Bodies oscillate cyclically in synchronized cultures of Neuro 2A cells. When the cultures reached 60–70% confluence, the medium was replaced with a fresh one containing only 0.25% serum, condition in which the cell cycle is arrested (see M&M). The following day they were synchronized with dexamethasone and fixed every 4 h between 8 and 68 h post-synchronization. The cells fixed on cover slips were treated with two antibodies by ICC, anti-GE-1/HEDLS (red) and anti-DDX6 (green), recognized PB markers. In addition, the nuclei were stained with dapi (blue). Then they were analyzed by epifluorescence microscopy and pictures were taken with a CCD camera. On the left are shown the post-synchronization time-points that are illustrated and on top the names of the markers. The images were analyzed with ImageJ and three parameters were quantified: number (per field, it was normalized considering that the

(Continued)

FIGURE 1 | Continued
field was completely covered with cells), average signal intensity and the average area of the PBs. These quantifications are shown in the right panel. The Kruskall–Wallis test followed by Dunn's multiple comparison test was used to determine whether the changes over time were statistically significant. MetaCycle was used to assess whether the time series of data showed rhythmicity. These analyses are presented in **Table 1** and **Supplementary Tables S5–S10**, all three parameters showed cyclic changes with the two markers. With the period, phase and amplitude values obtained by MetaCycle, the data were adjusted to a cosine-fitted curve (CFC). In the case of the PB number, the curve obtained when considering the PBs detected with the two antibodies (colocalization) is also shown.

Cells were fixed every 4 h for 68 h post-synchronization for immunocytochemistry analysis.

Immunocytochemistry

Immunocytochemistry (ICC) was achieved according a protocol described by Kedersha and colleagues for analyzing PBs (Kedersha and Anderson, 2007). Briefly, Neuro 2a cells were washed twice with PBS, fixed with paraformaldehyde 4% for 15 min., permeabilized with -20°C methanol for 10 min., and incubated 1 h in blocking solution (5% Horse serum-PBS). These steps were carried out at room temperature (RT). Then cells were incubated with a mouse monoclonal antibody against p70 S6 kinase α (H-9) (Santa Cruz Biotechnology), diluted 1:1000 in blocking solution, in a humidified chamber overnight at RT. This antibody recognizes p70 S6 kinase α in the nucleus and GE-1/HEDLS/EDC4 in cytoplasm, a known marker for PBs and has been widely used for studying this foci [reviewed in 20]. Then, cells were rinsed three times with PBS, followed by incubation with a polyclonal DyLight 549-AffiniPure donkey anti-mouse IgG secondary antibody (1:2000, Jackson ImmunoResearch Labs), diluted in the same blocking solution, 30 min at RT. Nuclei were stained with Dapi. Cells were rinsed three times with PBS and mounted on slices with mowiol (Sigma-Aldrich). In addition to anti-GE-1/HEDLS, anti-DDX6/P54/RCK (Bethyl Laboratories, 1:500 in blocking solution) was used in double immunolabeling experiments. This is another recognized PB marker (Kedersha and Anderson, 2007).

Image Detection and Analysis

Slices were visualized using an BX61 Fluorescence Microscope (Olympus) equipped with a UPLSAPO 60XO oil objective lens (NA 1.35) and U-T31 000v2 specific DAPI/Hoechs, U-TSP101para FITC, and U-T31014 Wide-band excitation set for Elphidium Bromide TRITC, Phenothrin Dil Chroma Filters. The images were acquired with a JAI® CV-M4+CL monochrome camera controlled by Cytovision® (Leica Biosystems). PBs were quantified according the procedure developed by Nissan and Parker (2008) for stress granules with modifications. The entire procedure was conducted using algorithms that guarantee an unbiased treatment of all pictures. Digital images of 1376 × 1038 pixels and 8 bits were processed with the ImageJ program as follow: *1)* Process menu > "Filters" > "Gaussian Blur" sigma radius 0.8 pix. *2)* Process menu > "Subtract background" (Rolling ball radius: 5 pix). *3)* Image > "Adjust" > "Threshold" 40 (red channel) or 35 (green channel). *4)* Analyze menu > "Analyze particles" > size 3–300 pix2, circularity 0.7-1. Importantly, the same threshold value was used in the analysis of all the images within each experiment, to ensure an unbiased comparison between time-points. P- bodies are considered circular, ∼300–500 nm in diameter (Cougot et al., 2012), for this reason we exclude particles without a circularity <0.7 (1 correspond to a perfect circle) or out of 3–300 pix^2 range. This pixel size range allows quantifying particles with a diameter of 200–2000 nm. The PBs observed in Neuro 2a cells presented an average diameter of 476 nm with this procedure. We were able to decrease the upper limit to a value closer to the largest particle found, even though it would not have affected the results. P-body number was normalized by area covered by cells, for that purpose, masks were created with Fiji ImageJ, and area occupied in each microphotograph was measured.

Statistical Analysis

Statistical analysis was performed using GraphPad Prism version 5.00 for Windows (GraphPad Software). Values are shown as mean ± SEM, unless otherwise indicated. The Kolmogorov-Smirnov's test was used to check for normality, and Barlett's test to check homogeneity of variances. Because non-normal distribution or homogeneity of variances were found, Kruskal–Wallis's test was used instead of ANOVA, followed by Dunn's multiple comparisons test; *p*-values $\leq$0.05 were considered as statistically significant. To evaluate periodicity in time-series data we employed MetaCycle (Wu et al., 2016), which is a R package that runs and integrates three algorithms: ARSER (Yang and Su, 2010), JTK_CYCLE (Hughes et al., 2010), and Lomb-Scargle (Glynn et al., 2006). The statistics applied with this analysis allow us to determine whether the data are periodic and, if so, their period, amplitude and phase. These parameters were applied to a Cosine function to plot the adjusted curves shown in the graph.

RESULTS

As mentioned in the Introduction, Jang and collaborators had shown important evidence that the number of PBs is regulated by the circadian clock (Jang et al., 2015). However, this study was limited to only two time-points, insufficient to describe a rhythm. Importantly, one of the time-points at which the number of PBs was analyzed was too close to synchronization (4 h), when the culture – and therefore the phenomenon studied – are still under the effect of the synchronizing agent (dexamethasone in this case). It is usual to start measuring at least 8 h after synchronization to analyze the rhythms independent of the effect of the agent used. We have also found, by using a database of circadian gene expression

TABLE 1 | PB temporal oscillations in Neuro 2a cells. PB number (normalized per field).

	DDX6		GE-1/HEDLS				DDX6		GE-1/HEDLS		
t(h)	**Mean**	**SEM**	**Mean**	**SEM**	***n***	**t(h)**	**Mean**	**SEM**	**Mean**	**SEM**	***n***
8	158.50	78.03	233.90	61.24	20	40	440.14	440.14	243.39	117.03	20
12	135.88	55.14	193.19	57.38	24	44	441.96	441.96	303.24	91.81	20
16	107.21	44.95	149.42	71.50	18	48	458.20	458.20	328.19	89.84	20
20	228.78	95.91	222.16	77.44	21	52	343.16	343.16	257.67	86.02	16
24	188.79	77.82	215.81	66.44	20	56	436.80	436.80	265.86	102.40	20
28	326.62	125.14	518.41	129.08	19	60	330.72	330.72	194.10	66.05	25
32	322.07	93.82	334.35	150.35	20	64	318.47	318.47	159.11	69.52	20
36	217.18	142.59	152.55	82.95	19	68	399.98	399.98	260.99	73.01	17

Statistical analysis

Kruskall-Wallis DDX6		Kruskall-Wallis GE-1/HEDLS	
P	**H**	***P***	**H**
P < 0.0001	171.50	P < 0.0001	132.30

MetaCycle (meta2d)1 DDX6				MetaCycle (meta2d)1GE-1/HEDLS			
P	**Period**	**Phase**	**Amp**	***P***	**Period**	**Phase**	**Amp**
5.32E-04	23.33	1.17	41.12	0.00	23.57	647	57.79

Signal intensity (a.u.)

	DDX6		GE-1/HEDLS				DDX6		GE-1/HEDLS		
t(h)	**Mean**	**SEM**	**Mean**	**SEM**	***n***	**t(h)**	**Mean**	**SEM**	**Mean**	**SEM**	***n***
8	39.48	2.18	57.93	3.20	20	40	45.56	2.60	58.90	3.59	20
12	39.61	2.02	58.50	2.62	24	44	46.41	1.73	61.00	2.15	20
16	37.94	1.63	53.21	2.19	15	48	46.49	2.02	60.72	1.91	20
20	41.27	2.86	57.84	3.83	21	52	45.19	1.78	59.37	2.54	16
24	39.75	1.70	56.28	2.01	20	56	46.64	3.46	59.72	3.96	20
28	40.08	1.66	59.68	2.63	19	60	46.97	2.78	60.23	3.12	25
32	41.83	1.52	58.10	2.02	20	64	47.14	3.13	59.63	4.29	20
36	40.15	2.19	55.31	2.76	19	68	47.31	2.28	62.19	3.42	17

Satistical analysis

Kruskall-Wallis DDX6		Kruskall-Wallis GE-1/HEDLS	
P	**H**	***P***	**H**
P < 0.0001	232.70	P < 0.0001	113.30

MetaCycle (meta2d)1 DDX6				MetaCycle (meta2d)1 GE-1/HEDLS			
P	**Period**	**Phase**	**Amp**	***P***	**Period**	**Phase**	**Amp**
1.85E-06	20.60	0.44	0.44	341E-07	19.93	7.22	1.34

Area (pixel^2)

	DDX6		GE-1/HEDLS				DDX6		GE-1/HEDLS		
t(h)	**Mean**	**SEM**	**Mean**	**SEM**	***n***	**t(h)**	**Mean**	**SEM**	**Mean**	**SEM**	***n***
8	10.70	2.36	16.12	2.38	20	40	14.95	2.41	16.56	2.81	20
12	11.80	2.02	16.72	1.75	24	44	16.19	1.84	17.97	1.83	20
16	10.37	2.15	13.41	1.82	15	48	15.25	1.86	17.88	1.80	20

(Continued)

TABLE 1 | Continued

	DDX6		GE-1/HEDLS				DDX6		GE-1/HEDLS		
t(h)	Mean	SEM	Mean	SEM	*n*	t(h)	Mean	SEM	Mean	SEM	*n*
20	12.39	2.44	16.28	2.73	21	52	13.89	1.65	16.67	1.84	16
24	10.97	1.30	14.60	1.74	20	56	16.07	3.37	17.53	3.46	20
25	11.19	1.81	16.98	1.90	19	60	15.39	2.47	17.35	2.38	25
32	12.25	1.27	15.78	1.56	20	64	16.07	2.79	17.90	3.19	20
36	11.07	1.92	14.21	1.74	19	68	16.05	1.90	18.63	2.73	17

Satistical analysis

Kruskall-Wallis DDX6		Kruskall-Wallis GE-1/HEDLS	
P	H	*P*	H
P < 0.0001	182.50	*P* < 0.0001	91.06

MetaCycle (meta2d)1 DDX6				MetaCycle (meta2d)1 GE-1/HEDLS			
P	Period	Phase	Amp	*p*	Period	Phase	Amp
141E-06	22.74	20.52	144	0.00	19.72	7.87	0.80

Note that the mean was calculated as the mean of the means of each micmphotograph. N indicates the number of microphotographs per time analyzed. Each picture contain an average of 23 cells per field.

[CircaDB, Pizarro et al., 2013], that two proteins involved in the nucleation of PBs, Tristetraprolin (TTP) and BRF-1 (Franks and Lykke-Andersen, 2007), present oscillations in the levels of their messengers in murine liver (**Supplementary Figures S1, S2**, from CircaDB). All this together led us to analyze whether PBs show oscillations over time.

In this work we analyze whether PBs present rhythms in cultures of Neuro 2A cells, which have already been used for circadian studies (Chilov et al., 2001; Margadant et al., 2007; Repouskou et al., 2010; Chang and Guarente, 2013). These cells were established from mouse neuroblastoma, so they grow continuously and do not stop dividing under normal culture conditions (10% FBS-MEM). For this reason we first test with which serum concentration the cells stop dividing and thus prevent the progress of the cell cycle from interfering with the determinations of the analyzed variables (see section "Materials and Methods"). When the cultures reached 60–70% confluence, the cell population was synchronized with dexamethasone for 1 h and subsequently maintained at 0.25% FBS-MEM until they were fixed at the indicated time-points. PBs were detected by ICC with an antibody recognizing the GE-1/HEDLS marker. Microphotographs were taken and the PBs were quantified with ImageJ (see section "Materials and Methods"). The number of PBs showed oscillations over time (**Supplementary Figure S3**). The determinations were made between 8 and 68 h post-synchronization, in that lapse two peaks and two valleys can be observed in the three parameters analyzed. In **Supplementary Figure S3A** are shown representative pictures of these time-points (left panel) and the same photos with the mask that was obtained with the quantification procedure used (right panel). **Supplementary Figure S3B** shows the result of quantifying the number of PBs normalized by the area occupied by cells, the average intensity of the signal obtained after subtracting the background, and the average area of the granules at the different times analyzed. The three variables analyzed showed a similar profile. All three parameters showed significant changes over time (Kruskall–Wallis test, **Supplementary Table S1** and **Supplementary Tables S2–S4** show Dunn's multiple comparison tests for the three parameters). The MetaCycle R package was used to determine whether the time series of data were rhythmic (Wu et al., 2016). This package applies statistical tests that determined that the parameters cycle with periods compatible with circadian rhythms, in addition to estimating amplitude and phase of oscillations (**Supplementary Table S1**). The number of PBs was the rhythm that showed the greatest amplitude. When the experiment was repeated, similar results were obtained. While the period of oscillations in signal intensity and area were comparable in the two experiments (signal intensity 24.17 vs. 22.81; area 23.34 vs. 22.46), the period of the number of PBs showed differences (30.52 vs. 23.15). In any case, taking into account that the variable is not being measured continuously and the sampling frequency (every 4 h), it is to be expected that the period cannot be determined precisely and the differences that are observed in the period estimations.

In order to corroborate with another marker the existence of the oscillations described in PBs, we performed double immunostaining experiments analyzing DDX6 [also known as P54/RCK, another recognized PB marker (Kedersha and Anderson, 2007)] together with GE-1/HEDLS. The cultures were synchronized and the same time-points were taken as in **Supplementary Figure S1**, although in this case two antibodies were used in the ICC. **Figure 1** and **Table 1** show that the number, signal intensity and area of PBs showed relatively similar profiles with both markers. All three variables, with both antibodies, showed statistically significant changes over time in the form of periodic oscillations of at least two cycles (Kruskall–Wallis test and MetaCycle, **Table 1**; **Supplementary Tables S5–S10**,

Dunn's multiple comparison tests. n = 16–24 pictures per time-point). In each microphotography there were 23.6 ± 9.1 nuclei (average ± SD); that is, between 378 and 566 cells were analyzed at each time-point. Remarkably, all three parameters showed higher levels in the second cycle when PBs were detected with anti-DDX6 (**Figure 1** and **Table 1**). The PB number was the variable that showed the greatest amplitude with the two markers. It was normalized by the surface occupied by the cells since several of them were not completely included in the pictures.

Considering this, when the PB number was divided by the number of nuclei, on average this coefficient was between 2.3 and 7.9 per cell when GE-1/HEDLS was used and between 2.7 and 10.8 with DDX6. The period estimated with the two antibodies was very similar, 23.57 h with anti-GE-1/HEDLS and 23.33 h with anti-DDX6. When only granules marked with both markers were considered, as expected the number decreased. Even so the behavior over time remained rhythmic (Fig. 1. p = 2.19E-11 by MetaCycle). When the signal intensity was analyzed, the overall values were different with each antibody, this is to be expected since they are different antibodies and fluorophores, although the time pattern was relatively similar but with greater amplitude for GE-1/HEDLS (**Figure 1** and **Table 1**). In the case of the PB area, as anticipated, the values were reduced since in general the overlap of the signal was not complete, which means that not all the pixels recognized with one antibody as a PB matched exactly with those detected by the other. However, the temporal behavior also showed to be statistically rhythmic (p = 5.3E-4). This experiment was repeated and showed similar results; therefore, these oscillations were demonstrated in 4 independent experiments with anti-GE-1/HEDLS and in 2 with anti-DDX6. In these repetitions minor changes in the phase and amplitude of the rhythms are observed, this is expected since the measurements were not made in a continuous way but with intervals of 4 h and taking different samples in each time-point; nevertheless the temporal profiles are similar in all the cases.

CONCLUSION

This work shows for the first time oscillations in the dynamics of PBs. These rhythms were evidenced both in the number, intensity levels of the marker used, and the area of these cytoplasmic ribonucleoprotein granules with two different markers. A previous study had shown differences in the number of PBs when comparing two time-points in U2OS cells, as well as that this difference disappeared by silencing a clock gene essential for the functioning of the circadian clock molecular mechanism (Jang et al., 2015). Taken together, these works indicate that PBs are modulated by circadian clocks. Interestingly, both we (manuscript submitted) and another group (Wang et al., 2019), have found that other type of mRNA granules, the stress granules, also have temporal variations in their number.

In this brief report we limit ourselves to presenting the phenomenon, we have not explored the mechanisms by which the rhythms described in PBs are generated. A plausible hypothesis is that the circadian clock control the levels of factors that can induce the formation of PBs. In fact, changes in the rate of translation of a marker of these foci, LSM1, suggested to Jang and colleagues that PBs could be controlled by the circadian clock (Jang et al., 2015). We searched the CircaDB database (Pizarro et al., 2013) for messengers of two other of these proteins, TTP and BRF1 (Franks and Lykke-Andersen, 2007), that oscillated in their levels, and in fact do so (**Supplementary Figures S1, S2**). Other proteins that induce the formation of PBs may also participate in the generation of the observed rhythms. In addition to changes in the concentration of these proteins, post-translational modifications that induce the phase transitions that form PBs have also been described. If any of these modifications are rhythmically controlled, this could also contribute to the phenomenon described.

It is currently postulated that PBs are membrane-free compartments where transcripts are stored (Hubstenberger et al., 2017; Standart and Weil, 2018). They have also been involved in translation silencing and mRNA degradation [discussed in Decker and Parker (2012), Ivanov et al. (2018)]. Since at the beginning of the century technologies were available to analyze the transcriptome and the proteome globally, circadian experiments were performed that demonstrated a significant number of genes (~50%) showed, contrary to expectations, a poor correlation between the abundance rhythms of their mRNA and protein (Reddy et al., 2006; Mauvoisin et al., 2014; Robles et al., 2014). The presence of many of these messengers in PBs, instead of in polysomes, could explain that even being abundant, their corresponding proteins would not be present in the same magnitude.

Considering the evidence suggesting that PBs store groups of messengers that participate in the regulation of specific pathways [mRNA regulons (Hubstenberger et al., 2017)], the fact that these foci are rhythmically regulated would contribute to understand how clocks can control a number of circadian rhythms at a post-transcriptional level.

AUTHOR CONTRIBUTIONS

MM, LS, and LP: acquisition, analysis and interpretation of data, making of the figures, revising the work, and design critically. EG-P: conception and design of the work, and manuscript writing. All authors contributed to the manuscript revision, and read and approved the submitted version.

FUNDING

The authors would like to acknowledge the support of the Agencia Nacional de Promoción Científica y Tecnológica (PICT 2013-2680), the Consejo Nacional de Investigaciones Científicas y Técnicas (CONICET), and the Universidad Nacional de Córdoba of Argentina for providing facilities and grants to carry out the research.

ACKNOWLEDGMENTS

The authors appreciate the technical assistance of Drs. Alejandra Trenchi, Susana Deheza, Gabriela Schachener, and the members of the "Centro de Microscopia Óptica y Confocal Avanzada de Coìrdoba (CEMINCO)", integrated to the "Sistema Nacional de Microscopia (SNM-MINCyT)" for microscopy assistant.

REFERENCES

Balsalobre, A., Brown, S. A., Marcacci, L., Tronche, F., Kellendonk, C., and Reichardt, H. M. (2000). Resetting of circadian time in peripheral tissues by glucocorticoid signaling. *Science* 289, 2344–2347. doi: 10.1126/science.289.5488.2344

Bass, J., and Lazar, M. A. (2016). Circadian time signatures of fitness and disease. *Science* 354, 994–999. doi: 10.1126/science.aah4965

Brengues, M., Teixeira, D., and Parker, R. (2005). Movement of eukaryotic mRNAs between polysomes and cytoplasmic processing bodies. *Science* 310, 486–489. doi: 10.1126/science.1115791

Chang, H. C., and Guarente, L. (2013). SIRT1 mediates central circadian control in the SCN by a mechanism that decays with aging. *Cell* 153, 1448–1460. doi: 10.1016/j.cell.2013.05.027

Chilov, D., Hofer, T., Bauer, C., Wenger, R. H., and Gassmann, M. (2001). Hypoxia affects expression of circadian genes PER1 and CLOCK in mouse brain. *FASEB J.* 15, 2613–2622. doi: 10.1096/fj.01-0092com

Cougot, N., Cavalier, A., Thomas, D., and Gillet, R. (2012). The dual organization of P-bodies revealed by immunoelectron microscopy and electron tomography. *J. Mol. Biol.* 420, 17–28. doi: 10.1016/j.jmb.2012.03.027

Courchaine, E. M., Lu, A., and Neugebauer, K. M. (2016). Droplet organelles? *EMBO J.* 35, 1603–1612. doi: 10.15252/embj.201593517

Decker, C. J., and Parker, R. (2012). P-bodies and stress granules: possible roles in the control of translation and mRNA degradation. *Cold Spring Harb. Perspect. Biol.* 4:a012286. doi: 10.1101/cshperspect.a012286

Franks, T. M., and Lykke-Andersen, J. (2007). TTP and BRF proteins nucleate processing body formation to silence mRNAs with AU-rich elements. *Genes Dev.* 21, 719–735. doi: 10.1101/gad.1494707

Glynn, E. F., Chen, J., and Mushegian, A. R. (2006). Detecting periodic patterns in unevenly spaced gene expression time series using Lomb-Scargle periodograms. *Bioinformatics* 22, 310–316. doi: 10.1093/bioinformatics/bti789

Green, C. B. (2018). Circadian posttranscriptional regulatory mechanisms in mammals. *Cold Spring Harb. Perspect. Biol.* 10:a030692. doi: 10.1101/cshperspect.a030692

Hubstenberger, A., Courel, M., Benard, M., Souquere, S., Ernoult-Lange, M., and Chouaib, R. (2017). P-Body purification reveals the condensation of repressed mRNA regulons. *Mol. Cell* 68, 144.e5–157.e5. doi: 10.1016/j.molcel.2017.09.003

Hughes, M. E., Hogenesch, J. B., and Kornacker, K. (2010). JTK-CYCLE: an efficient nonparametric algorithm for detecting rhythmic components in genome-scale data sets. *J. Biol. Rhythms* 25, 372–380. doi: 10.1177/0748730410379711

Ingelfinger, D., Arndt-Jovin, D. J., Luhrmann, R., and Achsel, T. (2002). The human LSm1-7 proteins colocalize with the mRNA-degrading enzymes Dcp1/2 and Xrnl in distinct cytoplasmic foci. *RNA* 8, 1489–1501.

Ivanov, P., Kedersha, N., and Anderson, P. (2018). Stress granules and processing bodies in translational control. *Cold Spring Harb. Perspect. Biol.* 11:a032813. doi: 10.1101/cshperspect.a032813

Jang, C., Lahens, N. F., Hogenesch, J. B., and Sehgal, A. (2015). Ribosome profiling reveals an important role for translational control in circadian gene expression. *Genome Res.* 25, 1836–1847. doi: 10.1101/gr.191296.115

Kedersha, N., and Anderson, P. (2007). Mammalian stress granules and processing bodies. *Methods Enzymol.* 431, 61–81. doi: 10.1016/s0076-6879(07)31005-7

Margadant, C., van Opstal, A., and Boonstra, J. (2007). Focal adhesion signaling and actin stress fibers are dispensable for progression through the ongoing cell cycle. *J. Cell Sci.* 120, 66–76. doi: 10.1242/jcs.03301

Mauvoisin, D., Wang, J., Jouffe, C., Martin, E., Atger, F., and Waridel, P. (2014). Circadian clock-dependent and -independent rhythmic proteomes implement distinct diurnal functions in mouse liver. *Proc. Natl. Acad. Sci. U.S.A.* 111, 167–172. doi: 10.1073/pnas.1314066111

Nagoshi, E., Brown, S. A., Dibner, C., Kornmann, B., and Schibler, U. (2005). Circadian gene expression in cultured cells. *Methods Enzymol.* 393, 543–557. doi: 10.1016/s0076-6879(05)93028-0

Nissan, T., and Parker, R. (2008). Analyzing P-bodies in *Saccharomyces cerevisiae Methods Enzymol.* 448, 507–520. doi: 10.1016/S0076-6879(08)02625-6

Pizarro, A., Hayer, K., Lahens, N. F., and Hogenesch, J. B. (2013). CircaDB: a database of mammalian circadian gene expression profiles. *Nucleic Acids Res.* 41, D1009–D1013. doi: 10.1093/nar/gks1161

Reddy, A. B., Karp, N. A., Maywood, E. S., Sage, E. A., Deery, M., and O'Neill, J. S. (2006). Circadian orchestration of the hepatic proteome. *Curr. Biol.* 16, 1107–1115. doi: 10.1016/j.cub.2006.04.026

Repouskou, A., Sourlingas, T. G., Sekeri-Pataryas, K. E., and Prombona, A. (2010). The circadian expression of c-MYC is modulated by the histone deacetylase inhibitor trichostatin A in synchronized murine neuroblastoma cells. *Chronobiol. Int.* 27, 722–741. doi: 10.3109/07420521003786800

Robles, M. S., Cox, J., and Mann, M. (2014). In-vivo quantitative proteomics reveals a key contribution of post-transcriptional mechanisms to the circadian regulation of liver metabolism. *PLoS Genet.* 10:e1004047. doi: 10.1371/journal.pgen.1004047

Schibler, U., Gotic, I., Saini, C., Gos, P., Curie, T., Emmenegger, Y., et al. (2015). Clock-talk: interactions between central and peripheral circadian oscillators in mammals. *Cold Spring Harb. Symp. Quant. Biol.* 80, 223–232. doi: 10.1101/sqb.2015.80.027490

Sfakianos, A. P., Whitmarsh, A. J., and Ashe, M. P. (2016). Ribonucleoprotein bodies are phased in. *Biochem. Soc. Trans.* 44, 1411–1416. doi: 10.1042/bst20160117

Sheth, U., and Parker, R. (2003). Decapping and decay of messenger RNA occur in cytoplasmic processing bodies. *Science* 300, 805–808. doi: 10.1126/science.1082320

Shin, Y., and Brangwynne, C. P. (2017). Liquid phase condensation in cell physiology and disease. *Science* 357:eaaf4382. doi: 10.1126/science.aaf4382

Standart, N., and Weil, D. (2018). P-Bodies: cytosolic droplets for coordinated mRNA storage. *Trends Genet.* 34, 612–626. doi: 10.1016/j.tig.2018.05.005

Takahashi, J. S. (2017). Transcriptional architecture of the mammalian circadian clock. *Nat. Rev. Genet.* 18, 164–179. doi: 10.1038/nrg.2016.150

Wang, R., Jiang, X., Bao, P., Qin, M., and Xu, J. (2019). Circadian control of stress granules by oscillating EIF2alpha. *Cell Death Dis.* 10:215. doi: 10.1038/s41419-019-1471-y

Wu, G., Anafi, R. C., Hughes, M. E., Kornacker, K., and Hogenesch, J. B. (2016). MetaCycle: an integrated R package to evaluate periodicity in large scale data. *Bioinformatics* 32, 3351–3353. doi: 10.1093/bioinformatics/btw405

Yang, R., and Su, Z. (2010). Analyzing circadian expression data by harmonic regression based on autoregressive spectral estimation. *Bioinformatics* 26, i168–i174. doi: 10.1093/bioinformatics/btq189

Zhang, R., Lahens, N. F., Ballance, H. I., Hughes, M. E., and Hogenesch, J. B. (2014). A circadian gene expression atlas in mammals: implications for biology and medicine. *Proc. Natl. Acad. Sci. U.S.A.* 111, 16219–16224. doi: 10.1073/pnas.1408886111

14

MeCP2 Deficiency Disrupts Kainate-Induced Presynaptic Plasticity in the Mossy Fiber Projections in the Hippocampus

Maria Laura Bertoldi[1,2], *Maria Ines Zalosnik*[1,2], *Maria Carolina Fabio*[3], *Susan Aja*[4], *German A. Roth*[1,2], *Gabriele V. Ronnett*[4,5†] *and Alicia L. Degano*[1,2*]

[1] Departamento de Química Biológica Ranwel Caputto, Facultad de Ciencias Químicas, Córdoba, Argentina, [2] Centro de Investigaciones en Química Biológica de Córdoba (CIQUIBIC), CONICET, Universidad Nacional de Córdoba, Córdoba, Argentina, [3] Instituto de Investigaciones Médicas Mercedes y Martin Ferreyra (INIMEC), CONICET, Córdoba, Argentina, [4] Center for Metabolism and Obesity Research, Johns Hopkins Medicine, Baltimore, MD, United States, [5] Department of Neuroscience, The Johns Hopkins University, School of Medicine, Baltimore, MD, United States

***Correspondence:**
Alicia L. Degano
adegano@fcq.unc.edu.ar;
adegano1@gmail.com

†Present address:
Gabriele V. Ronnett,
Janssen Research & Development, LLC, Spring House, PA, United States

Methyl cytosine binding protein 2 (MeCP2) is a structural chromosomal protein involved in the regulation of gene expression. Mutations in the gene encoding MeCP2 result in Rett Syndrome (RTT), a pervasive neurodevelopmental disorder. RTT is one of few autism spectrum disorders whose cause was identified as a single gene mutation. Remarkably, abnormal levels of MeCP2 have been associated to other neurodevelopmental disorders, as well as neuropsychiatric disorders. Therefore, many studies have been oriented to investigate the role of MeCP2 in the nervous system. In the present work, we explore cellular and molecular mechanisms affecting synaptic plasticity events *in vivo* in the hippocampus of MeCP2 mutant mice. While most studies addressed postsynaptic defects in the absence of MeCP2, we took advantage of an *in vivo* activity-paradigm (seizures), two models of MeCP2 deficiency, and neurobiological assays to reveal novel defects in presynaptic structural plasticity in the hippocampus in RTT rodent models. These approaches allowed us to determine that MeCP2 mutations alter presynaptic components, i.e., disrupts the plastic response of mossy fibers to synaptic activity and results in reduced axonal growth which is correlated with imbalanced trophic and guidance support, associated with aberrant expression of brain-derived neurotrophic factor and semaphorin 3F. Our results also revealed that adult-born granule cells recapitulate maturational defects that have been only shown at early postnatal ages. As these cells do not mature timely, they may not integrate properly into the adult hippocampal circuitry. Finally, we performed a hippocampal-dependent test that revealed defective spatial memory in these mice. Altogether, our studies establish a model that allows us to evaluate the effect of the manipulation of specific pathways involved in axonal guidance, synaptogenesis, or maturation in specific circuits and correlate it with changes in behavior. Understanding the mechanisms underlying the neuronal compromise caused by mutations in MeCP2 could provide information on the pathogenic mechanism of autistic spectrum disorders and improve our understanding of brain development and molecular basis of behavior.

Keywords: MeCP2, presynaptic plasticity, neurogenesis, activity-dependent gene expression, autism

INTRODUCTION

Rett syndrome (OMIM #312750) is one of the few ASDs of monogenic origin that results in mental retardation, motor dysfunction, seizures, and features of autism. In 1999, the main cause of RTT was shown to be mutations in the MeCP2 (Amir et al., 1999). This protein is a member of the family of methyl-CpG binding proteins that bind to gene promoters and regulate their expression (Nan et al., 1997). Alterations in this protein have been found in patients with learning disorders and associated neuropathologies, suggesting that this protein plays an important role in the development and maintenance of neuronal circuits. Understanding the pathological mechanisms that lead to this syndrome would be of great importance for knowing the bases of these disorders and for promoting the development of therapies.

Numerous studies in animal models of RTT indicate that MeCP2 contributes to the formation and maintenance of neuronal connectivity; MeCP2 deficiency affects neuronal maturation (Matarazzo et al., 2004; Palmer et al., 2008), axonal and dendritic morphology (Belichenko et al., 2008; Chapleau et al., 2009), axonal guidance events (Degano et al., 2009), regulates synapse formation and function, as well as synaptic plasticity (Asaka et al., 2006). Although RTT is considered a neurodevelopmental disorder, more recent studies have revealed that MeCP2 is also critical for the maintenance of mature neural networks and global cerebral anatomy during stages of postnatal brain development and in the adult brain (Ballas et al., 2012).

Importantly, it has been demonstrated that *in vitro* MeCP2 regulates gene expression induced by neuronal activity; activity increases MeCP2 phosphorylation (Chen et al., 2001; Martinowich et al., 2003), which leads to dynamic interaction with specific co-repressors, for instance NCoR (Lyst et al., 2013), modulating the expression of target genes like BDNF. Although there is strong evidence that MeCP2 mediates activity-dependent responses *in vivo* (Zhou et al., 2006; Ebert et al., 2013), few studies have explored the consequences of MeCP2 mutations on synaptic plasticity, after *in vivo* synaptic stimulation.

Furthermore, the vast majority of the studies in the field have been focused on the consequences of MeCP2 mutation/deficiency on postsynaptic components of neuronal circuitries, i.e., dendritic morphology and arborizations, as well as density and morphology of dendritic spines (Chapleau and Pozzo-Miller, 2008). This was reasonable, as early evidence from post-mortem studies in RTT patients supported the hypothesis that this was a disorder of dendritic refinement (Chahrour and Zoghbi, 2007). Therefore, most efforts have addressed the role of MeCP2 on dendritic function and development, while the implication of MeCP2 on the development and function of presynaptic components (axonal projections), also essential for proper neural connectivity, remains relatively unexplored. To this end, using the olfactory system as a neurodevelopmental model, we previously identified a novel function for MeCP2 in axonal guidance processes during the establishment of neuronal circuits, including axonal trajectory, axon fasciculation, pruning, and axonal targeting (Degano et al., 2009). Moreover, defects in these processes were more evident when synaptic activity was stimulated (in this case, after odorant exposure) (Degano et al., 2014).

The mouse hippocampus, a structure of great relevance in the pathophysiology of RTT (Chahrour and Zoghbi, 2007), displays two main events of presynaptic structural plasticity: adult neurogenesis at the DG, and dynamic changes in the size of the IPT, formed by granule cells MF (**Figure 1A**). Both forms of structural plasticity in the adult hippocampus correlate with improved performance in hippocampal-dependent learning tasks, and they are closely related to each other (Römer et al., 2011). It has been shown that exposure to an enriched environment or the induction of seizures activity favors adult neurogenesis in DG (Parent et al., 1997; Gray and Sundstrom, 1998; Lindvall et al., 2002), as well as the increase in the size of the IPT (Römer et al., 2011). Therefore, we proposed to use mouse models of RTT and a paradigm of seizures induction to investigate the cellular and molecular mechanisms involved in activity-dependent plasticity *in vivo* from the perspective of pre-synaptic components in the hippocampus from MeCP2-mutant mice.

In the present study, we report that inducing seizure activity in MeCP2-mutant animals reveals a novel role for MeCP2 in the structural plasticity of the MF-CA3 circuit. The lack of MeCP2 interferes with activity-dependent structural presynaptic plasticity in the hippocampus, affecting axonal growth/remodeling, the maturation of adult born neurons, as well as BDNF and Sema3F signaling. Likewise, we show that these plasticity defects correlate with a reduced performance in a spatial learning test (Barnes maze).

We propose that this is a model to study the causal relationships between structural alterations in the hippocampus and cognitive alterations present in mouse models of RTT. These studies may lay the foundations to establish a system that allows evaluating the effect of manipulating specific pathways involved in neural connectivity in a specific circuit and correlating it with changes in behavior. Moreover, these results may serve useful for approaching *in vivo*, in real-time studies for understanding the molecular basis of behavior in several neurodevelopmental or neurocognitive disorders.

MATERIALS AND METHODS

Mice

We used two RTT mouse models for these studies. (1) MeCP2-308 model (MUT), these animals carry a premature stop codon at amino acid 308, generating a truncated MeCP2 protein that lacks the C-terminal region (B6.129S-Mecp2 <tm1hzo>/J, Stock 005439, The Jackson Labs) (Shahbazian et al., 2002) and (2) MeCP2-Bird model (KO): these mice carry a conditional deletion in exons 3 and 4 of the Mecp2 gene causing the absence

Abbreviations: ASDs, autism spectrum disorders; BDNF, brain-derived neurotrophic factor; DG, dentate gyrus; GFAP, glial fibrillary acidic protein; IPT, hippocampal infrapyramidal tract; MeCP2; methyl-CpG 2 binding protein 2; MF, mossy fibers; RTT, Rett syndrome; Sema3F, semaphorin 3F; TrkB, tropomyosin-related kinase B.

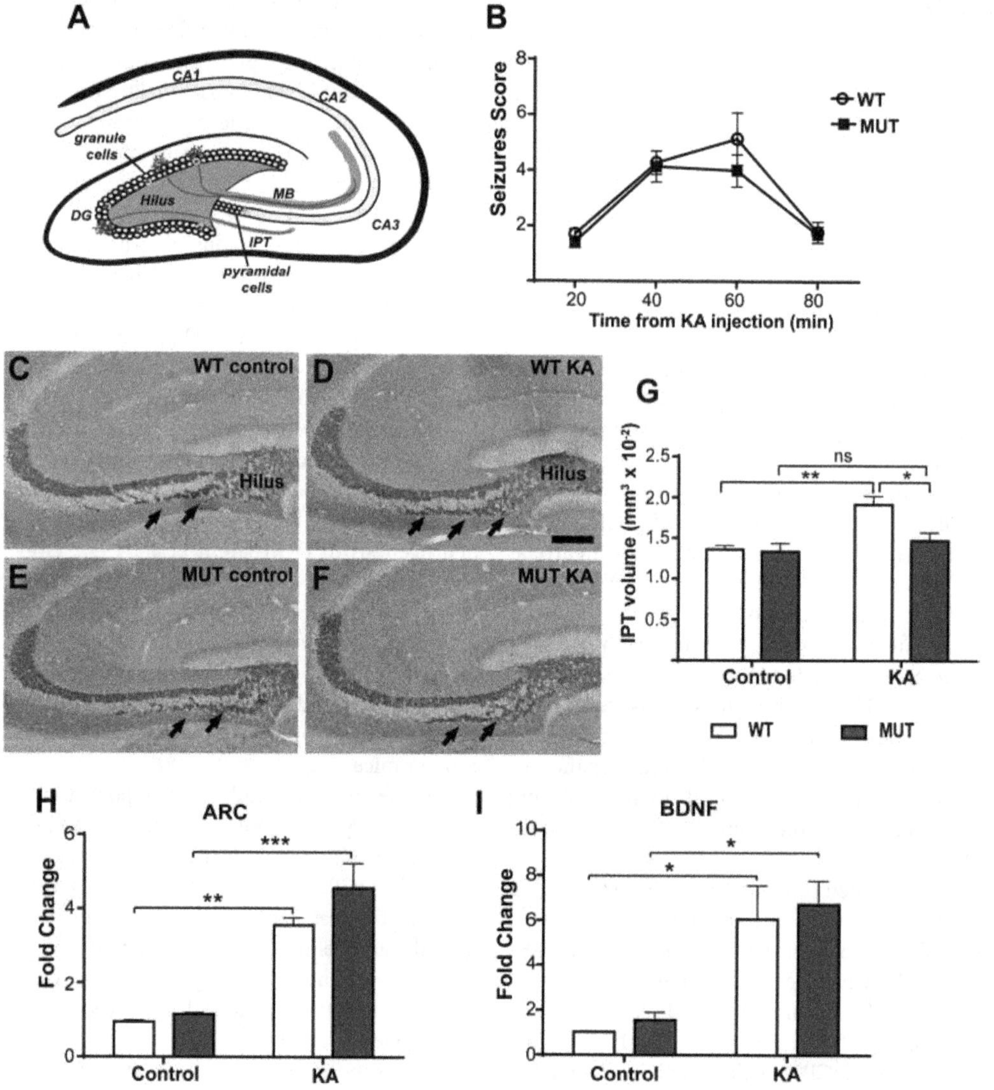

FIGURE 1 | KA-induced seizures failed to increase IPT size in a mouse model of MeCP2-308 mutation. **(A)** Hippocampal MF-CA3 circuit. The MF consist of the axons of the granule cells of the DG that project through the main tract (MT) in the lucid stratum or through the IPT located mainly in the stratum oriens. **(B)** Seizures activity over time after KA administration in MeCP2-308 MUT model. No differences in the development or severity of seizures were observed between WT and MUT mice in response to KA (n = 5 mice per experimental group, two-way ANOVA $p = 0.7023$, followed by Tukey's HSD test). **(C–F)** Representative images of IPT stained with anti-Synaptoporin in coronal hippocampal sections; IPT is indicated by black arrows. Two weeks after KA injection, WT mice **(D)** but not MUT mice **(F)** showed increased IPT size, in comparison with WT and MUT controls **(C,E)**. Scale bar: 200 μm. **(G)** Quantitative analysis of IPT volume in WT and MeCP2-308 MUT mice. KA-treated WT mice showed an increase in the IPT related to the controls; however, KA-treated MUT mice showed similar IPT size as MUT control. N = 4 mice per experimental group. **(H,I)** KA-induced gene expression: BDNF and Arc expression were determined by real-time RT-PCR from total hippocampus. Six hours after KA injection, a significant increase in the expression of the early activation genes Arc **(H)** and BDNF **(I)** was observed. Fold change was calculated in reference to the WT control group, which was normalized to 1. Results are represented as the ratio between the relative amount of the gene of interest and GAPDH. N = 4 mice per group. cDNA was prepared individually for each mouse and real-time RT-PCR reactions were run in duplicates for each mouse. Data analysis: two-way ANOVA followed by Tukey's HSD test. *$p < 0.05$; **$p < 0.01$; ***$p < 0.001$.

of this protein, starting at embryonic stages (B6.129P2(C)-Mecp2 <tm1.1Bird>/J, Stock 003890, The Jackson Labs) (Guy et al., 2001). Both colonies were maintained in a C57BL/6J background. All the experiments were performed using only hemizygous Mecp2 males (Mecp2 MUT or Mecp2 KO) and their corresponding WT male littermates as control. Animal procedures were fully reviewed and approved by the local animal committee (School of Chemistry, National University of Córdoba, Protocol 2018-832), which follows guidelines from the National Institute of Health.

In vivo Activity Paradigm

Male WT, KO, and MUT mice were genotyped following protocols provided by The Jackson Labs. Each mouse was administered with a single intraperitoneal (i.p.) injection of kainic acid (KA, 20 mg/kg, Sigma). As a control, the same volume of sterile PBS was injected (McLeod et al., 2013). Considering there are no reports of KA injection in the MUT and in order to provide similar seizure stimulus in WT and MUT mice, we performed several pilot experiments before selecting an adequate age for these experiments. At 6 weeks, the MUT mice were found to be resistant to KA, no convulsions were observed, nor an increase in the expression of activity-induced genes in hippocampus (i.e., BDNF or Arc measured by real-time PCR, data not shown). Conversely, 9-weeks-old MUT males showed similar kinetics and seizure activity as their respective WT littermates (**Figure 1B**). Therefore, since we observed differential sensitivity to KA at different ages in the MeCP2-308 model respect to WT littermates, we decided to use 9-weeks-old MUT males in our experiments for the purpose of using KA exposure as an *in vivo* stimulation paradigm. In the case of the KO, we used 6-weeks-old males, since the response to KA was already reported in the literature (McLeod et al., 2013). It is important to mention that the survival of the two mouse models is very different; male MUT mice live about a year (Shahbazian et al., 2002) while male KO mice survive about 10–12 weeks (Guy et al., 2001).

After KA injection, seizure response was recorded, which became evident after 20 min of injection. From the moment of KA injection, the animals were individually housed in separate boxes and monitored for several hours. The severity of the seizure response was graded according to the following scale: 0, similar to control; 1, increased respiratory rate; 2, in a state of "freezing" and with erratic contractions of the body; 3, straight and stiff tail with or without shaking; 4, the front legs begin to tremble; 5, straight and stiff tail along with tremor of front legs (once); 6, continuously shows straight and stiff tail along with front leg tremor (more than twice); 7, complete clonic tonic seizures, jumps; 8, death [adapted from McLeod et al. (2013)].

Immunohistochemistry

Whole brains were harvested from WT and Mecp2 MUT or KO mice after cardiac perfusion with ice-cold PBS and 4% paraformaldehyde (PFA; Sigma), embedded with Cryoplast (Biopack, Argentina) and serial coronal cryo-sections (20 μm) were obtained. For each brain, 12 numbered slides were used and each one carried six serial sections of the hippocampus. Thus, a fragment of the dorsal region of the hippocampus extending 240 μm along the rostro-caudal axis was represented on each slide (Römer et al., 2011). For BrdU labeling and IPT staining, we used a peroxidase method (ABC System, Vectastain, Vector Laboratories) with biotinylated anti-mouse and anti-rabbit antibodies (1:200; Vector Labs). Fluorescence IHC was performed according to our established protocols (Degano et al., 2009). Primary antibodies include synaptoporin (Synpr; 1:1000; Synaptic Systems), βIII tubulin (TUJ1; Covance; 1:1000), bromodeoxyuridine (BrdU; 1:1000; Roche), GFAP (1:250; Sigma), NeuN (1:1000, LSBio), doublecortin (DCX; 1:200; Santa Cruz), and phospho-TrkB receptor (pTrKB; 1:250; Millipore). Secondary antibodies include biotin donkey anti-rabbit or mouse (1:200, Vector Labs). Cy3 donkey anti-rabbit IgG (1:500), Alexa 545 anti-goat (1:1000), Alexa 488 donkey anti-rabbit, and mouse IgG or chicken (1:1000) were used to facilitate double or triple labeling (Jackson ImmunoResearch). Data were obtained from at least four animals from 3 L per genotype per time point. Images were collected using either a Zeiss Axioskop with a digital camera (Axiocam; Zeiss) or an Olympus FV1000 scanning confocal microscope equipped with a Kr/Ar laser.

Measurement of IPT Volume

Serial coronal sections were stained by IHC, using an antibody against the presynaptic vesicular protein: synaptoporin, enriched in MF (Singec et al., 2002). Images from hippocampus were obtained with an Axioplan microscope (Carl Zeiss) equipped with an Olympus XM10 camera. According to Römer et al. (2011), the IPT area was measured in each section, using the area measurement tool of the FIJI/Image J program (NIH). Then, the IPT volume was obtained for each slide, by multiplying the sum of the areas measured by the inverse of the sampling fraction (12) and by 20 (the thickness of the section in micrometers).

Cell Counts

In order to label proliferating cells, WT and MUT mice were i.p. injected with BrdU (50 mg/kg, Sigma) in 0.01 M PBS. For assessing KA-induced neurogenesis, different cohorts of dividing cells were labeled in a single day. Thus, three doses of BrdU (6 h apart) were injected on the 6th day after KA induction, since it was reported that the highest proliferative activity in DG is detected at 1 week from seizure induction (Burns and Kuan, 2005; Römer et al., 2011). The animals were perfused 2 days after BrdU administration; coronal cryosections were prepared and processed for IHC using anti-BrdU antibodies. Sections were analyzed with an Axioplan microscope (Carl Zeiss) equipped with an Olympus XM10 camera. BrdU-positive cells were analyzed and counted along the rostral–caudal extension of the granule cell layer of DG. The resulting numbers were then multiplied by 12 to obtain the estimated number of total cells per granule cell layer of DG (Römer et al., 2011).

In order to study the maturation of adult-born granule cells of DG, different cohorts of progenitor cells were labeled during 3 consecutive days: 5th, 6th, and 7th days after KA administration (temporal window of high proliferative activity), injecting two doses per day, separated by 7 h. The animals were then perfused 4 weeks after the last BrdU dose, enough time for the new neurons to reach the characteristic morphology of mature granule cells (Burns and Kuan, 2005).

Coronal sections were subjected to triple labeling IHC using: anti-BrdU, to visualize new DG cells and both anti-DCX and anti-neuronal nuclear protein (NeuN) that allows identifying immature and mature neurons, respectively. Triple labeling images (BrdU, DCX, and NeuN) were acquired using Olympus Fluoview 1000 and 1200 confocal microscopes, using a 60× objective. Only BrdU-positive cells located in the granule cell layer of DG were included in the analysis. The markers colocalization was analyzed through the entire *Z*-axis of each BrdU-positive cell (covering the whole cell soma) in single optical planes of 0.7 μm thickness. Total BrdU-positive cells were counted and their colocalization was analyzed with the neuronal markers in order to calculate the percentage of new mature and immature neurons for each animal.

Real-Time RT-PCR

Total RNA samples were prepared from five to six individual male mice per genotype per condition. Tissues were immediately frozen in liquid nitrogen and homogenized on dry ice. Total RNA was extracted with TRIzol reagent (Invitrogen) according to the manufacturer's protocol. Genomic DNA was digested with 1 unit of DNase I (Invitrogen). cDNA was produced using the mMLV reverse transcriptase (Promega) following standard protocols (Degano et al., 2014). Real-time PCR was carried out on an iCycler (Bio-Rad) by using a reaction mixture with SYBR Green as the fluorescent dye (Applied Biosystems), a 1/10 vol of the cDNA preparation as template, and 250 nM of each primer (Degano et al., 2009, 2014). Primer sequences for BDNF exon IX was obtained from Li et al. (2012). The cycle used for PCR was as follows: 95°C for 180 s (1 time); 95°C for 30 s, 60°C for 30 s, and 72°C for 30 s (40 times); and 95°C for 60 s (1 time). Samples were subjected to a melting-curve analysis to confirm the amplification specificity. The change in fluorescence of SYBR Green dye was monitored in every cycle and the threshold cycle (CT) was calculated above the background for each reaction. For each cDNA sample, a ratio between the relative amounts of target gene and GAPDH was calculated to compensate for variations in quantity or quality of starting mRNA, as well as for differences in reverse transcriptase efficiency. The fold change in the target gene relative to the GAPDH endogenous control gene was determined by: fold change = $2^{-\Delta(\Delta C_T)}$, where $\Delta C_T = C_{T,target} - C_{T,GAPDH}$ and $\Delta(\Delta C_T) = \Delta C_{T,KO} - \Delta C_{T,WT}$. RT-PCRs were run separately for each mouse in triplicate, and data were analyzed for statistical differences by two-way ANOVA using PRISM 6.0 software (GraphPad, San Diego, CA, United States).

Barnes Maze

Barnes maze test was used to evaluate the presence of cognitive deficits in spatial learning and memory of MeCP2 MUT mice in comparison with WT littermates. For this purpose, a Barnes maze for mice was built following the specifications reported by other authors (Rosenfeld and Ferguson, 2014). It consisted of a 92-cm diameter circular platform constructed from a white PVC slab. Twenty holes of 5 cm diameter were made in the perimeter (separated from each other by 7.5 and 2 cm from the edge of the platform). A black exit box 20 cm long, 9 cm high, and 9 cm wide, with a ramp inside it (escape hole), was placed under one of the holes in the platform. The circular platform was located 1 m high from the ground and over it, 1 m away, was illuminated with two white light bulbs of 150 W each. Visual signs consisting of panels with simple colored shapes (squares, triangles, stars) were mounted as visual cues around the room where the test was performed. All of the sessions were recorded using a 12-megapixel camera placed above the platform.

The Barnes maze use is similar to the radial arm and Morris maze but without diet restrictions and with lower physical stress for mice. Inside the maze, mice are motivated to escape from the illuminated and open platform toward a dark, small, and recessed chamber (escape box). In this experiment, we worked with 12 weeks MUT and WT mice, using the protocol of O'Leary and Brown (2013) as reference. The test consists of four steps divided into 4 days:

* Day 1. Habituation – It consisted in making the animal familiar with the environment, the platform, and the escape box. First, the animal was gently introduced into the escape box through the hole in the platform leading to it ("target" hole) and left there for 2 min. Then it was placed in the center of the platform for 30 s covered with a large transparent glass flask. After that period, the animal covered with the flask was guided to the target hole and the flask was located there for 3 min or until the animal enters the escape box. If after 3 min the animal did not enter the escape box, it was guided with the same flask to do so. Once inside the escape box, the animal was left there for 1 min and then it was returned to its usual cage.

* Day 2. Training – Each animal was subjected to three trainings (4 min each), separated from each other by a half-hour break. Every training began with the lights off above the platform and placing the animal in the center of the platform covered by a non-transparent container. Then, the 4-min counting starts, the lights above the platform were turned on and the container that covers the animal removed, allowing it to freely travel the entire platform. When the animal entered the escape box (located in the same hole of the platform in all trainings), the lights were immediately turned off and the mouse was left there for 1 min. In the event that after 4 min the animal has not entered the box, it was guided to it and once inside the box, the lights were turned off again, and the mouse left there for 1 min. In each training we recorded: the percentage of time that the animal spent in each quadrant of the platform, the first quadrant to which the animal was directed when discovered, the number of total explorations of the holes of the platform (considering exploration when the animal pokes its head through one of the holes in the platform), the number of explorations in each quadrant, the number of correct explorations in the target hole, and the latency of entry to the escape box.

* Day 3. Rest.

* Day 4. Memory test – In this case each animal was subjected to a single exposure on the platform that lasted 2 min and in which the escape box was removed. Again, the test started with the lights off and placing the animal in the center of the platform covered by a dark container. When the 2-min count started, lights were turned on and the container covering the animal was removed, allowing it to freely travel the entire platform. Again, the same parameters were recorded here as in the trainings except for the latency of entry to the escape box.

Statistical Analyses

All numerical analyses were performed using PRISM 6.0 software (GraphPad, San Diego, CA, United States). For all comparisons, two-way ANOVA was performed followed by Tukey's *post hoc* test, when appropriate. Differences were considered significantly different at a $p < 0.05$.

RESULTS

Kainic-Induced Seizures Failed to Increase the Size of the IPT in the Absence of MeCP2

To evaluate presynaptic structural plasticity in the absence of MeCP2 (i.e., adult neurogenesis and increase in the size of the IPT), we treated mice with KA to trigger seizures and robust neuronal activity, as shown by other authors (Ebert et al., 2013; Lyst et al., 2013). The animal models we use are from a C57BL6 background, which has a relatively high resistance to excitotoxic insults; therefore, they develop seizures in response to KA and neurogenesis is potentiated without leading to massive neuronal death (Schauwecker and Steward, 1997; Römer et al., 2011).

We generally used the MeCP2-308 mouse model (MUT) for these studies. Some of the experiments were replicated using MeCP2 Bird mouse models. MUT mice and their respective WT littermates were i.p. injected with KA or with sterile PBS (control), so we established four experimental groups: WT control, WT + KA, MUT control, and MUT + KA. In order to provide similar seizure stimulus in WT and MUT mice, we performed several pilot experiments before selecting an adequate developmental stage for this experiments (see the section "Materials and Methods"). A single KA dose was injected in 9-week-old MUT/WT mice, and seizure activity was assessed. **Figure 1** illustrates the average seizure activity at several time points after KA injection. MUT mice (**Figure 1B**) responded to KA with similar seizure activity as the WT, showing comparable kinetics and maximum average scores (MUT: 4 $\pm$ 1.29; WT: 5 $\pm$ 1.83; $p = 0.702$).

Two weeks after the KA injection, all animals were euthanized and perfused for morphometric analysis, according to Römer et al. (2011). These authors described that during this time window in C57BL/6 mice, the IPT reaches the greatest increase in volume in response to KA-induced seizures. Serial coronal cryosections of the dorsal hippocampus were subjected to IHC for MF labeling and the volume of the IPT was calculated (Römer et al., 2011). As expected, an increase in the IPT size was observed in the WT + KA group comparing with WT controls (**Figures 1C,D,G**). However, no change in the IPT size was observed between MUT control and MUT + KA mice (**Figures 1E–G**). Thus, after KA injection, only WT mice showed a significant increase in the IPT size [$F(1,17) = 4{,}858$; $p = 0.0416$].

To determine whether the lack of IPT growth in response to seizure activity in MeCP2 MUT mice was caused by defective neural activation in response to KA, the expression of activity-induced neuronal genes (Arc and BDNF) was evaluated. For this, new groups of mice from both RTT models were injected with KA and 6 h later, whole hippocampus were dissected from control and KA-injected MUT mice and WT littermates. The expression levels of Arc and BDNF were quantified by real-time RT-PCR. As shown in **Figures 1H,I**, MUT mice showed a significant increase in the expression of Arc and BDNF mRNA after 6 h of KA treatment in comparison with PBS-injected controls. Likewise, WT littermates showed an increase in Arc and BDNF mRNA levels in response to KA. Therefore, no significant differences were recorded between MUT mice and the WTs in terms of expression levels of Arc [$F(1.12) = 1.228$; $p = 0.2895$] and BDNF [$F(1,10) = 0.0034$; $p = 0.9521$] in response to KA stimulation. These results demonstrate that in MUT MeCP2 animals an increase in neuronal activity was induced in response to KA administration, similar in magnitude to that induced in WT animals.

It is important to report that the results shown so far were reproduced using a mouse model of MeCP2 deficiency (MeCP2 Bird model, KO) (**Figure 2**). KO mice responded to KA more severely than WT mice, showing higher seizure scores (KO: 6 $\pm$ 0.707; WT: 4 $\pm$ 0.316; $p < 0.05$); and the levels of KA-induced Arc and BDNF expression in these animals were similar to the WTs (**Figures 2A,C,D**). Nevertheless, KO mice also failed to show an increase of the IPT after seizure activity (**Figure 2B**).

Kainate-Induced Adult Neurogenesis and Survival of Adult-Born Neurons Are Not Affected in DG of MeCP2 Mutant Mice

It has been shown that the axons of adult-born neurons in DG contribute mainly to the plasticity of the IPT tract (Römer et al., 2011). Likewise, it has been reported that there is a significant rise in the number of new granule cells in the DG after seizure activity (Parent et al., 1997; Gray and Sundstrom, 1998; Scott et al., 1998; Parent and Lowenstein, 2002; Römer et al., 2011), supporting the idea that adult neurogenesis could be related to the increase of the IPT size. Therefore, we quantified the rate of adult neurogenesis in DG after KA administration. Nine-week-old MUT mice and WT littermates received a single i.p. injection of KA or PBS; 6 days later we labeled several cohorts of cell progenitors by i.p. BrdU injections. Animals were sacrificed 2 days later (8 days after KA injection), the dividing cells were labeled by IHC, and BrdU-positive cells were counted along the rostral–caudal extension of the granule cell layer of DG. Eight days after KA injection, a strong increase in the number of BrdU-positive cells was observed in the DG of KA-treated mice compared to the controls (**Figures 3A,B**). However, there were no significant differences in the neurogenic response to KA between the two genotypes [$F(1,8) = 0.2665$; $p = 0.6197$]. A significant increase in the number of dividing cells was observed in both WT and MUT KA-treated mice in comparison with their respective controls (**Figure 3C**). In addition, no significant differences were found between both genotypes in the basal numbers of BrdU-positive cells per DG (WT control: 1464 $\pm$ 103, MUT control: 1034 $\pm$ 61) ($p = 0.8169$). To confirm that DG dividing cells were neurons, we performed double labeling IHC for BrdU combined with the neuronal marker tubulin β-III (Tuj1) or with an astroglial cell marker (GFAP). Most BrdU$^+$ cells co-localized with the neuronal marker Tuj1, but not with GFAP. **Figures 3E,F** illustrate an example of this control, which was repeated for the samples analyzed. The data suggest that adult neurogenesis in DG is not affected by mutations in MeCP2, since a similar proliferative response was found in MUT and WT mice. However, it is possible that the survival of these new neurons is affected in the absence of MeCP2. For this purpose,

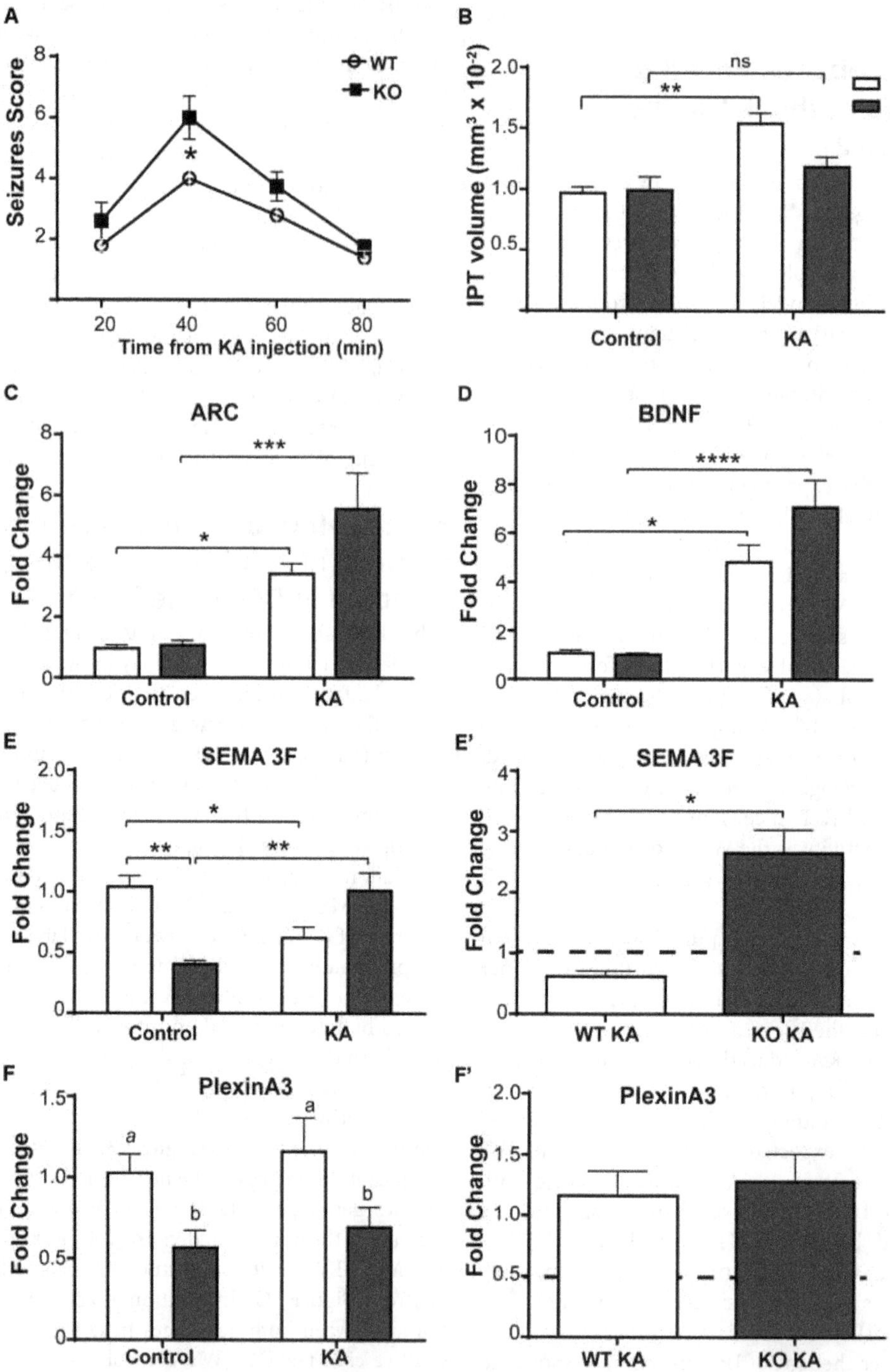

FIGURE 2 | KA-induced seizures failed to increase IPT size in a mouse model of MeCP2 deficiency. **(A)** Seizures activity over time after KA administration. Six-week-old MeCP2-Bird KO mice elicit significantly higher seizures scores than WT littermates, indicative of greater sensitivity to KA. $N = 4–5$ mice per experimental group, two-way ANOVA, followed by Tukey's HSD test, $^*p < 0.05$. **(B)** Quantitative analysis of IPT volume in WT and MeCP2-Bird KO mice. KA-treated WT mice showed an increase in the IPT volume with respect to controls; however, KA-treated KO mice showed similar IPT size as KO control. $N = 4$ mice per experimental group. **(C,D)** KA-induced neuronal gene expression: BDNF and Arc expression were quantified by real-time RT-PCR from total hippocampus. Six hours after KA injection, a significant increase in the expression of the early activation genes Arc **(C)** and BDNF **(D)** was observed. **(E,F)** Sema3F and Plexin A3 expression was assessed by real-time RT-PCR from total hippocampus. Two weeks after KA-seizures induction, a significant decrease in Sema3F was observed in KA-treated WT mice related to WT controls, whereas an opposite response was registered between KA-injected KO mice and KO controls. Basal Sema3F levels in KO mice were significantly lower than in the WT littermates **(E).** Regarding PlxnA3, no changes of expression were observed after KA treatment in WT or KO mice; however, PlxnA3 expression was significantly decreased in KO mice **(F)**. **(C–F)** Fold change was calculated in reference to the WT control group, which was normalized to 1. Results are represented as the ratio between the relative amount of the gene of interest and GAPDH. $N = 5$ mice per experimental group. cDNA was prepared

(Continued)

FIGURE 2 | Continued
individually for each mouse and real-time PCR reactions were run in duplicates for each mouse. Data analysis: two-way ANOVA followed by Tukey's HSD test, $*p < 0.05$; $**p < 0.01$; $***p < 0.001$. **(E′,F′)** In order to better evidence KA effect on each genotype, the expression levels generated by KA were re-calculated in relation to their respective control groups, WT or MUT. The dotted line on the Y-axis ($Y = 1$) represents the control values for each genotype. Mann–Whitney t-test with 95% confidence intervals, $*p < 0.05$.

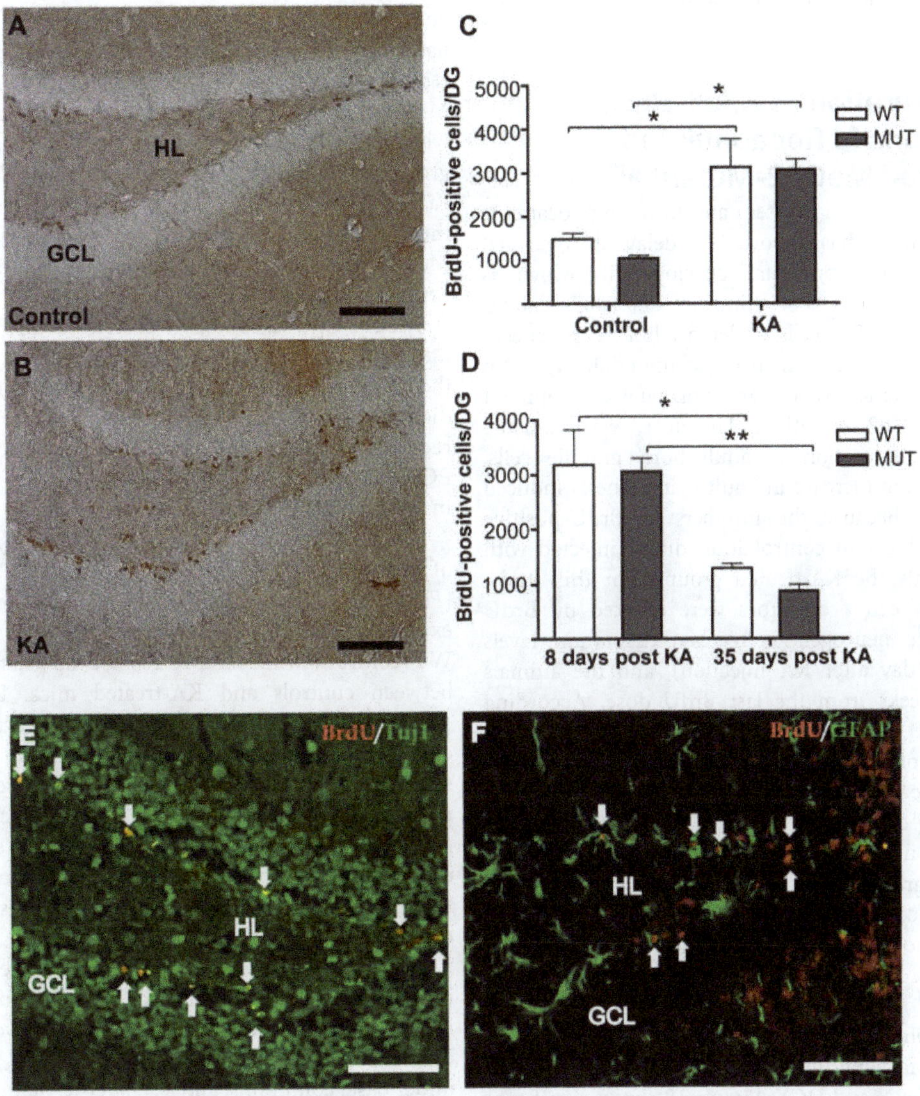

FIGURE 3 | Seizures induce similar rate of adult neurogenesis in WT and MeCP2-308 MUT mice. **(A,B)** IHC for BrDU labeling. Eight days after KA injection, a strong increase in the number of BrDU-positive cells was observed in DG from KA-treated mice **(B)** compared with control littermates **(A)**. Scale bar: 50 μm. GLC, granule cell layer; HL, hilus. **(C)** BrDU-positive cells per DG in KA-treated and controls WT and MUT mice. A single seizure episode induces an increase in the number of BrDU-positive cells that was detected in both WT and MUT mice, respective to their controls. **(D)** Quantification of BrdU-positive cells by DG in WT and MUT mice injected with KA. A similar decrease in the number of BrdU-positive cells was observed in the WT and MUT mice between days 8 and 35 post KA-induced activity. **(E,F)** Double labeling IHC for BrdU and neuronal or astroglial markers in hippocampus 8 days after KA administration. **(E)** Double labeling of newborn DG cells (BrdU in red, white arrows) and Tuj1 (green) a neuronal marker. **(F)** Double labeling of newborn DG cells (BrdU in red, white arrows) and GFAP (in green) labeling astroglial cells in hippocampus. Scale bar: 50 μm. $n = 3$ mice per each experimental group. Data analysis: two-way ANOVA followed by Tukey's HSD test, $*p < 0.05$; $**p < 0.01$.

we evaluated the proportion of KA-induced newborn DG cells ($BrdU^+$) that remained 5 weeks after the induction of seizure activity. **Figure 3D** illustrates the number of $BrdU^+$ cells per DG 8 days and 35 days after KA-induced seizures, when the new DG cells become mature neurons. At 35 days, $BrdU^+$ cells from WT mice decrease about 60% and in MUT 71% respect to day 8; therefore, no significant differences were detected between the genotypes in terms of $BrdU^+$ cell loss [$F(1,9) = 0.2091$;

$p = 0.5883$]. Also, no differences were detected in the absolute number of BrdU$^+$/DG cells between both genotypes at either 8 ($p = 0.9987$) or 35 ($p = 0.8383$) days after KA.

These observations suggest that the survival of the new DG neurons is not affected by MeCP2 mutation; therefore, we conclude that the lack of increase in the size of the IPT, registered 2 weeks after KA injection, was not due to a loss of new DG cells in MUT mice.

Defective Maturation of Adult-Born Granule Neurons Is Recapitulated in Kainate-Treated MeCP2-Mutant Mice

Previous work in the olfactory system and in the hippocampus from MeCP2-KO mice has reported a delay in neuronal maturation during early postnatal development, which is apparently compensated later on (Smrt et al., 2007; Palmer et al., 2008). Given that DG cells undergo adult neurogenesis, we wondered whether the new neurons of the adult organism recapitulate the defects shown in early postnatal development in a model of MeCP2 mutation. Therefore, we evaluated the percentage of maturation of adult born granule cells, taking advantage of the increase in adult neurogenesis induced by seizure activity. Because the numbers of BrdU-positive cells were extremely low in control individuals (injected with PBS), we report only the KA-treated groups. For this study, different cohorts of cell progenitors were marked by BrdU injections when the neurogenesis reached maximum levels (5th, 6th, and 7th day after KA injection), and the animals were perfused 4 weeks from the last BrdU dose. According to the literature, at that time adult-born DG neurons reach the characteristics of mature granule cells (Esposito, 2005). We performed triple immunofluorescence using three markers: anti-BrdU (dividing cells), anti-DCX as a marker of immature neurons, and the nuclear transcription factor NeuN, as a marker for mature granule cells (Esposito, 2005). All the BrdU-positive cells were counted and analyzed per animal sample, and we calculated the percentage of the adult-born neurons that reached maturity (BrdU$^+$ NeuN$^+$), the percentage of immature cells (BrdU$^+$ DCX$^+$) and at intermediate stage of maturation (BrdU$^+$ DCX$^+$ NeuN$^+$). **Figure 4A** illustrates examples of double and triple labeling for BrdU-positive cells and the neuronal markers NeuN and DCX. **Figure 4B** shows significant differences between WT and MeCP2 MUT mice [$F(2,21) = 13.73$; $p < 0.001$]; the percentage of new DG cells that reached maturity was significantly lower in MUT mice (MUT_{NeuN}: 86.39 ± 1.494%; WT_{NeuN}: 93.13 ± 0.762%). In addition, MUT mice showed a higher proportion of both immature cells (MUT_{DCX}: 3.85 ± 0.617%; WT_{DCX}: 1.41 ± 0.481%) and cells in transit to maturation ($MUT_{DCX+NeuN+}$: 9.76 ± 1.521%; $WT_{DCX+NeuN+}$: 5.46 ± 0.537%). Thus, MUT adult-born granule cells show abnormal maturation; immature cells accumulate at expense of lower numbers of mature cells.

These results indicate that mice carrying a mutated MeCP2 protein (MUT) show defective neuronal maturation in the adult hippocampus, similar to what was observed during early development in a different mouse model (Smrt et al., 2007).

Altered Expression of Activity-Induced Axon Guidance Molecules in the Context of MeCP2 Mutations

Using the olfactory system and MeCP2-deficient mice, we have demonstrated that axonal guidance defects were accompanied by alterations in the expression of Sema 3F and its receptor complex (PlexinA3 and Neuropilin-2). It has been demonstrated that this axonal guidance molecule regulates axonal growth, guidance, and targeting of hippocampal MF, acting as an inhibitor of axonal growth when combined with its receptor complex present in axons and inducing growth cone collapse (Bagri et al., 2003; Sahay et al., 2003; Riccomagno et al., 2012). Considering this background and the failure of the plastic response of IPT to seizure activity in MeCP2 MUT mice, we explored the Sema 3F pathway in our experimental conditions.

Methyl-CpG 2 binding protein 2 MUT mice and WT littermates were injected with KA or PBS and 2 weeks later the hippocampus of the different experimental groups were dissected. mRNA expression levels of Sema 3F gene and their two receptors (PlxnA3 and Npn-2) were quantified by real-time RT-PCR. **Figure 5** shows the expression levels of the genes analyzed in MUT and WT animals.

Regarding Sema 3F (**Figure 5A**), considerable differences of expression were detected between WT and MUT mice [$F(1,15) = 4.7$; $p < 0.05$]. A significant decrease of Sema3F expression was observed in WT mice + KA compared to WT controls, while in MUT mice no change was registered between controls and KA-treated mice. Likewise, the WT + KA mice presented significantly lower levels of Sema 3F compared to the MUT KA. For PlxnA3 (**Figure 5B**), no significant differences were registered between both genotypes, neither between controls and KA-treated mice [$F(1,14) = 1.327$; $p = 0.2687$]. Although there were no changes in the expression of Npn-2 in response to KA treatment (**Figure 5C**), we found a significant lower expression in the basal levels of Npn-2 in MUT mice [$F(1,14) = 8.072$; $p < 0.05$].

Figures 2E,F show the expression of the Sema 3F and PlxnA3 in KO and WT animals of the MeCP2Bird model after KA-induced seizures. In this animal model, we observed robust differences in Sema 3F expression between WT and KO mice under basal conditions, and also after KA-induced seizures.

Summarizing these observations, the lack of increase in IPT size after KA treatment, in the context of MeCP2 mutations, was accompanied by a deregulation in the expression levels of Sema 3F which, in concert with the receptor complex, exerts an important chemo-repulsive effect on hippocampal axons (Riccomagno et al., 2012).

BDNF Expression Induced by Neuronal Activity Is Deficient in Mecp2 Mutant Mice

In the hippocampus, neurotrophins levels are dynamically regulated by neuronal activity, and the modification of those levels can alter the growth and distribution of projections,

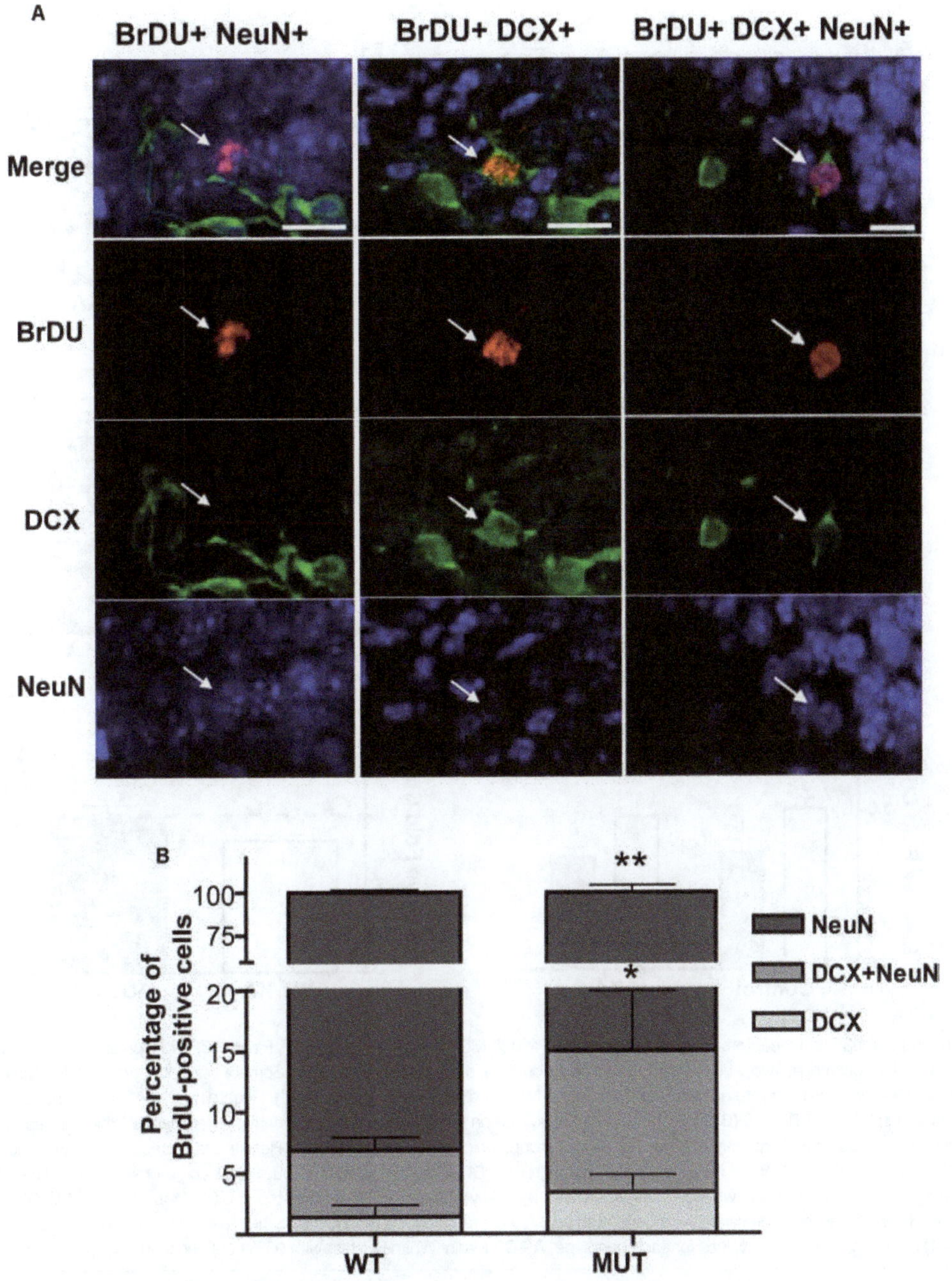

FIGURE 4 | Defective maturation is recapitulated in MeCP2 mutant adult-born granule neurons. **(A)** Triple IHC labeling of BrdU-positive cells and neuronal markers NeuN and DCX. Examples of BrDU-positive neurons in intermediate state of maturation that co-express both NeuN and DCX (right panel). Example of a mature neuron that only expresses NeuN (left panel) and an immature neuron that only expresses DCX (middle panel). The vertical panels are unique optical planes showing the three fluorescence channels separately and their overlapping in the upper panel. Scale bar: 15 μm. **(B)** Percentages of BrdU-positive cells in different stages of maturation in WT and MUT mice exposed to KA. 5 weeks after seizures, WT mice showed a high percentage of mature new granule cells (90%), while MUT mice presented significantly less mature cells and more immature cells. Each bar represents the mean ± standard error (SEM) of BrdU-positive cells co-localizing with the corresponding markers, normalized to the total number of BrdU-positive cells in each mouse. Each bar is subdivided to indicate the mean percentage of BrdU-positive cells at different states of maturation. n = 4–5 mice per experimental group. Data analysis: two-way ANOVA followed by Sidak's test, $*p < 0.05$; $**p < 0.01$.

and MF in particular. BDNF is normally expressed in most hippocampal neurons, including granule cells (Dieni et al., 2012; Isgor et al., 2015). This factor promotes the growth and orientation of granule cell axons *in vitro*, extends innervations of MF into CA3, and regulates its synaptic plasticity (Gómez-Palacio-Schjetnan and Escobar, 2008; Tamura et al., 2009; Römer et al., 2011; Schjetnan and Escobar, 2012). Also, it is now clear that MeCP2 is phosphorylated in response to synaptic activity,

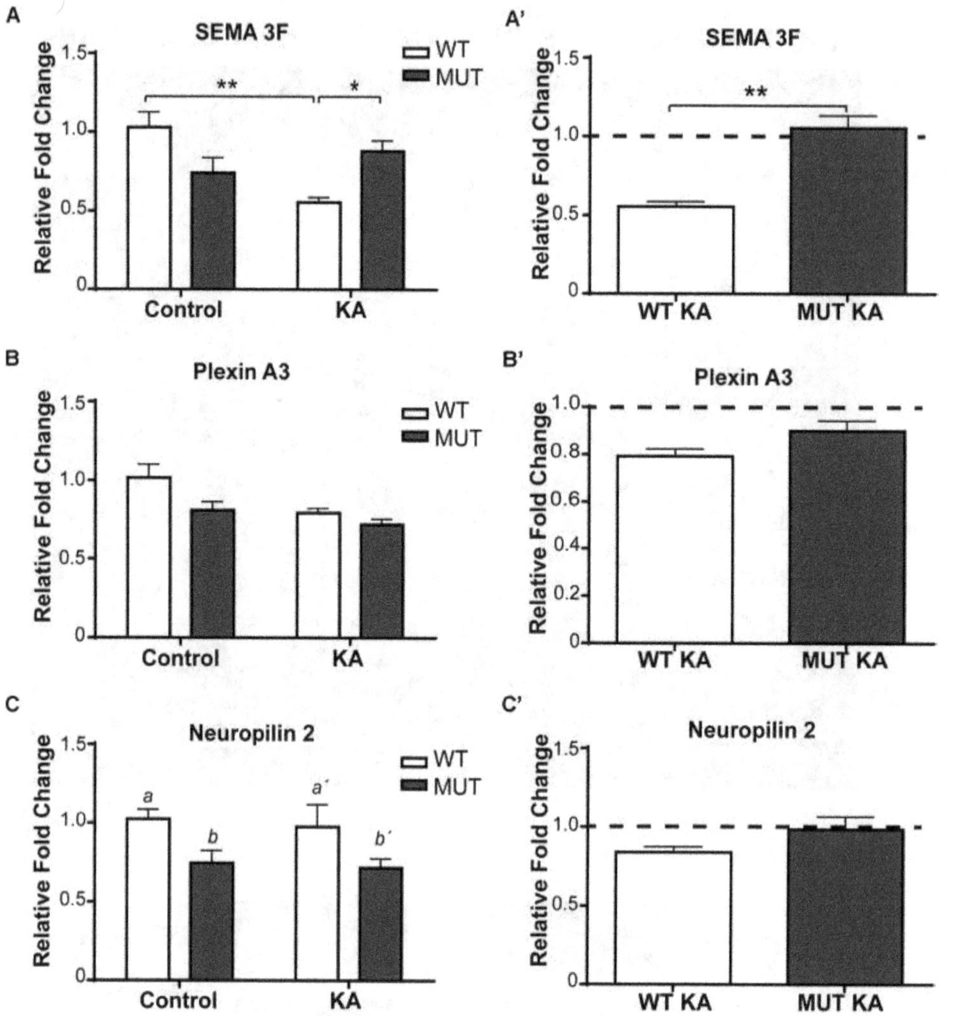

FIGURE 5 | Kainic-induced Sema3F and receptors levels in WT and MeCP2-308 MUT mice. **(A–C)** Sema3F, Plexin A3, and Npn-2 expression were assessed by real-time RT-PCR from total hippocampus. Two weeks after KA-seizures induction, a significant decrease in Sema3F was observed in KA-treated WT mice related to WT controls, whereas no differences were registered between KA-injected MUT and MUT control mice **(A,A′)**. Regarding PlxnA3, no changes of expression were observed after KA treatment in WT or MUT mice **(B,B′)**; however, Npn-2 expression in MUT mice was significantly lower than WT mice, independently of treatment **(C,C′)**. **(A–C)** Fold change was calculated in reference to the WT control group, which was normalized to 1. Results are represented as the ratio between the relative amount of the gene of interest and GAPDH. $N = 5$ mice per experimental group. cDNA was prepared individually for each mouse and real-time PCR reactions were run in duplicates for each mouse. Data analysis: two-way ANOVA followed by Tukey's HSD test, $^{*}p < 0.05$; $^{**}p < 0.01$; $^{***}p < 0.001$. **(A′–C′)** In order to better evidence KA effect on each genotype, the expression levels generated by KA were re-calculated in relation to their respective control groups, WT or MUT. The dotted line on the *Y*-axis ($Y = 1$) represents the control values for each genotype. **A′–C′:** Mann–Whitney *t*-test with 95% confidence intervals.

and that in this way, activity controls gene expression, i.e., BDNF production (Chen et al., 2001; Martinowich et al., 2003; Zhou et al., 2006). Although we have shown that BDNF levels increased similarly after 6 h of KA injection in both WT and MUT hippocampi (**Figure 1I**), we decided to evaluate BDNF expression after 2 weeks of treatment to determine whether BDNF expression correlates with the increase in IPT volume. As shown in **Figure 6A**, there was a significant difference between both genotypes in terms of BDNF expression [$F(1,13) = 10.61$; $p < 0.01$]. WT animals showed a moderate but significant increase in BDNF expression, 2 weeks after injection with KA. In contrast, in MUT mice BDNF expression remained unchanged between the control and the KA-treated group. Also, BDNF levels in MUT+KA animals were markedly lower than those of WT + KA mice (**Figure 6A**).

Considering that the effects of BDNF are largely mediated through its interaction with and the activation of the TrkB receptor, we proceeded to confirm our result by assessing the number of cells that express the phosphorylated TrkB receptor, as an indicator of BDNF action *in vivo* (Li et al., 2012; Helgager et al., 2014). For this, cryosections from the experimental groups were perfused after 2 weeks of KA treatment, when WT animals showed an increase in BDNF levels and in the size of the IPT in response to KA. Using IHC, we labeled pTrkB-positive cells and it became clear that the area with higher numbers of pTrkB-positive cells was the granule cell layer

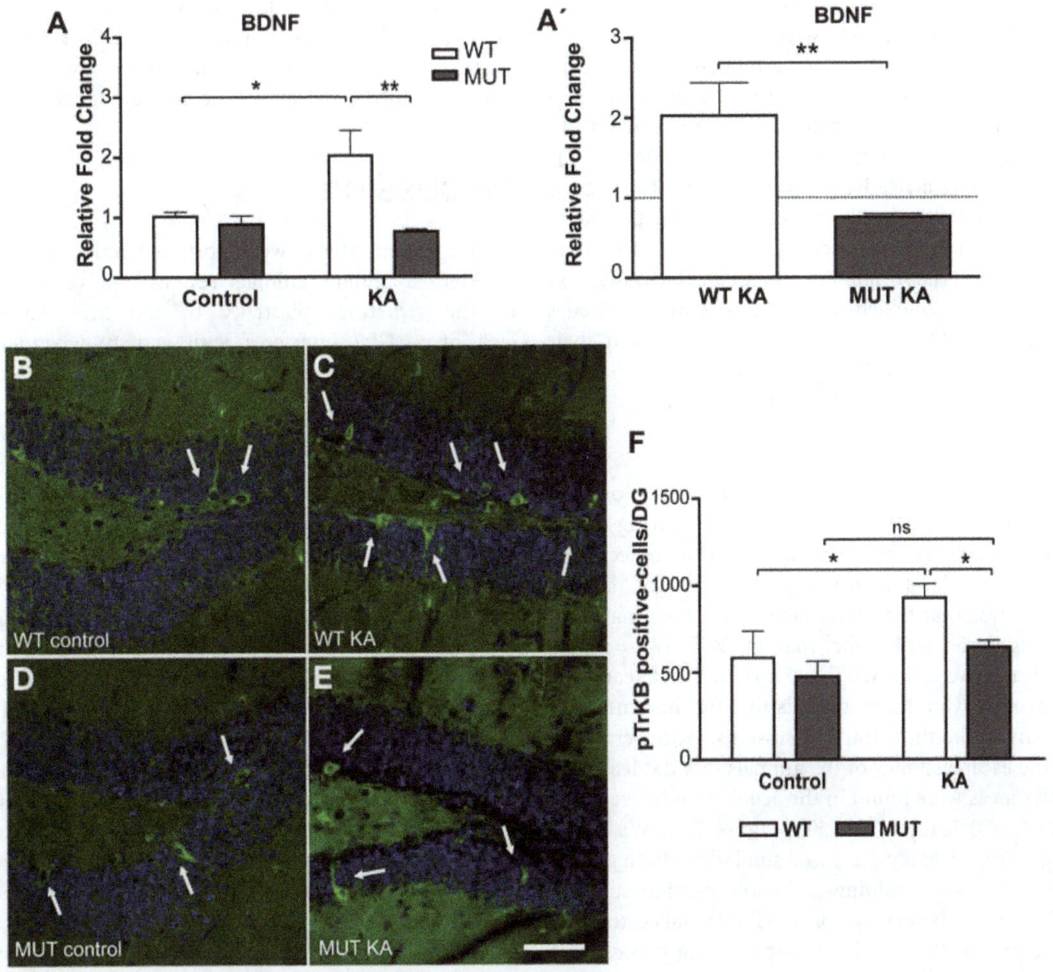

FIGURE 6 | Kainic-induced BDNF expression is deficient in MeCP2-308 MUT mice. **(A,A′)** BDNF expression was assessed by real-time RT-PCR from total hippocampus. **(A)** Two weeks after KA-seizures induction, a significant increase in BDNF was observed in KA-treated WT mice related to WT controls, whereas no differences were registered between KA-injected MUT and MUT control mice. Fold change was calculated in reference to the WT control group, which was normalized to 1. Results are represented as the ratio between the relative amount of the gene of interest and GAPDH. $N = 5$ mice per experimental group. cDNA was prepared individually for each mouse and real-time PCR reactions were run in duplicates for each mouse. **(A′)** In order to better evidence KA effect on each genotype, the expression levels generated by KA were re-calculated in relation to their respective control groups, WT or MUT. The dotted line on the Y-axis ($Y = 1$) represents the control values for each genotype. Data analysis: **(A)** two-way ANOVA followed by Tukey's HSD test, $^*p < 0.05$; $^{**}p < 0.01$. **(A′)** Mann–Whitney t-test with 95% confidence intervals, $^{**}p < 0{,}01$. **(B–E)** IHC- and pTrkB-positive cells quantification in DG. Two weeks after KA treatment, an increase in pTrkB-positive cells (white arrows) was observed in WT mice DG injected with KA **(C)** in comparison to KA-injected MUT mice **(E)** or control mice **(B,D)**. IHC labeling pTrkB (green) and Dapi (blue). Scale bar: 50 μm. **(F)** Quantification of pTrkB-positive cells per DG in WT and MUT mice injected with KA and control. A single seizure episode leads to an increase in the number of pTrkB-positive cells, detected 2 weeks after seizure activity only in WT mice. $n = 3$ mice per experimental group. Data analysis: two-way ANOVA followed by Tukey's HSD test, $^*p < 0.05$.

of the DG (**Figures 6B–E**). We found a significant difference between WT and MUT mice at 2 weeks after KA administration [$F(1,8) = 11.58$; $p < 0.01$]. While WT + KA showed a significant increase of pTrkB-positive cells in comparison with the controls, no significant differences were observed between treatments in MUT mice (**Figure 6F**). Again, the numbers of pTrkB-positive cells from the WT + KA were significantly higher than those of the MUT + KA.

Altogether, our results indicate that in WT animals, the growth of the IPT, detected at 2 weeks after KA seizure induction, is accompanied by an increase of BDNF expression. Conversely, no increase in the size of IPT is observed in MUT mice, which correlates with deficient BDNF expression in response to KA injection.

Mecp2 Mutant Mice Present Defects in Spatial Memory Evaluated Through the Barnes Maze Test

Given the defects found in activity-dependent plasticity of MF (IPT) in the dorsal region of MeCP2 MUT hippocampus and considering that this circuitry is mainly involved in the processing of spatial memory (Crusio et al., 1987; Crusio and Schwegler, 2005), we decided to assess spatial learning and memory abilities in these mice through their performance in the Barnes maze. It is estimated that, through successive training sessions, the improvement in performance to locate a hidden box to escape from aversive stimuli allows assessing learning processes and spatial memory in rodents (Rosenfeld and Ferguson, 2014). Considered less stressful for mice than water maze (Morris), the Barnes maze consists of a relatively simple design of a circular platform with several holes equally spaced around the perimeter edge. While one hole leads to an escape cage, the rest are blind. Slightly aversive stimuli (i.e., bright lights) provide the motivation to locate the escape cage, which is also flanked by visual cues (O'Leary and Brown, 2013). Therefore, MUT mice and their WT littermates were evaluated for spatial learning and memory according to their performance in the Barnes maze test.

Learning

The acquisition or learning of the escape box location was assessed by determining the escape latency during three successive training sessions; thus, the acquisition was reflected by lower escape latencies along the trainings. Interestingly, the first thing we noticed was that the percentage of MUT animals that did not learn was almost 20% higher than the WT (WT = 9.52% mice did not learn the task; MUT = 27.3% did not learn the task); "non-learners" were those animals that did not enter the escape box in any of the three training sessions. However, when we evaluated the escape latency of the animals that did learn, no significant differences were found in the acquisition between the groups [$F(6,117) = 0.744$; $p = 0.6150$] (**Figure 7A**). We found that the average escape latency decreased similarly in both groups throughout the successive trainings. This observation suggests that, although a higher percentage of MUT mice failed to learn the task, in the groups that did learn, the learning process was similar to that of the WT littermates.

Memory

Two days after the acquisition phase, we performed a final test of retention or memory, consisting of a single 2-min exposure on the platform, after removal of the escape box. In this spatial preference test the animal that remembers the maze will spend more time in the "target" quadrant, i.e., the quadrant where the escape box was previously located (O'Leary and Brown, 2013). The data showed a significant difference between genotypes [$F(1,36) = 14.81$; $p < 0.001$] (**Figure 7B**). While WT mice spent about 40% of the time in the target quadrant, MUT mice only spent an average of 24% of the total time in that quadrant (**Figure 7B**). Since the average percentage of time that a normal mouse will spend randomly in each quadrant of the platform during the test is about 25%, we can conclude that the MUT mice showed a failure in retaining the task learned during the acquisition phase.

These results were complemented by quantifying the percentage of snouts made by the animals in the target quadrant and in the escape hole with respect to the total snouts in the holes of the platform during the 2 min of the final memory test. The statistics showed a marked difference between WT and MUT MeCP2 [$F(1,38) = 22.7$; $p < 0.0001$]. WT mice explored the target quadrant and the escape hole significantly more than MUT mice (**Figures 7C,D**). Altogether, these results indicate that MeCP2 MUT mice do not show defects in the spatial learning process measured with the Barnes maze; however, they exhibit a marked failure in the spatial memory evaluated by the same test.

DISCUSSION

In the present study, we report that inducing seizure activity in MeCP2 mutant animals reveals a novel role for MeCP2 in the structural plasticity of the MF-CA3 circuit. The lack of MeCP2 interferes with activity-dependent structural presynaptic plasticity in the hippocampus, affecting axonal growth/remodeling, the maturation of adult born neurons, as well as BDNF and Sema3F signaling. Likewise, we show that these plasticity defects correlate with a reduced performance in a spatial learning test (Barnes maze).

Two central events in presynaptic structural plasticity have been described in mice and rat hippocampus: adult neurogenesis and dynamic changes in the size of the IPT, formed by DG granule cell axons. Both the formation of new DG neurons and the anatomy of the IPT are dynamically regulated in response to neurogenic stimuli, such as exposure to an enriched environment or the induction of epileptogenic activity (Parent and Lowenstein, 1997; Gray and Sundstrom, 1998; Lindvall et al., 2002; Belichenko et al., 2008; Römer et al., 2011). Although environmental enrichment may be a better physiological stimulus, it is not possible to ensure that any given animal receive similar stimulation. In the present study, we decided to treat animals with KA in order to trigger seizures and generate robust neuronal activity *in vivo*, as a way to provide controlled stimulation conditions, leading to more homogeneous activity. We based our experimental design on several reports using KA injections in different Rett mouse models, considering that those studies have established most of the activity-dependent responses described in the field (Ebert, 2013).

Most of our studies were developed in the MeCP2-308 (MUT) model which better resembles the human pathology; these mice express a mutated protein, their clinical evolution is progressive, and they survive for over a year. This is important because it permits experiments at more advanced ages and also avoids the results may be masked by near-death physiological conditions, as occurs with most of the studies performed in MeCP2 KO models (survival: 8–11 weeks). The original characterization of this mouse model revealed that MeCP2 MUT animals develop spontaneous seizures from 5 months of age (Moretti et al., 2005). However, there were no reports regarding the induction of seizures activity using this model. Here, we performed KA injection experiments in WT and MUT mice of 6, 9, and 12 weeks of age. Interestingly, 6 weeks old-MUT mice injected with KA did not develop seizures nor showed an increase in the expression of BDNF and Arc, in contrast to their WT littermates (data not shown) and MeCP2-KO mice (**Figure 2A**). Conversely, 12-weeks-old MUT mice were acutely sensitive to the KA doses that were just effective in 12-weeks-old WT mice (data not shown). Lastly, 9-weeks-old WT and MUT mice injected with KA showed similar levels of seizures activity and

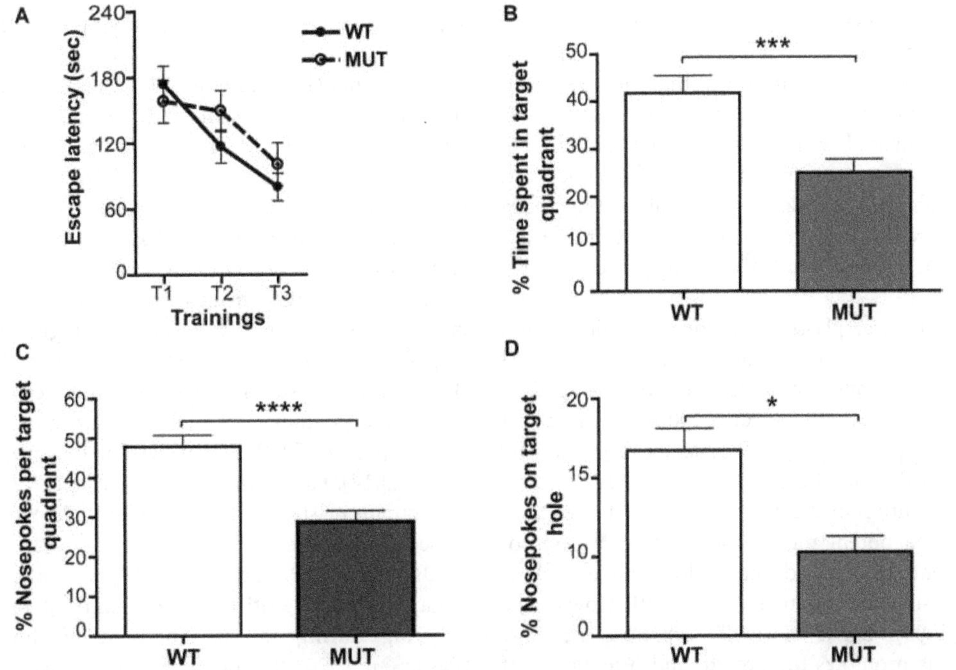

FIGURE 7 | Mecp2-mutant mice show defective spatial memory evaluated through the Barnes maze. **(A)** Learning: the acquisition was reflected by lower escape latencies along the trainings. For both experimental groups, a similar decrease in the escape latency time (measured in seconds) throughout the successive trainings was observed. n = 16-19 mice per experimental group. Data analysis: two-way ANOVA followed by Tukey's HSD test. **(B–D)** Memory: relative percentage of time spent and number of snouts made by the animals in the target quadrant and in the escape hole during the 2 min of the final memory test. **(B)** Percentage of time spent in target quadrant for WT and MUT mice. The analysis shows that WT mice spent significantly more time in the target quadrant than MUT mice. Percentage of snouts in the target quadrant holes **(C)** and in the escape hole **(D)** in relation to the total snouts performed in the holes of the platform in the 2 min of the final memory test. Both the percentage of snouts in the "target" quadrant **(C)** and in the escape hole **(D)** was significantly higher in WT mice when compared with the MUT. n = 16–19 mice per experimental group. Data analysis: Mann–Whitney t-test with 95% confidence interval. $^{*}p < 0.05$; $^{***}p < 0.001$; $^{****}p < 0.0001$.

increased expression of BDNF and Arc (**Figures 1B,H,I**). Thus, we found clear age-dependent differences in susceptibility to KA in MUT animals.

However, we observed no change in the IPT volume in 9-week-old MUT mice (**Figure 1G**), even though they showed increased neuronal activity in response to KA, similar in magnitude to that induced in WT animals (**Figures 1B,H,I**). These results suggest that the lack of IPT growth was not due to a defect in early neuronal activation in the hippocampus of MeCP2 MUT mice. We confirmed some of these results using another model MeCP2 Bird mice (KO). MeCP2 KO mice injected at 6 weeks of age showed greater sensitivity to KA than their WT counterparts (**Figure 2A**). This response is consistent with other author reports, using a different KO mouse model of MeCP2 (McLeod et al., 2013). When activity-induced gene expression was quantified after 6 h of KA, both WT and KO mice showed increased expression of BDNF and Arc (**Figures 2C,D**). However, only the WT mice of this model showed a significant increase in IPT size (**Figure 2B**), even though MeCP2 KO animals displayed higher seizures scores. Thus, using two different mouse models we show that even though similar seizure activity was recorded in every KA-injected animal and they show similar levels of hippocampal neural stimulation (measured as levels of activity-induced gene expression), no increase in the size of the IPT was detected in any of the models of MeCP2 deficiency (MUT or KO), indicating a deficit in the plastic IPT response to neuronal activity in the absence of normal MeCP2 function.

Since it has been demonstrated that the IPT size is dynamically influenced by an increase in neurogenesis (Römer et al., 2011), we evaluated adult neurogenesis in DG in response to KA. Our results showed that this process was not affected in MeCP2 MUT mice (**Figures 3A–C**), in agreement with previous work indicating that MeCP2 is not critical for neurogenesis (Smrt et al., 2007). The lack of IPT growth observed in MeCP2 MUT mice in response to KA would not be a consequence of a lower production of new granule cells in DG. However, it is possible that the survival of these new neurons is affected in the absence of MeCP2. In this sense, we observed that the proportion of new cells ($BrdU^{+}$) that remain 5 weeks in the DG after the induction of seizures activity was similar in WT and MUT mice (**Figure 3D**); therefore, the survival of the new DG neurons seems not to be affected by MeCP2 mutation. These results are also in agreement with older studies that found no signs of neurodegeneration or neuronal death in these models of MeCP2 deficiency (Moretti et al., 2005, 2006).

Interestingly, although neurogenesis was not affected in the absence of MeCP2, the new DG neurons displayed deficits in their ability to transition to a mature state (**Figure 4**). Our results show that mice carrying a mutated MeCP2 protein (MUT) have defects in the maturation of new neurons in adults, in a manner similar to that observed during early development in other RTT models (Matarazzo et al., 2004; Smrt et al., 2007; Palmer et al., 2008). The increase in adult neurogenesis induced by neuronal activity allowed us to show that this defect is recapitulated in the adult animal. The delay in maturation of DG newborn granule cells in adult animals suggests that, although in response to synaptic activity a similar number of new neurons are generated in the absence of MeCP2, they would not normally integrate into the circuit. This finding could have important implications in hippocampal-dependent learning processes, such as spatial memory tests.

Regarding the structural plasticity of the IPT tract, it has been proposed that this is the result of the coordinated increase of trophic factors and the decrease of chemo-repellant molecules (Bermúdez-Rattoni and Rekart, 2007). The levels of neurotrophins in the hippocampus are regulated dynamically by neuronal activity and the modification of these levels can alter the growth and distribution of the MF. Numerous studies have implicated BDNF as a potent modulator in many aspects of neuronal development (Huang and Reichardt, 2001), as well as in synaptic transmission and plasticity (Poo, 2001; Cowansage et al., 2010; Lu, 2003). BDNF normally expressed in most hippocampal neurons promotes the growth and orientation of the axons of granule cells *in vitro* and regulates the synaptic plasticity of MF (Gómez-Palacio-Schjetnan and Escobar, 2008; Tamura et al., 2009; Schjetnan and Escobar, 2012). In addition, MeCP2 has been shown to be phosphorylated in response to synaptic activity and regulates gene expression, in particular the production of BDNF (Chen et al., 2003; Martinowich et al., 2003). Our results demonstrate that in both WT and MeCP2 MUT animals, BDNF levels increase similarly in response to KA, at 6 h post injection. However, when we determined BDNF expression and pTrKB (an *in situ* indicator of endogenous BDNF protein; Li et al., 2012) at 2 weeks post-KA, we found it remains high in WT animals, but not in the MUT mice (**Figure 6F**). Thus, the IPT growth detected in WT animals was accompanied by an increase in the expression of BDNF; while in MeCP2 MUT mice, the lack of growth correlated with a poor change in BDNF expression. These results indicate that although the signaling events involved in the early neuronal response to seizure activity seems unaffected in the absence of MeCP2 (**Figure 1H**), we do detect a deficit of long-term BDNF support required for driving the axonal growth of MF in response to synaptic activity.

Given the importance of this neurotrophin, and considering that MeCP2 binds to one of BDNF promoters and regulates its expression, many studies have proposed a critical role for BDNF in the pathogenesis of RTT. In this sense, a general reduction in BDNF mRNA levels has been described in MeCP2 KO animal models (complete lack of protein) (Chang et al., 2006; Wang et al., 2006; Kobayashi, 2009; Li and Pozzo-Miller, 2014). However, it is interesting to note that those changes were reported when MeCP2 KO mice were already fully symptomatic (and with a life expectancy of 1–3 more weeks). In this sense, we found no differences in hippocampal BDNF expression between WT and MeCP2 KO 6-weeks-old mice under either basal or KA-treated conditions (**Figure 2D**), suggesting that BDNF expression in the absence of MeCP2 may be either associated to age or secondary to symptoms; this issue has been already noticed in our previous work and also discussed by other authors (Degano et al., 2014; Li and Pozzo-Miller, 2014). In contrast, in the present work, we show that in the MeCP2-308 mouse model, MUT mice in basal conditions show no differences in mRNA levels for BDNF in the hippocampus at either 9 or 11 weeks of age (**Figures 1I, 6A**). This observation was also reported in older and symptomatic MeCP2-308 MUT animals (Moretti et al., 2006). In addition, we observed that both WT and MUT groups responded with a similar increase in BDNF expression at 6 h post-KA (**Figure 1I**), although this response was not maintained over time in the MUT animals (**Figure 6A**). These results suggest a more complex relationship, and further studies are needed to clarify the role of BDNF in the absence of MeCP2 and in RTT pathogenesis (Li and Pozzo-Miller, 2014). Paradigms of *in vivo* synaptic activation combined with circuit plasticity and molecular tools may help to elucidate these relationships.

On the other hand, a body of evidence suggests that semaphorins are critical determinants of axonal growth and targeting during the development of the nervous system (Pasterkamp, 2012). Mice deficient in Sema 3F, Npn-2, or in PlexinA3 showed robust hypertrophy of the IPT tract (Cheng et al., 2001; Bagri et al., 2003; Riccomagno et al., 2012). Therefore, considering our previous reports revealing axonal guidance and Sema 3F deficits in MeCP2 KO mice (Degano et al., 2009), we focused in evaluating the Sema 3F pathway in the context of MeCP2 mutation. This molecule is involved in the growth, guidance, and target of hippocampal MFs (Bagri et al., 2003; Sahay et al., 2003), acting as an inhibitor of axonal growth and inducing their collapse (Riccomagno et al., 2012). In this sense, the response of WT mice injected with KA (**Figure 5A**) was in line to previous reports, which showed that WT mice exposed to seizure activity (using either KA or pilocarpine) display a decrease in mRNA Sema 3F levels between the 1st and 2nd week after seizures in CA3, CA1, and DG (Barnes et al., 2003; Cai et al., 2016); this decrease overlapped with the formation of new synapses in the MF-CA3 circuitry (Okazaki et al., 1995; Barnes et al., 2003). Thus, the reduction of Sema 3F expression induced by KA in WT animals (low chemo-repulsion) would promote a permissive milieu for MF growth, contributing to the dynamic increase in the size of the IPT registered after KA-induced seizures (Römer et al., 2011). Since both MUT and KO MeCP2 mice failed to show a decrease of Sema3F levels in response to KA (**Figures 2E,E′, 5A,A′**), we suggest that in these animals a local inhibitory environment for axonal growth is operating, which could account for the lack of IPT volume increase in the absence of normal MeCP2 expression.

It has been suggested that the process of structural plasticity shown by MF in response to synaptic activity involves a tightly regulated balance between growth factors and axonal guidance molecules (Bermúdez-Rattoni and Rekart, 2007). Here we report that an imbalanced expression of those crucial players might be responsible for the lack of MF growth in the absence of MeCP2 (**Figure 8**). Thus, after seizure activity, MeCP2 MUT and KO

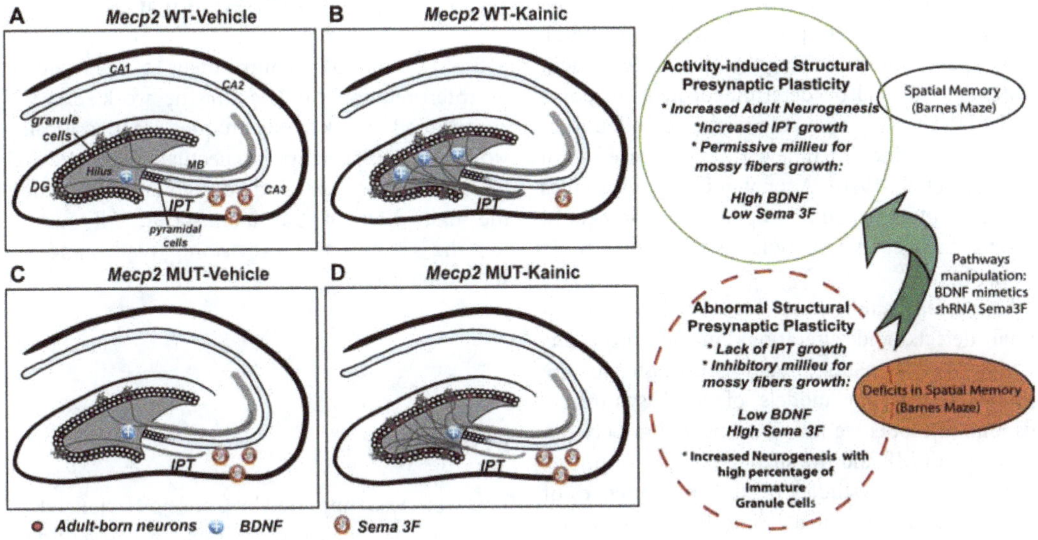

FIGURE 8 | Schematic summary of the activity-induced presynaptic plasticity regulated by MeCP2. In WT mice, seizures activity increases the level of neurogenesis, accompanied with higher levels of BDNF and lower of Sema3F, allowing IPT to grow **(A,B)**. Conversely, MUT animals show abnormal activity-dependent presynaptic plasticity characterized by the lack of IPT growth which correlates with imbalanced trophic and guidance support (BDNF and Sema3F abnormal levels). Although activity do increases the neurogenesis in MUT mice, adult born granule cells show developmental restraining and recapitulate maturational defects **(C,D)**. These results are in line with deficits in spatial memory observed in MUT mice. This study set the basis to establish a model to evaluate the effect of manipulating specific pathways involved in axonal guidance, synaptogenesis, and neuronal maturation to correlate with changes in behavior.

mice display an increase of the chemorepellant Sema 3F, which in concert with a deficient expression of the growth factor BDNF would generate an inhibitory environment for axonal growth.

In this study, we did not analyze the dendritic components of granule DG cells. However, in contrast to postmortem studies in RTT patients (Armstrong et al., 1995), the brains of symptomatic MeCP2-308 MUT mice did not show defects in dendritic arborizations in frontal cortex nor in the density of synapses or dendritic spines in CA1 area of hippocampus (Moretti et al., 2006). In addition, electrophysiological studies suggest that synaptic dysfunction precedes clinical symptoms; these were manifested as an increase in synaptic transmission and decreased LTD in the collateral synapses of Schaffer in this animal model (Moretti et al., 2006). Further studies using this animal model of MeCP2 mutation may define whether axonal components are the main substrate of these synaptic defects.

Presynaptic structural plasticity events have been correlated with improvements of performance in hippocampal-dependent learning tests (Römer et al., 2011). The considerable plasticity of the IPT has been observed early (Schwegler et al., 1990), and abundant evidence demonstrated the positive correlation between IPT size and animal performance in a great variety of behavioral tests of spatial memory (Lipp et al., 1988; Schwegler et al., 1990; Schöpke et al., 1991; Bernasconi-Guastalla et al., 1994; Laghmouch et al., 1997; Crusio and Schwegler, 2005; Delprato et al., 2015). Interestingly, deficits in radial maze performance were also associated with smaller IPT in a mouse model of Fragile-X Syndrome (Mineur et al., 2002). Therefore, we decided to evaluate spatial learning and memory of MeCP2 MUT mice through their ability to navigate the Barnes maze; it is estimated that the improvement in performance to locate an escape box to aversive stimuli, through successive training sessions, allows assessing learning processes and spatial memory in rodents. Previous studies showed that MeCP2-308 MUT mice (> 20 weeks of age = fully symptomatic) show learning and memory deficits in several hippocampal-dependent behavior paradigms (Morris water maze, fear contextual conditioning test, and long-term social memory) (Moretti et al., 2005, 2006). Our results indicate that earlier in development (12-weeks-old), 27% of MeCP2-308 MUT mice failed to learn the location of the exit box, compared with 10% of WT littermates. Interestingly, the MUT animals that learned the task had similar performance as the WTs during the trainings. Conversely, these MUT animals displayed clear spatial memory deficits, as they showed a marked failure in the retention of the acquired information evaluated by the same test (**Figures 7B–D**). It is important to emphasize that in this work we also revealed that failure in granule cells maturation recapitulates in each round of neurogenesis in the adult hippocampus, adding to the long-term circuitry dysfunction (**Figure 4**). Although it has not been demonstrated that memory *per se* is altered in patients, cognitive abnormalities are present in individuals with MeCP2 mutations, supporting the concept that the results obtained with the MeCP2-308 animal model would represent a correlate of cognitive deficits in RTT (Moretti et al., 2006).

Alterations of synaptic and axonal refinement have been implicated in the etiology of neurological diseases (Lewis and Levitt, 2002; Johnston, 2004; Pardo and Eberhart, 2007). Likewise, hippocampal MF synapses are important for spatial memory formation and consolidation (Nicoll and Schmitz, 2005; Bischofberger et al., 2006). Spatial learning and environmental enrichment result in an increase in the number, size, and complexity of the MF (Ramírez-Amaya et al., 2001;

Galimberti et al., 2006). In addition, the IPT presents a dramatic reorganization after induction of seizures (Cavazos et al., 1991). While the molecular pathways underlying the activity-dependent remodeling of MFs should still be determined, neurotrophins such as NGF and BDNF may play a role in the remodeling of MF in the normal brain, since their levels are increased with seizures activity (Zafra et al., 1990). Axonal guidance molecules including semaphorins, plexins, and neuropilins can also help to reconfigure MF after changes in activity levels (Holtmaat et al., 2003; Suto et al., 2010).

In light of the present studies, we propose that activity-dependent axonal defects and alterations in neurotrophins and guidance molecules signaling could contribute to the neurological defects present in models of RTT syndrome. Likewise, in this animal model we found a correlation between the structural plasticity of MF and the spatial memory response. This offers a powerful tool for studies on the consequences of MeCP2 mutation, since changes in a relatively simple neural circuit could be connected to changes in spatial memory defined from an animal behavioral test. Based on these studies, we establish a model that would allow to evaluate the effect of the manipulation of specific pathways involved in axonal guidance/synaptogenesis/neuronal maturation in a specific circuit in correlation with changes in spatial memory (**Figure 8**). This strategy may enable a better understanding of the factors that control synaptic activity-dependent remodeling in the normal brain and in disorders of connectivity, such as autism-related disorders.

AUTHOR CONTRIBUTIONS

MB, MZ, and MF contributed to the acquisition, analysis, or interpretation of data for the work. SA, GVR, and GAR contributed to key techniques and critically revised the work for important intellectual content. AD contributed to the conception and design of the study, and wrote the first draft of the manuscript. All authors contributed to the manuscript revision, read, and approved the submitted version.

FUNDING

This work was supported by Consejo Nacional de Investigaciones Científicas y Técnicas de la República Argentina (CONICET, to AD), Secretaria de Ciencia y Tecnología-Universidad Nacional de Córdoba (SeCyT-UNC, to AD), Agencia Nacional de Promoción Científica y Técnológica (FONCyT-PICT 2013 No. 106, to AD), International Society for Neurochemistry (ISN-CAEN, to AD and MB), and by a Research with the Daegu Gyeongbuk Institute of Science and Technology (DGIST) Convergence Science Center, funded by grant #10-BD-04 from Korean Ministry of Education, Science, and Technology (to SA and GVR).

REFERENCES

Amir, R. E., Van den Veyver, B. I, Wan, M., Tran, C. Q., Francke, U., and Zoghbi, H. Y. (1999). Rett syndrome is caused by mutations in X-linked MECP2, encoding methyl-CpG-binding protein 2. *Nat. Genet.* 23, 185–188. doi: 10.1038/13810

Armstrong, D., Dunn, J. K., Antalffy, B., and Trivedi, R. (1995). Selective dendritic alterations in the cortex of rett syndrome. *J. Neuropathol. Exp. Neurol.* 54, 195–201. doi: 10.1097/00005072-199503000-199503006

Asaka, Y., Jugloff, D. G. M., Zhang, L., Eubanks, J. H., and Fitzsimonds, R. M. (2006). Hippocampal synaptic plasticity is impaired in the Mecp2-null mouse model of Rett syndrome. *Neurobiol. Dis.* 21, 217–227. doi: 10.1016/j.nbd.2005.07.005

Bagri, A., Cheng, H. J., Yaron, A., Pleasure, S. J., and Tessier-Lavigne, M. (2003). Stereotyped pruning of long hippocampal axon branches triggered by retraction inducers of the semaphorin family. *Cell* 113, 285–299. doi: 10.1016/S0092-8674(03)00267-268

Ballas, N., Mandel, G., Nigam, A., Robinson, J. K., Du, F., Felice, C. A., et al. (2012). MeCP2 is critical for maintaining mature neuronal networks and global brain anatomy during late stages of postnatal brain development and in the mature adult brain. *J. Neurosci.* 32, 10021–10034. doi: 10.1523/jneurosci.1316-12.2012

Barnes, G., Puranam, R. S., Luo, Y., and McNamara, J. O. (2003). Temporal specific patterns of semaphorin gene expression in rat brain after kainic acid-induced status epilepticus. *Hippocampus* 13, 1–20. doi: 10.1002/hipo.10041

Belichenko, N. P., Belichenko, P. V., Li, H. H., Mobley, W. C., and Francke, U. (2008). Comparative study of brain morphology in Mecp2 mutant mouse models of Rett syndrome. *J. Comp. Neurol.* 508, 184–195. doi: 10.1002/cne.21673

Bermúdez-Rattoni, F., and Rekart, J. L. (2007). "SourceNeural Plasticity and Memory: From Genes to Brain Imaging," in *Presynaptic Structural Plasticity and Long-Lasting Memory: Focus on Learning-Induced Redistribution of Hippocampal Mossy Fibers*, ed. F. Bermúdez-Rattoni (Boca Raton FL: CRC Press/Taylor & Francis).

Bernasconi-Guastalla, S., Wolfer, D. P., and Lipp, H. P. (1994). Hippocampal mossy fibers and swimming navigation in mice: correlations with size and left-right asymmetries. *Hippocampus* 4, 53–63. doi: 10.1002/hipo.450040107

Bischofberger, J., Engel, D., Frotscher, M., and Jonas, P. (2006). Timing and efficacy of transmitter release at mossy fiber synapses in the hippocampal network. *Pflugers Arch. Eur. J. Physiol.* 453, 361–372. doi: 10.1007/s00424-006-0093-92

Burns, K. A., and Kuan, C. Y. (2005). Low of bromo- and iododeoxyuridine produce near-saturation labeling of adult proliferative populations in the dentate gyrus. *Eur. J. Neurosci.* 21, 803–807. doi: 10.1111/j.1460-9568.2005.03907.x

Cai, X., Long, L., Yang, L., Chen, Z., Ni, G., Qin, J., et al. (2016). Association between mossy fiber sprouting and expression of semaphorin-3f protein in dentate gyrus of hippocampus in lithium-pilocarpine-induced status epilepticus mouse model. *Neurol. Res.* 6412, 1–6. doi: 10.1080/01616412.2016.1243639

Cavazos, J. E., Golarai, G., and Sutula, T. P. (1991). Mossy fiber synaptic reorganization induced by kindling: time course of development, progression, and permanence. *J. Neurosci.* 11, 2795–2803. doi: 10.1523/jneurosci.11-09-02795.1991

Chahrour, M., and Zoghbi, H. Y. (2007). The story of rett syndrome: from clinic to neurobiology. *Neuron* 56, 422–437. doi: 10.1016/j.neuron.2007.10.001

Chang, Q., Khare, G., Dani, V., Nelson, S., and Jaenisch, R. (2006). The disease progression of Mecp2 mutant mice is affected by the level of BDNF expression. *Neuron* 49, 341–348. doi: 10.1016/j.neuron.2005.12.027

Chapleau, C. A., Calfa, G. D., Lane, M. C., Albertson, A. J., Larimore, J. L., Kudo, S., et al. (2009). Dendritic spine pathologies in hippocampal pyramidal neurons from Rett syndrome brain and after expression of Rett-associated MECP2 mutations. *Neurobiol. Dis.* 35, 219–233. doi: 10.1016/j.nbd.2009.05.001

Chapleau, C. A., and Pozzo-Miller, L. (2008). "Learning and memory: a comprehensive reference," in *Activity-Dependent Structural Plasticity of Dendritic Spines*, ed J. Byrne (Oxford: Elsevier)

Chen, R. Z., Akbarian, S., Tudor, M., and Jaenisch, R. (2001). Deficiency of methyl-CpG binding protein-2 in CNS neurons results in a Rett-like phenotype in mice. *Nat. Genet.* 27, 327–331. doi: 10.1038/85906

Chen, W. G., Chang, Q., Lin, Y., Meissner, A., West, A. E., Griffith, E. C., et al. (2003). Derepression of BDNF transcription involves calcium-dependent phosphorylation of MeCP2. *Science* 302, 885–889. doi: 10.1126/science.1086446

Cheng, H. J., Bagri, A., Yaron, A., Stein, E., Pleasure, S. J., and Tessier-Lavigne, M. (2001). Plexin-A3 mediates semaphorin signaling and regulates the development of hippocampal axonal projections. *Neuron* 32, 249–263. doi: 10.1016/S0896-6273(01)00478-470

Cowansage, K. K., LeDoux, J. E., and Monfils, M.-H. (2010). Brain-derived neurotrophic factor: a dynamic gatekeeper of neural plasticity. *Curr. Mol. Pharmacol.* 3, 12–29. doi: 10.2174/1874-470211003010012

Crusio, W. E., and Schwegler, H. (2005). Learning spatial orientation tasks in the radial-maze and structural variation in the hippocampus in inbred mice. *Behav. Brain Funct.* 1:3. doi: 10.1186/1744-9081-1-3

Crusio, W. E., Schwegler, H., and Lipp, H. P. (1987). Radial-maze performance and structural variation of the hippocampus in mice: a correlation with mossy fibre distribution. *Brain Res.* 425, 182–185. doi: 10.1016/0006-8993(87)90498-90497

Degano, A. L., Park, M. J., Penati, J., Li, Q., and Ronnett, G. V. (2014). MeCP2 is required for activity-dependent refinement of olfactory circuits. *Mol. Cell. Neurosci.* 59, 63–75. doi: 10.1016/j.mcn.2014.01.005

Degano, A. L., Pasterkamp, R. J., and Ronnett, G. V. (2009). MeCP2 deficiency disrupts axonal guidance, fasciculation, and targeting by altering Semaphorin 3F function. *Mol. Cell Neurosci.* 42, 243–254. doi: 10.1016/j.mcn.2009.07.009

Delprato, A., Bonheur, B., Algéo, M. P., Rosay, P., Lu, L., Williams, R. W., et al. (2015). Systems genetic analysis of hippocampal neuroanatomy and spatial learning in mice. *Genes Brain Behav.* 14, 591–606. doi: 10.1111/gbb.12259

Dieni, S., Matsumoto, T., Dekkers, M., Rauskolb, S., Ionescu, M. S., Deogracias, R., et al. (2012). BDNF and its pro-peptide are stored in presynaptic dense core vesicles in brain neurons. *J. Cell Biol.* 196, 775–788. doi: 10.1083/jcb.201201038

Ebert, D. H. (2013). Activity-dependent neuronal signalling and autism spectrum disorder. *Nature* 493, 327–337. doi: 10.1038/mp.2011.182

Ebert, D. H., Gabel, H. W., Robinson, N. D., Kastan, N. R., Hu, L. S., Cohen, S., et al. (2013). Activity-dependent phosphorylation of MeCP2 threonine 308 regulates interaction with NCoR. *Nature* 499, 341–345. doi: 10.1038/nature12348

Esposito, M. S. (2005). Neuronal differentiation in the adult hippocampus recapitulates embryonic development. *J. Neurosci.* 25, 10074–10086. doi: 10.1523/jneurosci.3114-05.2005

Galimberti, I., Gogolla, N., Alberi, S., Santos, A. F., Muller, D., and Caroni, P. (2006). Long-term rearrangements of hippocampal mossy fiber terminal connectivity in the adult regulated by experience. *Neuron* 50, 749–763. doi: 10.1016/j.neuron.2006.04.026

Gómez-Palacio-Schjetnan, A., and Escobar, M. L. (2008). In vivo BDNF modulation of adult functional and morphological synaptic plasticity at hippocampal mossy fibers. *Neurosci. Lett.* 445, 62–67. doi: 10.1016/j.neulet.2008.08.069

Gray, W. P., and Sundstrom, L. E. (1998). Kainic acid increases the proliferation of granule cell progenitors in the dentate gyrus of the adult rat. *Brain Res.* 790, 52–59. doi: 10.1016/S0006-8993(98)00030-34

Guy, J., Hendrich, B., Holmes, M., Martin, J. E., and Bird, A. (2001). A mouse Mecp2-null mutation causes neurological symptoms that mimic rett syndrome. *Nat. Genet.* 27, 322–326. doi: 10.1038/85899

Helgager, J., Huang, Y., and Mcnamara, J. (2014). Brain-derived neurotrophic factor but not vesicular zinc promotes TrkB activation within mossy fibers of mouse hippocampus in vivo. *J. Comp. Neurol.* 522, 3885–3899. doi: 10.1038/jid.2014.371

Holtmaat, A. J. G. D., Gorter, J. A., De Wit, J., Tolner, E. A., Spijker, S., Giger, R. J., et al. (2003). Transient downregulation of Sema3A mRNA in a rat model for temporal lobe epilepsy: a novel molecular event potentially contributing to mossy fiber sprouting. *Exp. Neurol.* 182, 142–150. doi: 10.1016/S0014-4886(03)00035-39

Huang, E. J., and Reichardt, L. F. (2001). Neurotrophins: roles in neuronal development and function. *Annu. Rev. Neurosci.* 24, 677–736. doi: 10.1146/annurev.neuro.24.1.677

Isgor, C., Pare, C., McDole, B., Coombs, P., and Guthrie, K. (2015). Expansion of the dentate mossy fiber-CA3 projection in the brain-derived neurotrophic factor-enriched mouse hippocampus. *Neuroscience* 288, 10–23. doi: 10.1016/j.neuroscience.2014.12.036

Johnston, M. V. (2004). Clinical disorders of brain plasticity. *Brain Dev.* 26, 73–80. doi: 10.1016/S0387-7604(03)00102-105

Kobayashi, K. (2009). Targeting the hippocampal mossy fiber synapse for the treatment of psychiatric disorders. *Mol. Neurobiol.* 39, 24–36. doi: 10.1007/s12035-008-8049-8045

Laghmouch, A., Bertholet, J. Y., and Crusio, W. E. (1997). Hippocampal morphology and open-field behavior in Mus musculus domesticus and Mus spretus inbred mice. *Behav. Genet.* 27, 67–73. doi: 10.1023/A:1025667426222

Lewis, D. A., and Levitt, P. (2002). Schizophrenia as a disorder of neurodevelopment. *Annu. Rev. Neurosci.* 25, 1–50. doi: 10.1146/annurev.neuro.25.112701.142754

Li, W., Calfa, G., Larimore, J., and Pozzo-Miller, L. (2012). Activity-dependent BDNF release and TRPC signaling is impaired in hippocampal neurons of Mecp2 mutant mice. *Proc. Natl. Acad. Sci. U.S.A.* 109, 17087–17092. doi: 10.1073/pnas.1205271109

Li, W., and Pozzo-Miller, L. (2014). BDNF deregulation in Rett syndrome. *Neuropharmacology* 76, 737–746. doi: 10.1016/j.neuropharm.2013.03.024

Lindvall, O., Elmer, E., Kokaia, Z., Nanobashvili, A., Kokaia, M., and Bengzon, J. (2002). Apoptosis and proliferation of dentate gyrus neurons after single and intermittent limbic seizures. *Proc. Natl. Acad. Sci. U.S.A.* 94, 10432–10437. doi: 10.1073/pnas.94.19.10432

Lipp, H. P., Schwegler, H., Heimrich, B., and Driscoll, P. (1988). Infrapyramidal mossy fibers and two-way avoidance learning: developmental modification of hippocampal circuitry and adult behavior of rats and mice. *J. Neurosci.* 8, 1905–1921. doi: 10.1523/jneurosci.08-06-01905.1988

Lu, B. (2003). Pro-region of neurotrophins: role in synaptic modulation. *Neuron* 39, 735–738. doi: 10.1016/S0896-6273(03)00538-535

Lyst, M. J., Ekiert, R., Ebert, D. H., Merusi, C., Nowak, J., Selfridge, J., et al. (2013). Rett syndrome mutations abolish the interaction of MeCP2 with the NCoR/SMRT co-repressor. *Nat. Neurosci.* 16, 898–902. doi: 10.1038/nn.3434

Martinowich, K., Hattori, D., Wu, H., Fouse, S., He, F., Hu, Y., et al. (2003). DNA methylation-related chromatin remodeling in activity-dependent bdnf gene regulation. *Science* 302, 890–893. doi: 10.1126/science.1090842

Matarazzo, V., Cohen, D., Palmer, A. M., Simpson, P. J., Khokhar, B., Pan, S. J., et al. (2004). The transcriptional repressor Mecp2 regulates terminal neuronal differentiation. *Mol. Cell. Neurosci.* 27, 44–58. doi: 10.1016/j.mcn.2004.05.005

McLeod, F., Ganley, R., Williams, L., Selfridge, J., Bird, A., and Cobb, S. R. (2013). Reduced seizure threshold and altered network oscillatory properties in a mouse model of Rett syndrome. *Neuroscience* 231, 195–205. doi: 10.1016/j.neuroscience.2012.11.058

Mineur, Y. S., Sluyter, F., De Wit, S., Oostra, B. A., and Crusio, W. E. (2002). Behavioral and neuroanatomical characterization of the Fmr1 knockout mouse. *Hippocampus* 12, 39–46. doi: 10.1002/hipo.10005

Moretti, P., Bouwknecht, J. A., Teague, R., Paylor, R., and Zoghbi, H. Y. (2005). Abnormalities of social interactions and home-cage behavior in a mouse model of Rett syndrome. *Hum. Mol. Genet.* 14, 205–220. doi: 10.1093/hmg/ddi016

Moretti, P., Levenson, J. M., Battaglia, F., Atkinson, R., Teague, R., Antalffy, B., et al. (2006). Learning and memory and synaptic plasticity are impaired in a mouse model of rett syndrome. *J. Neurosci.* 26, 319–327. doi: 10.1523/JNEUROSCI.2623-05.2006

Nan, X., Campoy, F. J., and Bird, A. (1997). MeCP2 is a transcriptional repressor with abundant binding sites in genomic chromatin. *Cell* 88, 471–481. doi: 10.1016/S0092-8674(00)81887-81885

Nicoll, R. A., and Schmitz, D. (2005). Synaptic plasticity at hippocampal mossy fibre synapses. *Nat. Rev. Neurosci.* 6, 863–876. doi: 10.1038/nrn1786

Okazaki, M. M., Evenson, D. A., and Victor Nadler, J. (1995). Hippocampal mossy fiber sprouting and synapse formation after status epilepticus in rats: Visualization after retrograde transport of biocytin. *J. Comp. Neurol.* 352, 515–534. doi: 10.1002/cne.903520404

O'Leary, T. P., and Brown, R. E. (2013). Optimization of apparatus design and behavioral measures for the assessment of visuo-spatial learning and memory of mice on the Barnes maze. *Learn. Mem.* 20, 85–96. doi: 10.1101/lm.028076.112

Palmer, A., Qayumi, J., and Ronnett, G. (2008). MeCP2 mutation causes distinguishable phases of acute and chronic defects in synaptogenesis and maintenance, respectively. *Mol. Cell. Neurosci.* 37, 794–807. doi: 10.1016/j.mcn.2008.01.005

Pardo, C. A., and Eberhart, C. G. (2007). Symposium: neurobiology of autism the neurobiology of autism. *Brain Pathol.* 17, 434–447. doi: 10.1111/j.1750-3639.2007.00102.x

Parent, J., and Lowenstein, D. (2002). Seizure-induced neurogenesis: Are more new neurons good for an adult brain? *Prog. Brain Res.* 135, 121–131. doi: 10.1016/S0079-6123(02)35012-X

Parent, J. M., and Lowenstein, D. H. (1997). Mossy fiber reorganization in the epileptic hippocampus. *Curr. Opin. Neurol.* 10, 103–109. doi: 10.1097/00019052-199704000-199704006

Parent, J. M., Yu, T. W., Leibowitz, R. T., Geschwind, D. H., Sloviter, R. S., and Lowenstein, D. H. (1997). Dentate granule cell neurogenesis is increased by seizures and contributes to aberrant network reorganization in the adult rat hippocampus. *J. Neurosci.* 17, 3727–3738. doi: 10.1523/jneurosci.17-10-03727.1997

Pasterkamp, R. J. (2012). Getting neural circuits into shape with semaphorins. *Nat. Rev. Neurosci.* 13, 605–618. doi: 10.1038/nrn3302

Poo, M. M. (2001). Neurotrophins as synaptic modulators. *Nat. Rev. Neurosci.* 2, 24–32. doi: 10.1038/35049004

Ramírez-Amaya, V., Balderas, I., Sandoval, J., Escobar, M. L., and Bermúdez-Rattoni, F. (2001). Spatial long-term memory is related to mossy fiber synaptogenesis. *J. Neurosci.* 21, 7340–7348. doi: 10.1523/jneurosci.21-18-07340.2001

Riccomagno, M. M., Hurtado, A., Wang, H., Macopson, J. G. J., Griner, E. M., Betz, A., et al. (2012). The RacGAP beta-chimaerin selectively mediates stereotyped hippocampal axonal pruning. *Cell* 149, 1594–1606. doi: 10.1016/j.cell.2012.05.018

Römer, B., Krebs, J., Overall, R. W., Fabel, K., Babu, H., Overstreet-Wadiche, L., et al. (2011). Adult hippocampal neurogenesis and plasticity in the infrapyramidal bundle of the mossy fiber projection: I. Co-regulation by activity. *Front. Neurosci.* 5:107. doi: 10.3389/fnins.2011.00107

Rosenfeld, C. S., and Ferguson, S. A. (2014). Barnes maze testing strategies with small and large rodent models. *J. Vis. Exp.* 26:e51194. doi: 10.3791/51194

Sahay, A., Molliver, M. E., Ginty, D. D., and Kolodkin, A. L. (2003). Semaphorin 3F is critical for development of limbic system circuitry and is required in neurons for selective CNS axon guidance events. *J. Neurosci.* 23, 6671–6680. doi: 10.1523/jneurosci.23-17-06671.2003

Schauwecker, P. E., and Steward, O. (1997). Genetic determinants of susceptibility to excitotoxic cell death: implications for gene targeting approaches. *Proc. Natl. Acad. Sci. U.S.A.* 94, 4103–4108. doi: 10.1073/pnas.94.8.4103

Schjetnan, A. G. P., and Escobar, M. L. (2012). In vivo BDNF modulation of hippocampal mossy fiber plasticity induced by high frequency stimulation. *Hippocampus* 22, 1–8. doi: 10.1002/hipo.20866

Schöpke, R., Wolfer, D. P., Lipp, H. -P., and Leisinger-Trigona, M. -C. (1991). Swimming navigation and structural variations of the infrapyramidal mossy fibers in the hippocampus of the mouse. *Hippocampus* 1, 315–328. doi: 10.1002/hipo.450010322

Schwegler, H., Crusio, W. E., and Brust, I. (1990). Hippocampal mossy fibers and radial-maze learning in the mouse: A correlation with spatial working memory but not with non-spatial reference memory. *Neuroscience* 109, 699–713. doi: 10.1016/0306-4522(90)90139-U

Scott, B. W., Wang, S., Burnham, W. M., De Boni, U., and Wojtowicz, J. M. (1998). Kindling-induced neurogenesis in the dentate gyrus of the rat. *Neurosci. Lett.* 248, 73–76. doi: 10.1016/S0304-3940(98)00355-353

Shahbazian, M. D., Young, J. I., Yuva-Paylor, L. A., Spencer, C. M., Antalffy, B. A., Noebels, J. L., et al. (2002). Mice with truncated MeCP2 recapitulate many Rett syndrome features and display hyperacetylation of histone H3. *Neuron* 35, 243–254. doi: 10.1016/S0896-6273(02)00768-767

Singec, I., Knoth, R., Ditter, M., Hagemeyer, C. E., Rosenbrock, H., Frotscher, M., et al. (2002). Synaptic vesicle protein synaptoporin is differently expressed by subpopulations of mouse hippocampal neurons. *J. Comp. Neurol.* 45, 103–203. doi: 10.1002/cne.10371

Smrt, R. D., Eaves-Egenes, J., Barkho, B. Z., Santistevan, N. J., Zhao, C., Aimone, J. B., et al. (2007). Mecp2 deficiency leads to delayed maturation and altered gene expression in hippocampal neurons. *Neurobiol. Dis.* 27, 77–89. doi: 10.1016/j.nbd.2007.04.005

Suto, F., Yoshida, Y., Tawarayama, H., Fujisawa, H., and Mitchell, K. J. (2010). Roles of Semaphorin-6B and Plexin-A2 in lamina-restricted projection of hippocampal mossy fibers. *J. Neurosci.* 30, 7049–7060. doi: 10.1523/jneurosci.0073-10.2010

Tamura, M., Tamura, N., Ikeda, T., Koyama, R., Ikegaya, Y., Matsuki, N., et al. (2009). Influence of brain-derived neurotrophic factor on pathfinding of dentate granule cell axons, the hippocampal mossy fibers. *Mol. Brain.* 2:2. doi: 10.1186/1756-6606-2-2

Wang, Q., Ogier, M., Wang, H., Katz, D. M., Hellard, D., Smith, C., et al. (2006). Dysregulation of brain-derived neurotrophic factor expression and neurosecretory function in Mecp2 null Mice. *J. Neurosci.* 26, 10911–10915. doi: 10.1523/jneurosci.1810-06.2006

Zafra, F., Hengerer, B., Leibrock, J., Thoenen, H., and Lindholm, D. (1990). Activity dependent regulation of BDNF and NGF mRNAs in the rat hippocampus is mediated by non-NMDA glutamate receptors. *EMBO J.* 9, 3545–3550. doi: 10.1038/SJ.BJP.0706310

Zhou, Z., Hong, E. J., Cohen, S., Zhao, W. N., Ho, H. Y., Schmidt, L., et al. (2006). Brain-specific phosphorylation of MeCP2 regulates activity-dependent bdnf transcription, dendritic growth, and spine maturation. *Neuron* 52, 255–269. doi: 10.1016/j.neuron.2006.09.037

15

Expression of Non-visual Opsins Opn3 and Opn5 in the Developing Inner Retinal Cells of Birds: Light-Responses in Müller Glial Cells

Maximiliano N. Rios[1,2†], *Natalia A. Marchese*[1,2†] *and Mario E. Guido*[1,2*]

[1] *Centro de Investigaciones en Química Biológica de Córdoba (CIQUIBIC), CONICET, Facultad de Ciencias Químicas, Universidad Nacional de Córdoba, Córdoba, Argentina,* [2] *Departamento de Química Biológica "Ranwel Caputto," Facultad de Ciencias Químicas, Universidad Nacional de Córdoba, Córdoba, Argentina*

Correspondence:
Mario E. Guido
mguido@fcq.unc.edu.ar
† These authors have contributed equally to this work

The avian retina is composed of different types of photoreceptors responsible for image and non-image forming tasks: the visual photoreceptor cells (cones and rods), the melanopsin-expressing intrinsically photoresponsive retinal ganglion cells (ipRGCs) and horizontal cells. Furthermore, the non-visual opsins Opn3 (encephalopsin/panaopsin) and Opn5 (neuropsin) have been shown to be expressed in the vertebrate inner retina, responding to blue (BL) and UV light, respectively. Here we investigated the expression and localization of Opn3 and Opn5 in the developing chick retina at different embryonic days (E) as well as in primary cultures of retinal Müller glial cells (MCs). Opn3 and Opn5 mRNAs and proteins appeared as early as E10 although traces of Opn3- and Opn5-like proteins were seen earlier by E7 in the forming RGC layer and in glial cells extending throughout the developing nuclear layer. Later on, at postnatal days 1–10 (PN1–10) a significant expression of Opn3 was observed in inner retinal cells and processes in plexiform layers, together with expression of the glial markers glutamine synthetase (GS) and the glial fibrillary acidic protein (GFAP). Opn3 and Opn5 were found to be expressed in primary MC cultures prepared at E8 and kept for 2 weeks. In addition, significant effects of BL exposure on Opn3 expression and subcellular localization were observed in MCs as BL significantly increased its levels and modified its nuclear location when compared with dark controls, through a mechanism dependent on protein synthesis. More importantly, a subpopulation of MCs responded to brief BL pulses by increasing intracellular Ca^{2+} levels; whereas light-responses were completely abolished with the retinal bleacher hydroxylamine pretreatment. Taken together, our findings show that these two opsins are expressed in inner retinal cells and MCs of the chicken retina at early developmental phases and remain expressed in the mature retina at PN days. In addition, the novel photic responses seen in MCs may suggest another important role for the glia in retinal physiology.

Keywords: retina, opsin, Müller cells, blue light, retinal ganglion cells, calcium, development

INTRODUCTION

Opsins are photosensitive pigments that bind a retinaldehyde chromophore to form a light-sensitive G protein-coupled receptor able to sense specific wavelength ranges. The vertebrate retina contains a number of different opsins responsible for the photoreception involved in visual functions such as image- and non-image forming tasks (Guido et al., 2010; Meister and Tessier-Lavigne, 2013; Diaz et al., 2016). Classical photoreceptor cells (PRCs) - cones and rods - are responsible for color (diurnal) and black and white (nocturnal) vision, respectively (Meister and Tessier-Lavigne, 2013). PRCs connect through the outer plexiform layer (OPL) to the inner nuclear layer (INL), comprising horizontal cells (HCs), bipolar and amacrine cells, and the INL cells connect with the retinal ganglion cells (RGCs) through the inner plexiform layer (IPL). RGC axons form the optic nerve and send visual information to the brain (Meister and Tessier-Lavigne, 2013). The retina contains diverse types of glial cells, the most abundant being the Müller glial cells (MCs) that extend throughout the inner retina. MCs are responsible for several important physiological activities, both during and after development, significantly contributing to homeostasis and even to more complex processes such as neuronal regeneration (Jorstad et al., 2017; Subirada et al., 2018).

In recent decades, a subpopulation of RGCs expressing the non-visual photopigment melanopsin (Opn4) (Provencio et al., 1998, 2000) was characterized as intrinsically photosensitive RGCs (ipRGCs) in the rodent retina (Hattar et al., 2002). These cells projecting to different brain areas were shown to be involved in setting the biological clock, controlling pupillary light reflexes, suppressing pineal melatonin and other activities (Berson, 2003; Guido et al., 2010; Ksendzovsky et al., 2017; Lazzerini Ospri et al., 2017). It was reported that ipRGCs are also present in chick retina (Contin et al., 2006, 2010; Diaz et al., 2014, 2017) and that they may participate in the regulation of diverse non-visual functions, as observed in blind chicks (Valdez et al., 2012, 2013, 2015). In birds, as well as in other non-mammalian vertebrates, there are two Opn4 genes, the *Xenopus* (Opn4x) and the mammalian (Opn4m) orthologs (Bellingham et al., 2006). Both proteins are expressed in RGCs of chicks very early in development at embryonic day (E) 8 (Verra et al., 2011) while Opn4x is also strongly expressed in HCs by E15 and at later stages (Verra et al., 2011; Morera et al., 2016). Opn4x confers photosensitivity on these HCs (Morera et al., 2016), likely contributing to lateral interaction with PRCs and cooperating with ipRGCs in non-visual activities.

A number of other non-visual opsins/photoisomerases have been reported to be present in the inner retina of mammals such as neuropsin (Opn5) (Tarttelin et al., 2003; Kojima et al., 2011; Nieto et al., 2011) and encephalospin/panaopsin (Opn3) (Halford et al., 2001b). Both opsins are also present in the post-hatching chick retina and brain, specifically in HCs, hypothalamus, and cerebellum (Yamashita et al., 2010; Kato et al., 2016). Furthermore, the putative photoisomerase retinal G protein-coupled receptor (RGR) was shown to be expressed in the inner retina of birds and particularly in Opn4x (+) ipRGCs to modulate retinaldehyde levels in the light, thus maintaining the balance of inner retinal retinoid pools (Diaz et al., 2017).

The goal of the current work was to investigate the onset of expression of the non-visual opsins Opn3 and Opn5 during development in the embryonic chick retina and in primary cultures of MCs. To this end, we first examined the expression of Opn3 and Opn5 at the mRNA and protein levels in whole developing retina at different embryonic (E) stages and in primary MC cultures of E8 retinas. Finally, we evaluated the effect of light exposure on Opn3 expression in retinal cells and the potential photic responses of MCs in culture by Ca^{+2} fluorescence imaging.

MATERIALS AND METHODS

Animal Handling

For the different studies performed, chicken embryos (*Gallus gallus domesticus*) (Avico) at different E and at postnatal day 1 (PN1) were used as previously described in Diaz et al. (2016). Eggs were incubated at 37°C with 60% of humid atmosphere (Yonar®Incubators). Chickens were sacrificed by decapitation. All experiments were performed in accordance with the Use of Animals in Ophthalmic and Vision Research of ARVO, approved by the local animal care committee (School of Chemistry, National University of Córdoba; Exp.15-99-39796) and CICUAL (Institutional Committee for the Care and Use of Experimental Animals).

Retinal Fixation and Sectioning

After enucleation, eyes were hemisected equatorially and the gel vitreous was removed from the posterior eyecup. Samples were fixed for 30 min at 20°C in 4% paraformaldehyde plus 3% sucrose in 0.1 M phosphate buffer, pH 7.4, as described in Diaz et al. (2016). Fixed samples were washed three times in phosphate-buffered saline (PBS; 0.05 M phosphate buffer, 195 mM NaCl, pH 7.4), cryo-protected in PBS plus 30% sucrose, soaked in embedding medium (O.C.T. Compound, Tissue-Tek) for 10 min, and freeze-mounted onto aluminium sectioning blocks. Transverse sections nominally 14 μm thick were cut consistently from the posterior pole of the eye, near the dorsal portion of the pecten, and thaw-mounted on Super-Frost glass slides (Fisher Scientific). Sections were air-dried and stored at −20°C until use.

Primary Cultures of Müller Glial Cells

Primary cultures of MCs were purified from neural chick E8 retinas dissected in ice-cold Ca^{+2}–Mg^{+2}-free Tyrode's buffer containing 25 mM glucose as previously reported (Loiola and Ventura, 2011; Lopez-Colome et al., 2012; Diaz et al., 2014, 2016; Freitas et al., 2016). Briefly, cells were treated with papain (P3125 Sigma–Aldrich) for 25 min at 37°C and deoxyribonuclease I (18047-019 Invitrogen) and rinsed with fetal bovine serum (FBS) 10% and Dulbecco's modified Eagle's medium (DMEM). After dissociation, the cells in suspension were seeded in Petri dishes and grown in DMEM supplemented with 10% FBS for at least 1 week; then, cultures were replicated using trypsin in new

Petri dishes and allowed to grow for another week in DMEM supplemented with 10% FBS at 37°C under constant 5% CO_2-air flow in a humid atmosphere.

Light Treatment in Primary Cultures of Retinal Cells

Primary cultures of MCs were pre-incubated with 9-*cis*-retinal 0.6 μM for 1 h in DMEM. Cultures were then divided into three groups: darkness control (dark), blue light (BL) stimulation (470–490 nm, peak at 480 nm) for 1 h (BL 1 h, LED of 68 μW/cm^2), and darkness condition for 1 h after the BL stimulation (1 h post-BL). In some experiments, cells were treated with 50 μg/mL cycloheximide (CHD) (Sigma–Aldrich) to inhibit protein synthesis, for 1 h before BL stimulation or at the beginning of the BL stimulus for the 1 h post-BL group. Cells were used for immunocytochemistry and protein purification.

Immunohistochemistry

Retinal sections were fixed with 4% paraformaldehyde, washed in PBS for 10 min, and permeabilized with Triton 100 0.1% for 15 min according to Diaz et al. (2016) with modifications. Samples were subsequently treated with blocking buffer [PBS supplemented with 3% bovine serum albumin (BSA) 0.1% Tween 20, and 0.1% $NaNO_3$] for 40 min and incubated overnight at 4°C with the respective antibodies as indicated in **Supplementary Table 1**. The retinal sections were rinsed three times in washing buffer (PBS with Tween 20 0.1%) and finally incubated with secondary antibodies (Jackson Dylight^{TM} 488-conjugated AffiniPure Donkey Anti-Mouse or Dylight^{TM} 549-conjugated AffiniPure Donkey Anti-Rabbit at 1:1000 dilution) for 1 h at room temperature (RT). The samples were also incubated with 4′,6-diamidino-2-phenylindole (DAPI) stain (3 μM). Coverslips were finally washed thoroughly and visualized by confocal microscopy (FV1200; Olympus, Tokyo, Japan).

Western Blot

Homogenates of chick embryonic retinas and primary MCs cultures were resuspended in RIPA buffer [50 mM Tris-HCl, pH 8.0, with 150 mM sodium chloride, 1.0% Igepal (NP-40), 0.5% sodium-deoxycholate, and 0.1% sodium dodecyl sulfate] containing protease inhibitors (Sigma–Aldrich) and processed for western blot (WB) according to Verra et al. (2011) and Nieto et al. (2011). Homogenates were resuspended in sample buffer and separated by SDS-gel electrophoresis on 12% polyacrylamide gels (50 mg total protein/lane), transferred onto Polyvinylidenefluoride (PVDF) membranes, blocked for 1 h at RT with 5% BSA in PBS, and then incubated overnight at 4°C with specific antibodies (**Supplementary Table 1**) in the incubation buffer (3% BSA, 0.1% Tween 20, 1% glycine, 0.02% sodium azide in PBS). Membranes were washed three times for 15 min each in washing buffer (0.1% Tween 20 in PBS) and incubated with the corresponding secondary antibody in the incubation buffer during 1 h at RT followed by three washes with washing buffer for 15 min each. Membranes were scanned using an Odyssey IR Imager (LI-COR Biosciences). After incubation with the specific antibodies, membranes were stripped with NaOH 1 M for 5 min and incubated in blocking buffer containing α-tubulin antibody.

Immunocytochemistry

Cultured cells were fixed for 15 min in 4% paraformaldehyde in PBS and washed in PBS, treated with blocking buffer (3% BSA, 0.1% Tween 20, 1% glycine, 0.02% sodium azide in PBS), and incubated overnight with the primary antibodies (**Supplementary Table 1**). They were then rinsed in PBS and incubated with secondary antibodies from Jackson (1:1000) for 1 h at RT. Samples were incubated with DAPI (3 μM). Coverslips were finally washed thoroughly and visualized by confocal microscopy (FV1200; Olympus, Tokyo, Japan) (Morera et al., 2012).

RNA Isolation and RT-PCR

Total RNA from whole retina and MC cultures was extracted following the method of Chomczynski and Sacchi using the TRIzol^{TM} kit for RNA isolation (Invitrogen). RNA integrity was checked and quantified by UV spectrophotometry (Epoch Microplate Spectrophotometer, Biotek). Finally, 2 μg of total RNA was treated with DNAse (Promega) to eliminate contaminating genomic DNA. cDNA was synthesized with M-MLV (Promega) using Random Primers (Promega) as previously described in Diaz et al. (2016).

The oligonucleotide sequences used for PCR from the *G. gallus* sequences were as follows:

Opn3:

Forward GCCTCTTCGGGATCGTTTCA
Reverse ATGTGATAGCCCGCCAAGAC

Opn5:

Forward GACTTAAAGCTGCGGTGCTC
Reverse TCCCAGAGTTGAAAGAATCCCAAT

TATA-binding protein (*TBP*):

Forward TGGCACACGAGTAACAAGAG
Reverse CCTTGAGCGTCAGGGAAATAG

Polymerase Chain Reaction

Initial denaturation step of 1 min at 94°C, 35 cycles of 60 s at 94°C, 50 s at 60–65°C, 90 s at 72°C, and a final 5 min elongation step at 72°C. Amplification products were separated by 2% agarose gel electrophoresis and visualized by ethidium bromide or sybersafe (Invitrogen^{TM}) staining.

Calcium Imaging by Calcium Orange AM Fluorescence Microscopy

Cells were grown in an 8-well Lab-Tek recording chamber (Nunc^{TM}, NY, United States) in a colorless DMEM (GIBCO). On the day of the experiment, MCs were incubated with 0.1% of pluronic acid F-127 and the Ca^{2+} indicator dye

Calcium Orange AM 5 μM (Invitrogen–Molecular Probes) in a colorless DMEM for 1 h at 37°C, under darkness condition. The fluorescence imaging technique was performed by using the Ca^{2+}-sensitive indicator excited at 543 nm with a laser coupled to a confocal microscope (Olympus FluoView-1000). The emitted fluorescence was captured every 2 s, using a PlanApo N 60 × Uplan SApo oil-immersion objective (NA: 1.42; Olympus). The 12 bit 4 × 4 binned fluorescence images for each photo were used to quantify fluorescence levels in the cells using ImageJ; the mean fluorescence intensity in each cell was background-corrected by subtracting the mean fluorescence of an area with no cells (only cells showing positive fluorescence pre-stimuli were considered for the analysis). The mean intensity of individual cells was measured in each captured image series. Changes in fluorescence levels were quantified as the ratio between each relative intensity level measured after a BL stimulus of 68 $\mu W/cm^2$ for 20 s (F) and the mean of intensities of serial pictures before stimulation (F_o), the same measurements were quantified in the background to correct F/F_o for each cell, as described in Morera et al. (2016). Fluorescence intensities during stimulation were not considered for the analyses and are shown as arbitrary values of $F/F_o = 1$. In some experiments, MC cultures were treated with 30 mM hydroxylamine (Taurus) for 1 h in DMEM to block the retinal binding to opsins or treated with 2 μM Ionomycin (Sigma–Aldrich) as positive control. HEK-293 cells, that do not express non-visual opsins, were used as negative controls and stimulated with a BL pulse or Ionomycin. Values of F/F_o are not linearly related to changes in $[Ca^{+2}]_i$ but are intended to provide a qualitative indication of variations in $[Ca^{+2}]_i$. No significant vehicle effects or changes in focus were detected. Responses were considered significant when the ratio at the peak differed from the baseline levels by at least 20%.

MTT Assay

Mcs enriched cultures were replicated in 96-well plates and grown for 4 days at 37°C. Cells were divided into two groups: dark and BL for 1 h. Cells in darkness were used as basal controls. After treatment, the medium was removed and replaced by 10% FBS in DMEM and cells were kept in darkness for 24 h at 37°C. Then, 10 μL of MTT reagent (5 mg/mL; Sigma) was added to each well, plates were further incubated for 2 h at 37°C as described by Wagner et al. (2018) followed by addition of 100 μL of DMSO:isopropanol (1:1, v/v) and incubation for a few minutes at RT, protected from light. Samples were analyzed at a wavelength of 570 nm with a reference at 650 nm in an Epoch Microplate Spectrophotometer.

Statistics

Statistical analyses involved a *t*-test or one-way analysis of variance (ANOVA) followed by Bonferroni *post hoc* comparison when appropriate. Otherwise, when normal distribution or homogeneity of residuals was infringed, Mann–Whitney (M–W) or Kruskal–Wallis (K–W) tests were used with pairwise comparisons performed by the Dunn's test when appropriate. In all cases significance was considered at $p < 0.05$.

RESULTS

To investigate expression of Opn3 and Opn5 in the developing retina of chickens, we evaluated their expression at different embryonic stages in the whole retina and in primary cultures of MCs at early embryonic days. BL-driven responses in MCs were assessed by WB, immunochemistry, and Ca^{+2} fluorescence imaging.

Expression of Opn3 and Opn5 in the Developing Retina

Figures 1, 2 show that Opn3 and Opn5 mRNAs (**Figure 1A**) and proteins (**Figures 1B–F, 2D**) from samples of the whole developing retina collected at different embryonic days appeared as early as E10. However, traces of Opn3- and Opn5-like proteins were also seen earlier by E7 mainly in the first-appearing cells in the RGC layer and extending throughout the developing nuclear layer (**Figures 1E,F, 2D**). A significant effect of developmental time for Opn3 expression along the embryonic stages up to PN1 was found ($p < 0.05$ by K–W test) (**Figure 1C**) whereas *post hoc* comparisons indicated that levels of Opn3 protein at PN1 differed from those at E10. By contrast, no significant differences were observed in Opn5 expression across time examined from E10 to PN1 (**Figure 1D**). Controls of antibody specificity against Opn3 and Opn5 proteins are shown in **Supplementary Figures 1, 2**, respectively.

In later stages (PN10), positive immunoreactivity for Opn3-like protein was observed in inner retinal cells and plexiform layers in close proximity to the glial marker glutamine synthetase (GS) (**Figure 2D**). As shown in **Figure 2**, the glial fibrillary acidic protein (GFAP) marker was detectable by WB in samples of the whole retina as early as E10 whereas GS was visualized at a later stage (E15 and later on); nevertheless, GS-like protein was observed as early as E7 by IHC (**Figure 2D**), when Opn3 and Opn5 were also visualized.

A significant temporal effect on GS expression along development was visualized ($p < 0.05$ by K–W test) with the highest GS levels at PN1 ($p < 0.01$) compared with those at E10 (**Figure 2B**). Also, there was a significant temporal effect for GFAP expression along the embryonic days ($p < 0.05$ by K–W test). Pairwise comparisons revealed that GFAP levels at PN1 ($p < 0.0001$) differed from those at E10 (**Figure 2C**).

Expression of Opn3 and Opn5 in Müller Glial Cell Primary Cultures. Light Effects

We next investigated expression of Opn3 and Opn5 early in development, in primary cultures highly enriched in MCs prepared at E8 and kept for 2 weeks. Glial cell cultures exhibited the typical glial morphology and expressed higher levels of the characteristic glial marker GFAP by WB [median value, in arbitrary units, 1.20 vs. 0.89 in MCs and total retina (TR) cultures, respectively, **Figure 3A**], and showed positive

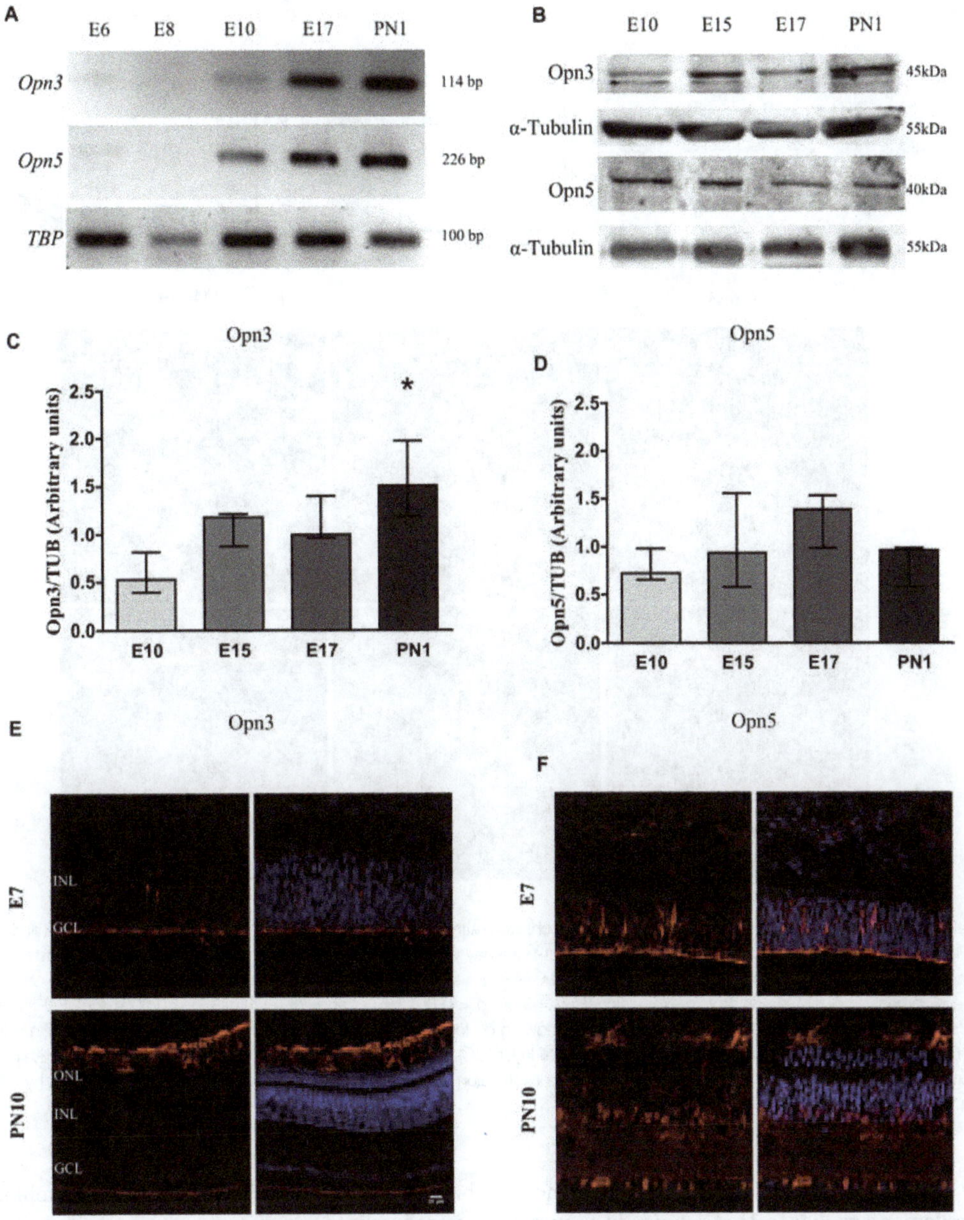

FIGURE 1 | Temporal profiles of Opn3 and Opn5 expression in the developing chicken retina. **(A)** Analysis of *Opn3* and *Opn5* mRNA expression (with *TBP* as housekeeping gene) in the whole chicken retina from embryonic day 6 (E6) to post-natal day 1 (PN1). **(B–D)** Analysis of protein expression of Opn3 and Opn5 in the whole chicken retina from E10 to PN1 by WB. **(B)** Immunoblots show two bands of ~43–45 kDa for Opn3 protein, whereas a single band was observed at ~40 kDa for Opn5 protein. **(C)** The histogram shows the median with range for Opn3 levels in the whole chicken retina from E10 to PN1. The K–W test revealed a significant effect of developmental stage [$H_{(3)} = 8.13$, *$p < 0.05$], *Values at PN1 differ from those at E10 stage (n = 3/group). **(D)** The graph shows the median with range for Opn5 levels in the whole chicken retina from E10 to PN1. The K–W test revealed no significant effect of development [$H_{(3)} = 3.97$, $p > 0.05$ (n = 3/group)]. **(E,F)** Immunohistochemical labeling of Opn3- and Opn5-like proteins, respectively, in retinal sections at E7 and PN10. Opn3- and Opn5-like proteins are stained in red and DAPI in blue. Retinal sections were visualized by confocal microscopy at 60× magnification. Scale bar = 20 μm.

immunoreactivity for the glial markers GS and Vimentin by ICC (**Figures 3B, 4C**). Double immunolabeling for Opn3- and Opn5-like proteins together with the glial marker GS was observed in MCs cultures (**Figure 3B**). It is noteworthy that both opsins exhibited a particular subcellular pattern of labeling in GS (+) MCs (merge). Immunoreactivity for the two photopigments was seen in the whole cell with some nuclear staining; similar subcellular distribution has been reported in different cell lines as described in The Human Protein Atlas[1].

In another series of experiments, MCs cultures were exposed to BL of 68 $\mu W/cm^2$ for 1 h (BL), other cultures were later returned to the dark for 1 h (1 h post-BL), and controls

[1]https://www.proteinatlas.org/ENSG00000054277-OPN3/cell#human

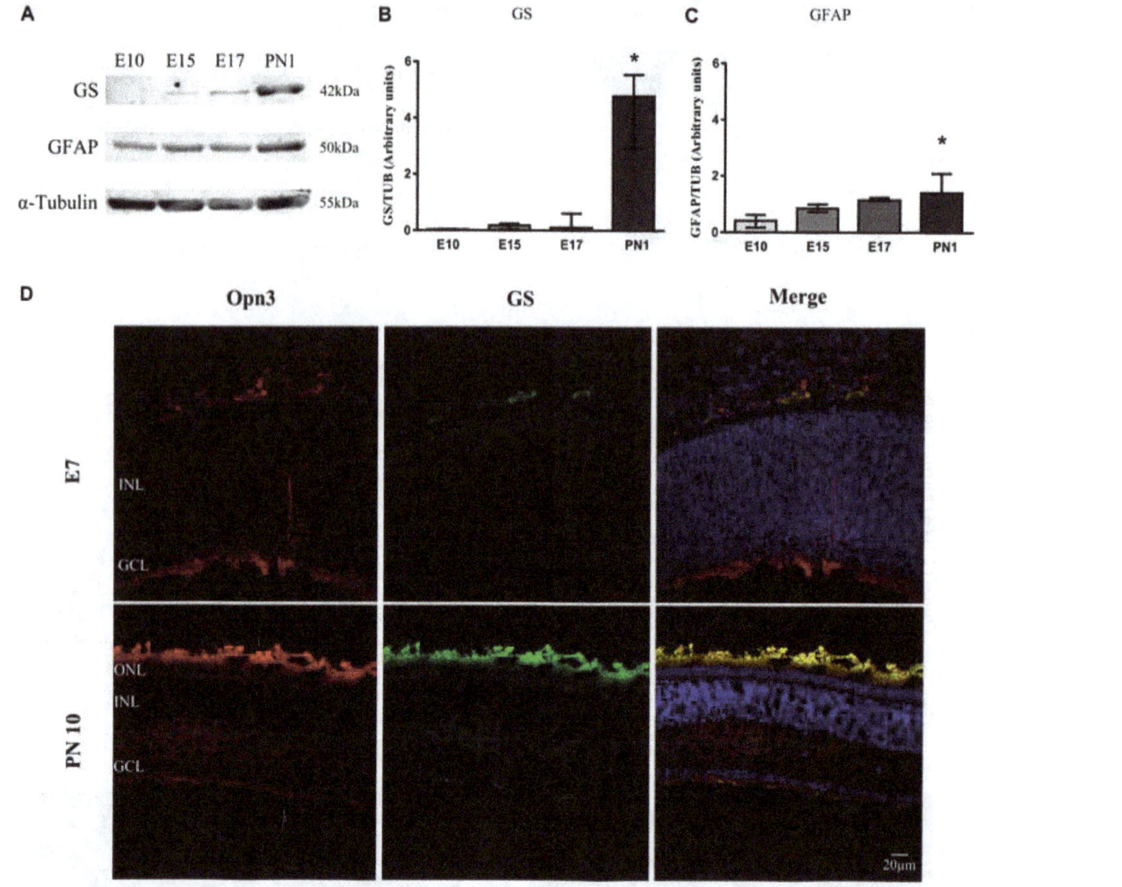

FIGURE 2 | Temporal profile of Müller glial cells markers in the developing chicken retina. **(A)** Analysis of glutamine synthetase (GS) and glial fibrillary acidic protein (GFAP) levels of whole chicken retinas from embryonic day 10 (E10) to post-natal day 1 (PN1) assessed by WB; immunoblots show bands at ~42 and 50 kDa, respectively. **(B,C)** The histograms show the median with range of GS and GFAP levels in the whole chicken retina from E10 to PN1. The K–W test revealed a significant effect of development on glial markers' protein expression [$H_{(3)} = 9.36, p < 0.001$ for GS and $H_{(3)} = 10.38, p < 0.0001$ for GFAP]. PN1 values differ from those at E10 stage (*$p < 0.05$, $n = 3$/group). **(D)** Immunohistochemistry showing co-localization of Opn3- (red) and GS-like proteins (green) in the chicken retina at E7 and PN10. At E7 Opn3-like protein is localized mainly in the ganglion cell layer (GCL) with low GS expression. In the PN10 stage, Opn3-like protein shows a more ubiquitous localization in the inner nuclear layer (INL) and an increase in the expression with GS at the GCL. Retina sections were visualized by confocal microscopy at 60× magnification. Scale bar = 20 μm.

maintained in the dark for different pharmacological treatments (**Figure 4** and **Supplementary Figure 3**). As shown in **Figure 4**, BL exposure significantly increased the levels of Opn3 protein in the MCs cultures (**Figures 4A,B**) as seen in 1 h BL or 1 h post-BL cultures compared with dark controls. The one-way ANOVA revealed a significant effect of light condition on Opn3 levels (dark, BL 1 h, and 1 h post-BL) ($p < 0.01$). *Post hoc* comparisons indicated that Opn3 levels for 1 h BL and 1 h post-BL conditions differed from controls maintained in the dark ($p < 0.05$).

In addition, BL exposure caused a notable change in the intracellular localization of this opsin as shown in **Figure 4C**. As denoted with white arrowheads and further magnified in the insets (**Figure 4C**), immunoreactivity associated to Opn3 was distributed all through the cellular body and nuclei of both dark conditions (dark control and 1 h dark post-BL) whereas for BL-treated cultures, a diminished nuclear localization and a higher immunoreactivity in processes resembling proto-end feet were visualized.

In further experiments carried out in the presence of the protein synthesis inhibitor CHD shown in **Supplementary Figure 3**, it was demonstrated that if protein synthesis is blocked, no light induction is observed in 1 h BL- or 1 h post-BL-treated cultures with similar protein levels to those found in the dark (**Supplementary Figures 3A,B**). Results strongly suggest that such mechanism depends on the *de novo* synthesis of protein. The K–W test revealed that there was no significant effect on Opn3 expression under the different light conditions examined with CHD pretreatment. In addition, **Supplementary Figure 3C** shows that Opn3 immunolabeling remained concentrated in nuclear compartments and all through the cell body in cultures treated with CHD, even after BL exposure (**Supplementary Figure 3C**) and no re-localization of Opn3-like

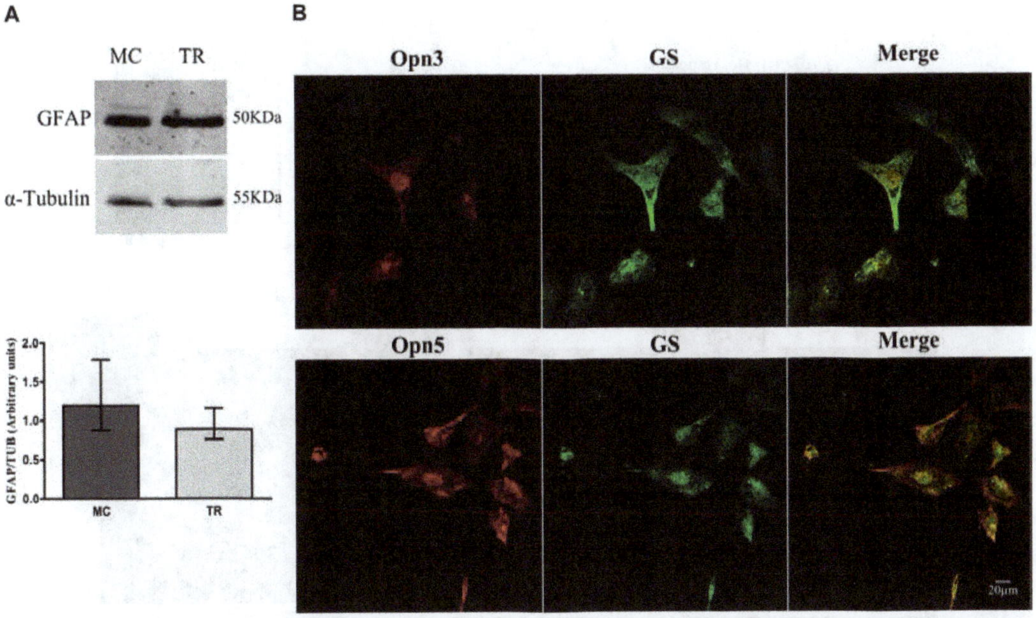

FIGURE 3 | Characterization of primary cultures of Müller glial cells. **(A)** Analysis of GFAP levels by WB in primary cultures of Müller glial cells and of total retina (TR) prepared at E8, immunoblots show bands at ~50 kDa. The histograms show the median with range for GFAP levels in primary cultures of MC and TR (n = 4/group). Primary cultures were highly enriched in Müller glial cells as defined by morphological cell identification (non-neuron-like morphology) and glial marker expression. **(B)** Primary cultures of Müller cells were labeled for Opn3- or Opn5- (red) and GS-like proteins (green) and visualized by confocal microscopy. Müller cells showed ubiquitous and generalized localization of Opn3 and Opn5. Scale bar = 20 μm.

immunofluorescence was observed in any illumination condition (dark, BL, or 1 h post-BL).

In another series of control experiments, and to discard any deleterious effect of bright BL exposure in retinal cell cultures, cell viability by MTT in dark or photic-exposed cells to BL for 1 h was assessed 24 h after the stimulus (**Supplementary Figure 4**). No significant differences were found in cell viability according to MTT absorbance of MCs cultures between dark and 1 h BL conditions.

Light Responses in Primary Müller Glial Cell Cultures

For all retinal photoreceptors characterized, a common feature found leading to intrinsic photosensitivity is related to significant changes in intracellular Ca^{2+} levels differentially causing cell hyperpolarization or depolarization, respectively (Qiu et al., 2005; Sekaran et al., 2005; Contin et al., 2010; Nieto et al., 2011; Morera et al., 2016; Diaz et al., 2017). Taking these observations into consideration, and in order to test whether primary MCs cultures expressing non-visual opsins (shown in **Figures 3, 4** and **Supplementary Figure 3**) may respond to BL, we assessed changes in intracellular Ca^{2+} levels by fluorescent imaging with calcium orange in cell cultures after photic stimulation. At first, when MCs cultures were exposed to brief light pulses of white (1000 lux), red or BL of 68 μWatt for 10 s, no responses were evoked (data not shown); however, a BL pulse of 20 s was able to promote significant increases (>20%) in relative intracellular Ca^{2+} levels in individual MCs (**Figures 5A,B**). Moreover, **Figure 5C** shows the light-evoked responses in Ca^{2+} fluorescence for the subpopulation displaying ≥20% increase responses, with the dark blue recording representing the average of all evoked responses. In this subset of glial cells, positive light responses to a 20 s BL pulse persisted for several minutes, ranging from 100 to 300 s. In addition, the Ca^{+2} ionophore ionomycin (2 μM) was used as a positive control in MCs, promoting an acute and transient peak of Ca^{+2} increase as indicated in the inset of **Figure 5C**. As shown in **Figures 5E,F**, 41.40% of cells in the culture did not respond to BL stimulation at the intensity applied (**Figure 5E**, black circles); however, 58.60% of cells left did respond according to the following distribution: 14% of cells did respond, showing a 10–20% increase in Ca^{2+} fluorescence levels over the basal threshold (**Figures 5E,F**, green squares), while another subpopulation of cells (~44.80%) responded with an increase in Ca^{2+} levels >20% (**Figures 5E,F**, blue triangles). It is known that most opsin photopigments identified used a vitamin A-derivative retinaldehyde as chromophore (Diaz et al., 2016). To further investigate the specificity of the BL responses observed in MCs cultures, in other series of control experiments, we proceeded to bleach the retinaldehyde by pretreating cultures with hydroxylamine before BL stimulation. As shown in **Figure 5D**, light-responses associated to changes in intracellular Ca^{2+} were completely abolished with the retinal bleacher hydroxylamine (30 mM) pretreatment, resulting in 87.5% of non-responding cells. Relative fluorescent Ca^{2+} levels (ΔF) analysis indicates significant different responses of the higher than 20% increase subpopulation and ionomycin stimulated group compared with

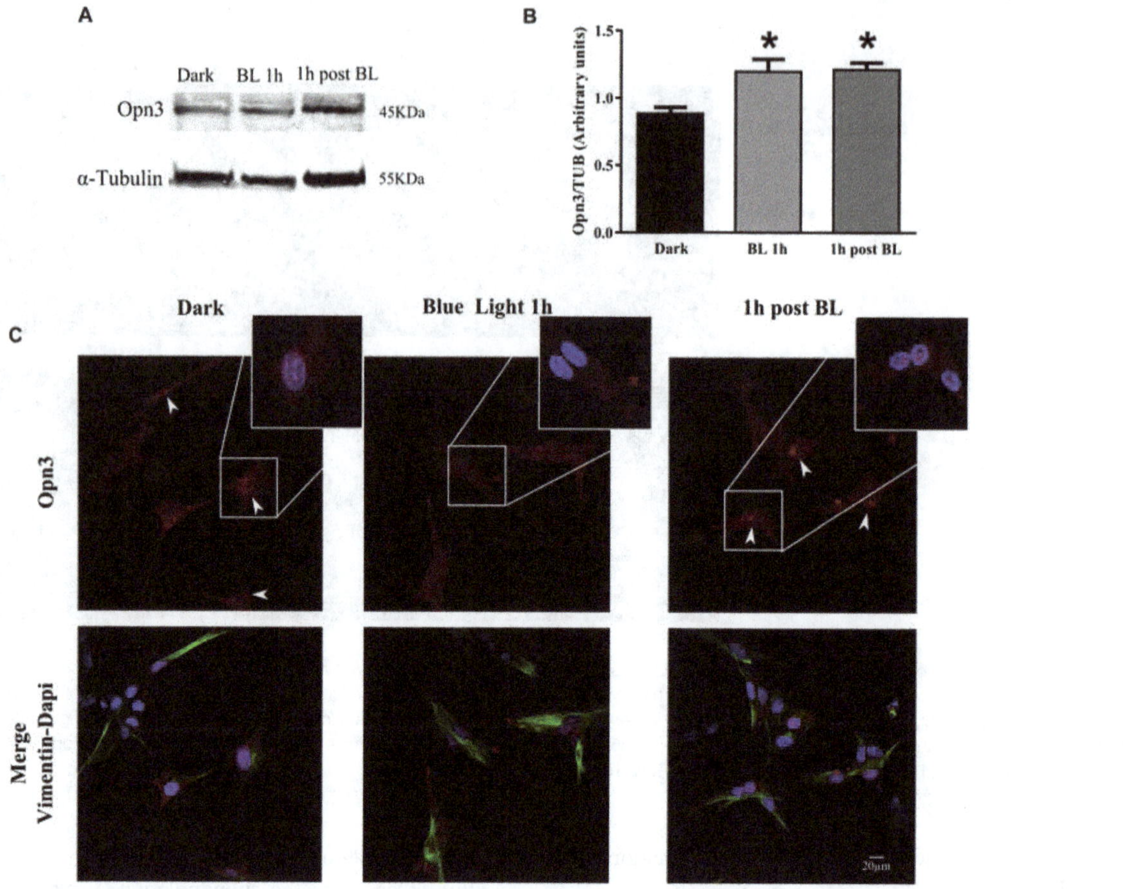

FIGURE 4 | Effect of blue light on Opn3 protein in primary cultures of Müller glial cells. **(A)** Analysis of Opn3 protein in Müller cells at different light conditions by WB. Immunoblots show two bands of ~43–45 kDa for Opn3 protein in the three experimental conditions: dark, blue light for 1 h (BL 1 h), and 1 h post-BL. **(B)** The histograms show the media ± SEM of Opn3 levels in the three illumination conditions. Increased Opn3 protein levels in Müller glial cells cultures were observed for 1 h of BL stimulation and 1 h after BL exposure over the dark control [*$p < 0.01$ by one-way ANOVA $F_{(2,9)} = 8.48$, $n = 3$–5/group]. **(C)** Localization of Opn3 immunoreactivity in Müller cell cultures by ICC for Opn3 (red), the intermedium filament marker Vimentin (green), and DAPI (blue), further magnified in the insets. Opn3-like protein was localized in inner cellular membranes with a strong labeling surrounding the nucleus in darkness and 1 h post-BL conditions, where nuclear accumulations were detected (see insets for higher magnification). By contrast, cell cultures exposed to BL for 1 h did not show substantial nuclear-like accumulation of Opn3 immunofluorescence. Scale bar = 20 μm.

fluorescence values in non-responding retinal MCs ($p < 0.0001$ by ANOVA, **Figure 5E**).

Although not all glial cells in the cultures responded to light in the experimental conditions tested, other controls were carried out to assess the specificity of the observed photic responses, by assessing Ca^{2+} fluorescence imaging in HEK-293 cells exposed to bright BL (68 $\mu W/cm^2$) (**Supplementary Figure 5**). No BL responses were found in any cell of the cultures exposed to different intensities and durations (data not shown). HEK-293 cells not expressing Opn3 and Opn5 [our results, Yamashita et al. (2010) and Sugiyama et al. (2014) were unable to respond to BL under the experimental conditions tested (light blue lines; average: dark blue) but did so in the presence of 2 μM ionomycin (orange lines, average: red) (**Supplementary Figure 5A**)]. This pharmacological treatment, known to promote the intracellular mobilization of Ca^{+2}, did elicit significant increases in the Ca^{2+} indicator fluorescence (**Supplementary Figure 5B**).

DISCUSSION

In addition to the cone and rod photopigments (Opn1 and Opn2) involved in purely visual functions relating to day/night vision and image forming processes, a wide range of non-visual opsins has been characterized in vertebrates over the last decades whose functions are not fully known (Peirson et al., 2009; Guido et al., 2010; Nagata et al., 2010; Terakita and Nagata, 2014; Leung and Montell, 2017; Dalesio et al., 2018); among these, Opn3, Opn4, and Opn5 are the most recently identified. In addition to mammals and other vertebrates (Bertolesi et al., 2014), ipRGCs expressing Opn4x and Opn4m were also shown to be present in chick retina (Contin et al., 2006, 2010; Diaz et al., 2014, 2016), appearing very early in development at E8 (Verra et al., 2011). Opn4x is also strongly expressed in HCs by E15 and at later stages (Verra et al., 2011; Morera et al., 2016), conferring photosensitivity on these HCs through a photocascade involving the Gq protein, activation

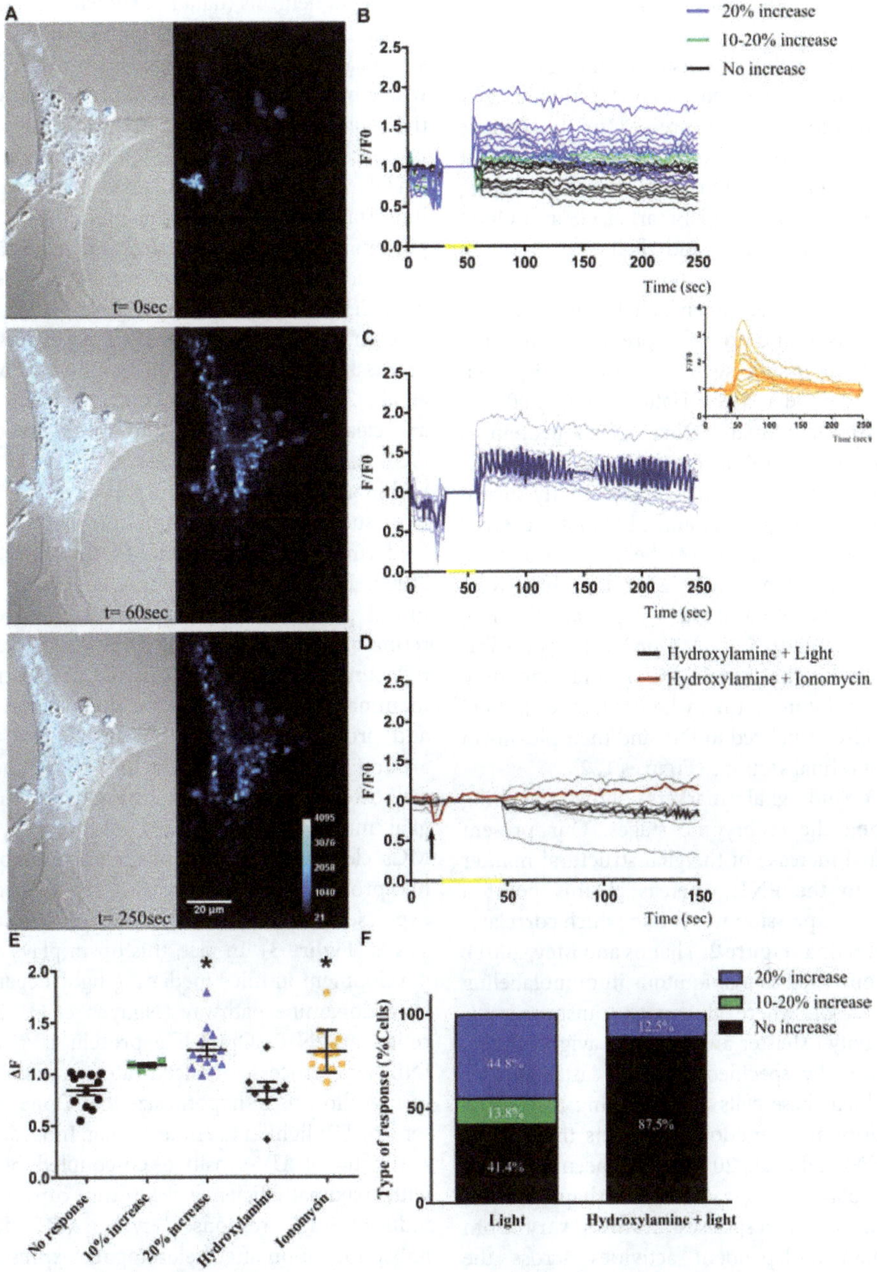

FIGURE 5 | Blue light-induced changes in intracellular Ca^{2+} levels in Müller glial cells. **(A)** Representative Müller glial cells kept in culture for 2 weeks loaded with Calcium Orange AM and displaying a significant increase in intracellular Ca^{2+} fluorescence levels after a blue light pulse (BL) of 20 s and visualized at 60 and 250 s (left panels). The Ca^{2+} response is shown in a pseudo color scale with the highest response in white (right panels). Scale bar = 20 µm. **(B)** Graphical representation showing the F/F_o ratio for different Ca^{2+} responses in Müller glial cells when exposed to a single brief BL pulse of 68 µW/cm^2 for 20 s (yellow mark). Responses are divided into: (i) cells that did not respond to BL (black lines); (ii) cells that responded with fluorescence increase between 10–20% to BL (green lines); (iii) cells that responded with an increase in fluorescence >20% to BL (blue lines). **(C)** Graphical representation of the F/F_o ratio for changes in fluorescence levels in cells that responded with 20% increase in fluorescence to the BL stimulus (yellow mark). The dark blue line represents the average response of photosensitive cells. Inset shows Müller glial cells responses to ionomycin stimulation (2 µM) (arrow). **(D)** Graphical representation indicating the F/F_o ratio for the changes in fluorescence levels in cells pre-treated with the retinal bleacher hydroxylamine (30 mM) and stimulated with BL pulse (yellow mark; gray lines) and the ionophore ionomycin (2 µM) (arrow; red line). **(E)** Graphical representation of relative fluorescent Ca^{2+} levels (ΔF) in Müller glial cells when exposed to a single brief BL pulse: black, cells that did not respond to BL; green, cells that responded with a fluorescence increase between 10 and 20% to BL; blue, cells that responded with an increase in fluorescence >20% to BL; gray, cells pre-treated with the retinal bleacher hydroxylamine (30 mM); and orange, cells stimulated with ionomycin (2 µM). The graph shows individual values with the media ± SEM. A one-way ANOVA revealed a significant effect of treatment of light or ionomycin [$F_{(4,46)} = 10.63$, $^*p < 0.0001$) compared with the no-increase in Ca^{2+} levels group (51 cells from eight independent experiments). **(F)** Graphical representation for the percentage of each type of response in Müller glial cells pre-treated or not with hydroxylamine. The Ca^{2+} increase triggered by the brief BL pulse is abolished with the retinal bleacher, suggesting an opsin-mediated response.

of phospholipase C, Ca^{2+} mobilization, and GABA release (Morera et al., 2016).

Here, we demonstrate that the non-visual opsins Opn3 and Opn5 are expressed in inner retinal cells of chick retina at early phases of development and remain expressed in the mature retina at PN1 and PN10. Moreover, our results indicate that these opsins are expressed particularly in glial cells, considering the similar expression pattern of the glial marker GS and Opn3 in the developing and mature retina and their expression in enriched MCs cultures.

Opn3 was originally designated as encephalopsin and then as panopsin, since it was found to be expressed within the retina and in extra-retinal tissues such as brain, testis, liver, and lung (Blackshaw and Snyder, 1999; Halford et al., 2001a,b; Tarttelin et al., 2003). In the human retina, Opn3 protein is expressed in the different neural layers including the GCL (Halford et al., 2001a); in the chick, it was more recently shown that two Opn3-related proteins (cOpn3 and cTMT) are present in PN retinal HCs, hypothalamus, and cerebellum (Kato et al., 2016). Here, we found that Opn3 mRNA and protein were detected in the whole chick retina at early stages around E7–10 up to PN1 and PN10 (**Figures 1, 2**). Opn3 expression was localized at first in cells of the forming GCL and extending throughout the inner developing retina; whereas later on, Opn3 immunoreactivity was also visualized in INL and their plexiform layers (IPL and OPL) of retinal sections (**Figures 1, 2**).

Remarkably, Opn3 and glial markers show matching expression curves along the embryonic stages. Our present results indicate a gradual increase of the glial structural marker GFAP expression up to the PN1; whereas at this point a substantial increase in GS expression was found which correlates with a functional visual retina (**Figure 2**; Thanos and Mey, 2001). In fact, GS at PN10 is observed as a ubiquitous immunolabeling at the ONL, IPL, and GCL where glutamate transmission is essential for retinal activity (Meister and Tessier-Lavigne, 2013). In this sense, MCs are fully specified near the last stages of development, along which these cells are becoming mature by establishing their polarity and functional domains throughout the retinal layers (MacDonald et al., 2017). It has been proposed that synaptic activity plays a crucial role in shaping these functional domains, as Ca^{+2} responses in MCs vary from acetylcholine- to glutamate-dependent activities across the developmental stages (Rosa et al., 2015; MacDonald et al., 2017). Interestingly, we observed similar distribution patterns of Opn3 and GS in the chicken strongly predicting non-visual opsin expression by MCs. In fact, this was later confirmed in primary cultures of MCs, prepared at E8 and kept for 2 weeks, showing co-expression of GS/vimentin and Opn3/Opn5 (**Figures 3, 4**).

The presence of Opn3 in extra ocular tissue has been related to the light-driven regulation of different functions (Koyanagi et al., 2013) such as wound healing responses (Castellano-Pellicena et al., 2018) and pigmentation of melanocytes (Regazzetti et al., 2018). Although the precise role of Opn3 in the developing and mature retina of birds is still unknown, it is noteworthy that levels of Opn3 protein and its intracellular localization are highly regulated by light in MCs (**Figure 4** and **Supplementary Figure 3**), neurons (data not shown), and melanocytes (Ozdeslik et al., 2019). Particularly, Opn3 protein levels in MCs were significantly induced by light exposure (1 h BL or 1 h post-BL) with a marked modification in protein pattern location, in which the immunolabeling associated to Opn3 substantially decreased in the cellular nuclei in the light condition and it was recovered 1 h later in the dark after BL exposure (**Figure 4**). In addition, it is important to remark that this mechanism of light induction and protein intracellular re-localization of Opn3 protein is dependent on *de novo* synthesis of protein as clearly observed after treatment with CHD (**Supplementary Figure 3**).

Opn5 mRNA was found to be expressed in mouse testis, brain, and eye, as well as in human retina and brain (Tarttelin et al., 2003). Whereas in the rat, Opn5 mRNA and protein are clearly expressed in the retina, specifically in INL and GCL cells and in IPL processes (Nieto et al., 2011); moreover, within the human and mice retina Opn5 is particularly seen in a subset of non-rod/non-cone retinal neurons and in the epidermal and muscle cells of the outer ears (Kojima et al., 2011). In the chicken, it was shown to be expressed in the pineal gland and in neurons of the INL and GCL of the retina of post-hatching chicks at PN14 (Yamashita et al., 2010), reflecting a similar retinal distribution in mammalian and non-mammalian retinas. Here we demonstrated that Opn5 mRNA and protein appeared very early in the developing retina at around E7–10, particularly in cells of the forming GCL and cells extending throughout the immature inner retina, resembling glial morphology (**Figure 1**). Moreover, primary cultures of MCs clearly exhibited a positive immunoreactivity for Opn5-like protein, further supporting the idea that this opsin is also expressed in retinal cells and MC cultures at early developmental stages (**Figure 3**). In fact, this opsin plays a key role during eye development in mice mediating light-dependent vascularization by a dopamine pathway (Nguyen et al., 2019). In the mature retina at PN10, Opn5-like protein is visualized in the GCL, INL, and processes concentrated at the IPL and OPL. These results allow us to hypothesize that Opn5 may play a key role in sensing UV light in the inner retina. Indeed, this opsin constitutes a functional UV-sensitive Gi-coupled bistable photopigment with maximal efficiency ~420 nm, capable of conferring light-induced Ca^{2+} responses, cyclic AMP decrease, and MAPK phosphorylation after heterologous expression in HEK-293 cells (Sugiyama et al., 2014). In birds, apart from its potential role in the retina, Opn5 is involved in the photoreception required for seasonal reproduction, presumably acting as a deep brain photoreceptor molecule (Nakane et al., 2010; Yamashita et al., 2010). In mammals, Opn5 has been reported to be directly and specifically involved in the photic synchronization of the retinal clock (Buhr et al., 2015) and more recently to be associated with photoentrainment and phase shifting to UV light (Ota et al., 2018). However, in triple knockout mice lacking essential components of phototransduction signaling for rods, cones, and ipRGCs, minimal responses were observed following UV light stimulation, suggesting a very limited role for Opn5 in driving excitatory photic responses within the mouse retina (Hughes et al., 2016).

In order to have an active opsin photopigment, the PRC requires a vitamin A derivative available to work as chromophore since it is known that for most photopigments characterized such chromophores are retinoids that can be recycled in the retina itself or in the adjacent retinal pigment epithelium (Diaz et al., 2016, 2017; Morera et al., 2016). In this connection, the putative photoisomerase RGR found to be expressed in the inner chicken retina (Bailey and Cassone, 2004) and particularly in ipRGCs early in development is likely to be used by the different opsins (Opn3, 4, and 5) for the purpose of modulating retinaldehyde levels in light and thus keeping the balance of inner retinal retinoid pools (Diaz et al., 2016). Initially identified in bovine retinal pigment epithelium (Jiang et al., 1993), RGR was subsequently found within the retina in RGCs and/or MCs (Pandey et al., 1994; Hao and Fong, 1996, 1999; Chen et al., 2001a,b; Maeda et al., 2003; Bailey and Cassone, 2004; Wenzel et al., 2005; Diaz et al., 2017). It thus appears more likely that RGR enhances the classical and ipRGC visual cycles rather than forming part of an alternative photic visual cycle (Wenzel et al., 2005; Radu et al., 2008; Diaz et al., 2017).

Retinal Müller Glial Cells as Light-Sensors: Ca^{2+} Responses Triggered by Light Stimulation

Here we show for the first time that primary cultures of embryonic MCs expressing typical markers for glia also display the expression of Opn3- and Opn5-like proteins (**Figure 3**). Similar results were observed in retinal sections having double immunolabeling for Opn3 and the glial marker GS (**Figure 2**). Additionally Opn3 levels and cellular localization are modified by BL stimulation by a mechanism dependent on protein synthesis (**Figure 4** and **Supplementary Figure 3**). The question arising from these observations is whether these opsin-expressing glial cells respond to light. One known characteristic of vertebrate photosensitivity to PRCs, ipRGCs, and Opn4x-expressing HCs is the change in intracellular Ca^{2+} levels after light exposure, differentially causing cell hyperpolarization or depolarization, respectively, in avian and mammalian retinal cells (Qiu et al., 2005; Sekaran et al., 2005; Contin et al., 2010; Nieto et al., 2011; Meister and Tessier-Lavigne, 2013; Morera et al., 2016; Diaz et al., 2017). MCs primary cultures showed distinct and specific increases in somatic Ca^{+2} responses to a brief light stimulus for at least 20 s at the blue range wavelength (~480 nm) (**Figure 5**) compared with basal values at dark conditions or cultures subject to shorter light exposure times and different wavelengths (red, white) (data not shown). Furthermore, three different subpopulations of cells were observed in the MCs primary cultures in terms of responses to BL: 41% of the population showed no response, whereas the 59% remaining displayed detectable BL responses; most of them responding with a >20% average increase in fluorescence. This latter segment of the population exhibited lasting responses to brief light pulses of at least 20 s, persisting for at least 100–300 s. In agreement with this, the photic responses involving Ca^{+2} mobilization were lost when cells were pretreated with hydroxylamine a retinaldehyde bleacher as previously shown in intrinsically photosensitive HCs strongly indicating that this phenomenon requires an active chromophore (Morera et al., 2016). Even though most cells expressed Opn3, only ~60% of them responded to light with Ca^{+2} increase, the remaining percentage may not have functional opsins in their membrane; need longer time of exposure, higher BL intensities, or might be activating a different signaling pathway, i.e., related to cyclic nucleotides as it has been previously described by Koyanagi et al. (2013). Indeed, in *ex vivo* conditions there is only a percentage of MCs that show Ca^{+2} increase in response to the neuronal activation observed after light or electric stimulation (Newman, 2005). In line with our results the human MCs line MIO-M1 was shown to express a number of different opsins and to respond to repetitive stimulation with 480 nm light (Hollborn et al., 2011). In isolated rat retina, Ca^{+2} increases in glial cells were evoked by light-induced neuronal activity, suggesting a neuron-to-glia signaling in the retina mediated by ATP release (Newman, 2005). In MCs of the adult guinea pig retina, light stimulation evoked two differential Ca^{+2} responses (Rillich et al., 2009) probably an indication that retinal light stimulation causes glial activation by alterations in both the membrane potential and ATP-mediated mechanisms. However, our results clearly show direct Ca^{+2} responses to BL stimulation by MCs in primary cultures free of other types of retinal cells. Since Opn3 responds specifically to BL in a wavelength range peaking at 480 nm whereas Opn5 has been reported to respond to UV stimulation at 380 nm in the dark, we assumed that Opn5 would not be selectively activated by the experimental conditions applied (BL in dark adapted cells) (Kojima et al., 2011; Yamashita et al., 2014). Nevertheless, we cannot discard that the edges of the action spectra for lights centered at 480 nm could stimulate Opn5 in the violet/UV range as reported. Further experiments will be required to fully understand the role of retinal glial cells under physiological conditions and photic stimulation in the context of the entire retina. In this connection, Ca^{+2} increase in MCs has been linked to ATP release (Newman, 2003), extracellular H^{+} flux (Tchernookova et al., 2018), and potentially D-serine release (Metea and Newman, 2006), to regulate retinal neurotransmission. In addition, MCs may play a role in non-visual processes regulated by light such as the setting of the biological clock as well as in optical and visual functions acting as living optic fibers or enhancers of human vision acuity (MacDonald et al., 2017). Along these lines it has recently been demonstrated that a cell-autonomous clock present in SCN astrocytes may drive circadian behavior in mammals (Brancaccio et al., 2019).

Overall, we show that the two studied non-visual opsins are present in the inner retina of chicks from very early developmental stages to PN before there is any sign of vision. Their expression was found to be present in inner retinal cells including MCs kept in culture for several days. It is therefore likely that these opsins contribute with Opn4m and x to the detection of light and thus to regulation of the diverse activities required for the adequate development of the eye and functioning of the avian retina. Moreover, we demonstrated that MCs were affected by BL stimulation in terms of Opn3 protein and its intracellular localization as previously reported for the immunoreactivity of Opn4 and Opn5 in the retina of rats exposed to continuous light of low intensity (Benedetto et al., 2017). In addition, similar results were found in primary cultures of Opn3 (+) retinal neurons of chick embryos exposed to BL and displaying marked changes in protein levels and intracellular localization (data not shown). More important, MCs expressing non-visual opsins appear to be able to sense BL in the inner retina by increasing intracellular levels of Ca^{2+}, novel events that presumably affect cell to cell interaction and glia to neuron communication, while increasing levels of Opn3 in the whole cell, thus preparing the inner retina and its circuits for the light exposure times.

AUTHOR CONTRIBUTIONS

MR, NM, and MG designed the research, and analyzed and discussed the data. MR and NM performed the research. MG contributed to the new reagents, analytic tools and wrote the manuscript.

FUNDING

This work was supported by the Agencia Nacional de Promoción Científica y Técnica (FONCyT, PICT 2013 No. 021 and PICT 2016 No. 187), the Consejo Nacional de Investigaciones Científicas y Tecnológicas de la República Argentina (CONICET) (PIP 2014), and the Secretaría de Ciencia y Tecnología de la Universidad Nacional de Córdoba (SeCyT-UNC).

REFERENCES

Bailey, M. J., and Cassone, V. M. (2004). Opsin photoisomerases in the chick retina and pineal gland: characterization, localization, and circadian regulation. *Invest. Ophthalmol. Vis. Sci.* 45, 769–775.

Bellingham, J., Chaurasia, S. S., Melyan, Z., Liu, C., Cameron, M. A., Tarttelin, E. E., et al. (2006). Evolution of melanopsin photoreceptors: discovery and characterization of a new melanopsin in nonmammalian vertebrates. *PLoS Biol.* 4:e254. doi: 10.1371/journal.pbio.0040254

Benedetto, M. M., Guido, M. E., and Contin, M. A. (2017). Non-Visual photopigments effects of constant light-emitting diode light exposure on the inner retina of wistar rats. *Front. Neurol.* 8:417. doi: 10.3389/fneur.2017.00417

Berson, D. M. (2003). Strange vision: ganglion cells as circadian photoreceptors. *Trends Neurosci.* 26, 314–320. doi: 10.1016/S0166-2236(03)00130-9

Bertolesi, G. E., Hehr, C. L., and McFarlane, S. (2014). Wiring the retinal circuits activated by light during early development. *Neural Dev.* 9:3. doi: 10.1186/1749-8104-9-3

Blackshaw, S., and Snyder, S. H. (1999). Encephalopsin: a novel mammalian extraretinal opsin discretely localized in the brain. *J. Neurosci.* 19, 3681–3690. doi: 10.1523/jneurosci.19-10-03681.1999

Brancaccio, M., Edwards, M. D., Patton, A. P., Smyllie, N. J., Chesham, J. E., Maywood, E. S., et al. (2019). Cell-autonomous clock of astrocytes drives circadian behavior in mammals. *Science* 363, 187–192. doi: 10.1126/science.aat4104

Buhr, E. D., Yue, W. W., Ren, X., Jiang, Z., Liao, H. W., Mei, X., et al. (2015). Neuropsin (OPN5)-mediated photoentrainment of local circadian oscillators in mammalian retina and cornea. *Proc. Natl. Acad. Sci. U.S.A.* 112, 13093–13098. doi: 10.1073/pnas.1516259112

Castellano-Pellicena, I., Uzunbajakava, N. E., Mignon, C., Raafs, B., Botchkarev, V. A., and Thornton, M. J. (2018). Does blue light restore human epidermal barrier function via activation of opsin during cutaneous wound healing? *Lasers Surg. Med.* 51, 370–382. doi: 10.1002/lsm.23015

Chen, P., Hao, W., Rife, L., Wang, X. P., Shen, D., Chen, J., et al. (2001a). A photic visual cycle of rhodopsin regeneration is dependent on Rgr. *Nat. Genet.* 28, 256–260. doi: 10.1038/90089

Chen, P., Lee, T. D., and Fong, H. K. (2001b). Interaction of 11-cis-retinol dehydrogenase with the chromophore of retinal g protein-coupled receptor opsin. *J. Biol. Chem.* 276, 21098–21104. doi: 10.1074/jbc.M010441200

Contin, M. A., Verra, D. M., and Guido, M. E. (2006). An invertebrate-like phototransduction cascade mediates light detection in the chicken retinal ganglion cells. *FASEB J.* 20, 2648–2650. doi: 10.1096/fj.06-6133fje

Contin, M. A., Verra, D. M., Salvador, G., Ilincheta, M., Giusto, N. M., and Guido, M. E. (2010). Light activation of the phosphoinositide cycle in intrinsically photosensitive chicken retinal ganglion cells. *Invest. Ophthalmol. Vis. Sci.* 51, 5491–5498. doi: 10.1167/iovs.10-5643

Dalesio, N. M., Barreto Ortiz, S. F., Pluznick, J. L., and Berkowitz, D. E. (2018). Olfactory, taste, and photo sensory receptors in non-sensory organs: it just makes sense. *Front. Physiol.* 9:1673. doi: 10.3389/fphys.2018.01673

Diaz, N. M., Morera, L. P., and Guido, M. E. (2016). Melanopsin and the non-visual photochemistry in the inner retina of vertebrates. *Photochem. Photobiol.* 92, 29–44. doi: 10.1111/php.12545

Diaz, N. M., Morera, L. P., Tempesti, T., and Guido, M. E. (2017). The visual cycle in the inner retina of chicken and the involvement of retinal g-protein-coupled receptor (RGR). *Mol. Neurobiol.* 54, 2507–2517. doi: 10.1007/s12035-016-9830-35

Diaz, N. M., Morera, L. P., Verra, D. M., Contin, M. A., and Guido, M. E. (2014). Early appearance of nonvisual and circadian markers in the developing inner retinal cells of chicken. *Biomed. Res. Int.* 2014:646847. doi: 10.1155/2014/646847

Freitas, H. R., Ferraz, G., Ferreira, G. C., Ribeiro-Resende, V. T., Chiarini, L. B., do Nascimento, J. L., et al. (2016). Glutathione-induced calcium shifts in chick retinal glial cells. *PLoS One* 11:e0153677. doi: 10.1371/journal.pone.0153677

Guido, M. E., Garbarino-Pico, E., Contin, M. A., Valdez, D. J., Nieto, P. S., Verra, D. M., et al. (2010). Inner retinal circadian clocks and non-visual photoreceptors: novel players in the circadian system. *Prog. Neurobiol.* 92, 484–504. doi: 10.1016/j.pneurobio.2010.08.005

Halford, S., Bellingham, J., Ocaka, L., Fox, M., Johnson, S., Foster, R. G., et al. (2001a). Assignment of panopsin (OPN3) to human chromosome band 1q43 by in situ hybridization and somatic cell hybrids. *Cytogenet. Cell Genet.* 95, 234–235. doi: 10.1159/000059351

Halford, S., Freedman, M. S., Bellingham, J., Inglis, S. L., Poopalasundaram, S., Soni, B. G., et al. (2001b). Characterization of a novel human opsin gene with wide tissue expression and identification of embedded and flanking genes on chromosome 1q43. *Genomics* 72, 203–208. doi: 10.1006/geno.2001.6469

Hao, W., and Fong, H. K. (1996). Blue and ultraviolet light-absorbing opsin from the retinal pigment epithelium. *Biochemistry* 35, 6251–6256. doi: 10.1021/bi952420k

Hao, W., and Fong, H. K. (1999). The endogenous chromophore of retinal G protein-coupled receptor opsin from the pigment epithelium. *J. Biol. Chem.* 274, 6085–6090. doi: 10.1074/jbc.274.10.6085

Hattar, S., Liao, H. W., Takao, M., Berson, D. M., and Yau, K. W. (2002). Melanopsin-containing retinal ganglion cells: architecture, projections, and intrinsic photosensitivity. *Science* 295, 1065–1070. doi: 10.1126/science.1069609

Hollborn, M., Ulbricht, E., Rillich, K., Dukic-Stefanovic, S., Wurm, A., Wagner, L., et al. (2011). The human muller cell line MIO-M1 expresses opsins. *Mol. Vis.* 17, 2738–2750.

Hughes, S., Rodgers, J., Hickey, D., Foster, R. G., Peirson, S. N., and Hankins, M. W. (2016). Characterisation of light responses in the retina of mice lacking principle components of rod, cone and melanopsin phototransduction signalling pathways. *Sci. Rep.* 6:28086. doi: 10.1038/srep28086

Jiang, M., Pandey, S., and Fong, H. K. (1993). An opsin homologue in the retina and pigment epithelium. *Invest. Ophthalmol. Vis. Sci.* 34, 3669–3678.

Jorstad, N. L., Wilken, M. S., Grimes, W. N., Wohl, S. G., VandenBosch, L. S., Yoshimatsu, T., et al. (2017). Stimulation of functional neuronal regeneration from muller glia in adult mice. *Nature* 548, 103–107. doi: 10.1038/nature23283

Kato, M., Sugiyama, T., Sakai, K., Yamashita, T., Fujita, H., Sato, K., et al. (2016). Two opsin 3-related proteins in the chicken retina and brain: a TMT-Type opsin 3 is a blue-light sensor in retinal horizontal cells, hypothalamus, and cerebellum. *PLoS One* 11:e0163925. doi: 10.1371/journal.pone.0163925

Kojima, D., Mori, S., Torii, M., Wada, A., Morishita, R., and Fukada, Y. (2011). UV-sensitive photoreceptor protein OPN5 in humans and mice. *PLoS One* 6:e26388. doi: 10.1371/journal.pone.0026388

Koyanagi, M., Takada, E., Nagata, T., Tsukamoto, H., and Terakita, A. (2013). Homologs of vertebrate Opn3 potentially serve as a light sensor in nonphotoreceptive tissue. *Proc. Natl. Acad. Sci. U.S.A.* 110, 4998–5003. doi: 10.1073/pnas.1219416110

Ksendzovsky, A., Pomeraniec, I. J., Zaghloul, K. A., Provencio, J. J., and Provencio, I. (2017). Clinical implications of the melanopsin-based non-image-forming visual system. *Neurology* 88, 1282–1290. doi: 10.1212/WNL.0000000000003761

Lazzerini Ospri, L., Prusky, G., and Hattar, S. (2017). Mood, the circadian system, and melanopsin retinal ganglion cells. *Annu. Rev. Neurosci.* 40, 539–556. doi: 10.1146/annurev-neuro-072116-31324

Leung, N. Y., and Montell, C. (2017). Unconventional roles of opsins. *Annu. Rev. Cell Dev. Biol.* 33, 241–264. doi: 10.1146/annurev-cellbio-100616-2

Loiola, E. C., and Ventura, A. L. (2011). Release of ATP from avian muller glia cells in culture. *Neurochem. Int.* 58, 414–422. doi: 10.1016/j.neuint.2010.12.019

Lopez-Colome, A., Martinez-Lozada, Z., Guillem, A. M., Lopez, E., and Ortega, A. (2012). Glutamate transporter-dependent mTOR phosphorylation in muller glia cells. *ASN Neuro.* 4:e00095. doi: 10.1042/AN20120022

MacDonald, R. B., Charlton-Perkins, M., and Harris, W. A. (2017). Mechanisms of muller glial cell morphogenesis. *Curr. Opin. Neurobiol.* 47, 31–37. doi: 10.1016/j.conb.2017.08.005

Maeda, T., Van Hooser, J. P., Driessen, C. A., Filipek, S., Janssen, J. J., and Palczewski, K. (2003). Evaluation of the role of the retinal G protein-coupled receptor (RGR) in the vertebrate retina in vivo. *J. Neurochem.* 85, 944–956. doi: 10.1046/j.1471-4159.2003.01741.x

Meister, M., and Tessier-Lavigne, M. (2013). "Low-level visual processing: the retina," in *Principles of Neural Science*, 5th Edn, eds J. H. S. Eric, R. Kandel, T. M. Jessell, S. A. Siegelbaum, and A. J. Hudspeth (New York, NY: The McGraw-Hill Companies Inc.).

Metea, M. R., and Newman, E. A. (2006). Calcium signaling in specialized glial cells. *Glia* 54, 650–655. doi: 10.1002/glia.20352

Morera, L. P., Diaz, N. M., and Guido, M. E. (2012). A novel method to prepare highly enriched primary cultures of chicken retinal horizontal cells. *Exp. Eye Res.* 101, 44–48. doi: 10.1016/j.exer.2012.05.010

Morera, L. P., Diaz, N. M., and Guido, M. E. (2016). Horizontal cells expressing melanopsin x are novel photoreceptors in the avian inner retina. *Proc. Natl. Acad. Sci. U.S.A.* 113, 13215–13220. doi: 10.1073/pnas.1608901113

Nagata, T., Koyanagi, M., and Terakita, A. (2010). "Molecular evolution and functional diversity of opsin-based photopigments," in *Photobiological Sciences Online*, eds J. Lee, and K. Smith (Osaka: Osaka City University).

Nakane, Y., Ikegami, K., Ono, H., Yamamoto, N., Yoshida, S., Hirunagi, K., et al. (2010). A mammalian neural tissue opsin (opsin 5) is a deep brain photoreceptor in birds. *Proc. Natl. Acad. Sci. U.S.A.* 107, 15264–15268. doi: 10.1073/pnas.1006393107

Newman, E. A. (2003). Glial cell inhibition of neurons by release of ATP. *J. Neurosci.* 23, 1659–1666. doi: 10.1523/jneurosci.23-05-01659.2003

Newman, E. A. (2005). Calcium increases in retinal glial cells evoked by light-induced neuronal activity. *J. Neurosci.* 25, 5502–5510. doi: 10.1523/JNEUROSCI.1354-05.2005

Nguyen, M. T., Vemaraju, S., Nayak, G., Odaka, Y., Buhr, E. D., Alonzo, N., et al. (2019). An opsin 5-dopamine pathway mediates light-dependent vascular development in the eye. *Nat. Cell Biol.* 21, 420–429. doi: 10.1038/s41556-019-0301-x

Nieto, P. S., Valdez, D. J., Acosta-Rodriguez, V. A., and Guido, M. E. (2011). Expression of novel opsins and intrinsic light responses in the mammalian retinal ganglion cell line RGC-5. presence of OPN5 in the rat retina. *PLoS One* 6:e26417. doi: 10.1371/journal.pone.0026417

Ota, W., Nakane, Y., Hattar, S., and Yoshimura, T. (2018). Impaired circadian photoentrainment in Opn5-null mice. *Science* 6, 299–305. doi: 10.1016/j.isci.2018.08.010

Ozdeslik, R. N., Olinski, L. E., Trieu, M. M., Oprian, D. D., and Oancea, E. (2019). Human nonvisual opsin 3 regulates pigmentation of epidermal melanocytes through functional interaction with melanocortin 1 receptor. *Proc. Natl. Acad. Sci. U.S.A.* 116, 11508–11517. doi: 10.1073/pnas.1902825116

Pandey, S., Blanks, J. C., Spee, C., Jiang, M., and Fong, H. K. (1994). Cytoplasmic retinal localization of an evolutionary homolog of the visual pigments. *Exp. Eye Res.* 58, 605–613. doi: 10.1006/exer.1994.1055

Peirson, S. N., Halford, S., and Foster, R. G. (2009). The evolution of irradiance detection: melanopsin and the non-visual opsins. *Philos. Trans. R. Soc. Lond. B Biol. Sci.* 364, 2849–2865. doi: 10.1098/rstb.2009.0050

Provencio, I., Jiang, G., De Grip, W. J., Hayes, W. P., and Rollag, M. D. (1998). Melanopsin: an opsin in melanophores, brain, and eye. *Proc. Natl. Acad. Sci. U.S.A.* 95, 340–345. doi: 10.1073/pnas.95.1.340

Provencio, I., Rodriguez, I. R., Jiang, G., Hayes, W. P., Moreira, E. F., and Rollag, M. D. (2000). A novel human opsin in the inner retina. *J. Neurosci.* 20, 600–605. doi: 10.1523/jneurosci.20-02-00600.2000

Qiu, X., Kumbalasiri, T., Carlson, S. M., Wong, K. Y., Krishna, V., Provencio, I., et al. (2005). Induction of photosensitivity by heterologous expression of melanopsin. *Nature* 433, 745–749. doi: 10.1038/nature03345

Radu, R. A., Hu, J., Peng, J., Bok, D., Mata, N. L., and Travis, G. H. (2008). Retinal pigment epithelium-retinal G protein receptor-opsin mediates light-dependent translocation of all-trans-retinyl esters for synthesis of visual chromophore in retinal pigment epithelial cells. *J. Biol. Chem.* 283, 19730–19738. doi: 10.1074/jbc.M801288200

Regazzetti, C., Sormani, L., Debayle, D., Bernerd, F., Tulic, M. K., De Donatis, G. M., et al. (2018). Melanocytes sense blue light and regulate pigmentation through opsin-3. *J. Invest. Dermatol.* 138, 171–178. doi: 10.1016/j.jid.2017.07.833

Rillich, K., Gentsch, J., Reichenbach, A., Bringmann, A., and Weick, M. (2009). Light stimulation evokes two different calcium responses in muller glial cells of the guinea pig retina. *Eur. J. Neurosci.* 29, 1165–1176. doi: 10.1111/j.1460-9568.2009.06682.x

Rosa, J. M., Bos, R., Sack, G. S., Fortuny, C., Agarwal, A., Bergles, D. E., et al. (2015). Neuron-glia signaling in developing retina mediated by neurotransmitter spillover. *eLife* 4:e09590. doi: 10.7554/eLife.09590

Sekaran, S., Lupi, D., Jones, S. L., Sheely, C. J., Hattar, S., Yau, K. W., et al. (2005). Melanopsin-dependent photoreception provides earliest light detection in the mammalian retina. *Curr. Biol.* 15, 1099–1107. doi: 10.1016/j.cub.2005.05.053

Subirada, P. V., Paz, M. C., Ridano, M. E., Lorenc, V. E., Vaglienti, M. V., Barcelona, P. F., et al. (2018). A journey into the retina: muller glia commanding survival and death. *Eur. J. Neurosci.* 47, 1429–1443. doi: 10.1111/ejn.13965

Sugiyama, T., Suzuki, H., and Takahashi, T. (2014). Light-induced rapid Ca(2)(+) response and MAPK phosphorylation in the cells heterologously expressing human OPN5. *Sci. Rep.* 4:5352. doi: 10.1038/srep05352

Tarttelin, E. E., Bellingham, J., Hankins, M. W., Foster, R. G., and Lucas, R. J. (2003). Neuropsin (Opn5): a novel opsin identified in mammalian neural tissue. *FEBS Lett.* 554, 410–416. doi: 10.1016/s0014-5793(03)01212-2

Tchernookova, B. K., Heer, C., Young, M., Swygart, D., Kaufman, R., Gongwer, M., et al. (2018). Activation of retinal glial (Muller) cells by extracellular ATP induces pronounced increases in extracellular H+ flux. *PLoS One* 13:e0190893. doi: 10.1371/journal.pone.0190893

Terakita, A., and Nagata, T. (2014). Functional properties of opsins and their contribution to light-sensing physiology. *Zoolog. Sci.* 31, 653–659. doi: 10.2108/zs140094

Thanos, S., and Mey, J. (2001). Development of the visual system of the chick. II. mechanisms of axonal guidance. *Brain Res. Brain Res. Rev.* 35, 205–245.

Valdez, D. J., Garbarino-Pico, E., Diaz, N. M., Silvestre, D. C., and Guido, M. E. (2012). Differential regulation of arylalkylamine N-acetyltransferase activity in chicken retinal ganglion cells by light and circadian clock. *Chronobiol. Int.* 29, 1011–1020. doi: 10.3109/07420528.2012.707160

Valdez, D. J., Nieto, P. S., Della Costa, N. S., Schurrer, C., and Guido, M. E. (2015). Circadian control of the pupillary light responses in an avian model of blindness, the GUCY1* chickens. *Invest. Ophthalmol. Vis. Sci.* 56, 730–737. doi: 10.1167/iovs.14-15481

Valdez, D. J., Nieto, P. S., Diaz, N. M., Garbarino-Pico, E., and Guido, M. E. (2013). Differential regulation of feeding rhythms through a multiple-photoreceptor system in an avian model of blindness. *FASEB J.* 27, 2702–2712. doi: 10.1096/fj.12-222885

Verra, D. M., Contin, M. A., Hicks, D., and Guido, M. E. (2011). Early onset and differential temporospatial expression of melanopsin isoforms in the developing chicken retina. *Invest. Ophthalmol. Vis. Sci.* 52, 5111–5120. doi: 10.1167/iovs.11-75301

Wagner, P. M., Sosa Alderete, L. G., Gorne, L. D., Gaveglio, V., Salvador, G., Pasquare, S., et al. (2018). Proliferative glioblastoma cancer cells exhibit persisting temporal control of metabolism and display differential temporal drug susceptibility in chemotherapy. *Mol. Neurobiol.* 56, 1276–1292. doi: 10.1007/s12035-018-1152-3

Wenzel, A., Oberhauser, V., Pugh, E. N. Jr., Lamb, T. D., Grimm, C., Samardzija, M., et al. (2005). The retinal G protein-coupled receptor (RGR) enhances isomerohydrolase activity independent of light. *J. Biol. Chem.* 280, 29874–29884. doi: 10.1074/jbc.M503603200

Yamashita, T., Ohuchi, H., Tomonari, S., Ikeda, K., Sakai, K., and Shichida, Y. (2010). Opn5 is a UV-sensitive bistable pigment that couples with Gi subtype of G protein. *Proc. Natl. Acad. Sci. U.S.A.* 107, 22084–22089. doi: 10.1073/pnas.1012498107

Yamashita, T., Ono, K., Ohuchi, H., Yumoto, A., Gotoh, H., Tomonari, S., et al. (2014). Evolution of mammalian Opn5 as a specialized UV-absorbing pigment by a single amino acid mutation. *J. Biol. Chem.* 289, 3991–4000. doi: 10.1074/jbc.M113.514075

16

The Complex Interactions Between Obesity, Metabolism and the Brain

Romina María Uranga[1,2] and Jeffrey Neil Keller[3]**

[1] Instituto de Investigaciones Bioquímicas de Bahía Blanca, Universidad Nacional del Sur-Consejo Nacional de Investigaciones Científicas y Técnicas, Bahía Blanca, Argentina, [2] Departamento de Biología, Bioquímica y Farmacia, Universidad Nacional del Sur, Bahía Blanca, Argentina, [3] Pennington Biomedical Research Center, Louisiana State University System, Baton Rouge, LA, United States

****Correspondence:***
Romina María Uranga
ruranga@inibibb-conicet.gob.ar;
ruranga@criba.edu.ar
Jeffrey Neil Keller
jeffrey.keller@pbrc.edu

Obesity is increasing at unprecedented levels globally, and the overall impact of obesity on the various organ systems of the body is only beginning to be fully appreciated. Because of the myriad of direct and indirect effects of obesity causing dysfunction of multiple tissues and organs, it is likely that there will be heterogeneity in the presentation of obesity effects in any given population. Taken together, these realities make it increasingly difficult to understand the complex interplay between obesity effects on different organs, including the brain. The focus of this review is to provide a comprehensive view of metabolic disturbances present in obesity, their direct and indirect effects on the different organ systems of the body, and to discuss the interaction of these effects in the context of brain aging and the development of neurodegenerative diseases.

Keywords: obesity, overweight, metabolic dysfunction, brain, weight loss

OBESITY

Obesity is often considered to result from excessive calorie consumption (food intake) and/or insufficient or inadequate calorie expenditure (metabolic and physical activity) (**Figure 1**). Obesity is a complex and chronic non-communicable disease that affects more than a third of the world's population (Hruby and Hu, 2015). It has been shown that obesity in middle age is able to shorten life expectancy by 4–7 years (Peeters et al., 2003). A major problem with obesity is the diverse set of health associated complications it promotes including hypertension, diabetes, increased cardiovascular risk, and cancer (Calle et al., 2003). The most commonly utilized tool used for measuring obesity today is the body mass index (BMI), defined as a person's weight in kilograms divided by his or her height in meters squared. By convention, a person with a BMI of less than 25.0 is considered non-obese or "normal," a person with a BMI between 25.0 and 29.9 is defined as overweight, and a person with a BMI of 30 or more is considered obese. A BMI of more than 40.0 deserves particular attention since it represents morbid obesity (also known as severe or extreme obesity). This index provides a reasonable estimate of body fat, and it is more accurate than skinfold measurements. However, the use of BMI has certain limitations, because it does not distinguish between lean and fat mass, nor does it indicate anything about fat distribution. In this sense, computed tomography or magnetic resonance imaging are the most accurate methods to measure the amount of visceral fat. Unfortunately, these tests are expensive and require sophisticated equipment. Waist circumference, a more straightforward but more reliable method to measure abdominal adiposity, has become an increasingly important tool for classifying obesity (Hu, 2007). Numerous studies have shown that many obesity-related risk factors depend mainly on fat body distribution rather than excess weight *per se*. Hence, it is important to take into account how body fat is distributed in an individual, for example, between subcutaneous versus visceral (or intra-abdominal) fat. It is important to note that visceral fat, but not subcutaneous fat, is more associated with metabolic syndrome, which is further discussed below.

Adipose Deposition

Adipose tissue is a complex, specialized, multicellular organ able to influence the function of almost all other organs. It is a loose connective tissue composed mostly of adipocytes, but which also contains the stromal-vascular fraction of cells (vascular endothelial cells, preadipocytes, and fibroblasts) as well as macrophages. Adipose tissue is very heterogeneous and, anatomically, consists of different fat depots with unique characteristics. This mentioned heterogeneity in adipose tissue is not only from an anatomical point of view but also from the characteristics of the tissue expansion, the regulation of lipid metabolism and also the pattern of secreted factors (collectively called "adipokines") in a particular fat depot. All these characteristics bring with them metabolic consequences that impact the whole body, including the brain. It is known that each anatomical fat depot has a particular physiological role, which implies having specific metabolic and hormonal characteristics. As aforementioned, there is strong evidence showing that some fat depots are more robustly associated with disease development and outcomes.

In mammals, adipose tissue forms *in utero* just before birth and throughout life. Moreover, the continuous generation of new adipocytes has been shown in adult humans (Spalding et al., 2008). Unfortunately, little is known about adipocyte development. However, the study of adipose stem cell biology results extremely important for understanding adipose tissue development, expansion, migration, and maintenance. Adipose tissue is classified as white adipose tissue (WAT) and brown adipose tissue (BAT). These two main classes are molecularly and functionally different. WAT serves majorly as an energy store whereas BAT dissipates energy generating heat. WAT is spread throughout the body as subcutaneous and visceral fat. Subcutaneous WAT (sWAT) is a fat layer under the skin, with major depots in the upper and lower body. The upper body subcutaneous fat consists of superficial and deep abdominal fat, extremity fat, and, in the case of females, breast fat, whereas the lower body subcutaneous fat is mainly in the gluteofemoral region (Jensen, 2008; Kwok et al., 2016). Visceral WAT (vWAT) is around vital organs within the abdominal cavity and rib cage. Its major depots are the omental, mesenteric, epicardial, and mediastinal (Kwok et al., 2016). Numerous differences between sWAT and vWAT have been reported. For example, sWAT is heterogeneous and is composed mainly of unilocular adipocytes together with small multilocular adipocytes whereas vWAT looks more uniform and is composed mainly of large unilocular adipocytes (Tchernof et al., 2006; Tchkonia et al., 2007). It is believed that while increased sWAT deposition (known as a pear-shaped fat distribution) might protect against metabolic dysfunction, the increase in vWAT (known as an apple-shaped fat distribution) might increase the risk of metabolic disease (Grauer et al., 1984; Snijder et al., 2003a,b). Indeed, vWAT has been demonstrated to expand majorly by hypertrophy of preexisting adipocytes while sWAT expands by hyperplasia, i.e., the increase of the number of progenitor cells and subsequent differentiation. It is important to highlight that bigger hypertrophic adipocytes are usually associated with metabolic dysfunction. In line with this, very important in terms of metabolic disease is the fact that vWAT adipocytes are metabolically (i.e., lipolytically) more active than sWAT adipocytes, thus releasing more free fatty acids to the bloodstream (Wajchenberg, 2000; Hajer et al., 2008). vWAT is also associated with the release of pro-inflammatory adipokines (Fontana et al., 2007) and this would explain, at least partially, why central obesity is strongly linked with metabolic complications such as type-2 diabetes mellitus and cardiovascular disease, and many others caused by elevated free fatty acids (Jensen, 2008). Indeed, this characteristic of being metabolically less active than vWAT makes of sWAT a very important source of free fatty acids during food deprivation. It is important to highlight at this point that vWAT mass but not sWAT mass correlates with the development of insulin resistance (Chowdhury et al., 1994; Wajchenberg, 2000; Hoffstedt et al., 2018). A plethora of studies argue in favor of women better distributing fat in the periphery (compared to men having more central obesity) and thus having better metabolic health (Kwok et al., 2016).

Interesting experiments with transplantation of adipose tissue have been performed in animals, and they have been very useful for assessing the different functions and metabolic properties of the different fat depots. For example, transplantation of subcutaneous fat from donor mice into visceral fat site of recipient mice has shown to confer metabolic benefits in the latter, namely decrease in body weight and total fat, improvement of insulin sensitivity, and lowering of both insulinemia and glycemia (Tran et al., 2008). Unexpectedly, intraperitoneal transplantation of visceral fat from lean mice showed to improve insulin sensitivity, suggesting that the metabolic performance of a certain fat depot is more important as a metabolic risk factor than the anatomical location or the amount of fat itself (Konrad et al., 2007; Kwok et al., 2016). On the other hand, transplantation of visceral fat or subcutaneous fat into subcutaneous fat site has not shown to cause any alterations in body weight or metabolic profile, so it seems there are both donor and recipient site-specific factors that intervene in the final outcome (Tran et al., 2008). Other experiments have shown similar results in both autologous as well as heterotransplantation of subcutaneous fat into the intraabdominal cavity of diet-induced obese animals. In both cases, transplanted adipocytes showed to diminish their size, and insulin sensitivity, as well as serum lipid profile, showed to be improved, correcting almost all the metabolic parameters altered by obesity (Foster et al., 2013; Torres-Villalobos et al., 2016). Interestingly, transplantation of brown adipose tissue to the visceral cavity has also demonstrated to prevent weight gain and improve carbohydrate metabolism in high-fat diet-induced obese animals (Townsend and Tseng, 2012). All this evidence strongly suggests that fat cells from different depots do have different characteristics and thus can play protective or detrimental roles in metabolism.

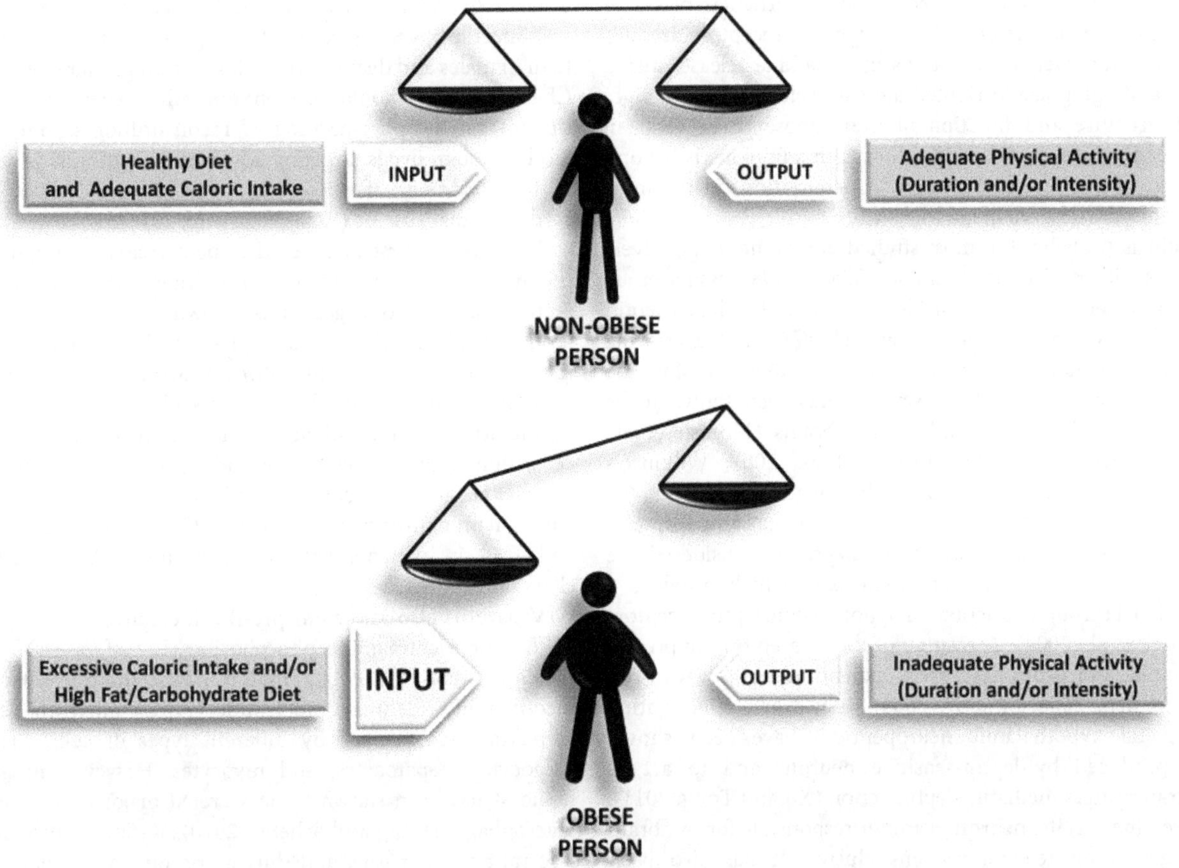

FIGURE 1 | Scheme depicting how the imbalance between the input and the output leads to obesity as a final outcome.

Obesity and Peripheral Health

Obesity is known as a chronic low-grade inflammatory disorder that results a triggering factor for many other metabolic and inflammatory disturbances. The obesity-linked inflammatory response includes many components of the classical inflammatory response, namely augmented secretion of circulating inflammatory factors, recruitment of leukocytes to inflamed tissues and organs, and activation of these leukocytes. However, the metainflammation observed in obesity has distinctive characteristics. For example, it is known that the chronic low-grade inflammation ends affecting the metabolic homeostasis in the long-term. Also, the multi-organ affection observed as the result of obesity-associated inflammation results to be unique (Lumeng and Saltiel, 2011). Adipose tissue, which was primarily thought to be a mere storage depot for triglycerides, is now considered an immune organ playing a vital role as a primary *in vivo* site of inflammation in obesity. Indeed, adipose tissue also plays a critical endocrine role due to the ever-increasing number of adipocyte-derived secretory factors that have been described.

Obesity, Adipokines, and Peripheral Inflammation

Substantial evidence supports that many of the circulating adipokines might be responsible for the peripheral inflammation observed in obese patients, including tumor necrosis factor α (TNFα), leptin, and various interleukins, among others. Importantly, the dysregulation of the adipokine secretion pattern has been linked to obesity and all the obesity-related metabolic disturbances such as cardiovascular disease, hypertension, type-2 diabetes, etc. Moreover, changes in either the amount or the quantity of the secreted adipokines are able to affect the various organ systems of the body vital for energy homeostasis. It is important to note that the weight loss-associated normalization of the adipokine secretion pattern is linked to the consequent normalization of different metabolic parameters, reinforcing the idea that adipokines are critical for the whole body metabolic homeostasis.

It is important to highlight that although secreted by adipose tissue, adipokines (except for leptin) are not solely secreted by adipocytes. Leukocytes, almost half of the non-adipocytes cell fraction in adipose tissue, are the source of classic adipokines such as IL-1, TNFα, visfatin, and resistin. Many other adipokines are produced and secreted by both adipocytes and leukocytes, such as adiponectin and IL-6. All fat depots are able to release adipose hormones, but visceral fat is considered to be the primary source of them. It has also been demonstrated that each fat depot has a particular pattern of adipokine expression (Dodson et al., 2014; Zhang et al., 2014). Interestingly, it has been shown that adipokines are also released by some particular places of the central nervous system where adipokine receptors are also expressed. Nonetheless, alterations of adipokine release during obesity and aging are attributed almost exclusively to changes in the structure and function of the adipose tissue (Kiliaan et al., 2014). A detailed description of each adipokine is beyond the scope of this review, but a few generalizations of the most important ones deserve mention.

Leptin is probably the most studied adipokine. It positively correlates with BMI (Friedman and Halaas, 1998; Lissner et al., 1999); however, obesity is considered a state of reduced leptin function. It is produced peripherally by WAT but exerts the bulk of its metabolic functions centrally, after crossing the blood brain barrier (BBB). However, it has been shown to be produced both in rodent and human brains (Morash et al., 1999; Wiesner et al., 1999; Brown et al., 2007; Wilkinson et al., 2007). It is well known that leptin action in the hypothalamus maintains body weight homeostasis in response to changes in the nutritional status. Leptin is considered the principal regulator of the "brain-gut-axis," which provides a satiety signal through its action on hypothalamic leptin receptors (Konturek et al., 2004). Activation of these receptors suppresses food intake and promotes energy expenditure pathways (Tilg and Moschen, 2006; Simerly, 2008). It is worth highlighting that several hypothalamic neuropeptides have been shown to be produced by leptin-sensitive neurons and to act as neurotransmitters mediating leptin action (Xu and Tong, 2011). However, the specific neurotransmitter responsible for midbrain leptin action on feeding remains elusive. It has also been shown that leptin is able to regulate numerous inflammatory and immune processes, including cytokine expression and cell proliferation and death (O'Rourke, 2010). Very importantly, experiments of leptin receptor restoration in the brain of mice which completely lack the receptor function have shown the normalization of the metabolic parameters (de Luca et al., 2005). Interestingly, leptin signaling has also been suggested to be one of the circulating factors connecting obesity and the consequent reproductive dysfunction, being the reproduction defects reverted by pharmacological administration of leptin (Tong and Xu, 2012).

Adiponectin is an adipokine with insulin-sensitizing and anti-inflammatory effects produced exclusively by adipose tissue and suggested to be a visceral adiposity marker, due to the fact that several studies in humans have shown that visceral adipocytes secret more adiponectin than subcutaneous adipocytes (Lenchik et al., 2003; Ryan et al., 2003; Matsuzawa, 2007; Drolet et al., 2009). It exists as trimers, hexamers, and high-molecular-weight (HMW) multimeric complexes (Rutkowski and Scherer, 2014). Recent data indicate that the HMW complexes have predominant action in metabolic tissues (Achari and Jain, 2017). Unlike the majority of adipokines, adiponectin plasma levels correlate inversely with obesity, insulin resistance, and type-2 diabetes mellitus (Hotta et al., 2001; Kondo et al., 2002; Deng and Scherer, 2010). However, the decreased level of adiponectin in obesity is not clear yet. Physiological functions of adiponectin in the brain have been related majorly to food intake, energy expenditure, lipid and glucose metabolism, and body weight control (Kubota et al., 2007; Wen et al., 2010; Park et al., 2011). Interestingly, adiponectin physiological levels are generally higher in females than in males and decrease in both sexes as age increases (Ng and Chan, 2017). It should be mentioned that several studies have shown that the pharmacological reconstitution of adiponectin levels through drugs targeting adiponectin synthesis would help in the treatment of obesity and the associated diabetes and cardiovascular disease (Achari and Jain, 2017).

Resistin was first discovered to be secreted by adipocytes in rodents. However, in humans, it is predominantly expressed and secreted by macrophages. It is known that increased resistin levels are linked to the development of insulin resistance, diabetes mellitus, and cardiovascular disease. Moreover, resistin would promote endothelial dysfunction, vascular smooth muscle cell proliferation, arterial inflammation, and the generation of foam cells, thus contributing to the pathogenesis of atherosclerosis (Park et al., 2017). Circulating levels of resistin correlate directly with inflammatory markers such as C-reactive protein, TNFα, and IL-6 in patients with different metabolic disturbances (Park and Ahima, 2013).

Visfatin is also known as pre-B cell colony-enhancing factor (PBEF) or nicotinamide phosphoribosyltransferase (NAMPT), the latter due to the fact that it is the limiting enzyme in nicotinamide adenine dinucleotide (NAD) biosynthesis. This adipokine is expressed by different types of cells, including adipocytes, hepatocytes, and myocytes. However, in adipose tissue, it has been shown to be secreted majorly by infiltrating macrophages (Deng and Scherer, 2010). Visfatin is produced by visceral adipose tissue, and thus its production is increased in abdominal obesity. Interestingly, visfatin has been demonstrated to bind to insulin receptor and mimic insulin hypoglycemic effects, i.e., decreasing glucose release from the liver and increasing glucose uptake and utilization by peripheral tissues (Singla et al., 2010).

Apelin has been relatively recently classified as an adipokine since although it is produced and secreted by adipocytes, it is also expressed (together with its receptor) in the central nervous system and the cardiovascular system. Apelin has been related to the regulation of blood pressure, food intake, cell proliferation, and angiogenesis (Castan-Laurell et al., 2011). *In vitro* as well as *in vivo* studies have shown a strong relationship between apelin and insulin (Boucher et al., 2005). Moreover, apelin has been suggested to be the last protection before the appearance of obesity-associated metabolic disorders such as insulin resistance, type-2 diabetes, or cardiovascular disease (Castan-Laurell et al., 2005).

IL-6 is a pro-inflammatory cytokine synthesized and secreted by several cell types, including adipocytes and immune cells. Not only does IL-6 participate in inflammatory responses but it also controls feeding behavior at a hypothalamic level (Stenlöf et al., 2003). IL-6 circulating levels have been systematically reported to be augmented in obesity, being visceral fat secretion an important source of IL-6 thus linking the enlarged visceral fat with the existence of systemic inflammation in obese patients (Fontana et al., 2007). Importantly, IL-6 levels have been reported to normalize in morbidly obese patients who underwent bariatric surgery (Illán-Gómez et al., 2012).

TNFα is an inflammatory adipokine whose levels are increased in adipose tissue and plasma of both obese rodents and humans (O'Rourke, 2010). It was the first inflammatory adipokine associated with the onset and progression of insulin resistance (Hotamisligil and Spiegelman, 1994). It was first thought to be secreted by adipocytes, but today it is accepted that the bulk of TNFα is secreted by adipose tissue-resident macrophages. It has been shown that high levels of TNFα and IL-6 suppress the transcription of adiponectin thus connecting the role of visceral fat accumulation in adiponectin decreased secretion in obesity (Suganami et al., 2005).

In summary, adipose tissue, as an immune and endocrine organ, produces a wide variety of soluble factors collectively called adipokines. These molecules were initially associated uniquely to metabolic activities, but today it is known that they regulate numerous physiological and physiopathological events. Adipokines have pro- and anti-inflammatory properties and are considered fundamental circulating factors mediating the cross-talk between different organs and metabolic systems, thus integrating the systemic metabolism with immunity.

Before leaving the topic of adipokines, it is important to note that while adipokines have been primarily studied in terms of their links to adipose tissue, it is well established that non-adipose tissues produce and release adipokines. For example, muscle is known to produce and release several cytokines which are also produced and released by adipose tissue (Trayhurn et al., 2011; Görgens et al., 2015; Leal et al., 2018). Similarly, the liver is known to be an organ that is very much involved in the contribution of overall circulating adipokine levels. For example, leptin, adiponectin, and resistin have been shown to be locally produced by the liver (Marra et al., 2005). It is therefore important to understand that even circulating adipokine levels, in obese and non-obese individuals, is the result of the shared contributions of adipokine production from multiple tissues.

Obesity and Peripheral Metabolic Changes

As mentioned, the obesity-associated increase in the adipose tissue mass is linked to a change in the adipokine secretion pattern, thus causing what is known as "metainflammation," which affects systemic metabolism. A common consequence of obesity is metabolic syndrome, a condition which is associated with pro-inflammatory states and which is considered to be a compilation of risk factors that predispose individuals to the development of cardiovascular disease and type-2 diabetes. The diagnosis of metabolic syndrome is made when any 3 of the 5 following risk factors are present: central obesity (enlarged waist circumference, defined according population-specific and country-specific criteria), high blood pressure (defined as systolic blood pressure $\geq$ 130 mm Hg or diastolic blood pressure $\geq$ 85 mm Hg), loss of glycemic control (elevated fasting glucose, defined as blood glucose > 100 mg/dl), low serum high-density lipoprotein (HDL) (defined as < 40 mg/dl in men and <50 mg/dl in women), and high serum triglycerides (defined as $\geq$ 150 mg/dl) (Lam and LeRoith, 2000). The existence of metabolic syndrome is well known to predispose an individual to diabetes and cardiovascular disease. It is important to know that metabolic syndrome also predisposes individuals to a number of other severe conditions including non-alcoholic fatty liver disease, non-alcoholic steatohepatitis, obstructive sleep apnea, and cancer, among others. Indeed, hyperleptinemia, hypoadiponectinemia, and insulin resistance are also widely linked to features of the metabolic syndrome.

Insulin resistance and type-2 diabetes mellitus are typical metabolic changes observed in obese patients. Insulin resistance implies impaired insulin-induced glucose uptake and metabolism in adipocytes and skeletal muscle, and impaired suppression of hepatic glucose production (Reaven, 1995). Insulin resistance is a key etiologic factor of type-2 diabetes but is also associated with a plethora of other pathophysiologic disorders including hypertension, hyperlipidemia, and atherosclerosis. Although several hypotheses about factors influencing insulin resistance coexist (including inflammation, mitochondrial dysfunction, hyperinsulinemia, lipotoxicity, oxidative stress, and endoplasmic reticulum stress), there is no consensus about a unifying mechanism for insulin resistance etiology (Ye, 2013). It is generally accepted that insulin resistance occurs first, with hyperinsulinemia as a pancreatic compensatory response, and after pancreatic failure to meet metabolic demands, hyperglycemia with hypoinsulinemia occurs. Importantly, central obesity precedes the development of insulin resistance, thus reinforcing the idea of visceral fat and its pro-inflammatory adipokines playing a key role in the pathophysiology of insulin resistance.

It is worth mentioning that although obesity is commonly associated with different metabolic abnormalities, 2–50% of obese adults are "metabolically healthy or metabolically normal" (the wide range is due to different criteria in the classification and also to the population studied) (Tiemann Luecking et al., 2015). The concept of "metabolically healthy obese" refers to obese people with normal metabolic risk profile (Karelis et al., 2005; Stefan et al., 2008). However, studies have previously shown that "metabolically healthy obese" individuals do have increased cardiovascular risk (Ärnloöv et al., 2010).

Effect of weight loss on metabolic endpoints of obesity

Reducing the amount of total body fat has been thought of as a strategy to diminish the impact of obesity and comorbidities on health. Weight loss interventions such as low-fat diets have been demonstrated to reduce many of the risk factors associated with obesity (Lee et al., 2011), as well as decrease all-cause mortality in obese adults. It is important to note that each reference to weight loss in this review is "intentional weight loss" and not involuntary weight loss. It is important to note that intentional weight reducing diets are routinely shown to be more effective in reducing blood pressure and improving dyslipidemia when combined with exercise (Schwingshackl et al., 2014). Interestingly, low-carbohydrate diets have been found to be more effective for reducing body weight than low-fat diets (Tobias et al., 2015). However, evidence supported by randomized controlled trials shows that most adults are unable to maintain weight loss (Wing and Phelan, 2005; Wadden et al., 2011; Ross et al., 2012). From this perspective, alternative approaches to diet-induced weight loss are needed, including the establishment of healthy eating and physical activity habits that may be more sustained over time. Bariatric surgery, also known as metabolic surgery, is associated with sustained weight loss, decreased cardiovascular risk factors and events, diminution in diabetes-linked microvascular complications, and improvement of obesity-associated comorbidities and overall survival (Christou et al., 2004; Sjöström et al., 2007; Sowemimo et al., 2007; Buchwald et al., 2009; Cummings and Rubino, 2018). Moreover, bariatric surgery has been shown to be superior to other weight loss-associated interventions in normalizing almost all the metabolic endpoints. However, studies with longer follow-up time (>5 years) are still needed, including studies that identify any potential long-term adverse effects following bariatric surgery (Busetto, 2014; Cummings and Rubino, 2018). Liposuction, which is mainly thought to remove subcutaneous fat without affecting visceral abdominal fat depot, is another common weight loss procedure. However, there is controversy about the impact of liposuction on obesity endpoints like insulin sensitivity. This controversy may be due in part to the fact that lipectomy of sWAT has been linked to the enlargement of vWAT (Benatti et al., 2012).

The complexity of weight loss in the elderly. As mentioned, there is a strong obesity-mortality association during adulthood. However, this association diminishes with age, and weight loss in older adults is not as beneficial as one might expect. Surprisingly, unintentional weight loss (more than 5% of body weight reduction in a year) in older adults is associated with increased morbidity and mortality (Gaddey and Holder, 2014). Although cachexia, i.e., the loss of muscle mass with or without fat loss, is thought to be the main responsible for these negative effects, the pathophysiology of unintentional weight loss remains unclear. It is well known that body composition changes with age, with fat mass gains until 65–70 years old, a characteristic peak in body weight around 60 years old, and gradual small decreases thereafter (Wallace and Schwartz, 2002). The ideal BMI in the elderly is considered (from a mortality point of view) to be of 25–30. At this point, it is worth to have in mind that although BMI in younger adults correlates quite well with total body fat, it does not in older adults and this might be an appropriate explication for the so-called "obesity paradox," according to which obese old individuals have lower mortality than lean. The main reason is that not only there is a continuous loss of body muscle with age (without loss in body fat), but also the height is reduced due to spine-shortening as a consequence of age-related bone disease. In this sense, as mentioned before, waist circumference is a better index of adiposity, mainly because it correlates with abdominal body fat, which is the main contributor to metabolic disorders. Moreover, inactivity in older adults is usually accompanied by a loss in body muscle mass, a condition which may go unnoticed but which brings several functional consequences in the long-term period. This condition is known as sarcopenic obesity, and together with degenerative joint disease, it leads to the incapability to perform activities of daily living. Thus the impairment in daily function finally causes the development of frailty phenotype (which is generally present in the elderly but is greatly increased with obesity) with disability as a final outcome (Han et al., 2011).

Many observational studies have linked weight loss with increased risk of mortality (Yaari and Goldbourt, 1998; Knudtson et al., 2005; Sørensen et al., 2005; Shea et al., 2011). There are several causes of unintentional weight loss in the elderly (Gaddey and Holder, 2014). Only intentional weight loss in older people seems to lead to some clinical benefits, mainly due to the fact that unintentional weight loss is often associated with underlying subclinical illnesses. However, since intentional weight loss is linked to muscle mass loss and decreased bone mass (Waters et al., 2013), it appears that diet-induced weight loss should be accompanied by a program of physical activity which can potentially inhibit the muscle and bone loss associated with diet-induced weight loss (Shea et al., 2011). Lifestyle interventions that include diet plus exercise components have been shown to lead to a 10% weight loss with changes in physical function and metabolism (Waters et al., 2013). However, the clinical significance of these observations as well as long-term consequences of weight loss remains unclear.

Obesity and Peripheral Lipid Changes

Dyslipidemia is very common in obesity, reaching almost 70% of obese patients. The lipid abnormalities usually observed in obese patients are high levels of serum triglycerides, free fatty acids, very low-density lipoproteins (VLDL), Apo B, and non-HDL cholesterol (Franssen et al., 2011; Bays et al., 2013). HDL-cholesterol levels are typically found to be low together with HDL dysfunction. Regarding LDL-cholesterol, although in the normal range, the size of LDL particles is unbalanced, with more small pro-atherogenic LDL particles rather than large ones. Lipid changes in obesity have been shown to be strongly dependent on body fat distribution. For example, visceral adipose tissue and upper body subcutaneous adipose tissue have been related to high triglyceride and HDL cholesterol levels and insulin resistance, whereas lower body subcutaneous adipose tissue has been related to a healthier lipid profile (Feingold and Grunfeld, 2018).

All these obesity-related lipid abnormalities are frequent observations in metabolic syndrome and typically associated with the pro-inflammatory state described before. An important link between obesity, metabolic syndrome, and dyslipidemia appears to be insulin resistance in peripheral tissues. It has been shown that the increase in circulating free fatty acids associated with obesity contributes to several metabolic disturbances being insulin resistance probably the most important (Karpe et al., 2011). It is important to highlight, however, that the increase in free fatty acids is not only a consequence of insulin resistance but also contributes to its development (Lam and LeRoith, 2000). There are several reasons for increased free fatty acids in obesity: (1) enlarged adipose tissue resistant to the antilipolytic effect of insulin; (2) increased liver fatty acid *de novo* synthesis (Jacome-Sosa and Parks, 2014; Björnson et al., 2016; Xiao et al., 2016); (3) increased uptake of triglyceride-rich lipoproteins by the liver (Yu and Ginsberg, 2005; Dash et al., 2015; Björnson et al., 2016; Xiao et al., 2016). This increased free fatty acid flux finally exceeds adipose tissue lipid storage capacity, and free fatty acids begin to accumulate in the liver, pancreas, skeletal muscle, and heart, a condition known as "ectopic lipid deposition" which has several pathologic consequences. Lipids result cytotoxic to cells other than adipocytes. For example, lipid deposition in the pancreas has been involved in the development of diabetes whereas lipid deposition in the skeletal muscle has been associated with insulin resistance. Moreover, lipid accumulation in the liver defines steatosis. The hypothesis of adipose tissue protecting against ectopic accumulation of lipids (working as a metabolic sink) has been supported by observations in animals and humans with lipodystrophy, where the absence of adipose tissue is associated with generalized lipid ectopic deposition and insulin resistance (O'Rourke, 2010).

Effect of weight loss on peripheral lipids

The effect of weight loss on peripheral lipid profile has been extensively assessed. Serum fasting and non-fasting triglyceride levels have been demonstrated to be reduced by weight loss (Chan et al., 2002; James et al., 2003). On average, a 3-kg weight loss represents a reduction of 15 mg/dl in triglyceride levels. Indeed, LDL levels are also usually decreased by weight loss, and HDL levels are usually increased: a 5- to 8-kg weight loss is associated with a decrease of 5 mg/dl in LDL and an increase of 2–3 mg/dl of HDL (Ebbert et al., 2014). However, considerable variability in the results has been observed, and the improvement of dyslipidemia is not always the final outcome. On the other hand, the type of weight-loss diet followed does impact on lipid profiles. It is still unclear which factors associated with weight loss are predictive of the change in lipid profile. Several studies have shown a poor correlation between lipid profile improvement and the degree of weight loss, and a threshold effect has been suggested when the lipid profile resulted improved with a minimal weight loss but when no further effects were observed with a larger weight loss (Kelly and Jones, 1986; Busetto et al., 2000).

Interestingly, metabolic surgery impacts positively on serum lipid levels as a consequence of weight loss. Normalization of serum lipid profile is a common observation after gastric bypass surgery. In a meta-analysis of 11 randomized clinical trials comparing surgical versus non-surgical treatment of morbid obesity, bariatric surgery was found to be associated with more significant weight loss, remission of metabolic syndrome, and improvement in lipid profiles with the consequent decrease in medication requirements (Gloy et al., 2013; Koliaki et al., 2017). A 5-year follow-up study compared patients who received medical therapy alone with patients who underwent surgical therapy. Surgical patients were found to achieve the greatest health benefits, with a more significant reduction in triglyceride levels and a more considerable increase in HDL with respect to patients who received medical treatment alone (Schauer et al., 2017). It is worth mentioning that the beneficial effects of bariatric surgery have been analyzed in the short-term period and up to 5 years after the intervention; however, the long-term effects remain elusive.

EFFECTS OF OBESITY-ASSOCIATED FAT DEPOSITION AND CIRCULATING FACTORS ON THE VARIOUS NON-CNS ORGANS OF THE BODY

Although the cause of obesity is mainly attributed to energy imbalance, the etiology of obesity is multifactorial, including genetic, psychological, economic, environmental, social, and physiological factors, only to cite some (Wright and Aronne, 2012). Whatever etiopathogenesis of obesity is considered, several organs are damaged as a consequence of the development of obesity, including the pancreas, liver, muscle, and the cardiovascular system. A brief outline of how ectopic fat deposition and the concomitant obesity-related circulating factors contribute to disease of each organ is provided (**Figure 2**).

Pancreas

The ectopic fat accumulation in the pancreatic gland is usually referred to as pancreatic steatosis. Intra- and interlobular adipocytes, acinar cell fat, as well as islet fat content have been found to be augmented in obesity (Pinnick et al., 2008; Lee et al., 2010). A close relationship between insulin resistance and pancreatic steatosis has been described. As it is known, pancreatic β-cells usually produce and release insulin to control glucose homeostasis. Under the condition of insulin resistance, pancreatic β-cells increase the production and release of insulin to maintain the normal glycemia. However, patients predisposed to type-2 diabetes fail to secrete enough insulin to meet the metabolic demand (due to insulin resistance in several tissues) and type-2 diabetes occurs (Poitout, 2004). Different stages in the development of type-2 diabetes have been well characterized. In the first stage, there is insulin hypersecretion, which allows for normal glycemic control. In contrast, during the second stage of type-2 diabetes, there is a failure of β-cells to secrete sufficient insulin for glycemic control, and thus hyperglycemia is manifest. However, it is a matter of debate whether dysfunction precedes or follows the loss of β-cells in obesity-linked diabetes mellitus (Alarcon et al., 2016). Whatever the origin of obesity-associated diabetes, there is a failure in insulin production and/or the secretory capacity of β-cells. Interestingly, *in vitro* studies have shown that β-cells have an exceptional capacity to synthesize significant amounts of insulin even in obesity-like conditions, and that this insulin is readily available for secretion. It is believed that fat accumulation in the pancreatic islets would be responsible for, at least in part, the decreased insulin secretion of the second stage of type-2 diabetes, since ectopic fat deposits in the pancreas have been reported to cause β-cell dysfunction, both directly through lipotoxicity exerted by free fatty acids and indirectly through activation of inflammatory pathways (Le et al., 2011; Pezzilli and Calculli, 2014). Moreover, evidence suggests that lipid toxicity to pancreatic β-cells is a long-term process and it takes around a decade before diabetes is diagnosed (Oakes et al., 1997). On the other hand, studies performed in morbidly obese humans have shown that obesity and peripheral insulin resistance are also associated with substantial changes in pancreatic metabolism and pancreatic blood flow, together

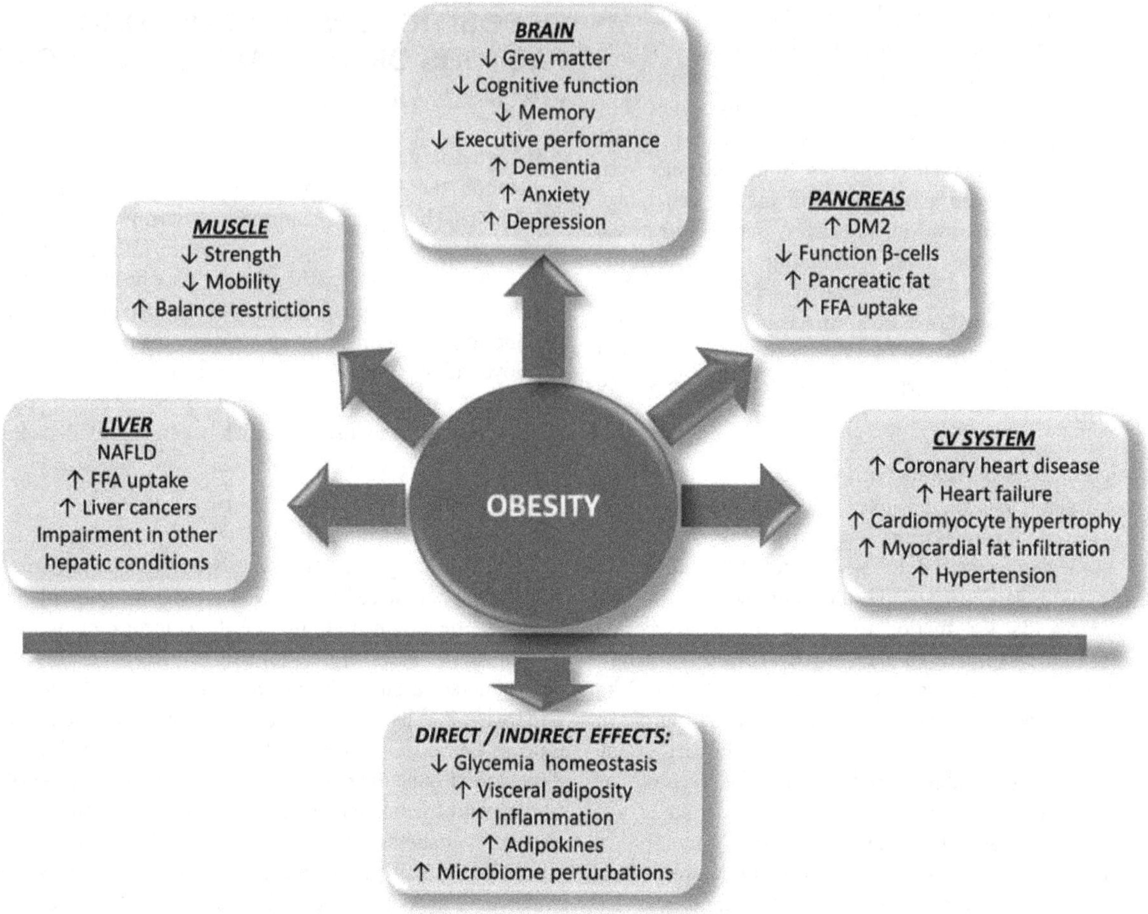

FIGURE 2 | Scheme showing the predicted impact of obesity on organ systems and the direct and indirect effects on health.

with β-cell dysfunction. Interestingly, as a consequence of insulin resistance in adipose tissue, increased free fatty acids have been shown to be delivered from the bloodstream in morbidly obese individuals, and these people clearly show a shift in the preferred pancreatic energy substrate, with lipid usage being predominant over glucose usage (Honka et al., 2014). The possibility of these observations (pancreatic metabolic shift and defect in blood flow) to be reverted by weight loss is still unclear.

In addition, the changes in circulating adipokines constitute an important link between the excessive adiposity in obesity, insulin resistance, and β-cell failure, mainly due to the fact that several adipokines have demonstrated to affect both the function and survival of β-cells thus deteriorating the function of the pancreas and contributing to acute and chronic pancreatitis as well as pancreatic cancer (Zhao et al., 2006; Gumbs, 2008). Leptin, adiponectin, resistin, and visfatin are the most important adipokines that would participate in the pathogenesis of pancreatic diseases (Biernacka and Małecka-Panas, 2015). Beyond the previously mentioned physiological roles of leptin, this adipokine has also been shown to reduce insulin secretion. It has also been demonstrated to regulate the inflammatory response, thus protecting the pancreas from some kinds of damage by reducing TNFα and increasing IL-4 production (Jaworek et al., 2002). Indeed, adiponectin has been shown to play anti-diabetic and anti-inflammatory roles. Regarding the role of adipokines and pancreatic disease, it is thought that the higher risk of acute pancreatitis in obese people would come from the increased adipokine-producer visceral fat in the surroundings of the pancreas (Biernacka and Małecka-Panas, 2015). However, the precise role of adipokines in acute and chronic pancreatitis, as well as in pancreatic cancer, is unclear yet and needs to be further investigated. Controversial results regarding the functions of leptin, visfatin, adiponectin, and resistin have been found.

In summary, obesity-linked type-2 diabetes is characterized by the decreased number and function of pancreatic β-cells. The impairment in β-cell function, as well as the number of β-cells, has been related to lipotoxicity (with the concomitant increased oxidative and endoplasmic reticulum stress) and the adipokine-induced inflammation processes (Halban et al., 2014).

Liver

Obesity has been involved as a risk factor at different stages of liver disease (Manne and Saab, 2014), not only causing non-alcoholic fatty liver disease (NAFLD) but also impairing the general state of patients with other preexisting conditions such as viral hepatitis. NAFLD is an important metabolic risk factor defined as a higher than 5% intracytoplasmic fat deposition in the hepatocyte in the absence of alcohol consumption, toxin exposure or viral disease (Tiniakos et al., 2010; Calvo et al., 2015). However, fat deposition is not the only observation of NAFLD, an inflammatory process coexists, with hepatocellular ballooning injury that can lead to fibrosis and cirrhosis (Brunt et al., 1999). Since triglycerides have been shown to accumulate in the liver through different manners, there is not a unique mechanism by which obesity could lead to NAFLD. Moreover, beyond the role of triglycerides, insulin resistance does have an important role in the development of fatty liver (Marchesini et al., 1999; Sanyal et al., 2001; Willner et al., 2001; Pagano et al., 2002). Free fatty acid uptake by the liver not only leads to hepatic steatosis but also produces hepatic toxicity by oxidative stress-dependent mechanisms (Manne and Saab, 2014). In this connection, it is thought that hepatic accumulation of triglycerides occurs first (hepatic steatosis or fatty liver) and then, since fatty liver is more prone to suffer oxidative injury, it evolves to steatohepatitis (Qureshi and Abrams, 2007).

The link between obesity and NAFLD has been explained by different hypotheses which take into consideration the portal hypothesis, the endocrine role of adipokines, and many observations from lipodystrophic states. It has been mentioned that visceral adipocytes constitute an important source of fatty acids and other factors entering the portal circulation (Qureshi and Abrams, 2007). The portal hypothesis supports the idea that the increased hepatic uptake of fatty acids coming from an enlarged visceral adipose tissue leads to decreased hepatic insulin clearance and thus increased circulating insulin. Indeed, fatty acids stimulate hepatic gluconeogenesis, triglyceride synthesis, and hepatic glucose output (by altering insulin signaling) (Kahn and Flier, 2000). On the other hand, adipokines are also involved in the development of NAFLD during obesity. For example, in addition to all the general effects of leptin, this adipokine has been shown to better liver enzymes and hepatic fat content, thus attenuating different manifestations of fatty liver in patients with lipoatrophy and metabolic syndrome (Lee et al., 2006). In obese NAFLD patients, leptin levels correlate with the severity of fatty liver, thus suggesting the presence of leptin resistance, probably due to a failure in leptin signaling. Low levels of adiponectin have been found in NAFLD patients, probably due to the concomitant high levels of IL-6 and TNFα found, both of which inhibit adiponectin expression. Therapy with adiponectin administration has shown to improve insulin resistance in animal models of obesity; however, in lipodystrophic animal cases, the complete reversal of insulin resistance requires the co-administration of leptin. Adipose tissue-derived TNFα and IL-6 cause the activation of Kupffer cells which leads to hepatic fibrogenesis. Moreover, TNFα has been shown to be also produced by the Kupffer cells, playing a key role in the pathogenesis of NAFLD (Qureshi and Abrams, 2007). Additionally, fatty liver, accompanied by insulin resistance and diabetes, is usually observed in lipodystrophic patients, where the fatty liver usually progresses to cirrhosis. Among different explanations proposed, reduced adiponectin and leptin levels are thought to be responsible for the presence of NAFLD in lipodystrophic individuals.

Not only has obesity been related to the development and progression of NAFLD, but also with the impairment of other hepatic conditions, being obesity considered as a strong risk factor for different liver cancers. Very interestingly, the mere losing weight of obese patients has been shown to be sufficient not only to improve the results of several hepatic treatments (Nobili et al., 2011) but also to increase insulin sensitivity and decrease hepatic triglyceride and free fatty acid uptake by liver (Viljanen et al., 2009; Manne and Saab, 2014).

Muscle

As a general picture, obesity is linked to functional limitations in muscle performance and increased probability of developing a functional disability related to strength, mobility, postural, and dynamic balance restrictions. It is known that obese people, regardless of age, have greater absolute maximum muscle strength in anti-gravity muscles compared to non-obese counterparts (this is valid only for lower limbs, since upper limb strength reveals no statistical difference between obese and normal-weight people) (Maffiuletti et al., 2007, 2008; Delmonico et al., 2009; Abdelmoula et al., 2012; Tomlinson et al., 2016). This observation has been interpreted as adiposity being a chronic overload stimulus for muscles, thus making muscles stronger and bigger. However, it is noteworthy that when muscular strength is normalized to total body mass, the obese people seem to be overall weaker than their lean control individuals. Notwithstanding, the existing literature shows considerable controversy on this matter (Tomlinson et al., 2016). For this reason, the real effect of obesity on skeletal muscle size, structure, and function remains elusive. Although there is no consensus regarding accurate measures of obesity-associated muscle damage or quality, it is worth mentioning that obesity does have been shown to generate a negative impact on skeletal musculature through adolescence to young and old adulthood (Blimkie et al., 1990; Rolland et al., 2004; Zoico et al., 2004; Maffiuletti et al., 2007, 2008). Obviously, the relevance for reduced muscle performance is higher for older people, as they are generally affected by reduced functional capacity. This includes impairments in walking, impaired ability to go up and downstairs, and difficulty with rising from chair or bed. Similarly, there is an augmented risk to suffer joint pathologies, such as knee osteoarthritis, due to joint overload and reduced muscle strength (Cooper et al., 1998; Rolland et al., 2009; LaRoche et al., 2011; Maden-Wilkinson et al., 2015). All these conditions represent a clear sign of poor quality of life for older people, which is worsened by obesity. Further work is needed to systematically investigate whether body fat percentage *per se* may be related to agonist muscle activation and antagonist co-activation and/or morphological and architectural muscle characteristics.

In connection to ectopic fat deposition, the accumulation of triglycerides intra-myocellularly and inter-myocellularly is known to cause lipotoxicity, insulin resistance, and impaired glucose metabolism. The increased flux of fatty acids to the myocyte appears to be the link between muscle fat infiltration and insulin resistance and altered glucose metabolism. It has been shown that when mitochondrial β-oxidation is overwhelmed due to an excess of free fatty acids entering the myocyte, metabolic intermediaries of fatty acids accumulate and finally impair insulin signaling (Moro et al., 2008; Ghosh, 2014). It has been shown that skeletal muscle fat infiltration, together with sarcopenia, is able to have not only metabolic consequences but also to impair the daily living, by diminishing mobility (Katsanos and Mandarino, 2011).

The effect of adipokines on the skeletal muscle has emerged as an important area of research. It has been shown that adipokines including leptin, adiponectin, visfatin, and resistin are able to affect muscle insulin sensitivity (Nicholson et al., 2018). There are several *in vitro* studies about the role of adipokines in the skeletal muscle metabolism and insulin sensitivity. However, those studies have been carried out mainly using rodent skeletal muscle cells that are known to have different fiber composition and different metabolic characteristics than human skeletal muscle cells. This may be the reason why reports about the role of adipokines in muscle function and insulin resistance result controversial.

Beyond the effect of inflammation-associated adipokines on skeletal muscle, it is worth mentioning that under obesity conditions, the muscle becomes an inflammatory organ itself, able to secrete several circulating factors (known as myokines) that can act in either autocrine, paracrine or endocrine manner, thus affecting the metabolism of both muscle and other organs. The muscle is able to secrete several hundred of factors in response to contraction, which became a whole new paradigm for understanding the communication between muscles and the various organ systems, including adipose tissue, liver, pancreas, and brain. It is worth to mention that some myokines exert their functions in the muscle itself and have been suggested to regulate skeletal muscle growth, repair, maintenance, and regeneration, in addition to mediating the health benefits of exercise (for review see Pedersen, 2013).

Cardiovascular System

Obesity, at the population level, has been considered as a risk factor for the development of cardiovascular diseases such as coronary heart disease and heart failure. Obesity-associated transition from asymptomatic subclinical left ventricle changes to overt dilated cardiomyopathy, irrespective of the coexistence of hypertension or diabetes mellitus, has been shown (Wong and Marwick, 2007). Importantly, body fat distribution has been found to be more important than total fat composition on left ventricle adaptations to obesity, with excessive visceral fat causing adverse hemodynamics, concentric left ventricle remodeling, lower cardiac output, and higher systemic vascular resistance. Lower-body subcutaneous fat has been found to cause eccentric left ventricle remodeling, higher cardiac output, and lower systemic vascular resistance, thus suggesting a protective role for subcutaneous adipose tissue, highlighting the importance of adipose tissue quality and function more than just the amount of body fat *per se* (Kim et al., 2016). In this regard, one hypothesis holds that the presence of insulin-sensitive subcutaneous adipose tissue protects the individual from ectopic accumulation of lipids and the development of metabolic syndrome (Kim et al., 2016). Cardiomyocyte hypertrophy and myocardial fat infiltration have also been demonstrated in obesity (Ommen and Lopez-Jimenez, 2013; Samanta et al., 2015). In this sense, obesity-triggered ectopic fat deposition is considered as a predictive risk factor for cardiovascular disease. The above mentioned ectopic fat accumulation in the liver and muscle (together with the associated inflammation) in particular constitutes a cardiovascular risk due to the associated insulin resistance and altered lipid and glucose metabolism. Fat surrounding the heart and blood vessels and within the renal sinus has been linked to local toxic effects by several lines of evidence. The damaging effect of ectopic fat in the cardiovascular system has been attributed to two main mechanisms: (1) fat deposition around the heart (pericardial or epicardial fat) and coronary arteries, (2) lipid accumulation within the cardiomyocyte. Pericardial, perivascular, pericoronary, and myocardial fat accumulation may lead to injury in blood vessels and heart directly by lipotoxicity and indirectly by cytokine secretion (Lim and Meigs, 2014). Fat in the neck is the only fat depot in the upper-body that is considered as an additional cardiovascular risk, and it has been found to positively correlate with insulin resistance, visceral fat content, and metabolic syndrome (Ben-Noun and Laor, 2003; Preis et al., 2010). Interestingly, pericardial fat has been proposed to play roles in support and mechanical purpose (for example, attenuation of vascular tension and torsion). However, this fat depot, when gets considerably enlarged in obesity conditions, represents a mechanical hindrance for the beating heart, thus altering cardiac size and performance (Iacobellis, 2009). In this connection, according to the Framingham Heart Study, pericardial fat is associated with coronary artery calcification and impaired cardiac function and conduction (Rosito et al., 2008). Accumulated fat around the coronary arteries and the heart appears to promote the atherosclerosis process, being associated with oxidative stress-related mechanisms. Myocardial fat accumulation has been associated with increased left ventricle mass, myocardiopathy and heart failure, mainly due to lipid-caused apoptosis of cardiomyocytes and the consequent cardiac dysfunction (Szczepaniak et al., 2003; Lim and Meigs, 2014).

A vast body of experimental, epidemiological, and clinical evidence supports the idea that obesity results harmful for both cardiovascular structure and function, mainly due to increased inflammation caused by deregulated adipokine production by a dysfunctional adipose tissue. In line with this, active endocrine and paracrine activity of cardiac ectopic fat depots within the cardiovascular system may be greatly responsible for insulin resistance and the atherosclerosis process. Moreover, leptin, adiponectin, resistin, visfatin, omentin, IL-1, IL-6, plasminogen activator inhibitor-1, and TNFα, among several other circulating factors, have been reported to signal to the myocardium through either paracrine or autocrine pathways (Iacobellis, 2015). Also, some anti-inflammatory factors secreted from perivascular fat (adiponectin, adrenomedullin, and omentin) have been demonstrated to play a key protective role in the regulation of the arterial vascular tone (vasodilation), decreasing oxidative stress, improving endothelial function, and increasing insulin sensitivity (Sacks and Fain, 2007; Piché and Poirier, 2018). It is important to highlight that secretion of pro-inflammatory adipokines is not only due to adipocyte secretion but also to secretion coming from adipose tissue-infiltrated macrophages (Chatterjee et al., 2009).

In summary, beyond the contribution of visceral fat-secreted adipokines to cardiovascular disease, the presence of cardiac ectopic fat does also contribute: firstly, due to mechanical functions, and secondly, due to cardiac ectopic fat-released adipokines which would link the ectopic cardiac fat depot, the vasculature, and the myocardium, thus playing key roles in the pathogenesis of cardiovascular disease.

THE "OBESE" BRAIN

This section of the review is dedicated exclusively to the brain in the context of obesity. We will approach this topic from a variety of perspectives, including the anatomical and functional changes observed in the brain of obese individuals, the effects of obesity-associated circulating factors on the brain, the effects of obesity-associated morbidities on the brain and, last but not least, the effects of obesity-associated inflammation on the brain.

Anatomical Aspects

Differences in both gray and white matter have been reported in obese individuals compared to their normal-weight counterparts. Regarding the gray matter, it has been shown that it is reduced in brain regions such as the hippocampus, prefrontal cortex, and other subcortical regions in the context of obesity (Stillman et al., 2017). Interestingly, these differences have been attributed exclusively to excessive adiposity, since they have been shown to be still present even after controlling obesity-associated conditions, including diabetes (Raji et al., 2009). Hippocampal atrophy is of particular importance since it has been related to Alzheimer's disease (AD) (Elias et al., 2000). Reduction in the volume of gray matter has been quite well established in several other brain regions of obese individuals using a variety of methodologies (Pannacciulli et al., 2006; Raji et al., 2009; Medic et al., 2016). There are studies reporting both obesity-associated reductions, as well as increases, in white matter in the context of obesity (Pannacciulli et al., 2006; Raji et al., 2009; Debette et al., 2010; Driscoll et al., 2012; van Bloemendaal et al., 2016).

Cognitive Function

Obesity and metabolic syndrome have undoubtedly been linked to deterioration in cognitive function. Moreover, clinical data have shown that obesity and diabetes mellitus are linked not only to cognitive decline but also to other brain disorders such as dementia, anxiety, and depression (Simon et al., 2006; Riederer et al., 2017; Sanderlin et al., 2017). Due to the difficulty to dissect the impact of each component of the obesity-associated altered metabolism on neuronal performance, it is assumed that brain structural changes, as well as the consequent cognitive impairment, are the result of the synergistic interplay between the different obesity-induced risk factors (Yaffe, 2007; Yates et al., 2012). Several models have been proposed that include the involvement of oxidative stress, inflammation, and abnormal brain lipid metabolism (Yates et al., 2012). Peripheral insulin resistance has been shown to be accompanied with cognitive decline, mainly in memory and executive performance (Heni et al., 2015; Mainardi et al., 2015; Cheke et al., 2017).

Several studies have reported that obesity in midlife is associated with increased risk of mild cognitive impairment, altered executive functioning and short-term memory, and dementia (Kivipelto et al., 2005; Cournot et al., 2006; Whitmer et al., 2008; Sabia et al., 2009; Nguyen et al., 2014). Similar results have been shown in studies carried out in animal models of high-fat diet-induced obesity (Murray et al., 2009; McNeilly et al., 2011; Nguyen et al., 2014). In contrast, the association between obesity late in life and cognitive function is less clear. A recent and important study of more than 10000 men and women, followed for up to 28 years, has examined the link between obesity and cognitive change. In this study, participants were assessed for BMI, waist circumference, signs of dementia, as well as cognitive decline (Singh-Manoux et al., 2018). This study identified that obesity (BMI $>$ 30) at age 50 years is a risk factor for dementia, whereas obesity was not a dementia risk factor at ages 60 and 70 years. This difference may be due to the fact that BMI starts to decline several years before the diagnosis of dementia (Singh-Manoux et al., 2018). These findings could explain, at least in part, the situation known as "obesity paradox" in which underweight older people consistently show an increased risk of dementia while people having normal BMI or even being overweight in the elderly do not.

Effects of Obesity-Associated Circulating Factors on the Brain

Vast epidemiological evidence supports a link between diabetes mellitus and cognitive dysfunction (Gudala et al., 2013; Koekkoek et al., 2015; Zhao et al., 2018). However, it should be mentioned that this association, as well as the severity of cognitive decline, may vary according to the type of diabetes and the age diabetes starts. Loss in glycemic control, evidenced by increased circulating HbA1c levels, has been found to be a risk factor for cognitive dysfunction, with behavioral and psychological manifestations (Sakurai et al., 2014). However, the Leiden 85-plus Study, which prospectively evaluated 599 individuals of ~85 years of age, reported that HbA1c concentrations were not associated with cognitive dysfunction (van den Berg et al., 2006). Clinical evidence has suggested that the duration of diabetes alone may not influence cognitive performance if glycemia is properly controlled over time (West et al., 2014). Interestingly, beyond the chronically high glucose levels, blood glucose peaks have been related to both cognitive impairment and increased risk of dementia (Geijselaers et al., 2015; Rawlings et al., 2017). Additionally, observational studies have shown beneficial effects of some glucose-lowering treatments on cognitive performance. For example, metformin has been shown to improve cognitive performance in US diabetic veterans (Orkaby et al., 2017).

Leptin deficiency has been linked to alterations in brain volume and structure, and these alterations have been shown to be reversed by external leptin administration (Matochik et al., 2005; London et al., 2011). Leptin has been shown to have a direct impact on the hypothalamic nuclei which are responsible for the production of both orexigenic and anorexigenic peptides

(Qi et al., 2004; Kishi and Elmquist, 2005). Indeed, leptin has been demonstrated to exert neurotrophic actions during the development of the hypothalamus, stimulating the growth of axons from the arcuate nucleus to other regions that control energy homeostasis, thus participating in the development of feeding circuits. Interestingly, this developmental activity of leptin has been shown to depend on timing and duration of leptin exposure (Bouret et al., 2004, 2012; Bouyer and Simerly, 2013; Kamitakahara et al., 2018). Leptin has also been related to presynaptic neurotransmitter release and postsynaptic neurotransmitter sensitivity, and to the processes of memory and cognition, especially to hypothalamic and hippocampal functions (Fewlass et al., 2004; Davidson et al., 2005; Harvey et al., 2005; Oomura et al., 2010). Alterations in hippocampal structure and function have been reported in animals with congenital leptin deficit, supporting a role for leptin in hippocampal development and function (Li et al., 2002; Dhar et al., 2014). Neurodegeneration, neurogenesis, synaptic plasticity as well as memory consolidation have been shown to be influenced by leptin action on the hippocampus (Doherty, 2011). Also, leptin has been shown to enhance cognition through the regulation of hippocampal function. Both *in vivo* and *in vitro* studies (the latter in hippocampal slices) have shown that exogenous leptin is able to induce long-term potentiation (Shanley et al., 2001; Wayner et al., 2004; Luo et al., 2015). Other *in vitro* studies have shown that leptin is able to induce synapse formation in cultured hippocampal neurons, thus providing a possible explanation for the long-term potentiation observed after leptin administration. Studies in humans have shown that high leptin levels are negatively correlated with late-in-life dementia risk (Harvey et al., 2005; Lieb et al., 2009). Moreover, leptin has been shown to reduce extracellular levels of amyloid beta peptide (Aβ; whose deposition is pathognomonic of AD) both *in vivo* and *in vitro* (Fewlass et al., 2004). For these reasons, the elevation of leptin has been suggested as a therapeutic alternative for dementia (Fewlass et al., 2004; Harvey et al., 2005; Irving and Harvey, 2013; McGregor and Harvey, 2018). Although animal studies are promising, further research is needed to assess whether these findings apply to human beings.

Due to undetectable levels of adiponectin in the cerebrospinal fluid (CSF), it was first thought that this hormone was not able to cross the BBB (Pan et al., 2006; Spranger et al., 2006). However, several studies have shown that intravenous injection of adiponectin leads to detectable levels of the hormone in the CSF of patients with unspecified neurological disorders (Kos et al., 2007; Kusminski et al., 2007; Neumeier et al., 2007). Indeed, as no HMW adiponectin has been detected in the CSF, it is now believed that only smaller forms of the adiponectin hormone can cross the BBB (Kusminski et al., 2007; Schulz et al., 2011). Thus, the origin of brain associated adiponectin is still a matter of debate. Adiponectin plasma levels correlate inversely with obesity, insulin resistance and type-2 diabetes mellitus (Hotta et al., 2001; Kondo et al., 2002), with adiponectin levels in the CSF being 1000-fold lower than the plasma levels (Kos et al., 2007; Kusminski et al., 2007). Adiponectin has been shown to regulate proliferation, neurogenesis, and branching of hippocampal neural stem cells (Zhang et al., 2011, 2016; Yau et al., 2014). Also, it has been shown to exert a neuroprotective role against Aβ-induced oxidative stress *in vitro* (Ng and Chan, 2017). Adiponectin deficiency in mice has shown to cause memory and spatial learning impairment, anxiety, and impaired fear conditioning, symptoms that are probably associated to the decreased synaptic protein levels, increased neuronal apoptosis and impaired insulin signaling found in those animals (Ng et al., 2016). Also, adiponectin-deficient mice have shown to suffer larger brain infarctions after ischemia and reperfusion compared with control animals, and adiponectin administration has shown to reduce the infarction size. Thus neuroprotective effects have been attributed to this adipokine (Nishimura et al., 2008). Adiponectin physiological levels are generally higher in females than in males and decrease in both sexes as age increases (Ng and Chan, 2017). However, among women, those with higher plasma levels of adiponectin have shown to exhibit poorer performance in language and global cognition and to coincide with greater mild cognitive impairment diagnosis (Wennberg et al., 2016). Nevertheless, more studies are necessary to conclusively affirm that higher adiponectin plasma level is a trustable predictor of cognitive decline. Patients with AD have been observed to have decreased levels of adiponectin in CSF, compared to those found in healthy controls or even to patients with mild cognitive impairment. However, adiponectin levels have been found to be increased in plasma of patients with mild cognitive impairment and AD, compared to that in controls. Thus, a loss of function of adiponectin signaling has been suggested to occur in the pathogenesis of AD (Waragai et al., 2017).

As mentioned before, the increased circulating levels of pro-inflammatory cytokines participate in obesity-induced systemic inflammation. This systemic inflammation may participate in the development of cognitive decline and dementia. For example, IL-1β and IL-6 have been shown to disrupt cognition- and memory-related neuronal circuits (Gemma and Bickford, 2007). Increased plasma levels of C-reactive protein and IL-6 have been identified in a meta-analysis performed by Koyama et al. (2013). Peripheral cytokines have been shown to induce local production of cytokines in the brain (Dantzer et al., 2008).

Effects of Obesity-Associated Morbidities on the Brain

It is important to highlight that all the obesity-associated morbidities mentioned before (cardiovascular disease, diabetes, atherosclerosis, etc.) do impact on brain health. Obesity-derived vascular problems, such as atherosclerosis and arteriosclerosis, which are systemic diseases, are known to affect the steady blood flow of vessels that feed the brain, thus contributing to cognitive impairment or even stroke, where large areas of the brain die due to the stop in the blood flow of a major brain artery caused by a blood clot. Vascular dementia has been shown to be caused by cerebrovascular disease, and compelling evidence has shown that cerebrovascular disease may be initiated by obesity (Gorelick et al., 2011; Zlokovic, 2011). However, many aspects of the association between obesity and cerebrovascular disease are still poorly defined. Also, epidemiological studies have shown that cardiovascular risk factors such as obesity, hypertension, diabetes, and low physical activity negatively affect brain performance (Wolf, 2012; Yano et al., 2014). A longitudinal study from Gustafson and coworkers has shown lower BBB integrity in overweight or obese individuals, compared to normal-weight controls (Gustafson et al., 2007). Similar evidence has been presented from rodent studies (Kanoski et al., 2010; Davidson et al., 2012). Indeed, irregular heartbeat conditions such as arrhythmia or atrial fibrillation, as well as obstructive sleep apnea (both highly prevalent in obese individuals), have been linked to increased risk of ischemic stroke and dementia development (Zhang et al., 2015). Interestingly, several studies have reported that obese people who survive to a first stroke event usually have improved subsequent cerebrovascular disease and mortality, as part of the previously mentioned "obesity paradox." This could come in line with the fact that obese people tend to suffer more lacunar-type of stroke, which is generally of faster recovery and better prognosis (Letra and Seiça, 2017).

Epidemiological studies have linked type-2 diabetes mellitus with cognitive impairment and dementia, with insulin resistance and hyperglycemia as the probable mechanistic links (Ott et al., 1996; Peila et al., 2002). Similarly, several cross-sectional studies have confirmed the association between insulin resistance and cognitive decline (van den Berg et al., 2006; Young et al., 2006; Ekblad et al., 2017). Hyperglycemia has been associated with poor cognitive outcomes both in cross-sectional studies (Yaffe et al., 2012) as well as in prospective studies (Prickett et al., 2015). A very recent 6-year follow-up study from Hong and coworkers has found that insulin resistance is associated with diminished cognitive performance in older individuals (Kong et al., 2018). Also, data from prospective studies have shown that individuals with type-2 diabetes exhibit poorer performance in information-processing speed, memory, attention, and executive function compared to controls (Hassing et al., 2004; van den Berg et al., 2010; Moheet et al., 2015). Longitudinal and cross-sectional studies have undoubtedly demonstrated a relationship between diabetes and mild/moderate cognitive dysfunction in type-2 diabetes, but less is known about the strength of association between diabetes and dementia. Systematic review and meta-analysis performed by Biessels and coworkers have shown an increase of 50–100% in the risk of dementia in people with type-2 diabetes, compared with people without diabetes (Biessels et al., 2006). However, the evidence is controversial, and further interventional studies are needed to evaluate the effect of controlling insulin resistance and diabetes on cognitive dysfunction.

Interestingly, obesity comorbidities have been shown to participate in the onset and progression of neurodegenerative diseases such as AD. The complete mechanisms by which obesity influences the risk of AD is not entirely clear yet. However, epidemiological studies have demonstrated that type-2 diabetes increases the risk of AD (Profenno et al., 2010). It is assumed that insulin resistance is a key causative factor for diabetes and it has been demonstrated that individuals with peripheral insulin resistance are more prone to develop AD and related pathologies (Sims-Robinson et al., 2010; Rasgon et al., 2011). Moreover, at the cellular and molecular level, insulin signaling has been demonstrated to interfere with Aβ degradation and deposition (Carro et al., 2002; Farris et al., 2003). Further, insulin deficiency has also been shown to promote tau phosphorylation, leading to the accumulation of neurofibrillary tangles (Schubert et al., 2003). Accumulating evidence has shown that the brain itself develops insulin resistance due to the impairment in the insulin pathway (Moloney et al., 2010; Talbot and Wang, 2014; Su et al., 2017). In line with this, *in vivo* experimental data have shown that insulin resistance modifies cognitive performance even in the absence of diabetes (Su et al., 2017). Moreover, insulin signaling impairment has been found in brains from AD patients (Talbot et al., 2012). Increased levels of amyloid proteins have been found in the plasma of obese individuals (Lee et al., 2009; Jahangiri et al., 2013). Also, higher expression levels of beta-amyloid precursor protein and tau, two pathognomonic features of AD, have been found in the hippocampus of morbidly obese patients, compared to non-obese controls (Mrak, 2009; Nguyen et al., 2014). On the other hand, numerous studies have demonstrated that high-fat diets contribute to the higher expression of AD markers in rodents (Studzinski et al., 2009; Puig et al., 2012; Koga et al., 2014). Indeed, uncontrolled diabetes has also been linked to the risk of developing AD (Xu et al., 2009).

Effects of Obesity-Associated Inflammation Within the Brain

Several aspects of brain function result affected by obesity-triggered inflammation. Periodic neuroinflammation is a necessary defense for the brain. However, when neuroinflammation becomes prolonged or uncontrolled (chronic neuroinflammation), it disrupts the normal protective barriers and leads to maladaptive synaptic plasticity and the development of different neurodegenerative disorders (Purkayastha and Cai, 2013). It has long been accepted that the BBB keeps blood inflammatory cells (monocytes and neutrophils) from getting into the brain. Therefore, microglia would be the only cells that mediate brain inflammation. However, it has become known that neutrophils and monocytes are able to infiltrate the injured brain and contribute to inflammation (Jeong et al., 2013). Astrocytes are known to produce anti-inflammatory factors that recruit monocytes, and neurons are able to both positively or negatively modulate anti-inflammatory response (Kim et al., 2010; Jeong et al., 2013). Thus, brain inflammation involves the coordinated efforts of several types of cells including microglia neutrophils, monocytes, astrocytes, and neurons.

Chronic neuroinflammation has been shown to impair adult hippocampal neurogenesis, and the blockade of neuroinflammation has demonstrated to restore it (Ekdahl et al., 2003; Monje et al., 2003). Also, impaired neurogenesis has been found in the hypothalamus of high-fat diet-fed rodents, probably due to the chronic neuroinflammatory response (Li et al., 2012). The complete mechanism is not fully understood, but stimulation of immune cells with the concomitant activation of the NF-kB pathway, and the release of interleukins and nitric oxide are thought to be involved (Purkayastha and Cai, 2013).

On the other hand, brain inflammation, mediated by inflammatory cells such as microglia and astrocytes, plays pivotal roles in regulating synaptic structure and function

(Mottahedin et al., 2017). Synaptic disorganization is an integral part of several neurological disorders (Ebrahimi-Fakhari and Sahin, 2015). Glial cells are thought to play a vital role in synaptic architecture and hence neuronal connectivity. For this reason, factors that affect glial cells during development may also have long-term consequences on the synapse performance. Accordingly, an interaction between synaptic disorganization and immune function has been linked with cognitive weakness (Delpech et al., 2015). The BBB is known to actively participate in the inflammatory events and, conversely, the obesity-associated chronic inflammation also influences the BBB. It has been suggested that the BBB disruption occurs well before the infiltration of immune cells to the site of inflammation. Once within the brain, these effector cells and their secreted factors act upon microglia, astrocytes, and pericytes, which are important components of the BBB, and collaborate to a further BBB disruption thus leading to neuronal damage (Sonar and Lal, 2018).

Chronic brain inflammation also has been linked to neurodegenerative disorders such as AD. Aβ peptide accumulation in the brain parenchyma and blood vessels has been shown to promote both acute and chronic inflammatory responses which are mediated by astrocytes and microglia and which may finally cause neurodegeneration. However, the role of inflammation in AD is controversial, because inflammation has been found to have a beneficial role in the early stages of the disease. Nevertheless, the chronic activation of the microglia has been linked to the increased generation of Aβ and also with tau phosphorylation (Meraz-Ríos et al., 2013). Overall, the inflammatory process in AD is characterized by changes in microglial morphology together with astrogliosis (increased number, size, and motility of astrocytes). Studies in rodent models have shown that neuroinflammation is linked to early stages in tauopathies, even preceding tangle formation (Yoshiyama et al., 2007). Although the neuronal death associated with inflammation makes it a potential risk factor in the pathogenesis of AD, whether brain inflammation is the cause of or a secondary phenomenon to this disorder is unclear yet. Obesity may serve as an amplifier or initiator of the chronic inflammation observed in AD patients, although further research is needed to clarify the specific contribution of obesity to the chronic brain inflammation observed at the onset and progression of AD.

CONCLUDING REMARKS

The causes and impact of obesity on overall health are far from linear and point to a complex set of interactions. The ultimate impact of obesity on an individual appears to be the summation of the effects of adipose-derived factors (adipokines, triglycerides, etc.) and indirect obesity effects (hypertension, glycemic dysregulation, etc.) and the physiology of the various organ systems of the body. Environmental factors and aging can accelerate or inhibit the effects of obesity on the various organ systems and tissues of the body, and this is an area of research that is rapidly expanding and identifying exciting results. Given the rapid increase in both obesity and aging in the populations of most Western societies, it will be critical to move obesity research into the realm of translational interventions, whereby the negative impacts of obesity on health are delayed or prevented in an increasingly elderly population.

AUTHOR CONTRIBUTIONS

RU and JK contributed to conception and design of the review and wrote the manuscript.

REFERENCES

Abdelmoula, A., Martin, V., Bouchant, A., Walrand, S., Lavet, C., Taillardat, M., et al. (2012). Knee extension strength in obese and nonobese male adolescents. *Appl. Physiol. Nutr. Metab.* 37, 269–275. doi: 10.1139/h2012-010

Achari, A. E., and Jain, S. K. (2017). Adiponectin, a therapeutic target for obesity, diabetes, and endothelial dysfunction. *Int. J. Mol. Sci.* 18:E1321. doi: 10.3390/ijms18061321

Alarcon, C., Boland, B. B., Uchizono, Y., Moore, P. C., Peterson, B., Rajan, S., et al. (2016). Pancreatic β-cell adaptive plasticity in obesity increases insulin production but adversely affects secretory function. *Diabetes* 65, 438–450. doi: 10.2337/db15-0792

Ärnloöv, J., Ingelsson, E., Sundstroöm, J., and Lind, L. (2010). Impact of body mass index and the metabolic syndrome on the risk of cardiovascular disease and death in middle-aged men. *Circulation* 121, 230–236. doi: 10.1161/CIRCULATIONAHA.109.887521

Bays, H. E., Toth, P. P., Kris-Etherton, P. M., Abate, N., Aronne, L. J., Brown, W. V., et al. (2013). Obesity, adiposity, and dyslipidemia: a consensus statement from the National Lipid Association. *J. Clin. Lipidol.* 7, 304–383. doi: 10.1016/j.jacl.2013.04.001

Benatti, F., Solis, M., Artioli, G., Montag, E., Painelli, V., Saito, F., et al. (2012). Liposuction induces a compensatory increase of visceral fat which is effectively counteracted by physical activity: a randomized trial. *J. Clin. Endocrinol. Metab.* 97, 2388–2395. doi: 10.1210/jc.2012-1012

Ben-Noun, L. L., and Laor, A. (2003). Relationship of neck circumference to cardiovascular risk factors. *Obes. Res.* 11, 226–231. doi: 10.1038/oby.2003.35

Biernacka, K., and Małecka-Panas, E. (2015). *Adipokines in Pancreatic Diseases.* Available at: http://www.pnmedycznych.pl/wp-content/uploads/2016/01/pnm_2015_8b_011-015.pdf (accessed April 15, 2015).

Biessels, G. J., Staekenborg, S., Brunner, E., Brayne, C., and Scheltens, P. (2006). Risk of dementia in diabetes mellitus: a systematic review. *Lancet Neurol.* 5, 64–74. doi: 10.1016/S1474-4422(05)70284-2

Björnson, E., Adiels, M., Taskinen, M.-R., and Borén, J. (2016). Kinetics of plasma triglycerides in abdominal obesity. *Curr. Opin. Lipidol.* 28, 11–18. doi: 10.1097/MOL.0000000000000375

Blimkie, C. J., Sale, D. G., and Bar-Or, O. (1990). Voluntary strength, evoked twitch contractile properties and motor unit activation of knee extensors in obese and non-obese adolescent males. *Eur. J. Appl. Physiol. Occup. Physiol.* 61, 313–318.

Boucher, J., Masri, B., Daviaud, D., Gesta, S., Guigné, C., Mazzucotelli, A., et al. (2005). Apelin, a newly identified adipokine up-regulated by insulin and obesity. *Endocrinology* 146, 1764–1771. doi: 10.1210/en.2004-1427

Bouret, S. G., Bates, S. H., Chen, S., Myers, M. G., and Simerly, R. B. (2012). Distinct roles for specific leptin receptor signals in the development of hypothalamic feeding circuits. *J. Neurosci.* 32, 1244–1252. doi: 10.1523/jneurosci.2277-11.2012

Bouret, S. G., Draper, S. J., and Simerly, R. B. (2004). Trophic action of leptin on hypothalamic neurons that regulate feeding. *Science* 304, 108–110. doi: 10.1126/science.1095004

Bouyer, K., and Simerly, R. B. (2013). Neonatal leptin exposure specifies innervation of presympathetic hypothalamic neurons and improves the metabolic status of leptin-deficient mice. *J. Neurosci.* 33, 840–851. doi: 10.1523/jneurosci.3215-12.2013

Brown, R., Imran, S. A., Belsham, D. D., Ur, E., and Wilkinson, M. (2007). Adipokine gene expression in a novel hypothalamic neuronal cell line: resistin-dependent regulation of fasting-induced adipose factor and SOCS-3. *Neuroendocrinology* 85, 232–241. doi: 10.1159/000104248

Brunt, E. M., Janney, C. G., Bisceglie, A. M., Neuschwander-Tetri, B. A., and Bacon, B. R. (1999). Nonalcoholic steatohepatitis: a proposal for grading and staging the histological lesions. *Am. J. Gastroenterol.* 94, 2467–2474. doi: 10.1111/j.1572-0241.1999.01377.x

Buchwald, H., Estok, R., Fahrbach, K., Banel, D., Jensen, M. D., Pories, W. J., et al. (2009). Weight and type 2 diabetes after bariatric surgery: systematic review and meta-analysis. *Am. J. Med.* 122, 248.e–256.e. doi: 10.1016/j.amjmed.2008.09.041

Busetto, L. (2014). Bariatric/metabolic surgery for the obese with Type 2 diabetes with BMI < 35 kg/m2: why caution is required. *Diabetes Manag.* 4, 123–130. doi: 10.2217/dmt.13.76

Busetto, L., Pisent, C., Rinaldi, D., Longhin, P. L., Segato, G., De Marchi, F., et al. (2000). Variation in lipid levels in morbidly obese patients operated with the LAP-BAND adjustable gastric banding system: effects of different levels of weight loss. *Obes. Surg.* 10, 569–577.

Calle, E. E., Rodriguez, C., Walker-Thurmond, K., and Thun, M. J. (2003). Overweight, obesity, and mortality from cancer in a prospectively studied cohort of U.S. adults. *N. Engl. J. Med.* 348, 1625–1638. doi: 10.1056/NEJMoa021423

Calvo, N., Beltrán-Debón, R., Rodríguez-Gallego, E., Hernández-Aguilera, A., Guirro, M., Mariné-Casadó, R., et al. (2015). Liver fat deposition and mitochondrial dysfunction in morbid obesity: an approach combining metabolomics with liver imaging and histology. *World J. Gastroenterol.* 21, 7529–7544. doi: 10.3748/wjg.v21.i24.7529

Carro, E., Trejo, J. L., Gomez-Isla, T., LeRoith, D., and Torres-Aleman, I. (2002). Serum insulin-like growth factor I regulates brain amyloid-β levels. *Nat. Med.* 8, 1390–1397. doi: 10.1038/nm793

Castan-Laurell, I., Boucher, J., Dray, C., Daviaud, D., Guigné, C., and Valet, P. (2005). Apelin, a novel adipokine over-produced in obesity: Friend or foe? *Mol. Cell. Endocrinol.* 245, 7–9. doi: 10.1016/J.MCE.2005.09.012

Castan-Laurell, I., Dray, C., Attané, C., Duparc, T., Knauf, C., and Valet, P. (2011). Apelin, diabetes, and obesity. *Endocrine* 40, 1–9. doi: 10.1007/s12020-011-9507-9

Chan, D. C., Watts, G. F., Barrett, P. H., Mamo, J. C. L., and Redgrave, T. G. (2002). *Markers of Triglyceride-Rich Lipoprotein Remnant Metabolism in Visceral Obesity.* Available at: https://pdfs.semanticscholar.org/f2a7/60b5c3b24a0cfec2e3e6ffc1188b70f7ef1c.pdf (accessed April 17, 2019).

Chatterjee, T. K., Stoll, L. L., Denning, G. M., Harrelson, A., Blomkalns, A. L., Idelman, G., et al. (2009). Proinflammatory phenotype of perivascular adipocytes: influence of high-fat feeding. *Circ. Res.* 104, 541–549. doi: 10.1161/CIRCRESAHA.108.182998

Cheke, L. G., Bonnici, H. M., Clayton, N. S., and Simons, J. S. (2017). Obesity and insulin resistance are associated with reduced activity in core memory regions of the brain. *Neuropsychologia* 96, 137–149. doi: 10.1016/j.neuropsychologia.2017.01.013

Chowdhury, B., Sjöström, L., Alpsten, M., Kostanty, J., Kvist, H., and Löfgren, R. (1994). A multicompartment body composition technique based on computerized tomography. *Int. J. Obes. Relat. Metab. Disord.* 18, 219–234.

Christou, N. V., Sampalis, J. S., Liberman, M., Look, D., Auger, S., McLean, A. P. H., et al. (2004). Surgery decreases long-term mortality, morbidity, and health care use in morbidly obese patients. *Ann. Surg.* 240, 416–423.

Cooper, C., Inskip, H., Croft, P., Campbell, L., Smith, G., McLaren, M., et al. (1998). Individual risk factors for hip osteoarthritis: obesity, hip injury, and physical activity. *Am. J. Epidemiol.* 147, 516–522.

Cournot, M., Marquie, J. C., Ansiau, D., Martinaud, C., Fonds, H., Ferrieres, J., et al. (2006). Relation between body mass index and cognitive function in healthy middle-aged men and women. *Neurology* 67, 1208–1214. doi: 10.1212/01.wnl.0000238082.13860.50

Cummings, D. E., and Rubino, F. (2018). Metabolic surgery for the treatment of type 2 diabetes in obese individuals LAGB Laparoscopic adjustable gastric banding NIH National Institutes of Health QALY Quality-adjusted life-year. *Diabetologia* 61, 257–264. doi: 10.1007/s00125-017-4513-y

Dantzer, R., O'Connor, J. C., Freund, G. G., Johnson, R. W., and Kelley, K. W. (2008). From inflammation to sickness and depression: when the immune system subjugates the brain. *Nat. Rev. Neurosci.* 9, 46–56. doi: 10.1038/nrn2297

Dash, S., Xiao, C., Morgantini, C., and Lewis, G. F. (2015). New insights into the regulation of chylomicron production. *Annu. Rev. Nutr.* 35, 265–294. doi: 10.1146/annurev-nutr-071714-034338

Davidson, T., Kanoski, S., Walls, E., and Jarrard, L. (2005). Memory inhibition and energy regulation. *Physiol. Behav.* 86, 731–746. doi: 10.1016/j.physbeh.2005.09.004

Davidson, T. L., Monnot, A., Neal, A. U., Martin, A. A., Horton, J. J., and Zheng, W. (2012). The effects of a high-energy diet on hippocampal-dependent discrimination performance and blood-brain barrier integrity differ for diet-induced obese and diet-resistant rats. *Physiol. Behav.* 107, 26–33. doi: 10.1016/j.physbeh.2012.05.015

de Luca, C., Kowalski, T. J., Zhang, Y., Elmquist, J. K., Lee, C., Kilimann, M. W., et al. (2005). Complete rescue of obesity, diabetes, and infertility in db/db mice by neuron-specific LEPR-B transgenes. *J. Clin. Invest.* 115, 3484–3493. doi: 10.1172/JCI24059

Debette, S., Beiser, A., Hoffmann, U., DeCarli, C., O'Donnell, C. J., Massaro, J. M., et al. (2010). Visceral fat is associated with lower brain volume in healthy middle-aged adults. *Ann. Neurol.* 68, 136–144. doi: 10.1002/ana.22062

Delmonico, M. J., Harris, T. B., Visser, M., Park, S. W., Conroy, M. B., Velasquez-Mieyer, P., et al. (2009). Longitudinal study of muscle strength, quality, and adipose tissue infiltration. *Am. J. Clin. Nutr.* 90, 1579–1585. doi: 10.3945/ajcn.2009.28047

Delpech, J.-C., Madore, C., Nadjar, A., Joffre, C., Wohleb, E. S., and Layé, S. (2015). Microglia in neuronal plasticity: Influence of stress. *Neuropharmacology* 96, 19–28. doi: 10.1016/j.neuropharm.2014.12.034

Deng, Y., and Scherer, P. E. (2010). Adipokines as novel biomarkers and regulators of the metabolic syndrome. *Ann. N. Y. Acad. Sci.* 1212, E1–E19. doi: 10.1111/j.1749-6632.2010.05875.x

Dhar, M., Wayman, G. A., Zhu, M., Lambert, T. J., Davare, M. A., and Appleyard, S. M. (2014). Leptin-induced spine formation requires TrpC channels and the CaM kinase cascade in the hippocampus. *J. Neurosci.* 34, 10022–10033. doi: 10.1523/JNEUROSCI.2868-13.2014

Dodson, M. V., Du, M., Wang, S., Bergen, W. G., Fernyhough-Culver, M., Basu, U., et al. (2014). Adipose depots differ in cellularity, adipokines produced, gene expression, and cell systems. *Adipocyte* 3, 236–241. doi: 10.4161/adip.28321

Doherty, G. H. (2011). Obesity and the ageing brain: could leptin play a role in neurodegeneration? *Curr. Gerontol. Geriatr. Res.* 2011:708154. doi: 10.1155/2011/708154

Driscoll, I., Beydoun, M. A., An, Y., Davatzikos, C., Ferrucci, L., Zonderman, A. B., et al. (2012). Midlife obesity and trajectories of brain volume changes in older adults. *Hum. Brain Mapp.* 33, 2204–2210. doi: 10.1002/hbm.21353

Drolet, R., Bélanger, C., Fortier, M., Huot, C., Mailloux, J., Légaré, D., et al. (2009). Fat depot-specific impact of visceral obesity on adipocyte adiponectin release in women. *Obesity* 17, 424–430. doi: 10.1038/oby.2008.555

Ebbert, J. O., Elrashidi, M. Y., and Jensen, M. D. (2014). Managing overweight and obesity in adults to reduce cardiovascular disease risk. *Curr. Atheroscler. Rep.* 16:445. doi: 10.1007/s11883-014-0445-x

Ebrahimi-Fakhari, D., and Sahin, M. (2015). Autism and the synapse. *Curr. Opin. Neurol.* 28, 91–102. doi: 10.1097/WCO.0000000000000186

Ekblad, L. L., Rinne, J. O., Puukka, P., Laine, H., Ahtiluoto, S., Sulkava, R., et al. (2017). Insulin resistance predicts cognitive decline: an 11-year follow-up of a nationally representative adult population sample. *Diabetes Care* 40, 751–758. doi: 10.2337/dc16-2001

Ekdahl, C. T., Claasen, J.-H., Bonde, S., Kokaia, Z., and Lindvall, O. (2003). Inflammation is detrimental for neurogenesis in adult brain. *Proc. Natl. Acad. Sci. U.S.A.* 100, 13632–13637. doi: 10.1073/pnas.2234031100

Elias, M. F., Beiser, A., Wolf, P. A., Au, R., White, R. F., and D'Agostino, R. B. (2000). The preclinical phase of alzheimer disease: a 22-year prospective study of the Framingham Cohort. *Arch. Neurol.* 57, 808–813.

Farris, W., Mansourian, S., Chang, Y., Lindsley, L., Eckman, E. A., Frosch, M. P., et al. (2003). Insulin-degrading enzyme regulates the levels of insulin, amyloid -protein, and the -amyloid precursor protein intracellular domain in vivo. *Proc. Natl. Acad. Sci. U.S.A.* 100, 4162–4167. doi: 10.1073/pnas.0230450100

Feingold, K. R., and Grunfeld, C. (2018). *Obesity and Dyslipidemia.* Available at: http://www.ncbi.nlm.nih.gov/pubmed/26247088 (accessed April 17, 2019).

Fewlass, D. C., Noboa, K., Pi-Sunyer, F. X., Johnston, J. M., Yan, S. D., and Tezapsidis, N. (2004). Obesity-related leptin regulates Alzheimer's Aβ. *FASEB J.* 18, 1870–1878. doi: 10.1096/fj.04-2572com

Fontana, L., Eagon, J. C., Trujillo, M. E., Scherer, P. E., and Klein, S. (2007). Visceral fat adipokine secretion is associated with systemic inflammation in obese humans. *Diabetes* 56, 1010–1013. doi: 10.2337/db06-1656

Foster, M. T., Softic, S., Caldwell, J., Kohli, R., DeKloet, A. D., and Seeley, R. J. (2013). Subcutaneous adipose tissue transplantation in diet-induced obese mice attenuates metabolic dysregulation while removal exacerbates it. *Physiol. Rep.* 1:e00015. doi: 10.1002/phy2.15

Franssen, R., Monajemi, H., Stroes, E. S. G., and Kastelein, J. J. P. (2011). Obesity and Dyslipidemia. *Med. Clin. North Am.* 95, 893–902. doi: 10.1016/j.mcna.2011.06.003

Friedman, J. M., and Halaas, J. L. (1998). Leptin and the regulation of body weight in mammals. *Nature* 395, 763–770. doi: 10.1038/27376

Gaddey, H. L., and Holder, K. (2014). Unintentional weight loss in older adults. *Am. Fam. Physician* 89, 718–722.

Geijselaers, S. L. C., Sep, S. J. S., Stehouwer, C. D. A., and Biessels, G. J. (2015). Glucose regulation, cognition, and brain MRI in type 2 diabetes: a systematic review. *Lancet Diabetes Endocrinol.* 3, 75–89. doi: 10.1016/S2213-8587(14)70148-2

Gemma, C., and Bickford, P. C. (2007). Interleukin-1beta and caspase-1: players in the regulation of age-related cognitive dysfunction. *Rev. Neurosci.* 18, 137–148.

Ghosh, S. (2014). Ectopic fat: the potential target for obesity management. *J. Obes. Metab. Res.* 1, 30–38. doi: 10.4103/2347-9906.123883

Gloy, V. L., Briel, M., Bhatt, D. L., Kashyap, S. R., Schauer, P. R., Mingrone, G., et al. (2013). Bariatric surgery versus non-surgical treatment for obesity: a systematic review and meta-analysis of randomised controlled trials. *BMJ* 347, f5934–f5934. doi: 10.1136/bmj.f5934

Gorelick, P. B., Scuteri, A., Black, S. E., DeCarli, C., Greenberg, S. M., Iadecola, C., et al. (2011). Vascular contributions to cognitive impairment and dementia. *Stroke* 42, 2672–2713. doi: 10.1161/STR.0b013e3182299496

Görgens, S. W., Eckardt, K., Jensen, J., Drevon, C. A., and Eckel, J. (2015). Exercise and regulation of adipokine and myokine production. *Prog. Mol. Biol. Transl. Sci.* 135, 313–336. doi: 10.1016/bs.pmbts.2015.07.002

Grauer, W. O., Moss, A. A., Cann, C. E., and Goldberg, H. I. (1984). Quantification of body fat distribution in the abdomen using computed tomography. *Am. J. Clin. Nutr.* 39, 631–637. doi: 10.1093/ajcn/39.4.631

Gudala, K., Bansal, D., Schifano, F., and Bhansali, A. (2013). Diabetes mellitus and risk of dementia: a meta-analysis of prospective observational studies. *J. Diabetes Investig.* 4, 640–650. doi: 10.1111/jdi.12087

Gumbs, A. A. (2008). Obesity, pancreatitis, and pancreatic cancer. *Obes. Surg.* 18, 1183–1187. doi: 10.1007/s11695-008-9599-3

Gustafson, D. R., Karlsson, C., Skoog, I., Rosengren, L., Lissner, L., and Blennow, K. (2007). Mid-life adiposity factors relate to blood-brain barrier integrity in late life. *J. Intern. Med.* 262, 643–650. doi: 10.1111/j.1365-2796.2007.01869.x

Hajer, G. R., van Haeften, T. W., and Visseren, F. L. J. (2008). Adipose tissue dysfunction in obesity, diabetes, and vascular diseases. *Eur. Heart J.* 29, 2959–2971. doi: 10.1093/eurheartj/ehn387

Halban, P. A., Polonsky, K. S., Bowden, D. W., Hawkins, M. A., Ling, C., Mather, K. J., et al. (2014). β-cell failure in type 2 diabetes: postulated mechanisms and prospects for prevention and treatment. *J. Clin. Endocrinol. Metab.* 99, 1983–1992. doi: 10.1210/jc.2014-1425

Han, T. S., Tajar, A., and Lean, M. E. J. (2011). Obesity and weight management in the elderly. *Br. Med. Bull.* 97, 169–196. doi: 10.1093/bmb/ldr002

Harvey, J., Shanley, L. J., O'Malley, D., and Irving, A. J. (2005). Leptin: a potential cognitive enhancer? *Biochem. Soc. Trans.* 33, 1029–1032. doi: 10.1042/BST20051029

Hassing, L. B., Grant, M. D., Hofer, S. M., Pedersen, N. L., Nilsson, S. E., Berg, S., et al. (2004). Type 2 diabetes mellitus contributes to cognitive decline in old age: a longitudinal population-based study. *J. Int. Neuropsychol. Soc.* 10, 599–607. doi: 10.1017/S1355617704104165

Heni, M., Kullmann, S., Preissl, H., Fritsche, A., and Häring, H.-U. (2015). Impaired insulin action in the human brain: causes and metabolic consequences. *Nat. Rev. Endocrinol.* 11, 701–711. doi: 10.1038/nrendo.2015.173

Hoffstedt, J., Amer, P., Hellers, G., and Lonnqvist', F. (2018). *Variation in Adrenergic Regulation of Lipolysis between Omental and Subcutaneous Adipocytes from Obese and Non-Obese Men.* Available at: www.jlr.org (accessed December 6, 2018).

Honka, H., Hannukainen, J. C., Tarkia, M., Karlsson, H., Saunavaara, V., Salminen, P., et al. (2014). Pancreatic metabolism, blood flow, and β-Cell function in obese humans. *J. Clin. Endocrinol. Metab.* 99, 981–990. doi: 10.1210/jc.2013-4369

Hotamisligil, G. S., and Spiegelman, B. M. (1994). Tumor necrosis factor alpha: a key component of the obesity-diabetes link. *Diabetes* 43, 1271–1278.

Hotta, K., Funahashi, T., Bodkin, N. L., Ortmeyer, H. K., Arita, Y., Hansen, B. C., et al. (2001). Circulating concentrations of the adipocyte protein adiponectin are decreased in parallel with reduced insulin sensitivity during the progression to type 2 diabetes in rhesus monkeys. *Diabetes* 50, 1126–1133.

Hruby, A., and Hu, F. B. (2015). The epidemiology of obesity: a big picture. *Pharmacoeconomics* 33, 673–689. doi: 10.1007/s40273-014-0243-x

Hu, F. B. (2007). Obesity and mortality: watch your waist, not just your weight. *Arch. Intern. Med.* 167, 875–876. doi: 10.1001/archinte.167.9.875

Iacobellis, G. (2009). Epicardial and pericardial fat: close, but very different. *Obesity* 17, 625–625. doi: 10.1038/oby.2008.575

Iacobellis, G. (2015). Local and systemic effects of the multifaceted epicardial adipose tissue depot. *Nat. Rev. Endocrinol.* 11, 363–371. doi: 10.1038/nrendo.2015.58

Illán-Gómez, F., Gonzálvez-Ortega, M., Orea-Soler, I., Alcaraz-Tafalla, M. S., Aragón-Alonso, A., Pascual-Díaz, M., et al. (2012). Obesity and inflammation: change in adiponectin, C-reactive protein, tumour necrosis factor-alpha and interleukin-6 after bariatric surgery. *Obes. Surg.* 22, 950–955. doi: 10.1007/s11695-012-0643-y

Irving, A. J., and Harvey, J. (2013). Leptin regulation of hippocampal synaptic function in health and disease. *Philos. Trans. R. Soc. B Biol. Sci.* 369:20130155. doi: 10.1098/rstb.2013.0155

Jacome-Sosa, M. M., and Parks, E. J. (2014). Fatty acid sources and their fluxes as they contribute to plasma triglyceride concentrations and fatty liver in humans. *Curr. Opin. Lipidol.* 25, 213–220. doi: 10.1097/MOL.0000000000000080

Jahangiri, A., Wilson, P. G., Hou, T., Brown, A., King, V. L., and Tannock, L. R. (2013). Serum amyloid A is found on ApoB-containing lipoproteins in obese humans with diabetes. *Obesity* 21, 993–996. doi: 10.1002/oby.20126

James, A. P., Watts, G., Barrett, H., Smith, D., Pal, S., Chan, D., et al. (2003). Effect of weight loss on postprandial lipemia and low density lipoprotein receptor binding in overweight men. *Metabolism* 52, 136–141. doi: 10.1053/META.2003.50032

Jaworek, J., Bonior, J., Pierzchalski, P., Tomaszewska, R., Stachura, J., Sendur, R., et al. (2002). Leptin protects the pancreas from damage induced by caerulein overstimulation by modulating cytokine production. *Pancreatology* 2, 89–99. doi: 10.1159/000055897

Jensen, M. D. (2008). Role of body fat distribution and the metabolic complications of obesity. *J. Clin. Endocrinol. Metab.* 93, 57–63. doi: 10.1210/jc.2008-1585

Jeong, H.-K., Ji, K., Min, K., and Joe, E.-H. (2013). Brain inflammation and microglia: facts and misconceptions. *Exp. Neurobiol.* 22, 59–67. doi: 10.5607/en.2013.22.2.59

Kahn, B. B., and Flier, J. S. (2000). Obesity and insulin resistance. *J. Clin. Invest.* 106, 473–481. doi: 10.1172/JCI10842

Kamitakahara, A., Bouyer, K., Wang, C. H., and Simerly, R. (2018). A critical period for the trophic actions of leptin on AgRP neurons in the arcuate nucleus of the hypothalamus. *J. Comp. Neurol.* 526, 133–145. doi: 10.1002/cne.24327

Kanoski, S. E., Zhang, Y., Zheng, W., and Davidson, T. L. (2010). The effects of a high-energy diet on hippocampal function and blood-brain barrier integrity in the rat. *J. Alzheimers Dis.* 21, 207–219. doi: 10.3233/JAD-2010-091414

Karelis, A. D., Faraj, M., Bastard, J.-P., St-Pierre, D. H., Brochu, M., Prud'homme, D., et al. (2005). The metabolically healthy but obese individual presents a favorable inflammation profile. *J. Clin. Endocrinol. Metab.* 90, 4145–4150. doi: 10.1210/jc.2005-0482

Karpe, F., Dickmann, J. R., and Frayn, K. N. (2011). Fatty acids, obesity, and insulin resistance: time for a reevaluation. *Diabetes* 60, 2441–2449. doi: 10.2337/db11-0425

Katsanos, C. S., and Mandarino, L. J. (2011). Protein metabolism in human obesity: a shift in focus from whole-body to skeletal muscle. *Obesity* 19, 469–475. doi: 10.1038/oby.2010.290

Kelly, T. M., and Jones, S. B. (1986). Changes in serum lipids after gastric bypass surgery. Lack of a relationship to weight loss. *Int. J. Obes.* 10, 443–452.

Kiliaan, A. J., Arnoldussen, I. A. C., and Gustafson, D. R. (2014). Adipokines: a link between obesity and dementia? *Lancet Neurol.* 13, 913–923. doi: 10.1016/S1474-4422(14)70085-7

Kim, J., Min, K.-J., Seol, W., Jou, I., and Joe, E. (2010). Astrocytes in injury states rapidly produce anti-inflammatory factors and attenuate microglial inflammatory responses. *J. Neurochem.* 115, 1161–1171. doi: 10.1111/j.1471-4159.2010.07004.x

Kim, S. H., Després, J. P., and Koh, K. K. (2016). Obesity and cardiovascular disease: friend or foe? *Eur. Heart J.* 37, 3560–3568. doi: 10.1093/eurheartj/ehv509

Kishi, T., and Elmquist, J. K. (2005). Body weight is regulated by the brain: a link between feeding and emotion. *Mol. Psychiatry* 10, 132–146. doi: 10.1038/sj.mp.4001638

Kivipelto, M., Ngandu, T., Fratiglioni, L., Viitanen, M., Kåreholt, I., Winblad, B., et al. (2005). Obesity and vascular risk factors at midlife and the risk of dementia and Alzheimer disease. *Arch. Neurol.* 62, 1556–1560. doi: 10.1001/archneur.62.10.1556

Knudtson, M. D., Klein, B. E. K., Klein, R., and Shankar, A. (2005). Associations with weight loss and subsequent mortality risk. *Ann. Epidemiol.* 15, 483–491. doi: 10.1016/j.annepidem.2004.12.003

Koekkoek, P. S., Kappelle, L. J., van den Berg, E., Rutten, G. E., and Biessels, G. J. (2015). Cognitive function in patients with diabetes mellitus: guidance for daily care. *Lancet Neurol.* 14, 329–340. doi: 10.1016/S1474-4422(14)70249-2

Koga, S., Kojima, A., Kuwabara, S., and Yoshiyama, Y. (2014). Immunohistochemical analysis of tau phosphorylation and astroglial activation with enhanced leptin receptor expression in diet-induced obesity mouse hippocampus. *Neurosci. Lett.* 571, 11–16. doi: 10.1016/j.neulet.2014.04.028

Koliaki, C., Liatis, S., le Roux, C. W., and Kokkinos, A. (2017). The role of bariatric surgery to treat diabetes: current challenges and perspectives. *BMC Endocr. Disord.* 17:50. doi: 10.1186/s12902-017-0202-6

Kondo, H., Shimomura, I., Matsukawa, Y., Kumada, M., Takahashi, M., Matsuda, M., et al. (2002). Association of adiponectin mutation with type 2 diabetes: a candidate gene for the insulin resistance syndrome. *Diabetes* 51, 2325–2328.

Kong, S. H., Park, Y. J., Lee, J.-Y., Cho, N. H., and Moon, M. K. (2018). Insulin resistance is associated with cognitive decline among older Koreans with normal baseline cognitive function: a prospective community-based cohort study. *Sci. Rep.* 8:650. doi: 10.1038/s41598-017-18998-0

Konrad, D., Rudich, A., and Schoenle, E. J. (2007). Improved glucose tolerance in mice receiving intraperitoneal transplantation of normal fat tissue. *Diabetologia* 50, 833–839. doi: 10.1007/s00125-007-0596-1

Konturek, S. J., Konturek, J. W., Pawlik, T., and Brzozowki, T. (2004). Brain-gut axis and its role in the control of food intake. *J. Physiol. Pharmacol.* 55(1 Pt 2), 137–154.

Kos, K., Harte, A. L., da Silva, N. F., Tonchev, A., Chaldakov, G., James, S., et al. (2007). Adiponectin and resistin in human cerebrospinal fluid and expression of adiponectin receptors in the human hypothalamus. *J. Clin. Endocrinol. Metab.* 92, 1129–1136. doi: 10.1210/jc.2006-1841

Koyama, A., O'Brien, J., Weuve, J., Blacker, D., Metti, A. L., and Yaffe, K. (2013). The role of peripheral inflammatory markers in dementia and Alzheimer's disease: a meta-analysis. *J. Gerontol. A Biol. Sci. Med. Sci.* 68, 433–440. doi: 10.1093/gerona/gls187

Kubota, N., Yano, W., Kubota, T., Yamauchi, T., Itoh, S., Kumagai, H., et al. (2007). Adiponectin stimulates AMP-activated protein kinase in the hypothalamus and increases food intake. *Cell Metab.* 6, 55–68. doi: 10.1016/j.cmet.2007.06.003

Kusminski, C. M., McTernan, P. G., Schraw, T., Kos, K., O'Hare, J. P., Ahima, R., et al. (2007). Adiponectin complexes in human cerebrospinal fluid: distinct complex distribution from serum. *Diabetologia* 50, 634–642. doi: 10.1007/s00125-006-0577-9

Kwok, K. H. M., Lam, K. S. L., and Xu, A. (2016). Heterogeneity of white adipose tissue: molecular basis and clinical implications. *Exp. Mol. Med.* 48:e215. doi: 10.1038/emm.2016.5

Lam, D. W., and LeRoith, D. (2000). *Metabolic Syndrome.* Available at: http://www.ncbi.nlm.nih.gov/pubmed/25905173 (accessed April 16, 2019).

LaRoche, D. P., Kralian, R. J., and Millett, E. D. (2011). Fat mass limits lower-extremity relative strength and maximal walking performance in older women. *J. Electromyogr. Kinesiol.* 21, 754–761. doi: 10.1016/j.jelekin.2011.07.006

Le, K.-A., Ventura, E. E., Fisher, J. Q., Davis, J. N., Weigensberg, M. J., Punyanitya, M., et al. (2011). Ethnic differences in pancreatic fat accumulation and its relationship with other fat depots and inflammatory markers. *Diabetes Care* 34, 485–490. doi: 10.2337/dc10-0760

Leal, L. G., Lopes, M. A., and Batista, M. L. Jr. (2018). Physical exercise-induced myokines and muscle-adipose tissue crosstalk: a review of current knowledge and the implications for health and metabolic diseases. *Front. Physiol.* 9:1307. doi: 10.3389/fphys.2018.01307

Lee, D., Sui, X., Artero, E. G., Lee, I.-M., Church, T. S., McAuley, P. A., et al. (2011). Long-term effects of changes in cardiorespiratory fitness and body mass index on all-cause and cardiovascular disease mortality in men. *Circulation* 124, 2483–2490. doi: 10.1161/CIRCULATIONAHA.111.038422

Lee, J. H., Chan, J. L., Sourlas, E., Raptopoulos, V., and Mantzoros, C. S. (2006). Recombinant methionyl human leptin therapy in replacement doses improves insulin resistance and metabolic profile in patients with lipoatrophy and metabolic syndrome induced by the highly active antiretroviral therapy. *J. Clin. Endocrinol. Metab.* 91, 2605–2611. doi: 10.1210/jc.2005-1545

Lee, Y., Lingvay, I., Szczepaniak, L. S., Ravazzola, M., Orci, L., and Unger, R. H. (2010). Pancreatic steatosis: harbinger of type 2 diabetes in obese rodents. *Int. J. Obes.* 34, 396–400. doi: 10.1038/ijo.2009.245

Lee, Y.-H., Martin, J. M., Maple, R. L., Tharp, W. G., and Pratley, R. E. (2009). Plasma Amyloid-β peptide levels correlate with adipocyte amyloid precursor protein gene expression in obese individuals. *Neuroendocrinology* 90, 383–390. doi: 10.1159/000235555

Lenchik, L., Register, T. C., Hsu, F. C., Lohman, K., Nicklas, B. J., Freedman, B. I., et al. (2003). Adiponectin as a novel determinant of bone mineral density and visceral fat. *Bone* 33, 646–651.

Letra, L., and Seiça, R. (eds) (2017). *Obesity and Brain Function.* Cham: Springer International Publishing.

Li, J., Tang, Y., and Cai, D. (2012). IKKβ/NF-κB disrupts adult hypothalamic neural stem cells to mediate a neurodegenerative mechanism of dietary obesity and pre-diabetes. *Nat. Cell Biol.* 14, 999–1012. doi: 10.1038/ncb2562

Li, X.-L., Aou, S., Oomura, Y., Hori, N., Fukunaga, K., and Hori, T. (2002). Impairment of long-term potentiation and spatial memory in leptin receptor-deficient rodents. *Neuroscience* 113, 607–615.

Lieb, W., Beiser, A. S., Vasan, R. S., Tan, Z. S., Au, R., Harris, T. B., et al. (2009). Association of plasma leptin levels with incident Alzheimer disease and MRI measures of brain aging. *JAMA* 302, 2565–2572. doi: 10.1001/jama.2009.1836

Lim, S., and Meigs, J. B. (2014). Links between ectopic fat and vascular disease in humans. *Arterioscler. Thromb. Vasc. Biol.* 34, 1820–1826. doi: 10.1161/ATVBAHA.114.303035

Lissner, L., Karlsson, C., Lindroos, A. K., Sjöström, L., Carlsson, B., Carlsson, L., et al. (1999). Birth weight, adulthood BMI, and subsequent weight gain in relation to leptin levels in Swedish women. *Obes. Res.* 7, 150–154.

London, E. D., Berman, S. M., Chakrapani, S., Delibasi, T., Monterosso, J., Erol, H. K., et al. (2011). Short-term plasticity of gray matter associated with leptin deficiency and replacement. *J. Clin. Endocrinol. Metab.* 96, E1212–E1220. doi: 10.1210/jc.2011-0314

Lumeng, C. N., and Saltiel, A. R. (2011). Inflammatory links between obesity and metabolic disease. *J. Clin. Invest.* 121, 2111–2117. doi: 10.1172/JCI57132

Luo, X., McGregor, G., Irving, A. J., and Harvey, J. (2015). Leptin induces a novel form of NMDA receptor-dependent LTP at hippocampal temporoammonic-CA1 synapses. *eNeuro* 2:ENEURO.0007-15.2015. doi: 10.1523/ENEURO.0007-15.2015

Maden-Wilkinson, T. M., McPhee, J. S., Jones, D. A., and Degens, H. (2015). Age-related loss of muscle mass, strength, and power and their association with mobility in recreationally-active older adults in the United Kingdom. *J. Aging Phys. Act.* 23, 352–360. doi: 10.1123/japa.2013-0219

Maffiuletti, N. A., Jubeau, M., Agosti, F., De Col, A., and Sartorio, A. (2008). Quadriceps muscle function characteristics in severely obese and nonobese adolescents. *Eur. J. Appl. Physiol.* 103, 481–484. doi: 10.1007/s00421-008-0737-3

Maffiuletti, N. A., Jubeau, M., Munzinger, U., Bizzini, M., Agosti, F., De Col, A., et al. (2007). Differences in quadriceps muscle strength and fatigue between lean and obese subjects. *Eur. J. Appl. Physiol.* 101, 51–59. doi: 10.1007/s00421-007-0471-2

Mainardi, M., Fusco, S., and Grassi, C. (2015). Modulation of hippocampal neural plasticity by glucose-related signaling. *Neural Plast.* 2015, 1–10. doi: 10.1155/2015/657928

Manne, V., and Saab, S. (2014). Impact of nutrition and obesity on chronic liver disease. *Clin. Liver Dis.* 18, 205–218. doi: 10.1016/j.cld.2013.09.008

Marchesini, G., Brizi, M., Morselli-Labate, A. M., Bianchi, G., Bugianesi, E., McCullough, A. J., et al. (1999). Association of nonalcoholic fatty liver disease with insulin resistance. *Am. J. Med.* 107, 450–455. doi: 10.1016/S0002-9343(99)00271-5

Marra, F., Aleffi, S., Bertolani, C., Petrai, I., and Vizzutti, F. (2005). Adipokines and liver fibrosis. *Eur. Rev. Med. Pharmacol. Sci.* 9, 279–284.

Matochik, J. A., London, E. D., Yildiz, B. O., Ozata, M., Caglayan, S., DePaoli, A. M., et al. (2005). Effect of leptin replacement on brain structure in genetically leptin-deficient adults. *J. Clin. Endocrinol. Metab.* 90, 2851–2854. doi: 10.1210/jc.2004-1979

Matsuzawa, Y. (2007). The metabolic syndrome and adipocytokines. *Expert Rev. Clin. Immunol.* 580, 2917–2921. doi: 10.1586/1744666X.3.1.39

McGregor, G., and Harvey, J. (2018). Food for thought: leptin regulation of hippocampal function and its role in Alzheimer's disease. *Neuropharmacology* 136, 298–306. doi: 10.1016/j.neuropharm.2017.09.038

McNeilly, A. D., Williamson, R., Sutherland, C., Balfour, D. J. K., and Stewart, C. A. (2011). High fat feeding promotes simultaneous decline in insulin sensitivity and cognitive performance in a delayed matching and non-matching to position task. *Behav. Brain Res.* 217, 134–141. doi: 10.1016/j.bbr.2010.10.017

Medic, N., Ziauddeen, H., Ersche, K. D., Farooqi, I. S., Bullmore, E. T., Nathan, P. J., et al. (2016). Increased body mass index is associated with specific regional alterations in brain structure. *Int. J. Obes.* 40, 1177–1182. doi: 10.1038/ijo.2016.42

Meraz-Ríos, M. A., Toral-Rios, D., Franco-Bocanegra, D., Villeda-Hernández, J., and Campos-Peña, V. (2013). Inflammatory process in Alzheimer's disease. *Front. Integr. Neurosci.* 7:59. doi: 10.3389/fnint.2013.00059

Moheet, A., Mangia, S., and Seaquist, E. (2015). Impact of diabetes on cognitive function and brain structure. *Ann. N. Y. Acad. Sci.* 1353, 60–71. doi: 10.1111/NYAS.12807

Moloney, A. M., Griffin, R. J., Timmons, S., O'Connor, R., Ravid, R., and O'Neill, C. (2010). Defects in IGF-1 receptor, insulin receptor and IRS-1/2 in Alzheimer's disease indicate possible resistance to IGF-1 and insulin signalling. *Neurobiol. Aging* 31, 224–243. doi: 10.1016/J.NEUROBIOLAGING.2008.04.002

Monje, M. L., Toda, H., and Palmer, T. D. (2003). Inflammatory blockade restores adult hippocampal neurogenesis. *Science* 302, 1760–1765. doi: 10.1126/science.1088417

Morash, B., Li, A., Murphy, P. R., Wilkinson, M., and Ur, E. (1999). Leptin gene expression in the brain and pituitary gland. *Endocrinology* 140, 5995–5998. doi: 10.1210/endo.140.12.7288

Moro, C., Bajpeyi, S., and Smith, S. R. (2008). Determinants of intramyocellular triglyceride turnover: implications for insulin sensitivity. *Am. J. Physiol. Metab.* 294, E203–E213. doi: 10.1152/ajpendo.00624.2007

Mottahedin, A., Ardalan, M., Chumak, T., Riebe, I., Ek, J., and Mallard, C. (2017). Effect of neuroinflammation on synaptic organization and function in the developing brain: implications for neurodevelopmental and neurodegenerative disorders. *Front. Cell. Neurosci.* 11:190. doi: 10.3389/fncel.2017.00190

Mrak, R. E. (2009). Alzheimer-type neuropathological changes in morbidly obese elderly individuals. *Clin. Neuropathol.* 28, 40–45.

Murray, A. J., Knight, N. S., Cochlin, L. E., McAleese, S., Deacon, R. M. J., Rawlins, J. N. P., et al. (2009). Deterioration of physical performance and cognitive function in rats with short-term high-fat feeding. *FASEB J.* 23, 4353–4360. doi: 10.1096/fj.09-139691

Neumeier, M., Weigert, J., Buettner, R., Wanninger, J., Schäffler, A., Mü, A. M., et al. (2007). Detection of adiponectin in cerebrospinal fluid in humans Downloaded from. *Am. J. Physiol. Endocrinol. Metab.* 293, 965–969. doi: 10.1152/ajpendo.00119.2007

Ng, R. C.-L., and Chan, K.-H. (2017). Potential neuroprotective effects of adiponectin in Alzheimer's disease. *Int. J. Mol. Sci.* 18:E592. doi: 10.3390/ijms18030592

Ng, R. C.-L., Cheng, O.-Y., Jian, M., Kwan, J. S.-C., Ho, P. W.-L., Cheng, K. K.-Y., et al. (2016). Chronic adiponectin deficiency leads to Alzheimer's disease-like cognitive impairments and pathologies through AMPK inactivation and cerebral insulin resistance in aged mice. *Mol. Neurodegener.* 11:71. doi: 10.1186/s13024-016-0136-x

Nguyen, J. C. D., Killcross, A. S., and Jenkins, T. A. (2014). Obesity and cognitive decline: role of inflammation and vascular changes. *Front. Neurosci.* 8:375. doi: 10.3389/fnins.2014.00375

Nicholson, T., Church, C., Baker, D. J., and Jones, S. W. (2018). The role of adipokines in skeletal muscle inflammation and insulin sensitivity. *J. Inflamm.* 15:9. doi: 10.1186/s12950-018-0185-8

Nishimura, M., Izumiya, Y., Higuchi, A., Shibata, R., Qiu, J., Kudo, C., et al. (2008). Adiponectin prevents cerebral ischemic injury through endothelial nitric oxide synthase–dependent mechanisms. *Circulation* 117, 216–223. doi: 10.1161/CIRCULATIONAHA.107.725044

Nobili, V., Carter-Kent, C., and Feldstein, A. E. (2011). The role of lifestyle changes in the management of chronic liver disease. *BMC Med.* 9:70. doi: 10.1186/1741-7015-9-70

Oakes, N. D., Bell, K. S., Furler, S. M., Camilleri, S., Saha, A. K., Ruderman, N. B., et al. (1997). Diet-induced muscle insulin resistance in rats is ameliorated by acute dietary lipid withdrawal or a single bout of exercise: parallel relationship between insulin stimulation of glucose uptake and suppression of long-chain fatty acyl-CoA. *Diabetes* 46, 2022–2028.

Ommen, S. R., and Lopez-Jimenez, F. (2013). Obesity and hypertrophic cardiomyopathy. *J. Am. Coll. Cardiol.* 62, 458–459. doi: 10.1016/j.jacc.2013.03.063

Oomura, Y., Aou, S., and Fukunaga, K. (2010). Prandial increase of leptin in the brain activates spatial learning and memory. *Pathophysiology* 17, 119–127. doi: 10.1016/j.pathophys.2009.04.004

Orkaby, A. R., Cho, K., Cormack, J., Gagnon, D. R., and Driver, J. A. (2017). Metformin vs sulfonylurea use and risk of dementia in US veterans aged=65 years with diabetes. *Neurology* 89, 1877–1885. doi: 10.1212/WNL.0000000000004586

O'Rourke, R. W. (2010). Inflammation in obesity-related disease. *Surgery* 145, 255–259. doi: 10.1016/j.surg.2008.08.038

Ott, A., Stolk, R. P., Hofman, A., Van Harskamp, F., Grobbee, D. E., and Breteler, M. M. B. (1996). *Association of Diabetes Mellitus and Dementia: The Rotterdam Study*. Available at: https://core.ac.uk/download/pdf/43310876.pdf (accessed April 19, 2019).

Pagano, G., Pacini, G., Musso, G., Gambino, R., Mecca, F., Depetris, N., et al. (2002). Nonalcoholic steatohepatitis, insulin resistance, and metabolic syndrome: Further evidence for an etiologic association. *Hepatology* 35, 367–372. doi: 10.1053/JHEP.2002.30690

Pan, W., Tu, H., and Kastin, A. J. (2006). Differential BBB interactions of three ingestive peptides: obestatin, ghrelin, and adiponectin. *Peptides* 27, 911–916. doi: 10.1016/j.peptides.2005.12.014

Pannacciulli, N., Del Parigi, A., Chen, K., Le, D. S., Reiman, E. M., and Tataranni, P. A. (2006). Brain abnormalities in human obesity: a voxel-based morphometric study. *Neuroimage* 31, 1419–1425. doi: 10.1016/j.neuroimage.2006.01.047

Park, H. K., and Ahima, R. S. (2013). Resistin in rodents and humans. *Diabetes Metab. J.* 37, 404–414. doi: 10.4093/dmj.2013.37.6.404

Park, H. K., Kwak, M. K., Kim, H. J., and Ahima, R. S. (2017). Linking resistin, inflammation, and cardiometabolic diseases. *Korean J. Intern. Med.* 32, 239–247. doi: 10.3904/kjim.2016.229

Park, S., Kim, D. S., Kwon, D. Y., and Yang, H. J. (2011). Long-term central infusion of adiponectin improves energy and glucose homeostasis by decreasing fat storage and suppressing hepatic gluconeogenesis without changing food intake. *J. Neuroendocrinol.* 23, 687–698. doi: 10.1111/j.1365-2826.2011.02165.x

Pedersen, B. K. (2013). Muscle as a secretory organ. *Compr. Physiol.* 3, 1337–1362. doi: 10.1002/cphy.c120033

Peeters, A., Barendregt, J. J., Willekens, F., Mackenbach, J. P., Al Mamun, A., Bonneux, L., et al. (2003). Obesity in adulthood and its consequences for life expectancy: a life-table analysis. *Ann. Intern. Med.* 138, 24–32.

Peila, R., Rodriguez, B. L., Launer, L. J., and Honolulu-Asia Aging Study. (2002). Type 2 diabetes, APOE gene, and the risk for dementia and related pathologies. *Diabetes* 51, 1256–1262. doi: 10.2337/DIABETES.51.4.1256

Pezzilli, R., and Calculli, L. (2014). Pancreatic steatosis: Is it related to either obesity or diabetes mellitus? *World J. Diabetes* 5, 415–419. doi: 10.4239/wjd.v5.i4.415

Piché, M.-E., and Poirier, P. (2018). Obesity, ectopic fat and cardiac metabolism. *Expert Rev. Endocrinol. Metab.* 13, 213–221. doi: 10.1080/17446651.2018.1500894

Pinnick, K. E., Collins, S. C., Londos, C., Gauguier, D., Clark, A., and Fielding, B. A. (2008). Pancreatic ectopic fat is characterized by adipocyte infiltration and altered lipid composition. *Obesity* 16, 522–530. doi: 10.1038/oby.2007.110

Poitout, V. (2004). β-cell lipotoxicity: burning fat into heat? *Endocrinology* 145, 3563–3565. doi: 10.1210/en.2004-0479

Preis, S. R., Massaro, J. M., Hoffmann, U., D'Agostino, R. B., Levy, D., Robins, S. J., et al. (2010). Neck circumference as a novel measure of cardiometabolic risk: the framingham heart study. *J. Clin. Endocrinol. Metab.* 95, 3701–3710. doi: 10.1210/jc.2009-1779

Prickett, C., Brennan, L., and Stolwyk, R. (2015). Examining the relationship between obesity and cognitive function: a systematic literature review. *Obes. Res. Clin. Pract.* 9, 93–113. doi: 10.1016/j.orcp.2014.05.001

Profenno, L. A., Porsteinsson, A. P., and Faraone, S. V. (2010). Meta-analysis of Alzheimer's disease risk with obesity. *Diabetes Relat. Disord. Biol. Psychiatry* 67, 505–512. doi: 10.1016/J.BIOPSYCH.2009.02.013

Puig, K. L., Floden, A. M., Adhikari, R., Golovko, M. Y., and Combs, C. K. (2012). Amyloid precursor protein and proinflammatory changes are regulated in brain and adipose tissue in a murine model of high fat diet-induced obesity. *PLoS One* 7:e30378. doi: 10.1371/journal.pone.0030378

Purkayastha, S., and Cai, D. (2013). Disruption of neurogenesis by hypothalamic inflammation in obesity or aging. *Rev. Endocr. Metab. Disord.* 14, 351–356. doi: 10.1007/s11154-013-9279-z

Qi, Y., Takahashi, N., Hileman, S. M., Patel, H. R., Berg, A. H., Pajvani, U. B., et al. (2004). Adiponectin acts in the brain to decrease body weight. *Nat. Med.* 10, 524–529. doi: 10.1038/nm1029

Qureshi, K., and Abrams, G. A. (2007). Metabolic liver disease of obesity and role of adipose tissue in the pathogenesis of nonalcoholic fatty liver disease. *World J. Gastroenterol.* 13, 3540–3553. doi: 10.3748/wjg.v13.i26.3540

Raji, C. A., Ho, A. J., Parikshak, N. N., Becker, J. T., Lopez, O. L., Kuller, L. H., et al. (2009). Brain structure and obesity. *Hum. Brain Mapp.* 31, 353–364. doi: 10.1002/hbm.20870

Rasgon, N. L., Kenna, H. A., Wroolie, T. E., Kelley, R., Silverman, D., Brooks, J., et al. (2011). Insulin resistance and hippocampal volume in women at risk for Alzheimer's disease. *Neurobiol. Aging* 32, 1942–1948. doi: 10.1016/J.NEUROBIOLAGING.2009.12.005

Rawlings, A. M., Sharrett, A. R., Mosley, T. H., Ballew, S. H., Deal, J. A., and Selvin, E. (2017). Glucose peaks and the risk of dementia and 20-year cognitive decline. *Diabetes Care* 40, 879–886. doi: 10.2337/dc16-2203

Reaven, G. M. (1995). Pathophysiology of insulin resistance in human disease. *Physiol. Rev.* 75, 473–486. doi: 10.1152/physrev.1995.75.3.473

Riederer, P., Korczyn, A. D., Ali, S. S., Bajenaru, O., Choi, M. S., Chopp, M., et al. (2017). The diabetic brain and cognition. *J. Neural Transm.* 124, 1431–1454. doi: 10.1007/s00702-017-1763-2

Rolland, Y., Lauwers-Cances, V., Cristini, C., van Kan, G. A., Janssen, I., Morley, J. E., et al. (2009). Difficulties with physical function associated with obesity, sarcopenia, and sarcopenic-obesity in community-dwelling elderly women: the EPIDOS (EPIDemiologie de l'OSteoporose) Study. *Am. J. Clin. Nutr.* 89, 1895–1900. doi: 10.3945/ajcn.2008.26950

Rolland, Y., Lauwers-Cances, V., Pahor, M., Fillaux, J., Grandjean, H., and Vellas, B. (2004). Muscle strength in obese elderly women: effect of recreational physical activity in a cross-sectional study. *Am. J. Clin. Nutr.* 79, 552–557. doi: 10.1093/ajcn/79.4.552

Rosito, G. A., Massaro, J. M., Hoffmann, U., Ruberg, F. L., Mahabadi, A. A., Vasan, R. S., et al. (2008). Pericardial fat, visceral abdominal fat, cardiovascular disease risk factors, and vascular calcification in a community-based sample. *Circulation* 117, 605–613. doi: 10.1161/CIRCULATIONAHA.107.743062

Ross, R., Lam, M., Blair, S. N., Church, T. S., Godwin, M., Hotz, S. B., et al. (2012). Trial of prevention and reduction of obesity through active living in clinical settings. *Arch. Intern. Med.* 172, 414–424. doi: 10.1001/archinternmed.2011.1972

Rutkowski, J. M., and Scherer, P. E. (2014). Isolation and quantitation of adiponectin higher order complexes. *Methods Enzymol.* 537, 243–259. doi: 10.1016/B978-0-12-411619-1.00013-6

Ryan, A. S., Berman, D. M., Nicklas, B. J., Sinha, M., Gingerich, R. L., Meneilly, G. S., et al. (2003). Plasma adiponectin and leptin levels, body composition, and glucose utilization in adult women with wide ranges of age and obesity. *Diabetes Care* 26, 2383–2388. doi: 10.2337/DIACARE.26.8.2383

Sabia, S., Kivimaki, M., Shipley, M. J., Marmot, M. G., and Singh-Manoux, A. (2009). Body mass index over the adult life course and cognition in late midlife: the Whitehall II Cohort Study. *Am. J. Clin. Nutr.* 89, 601–607. doi: 10.3945/ajcn.2008.26482

Sacks, H. S., and Fain, J. N. (2007). Human epicardial adipose tissue: a review. *Am. Heart J.* 153, 907–917. doi: 10.1016/j.ahj.2007.03.019

Sakurai, T., Kawashima, S., Satake, S., Miura, H., Tokuda, H., and Toba, K. (2014). Differential subtypes of diabetic older adults diagnosed with Alzheimer's disease. *Geriatr. Gerontol. Int.* 14, 62–70. doi: 10.1111/ggi.12250

Samanta, R., Pouliopoulos, J., Thiagalingam, A., Kovoor, P., and Bs, M. B. (2015). Role of adipose tissue in the pathogenesis of cardiac arrhythmias. *Heart Rhythm* 13, 311–320. doi: 10.1016/j.hrthm.2015.08.016

Sanderlin, A. H., Todem, D., and Bozoki, A. C. (2017). Obesity and Co-morbid conditions are associated with specific neuropsychiatric symptoms in mild cognitive impairment. *Front. Aging Neurosci.* 9:164. doi: 10.3389/fnagi.2017.00164

Sanyal, A. J., Campbell-Sargent, C., Mirshahi, F., Rizzo, W. B., Contos, M. J., Sterling, R. K., et al. (2001). Nonalcoholic steatohepatitis: association of insulin resistance and mitochondrial abnormalities. *Gastroenterology* 120, 1183–1192. doi: 10.1053/GAST.2001.23256

Schauer, P. R., Bhatt, D. L., Kirwan, J. P., Wolski, K., Aminian, A., Brethauer, S. A., et al. (2017). Bariatric surgery versus intensive medical therapy for diabetes — 5-year outcomes. *N. Engl. J. Med.* 376, 641–651. doi: 10.1056/NEJMoa1600869

Schubert, M., Brazil, D. P., Burks, D. J., Kushner, J. A., Ye, J., Flint, C. L., et al. (2003). Insulin receptor substrate-2 deficiency impairs brain growth and promotes tau phosphorylation. *J. Neurosci.* 23, 7084–7092.

Schulz, C., Paulus, K., and Lehnert, H. (2011). Adipocyte–brain: crosstalk. *Results Probl. Cell Differ.* 52, 189–201. doi: 10.1007/978-3-642-14426-4_16

Schwingshackl, L., Dias, S., and Hoffmann, G. (2014). Impact of long-term lifestyle programmes on weight loss and cardiovascular risk factors in overweight/obese participants: a systematic review and network meta-analysis. *Syst. Rev.* 3:130.

Shanley, L. J., Irving, A. J., and Harvey, J. (2001). Leptin enhances NMDA receptor function and modulates hippocampal synaptic plasticity. *J. Neurosci.* 21:RC186.

Shea, M. K., Nicklas, B. J., Houston, D. K., Miller, M. E., Davis, C. C., Kitzman, D. W., et al. (2011). The effect of intentional weight loss on all-cause mortality in older adults: results of a randomized controlled weight-loss trial. *Am. J. Clin. Nutr.* 94, 839–846. doi: 10.3945/ajcn.110.006379

Simerly, R. B. (2008). Hypothalamic substrates of metabolic imprinting. *Physiol. Behav.* 94, 79–89. doi: 10.1016/j.physbeh.2007.11.023

Simon, G. E., Von Korff, M., Saunders, K., Miglioretti, D. L., Crane, P. K., van Belle, G., et al. (2006). Association between obesity and psychiatric disorders in the US adult population. *Arch. Gen. Psychiatry* 63, 824–830. doi: 10.1001/archpsyc.63.7.824

Sims-Robinson, C., Kim, B., Rosko, A., and Feldman, E. L. (2010). How does diabetes accelerate Alzheimer disease pathology? *Nat. Rev. Neurol.* 6, 551–559. doi: 10.1038/nrneurol.2010.130

Singh-Manoux, A., Dugravot, A., Shipley, M., Brunner, E. J., Elbaz, A., Sabia, S., et al. (2018). Obesity trajectories and risk of dementia: 28 years of follow-up in the Whitehall II Study. *Alzheimers Dement.* 14, 178–186. doi: 10.1016/j.jalz.2017.06.2637

Singla, P., Bardoloi, A., and Parkash, A. A. (2010). Metabolic effects of obesity: a review. *World J. Diabetes* 1, 76–88. doi: 10.4239/wjd.v1.i3.76

Sjöström, L., Narbro, K., Sjöström, C. D., Karason, K., Larsson, B., Wedel, H., et al. (2007). Effects of bariatric surgery on mortality in swedish obese subjects. *N. Engl. J. Med.* 357, 741–752. doi: 10.1056/NEJMoa066254

Snijder, M. B., Dekker, J. M., Visser, M., Bouter, L. M., Stehouwer, C. D. A., Kostense, P. J., et al. (2003a). Associations of hip and thigh circumferences independent of waist circumference with the incidence of type 2 diabetes: the Hoorn study. *Am. J. Clin. Nutr.* 77, 1192–1197.

Snijder, M. B., Dekker, J. M., Visser, M., Yudkin, J. S., Stehouwer, C. D. A., Bouter, L. M., et al. (2003b). Larger thigh and hip circumferences are associated with better glucose tolerance: the Hoorn study. *Obes. Res.* 11, 104–111. doi: 10.1038/oby.2003.18

Sonar, S. A., and Lal, G. (2018). Blood-brain barrier and its function during inflammation and autoimmunity. *J. Leukoc. Biol.* 103, 839–853. doi: 10.1002/JLB.1RU1117-428R

Sørensen, T. I., Rissanen, A., Korkeila, M., and Kaprio, J. (2005). Intention to lose weight, weight changes, and 18-y mortality in overweight individuals without co-morbidities. *PLoS Med.* 2:e171. doi: 10.1371/journal.pmed.0020171

Sowemimo, O. A., Yood, S. M., Courtney, J., Moore, J., Huang, M., Ross, R., et al. (2007). Natural history of morbid obesity without surgical intervention. *Surg. Obes. Relat. Dis.* 3, 73–77. doi: 10.1016/j.soard.2006.10.017

Spalding, K. L., Arner, E., Westermark, P. O., Bernard, S., Buchholz, B. A., Bergmann, O., et al. (2008). Dynamics of fat cell turnover in humans. *Nature* 453, 783–787. doi: 10.1038/nature06902

Spranger, J., Verma, S., Göhring, I., Bobbert, T., Seifert, J., Sindler, A. L., et al. (2006). Adiponectin does not cross the blood-brain barrier but modifies cytokine expression of brain endothelial cells. *Diabetes* 55, 141–147.

Stefan, N., Kantartzis, K., Machann, J., Schick, F., Thamer, C., Rittig, K., et al. (2008). Identification and characterization of metabolically benign obesity in humans. *Arch. Intern. Med.* 168, 1609–1616. doi: 10.1001/archinte.168.15.1609

Stenlöf, K., Wernstedt, I., Fjällman, T., Wallenius, V., Wallenius, K., and Jansson, J.-O. (2003). Interleukin-6 levels in the central nervous system are negatively correlated with fat mass in overweight/obese subjects. *J. Clin. Endocrinol. Metab.* 88, 4379–4383. doi: 10.1210/jc.2002-021733

Stillman, C. M., Weinstein, A. M., Marsland, A. L., Gianaros, P. J., and Erickson, K. I. (2017). Body-brain connections: the effects of obesity and behavioral interventions on neurocognitive aging. *Front. Aging Neurosci.* 9:115. doi: 10. 3389/fnagi.2017.00115

Studzinski, C. M., Li, F., Bruce-Keller, A. J., Fernandez-Kim, S. O., Zhang, L., Weidner, A. M., et al. (2009). Effects of short-term Western diet on cerebral oxidative stress and diabetes related factors in APP × PS1 knock-in mice. *J. Neurochem.* 108, 860–866. doi: 10.1111/j.1471-4159.2008.05798.x

Su, F., Shu, H., Ye, Q., Wang, Z., Xie, C., Yuan, B., et al. (2017). Brain insulin resistance deteriorates cognition by altering the topological features of brain networks. *Neuroimage Clin.* 13, 280–287. doi: 10.1016/J.NICL.2016.12.009

Suganami, T., Nishida, J., and Ogawa, Y. (2005). A paracrine loop between adipocytes and macrophages aggravates inflammatory changes. *Arterioscler. Thromb. Vasc. Biol.* 25, 2062–2068. doi: 10.1161/01.ATV.0000183883.72263.13

Szczepaniak, L. S., Dobbins, R. L., Metzger, G. J., Sartoni-D'Ambrosia, G., Arbique, D., Vongpatanasin, W., et al. (2003). Myocardial triglycerides and systolic function in humans: in vivo evaluation by localized proton spectroscopy and cardiac imaging. *Magn. Reson. Med.* 49, 417–423. doi: 10.1002/mrm.10372

Talbot, K., and Wang, H.-Y. (2014). The nature, significance, and glucagon-like peptide-1 analog treatment of brain insulin resistance in Alzheimer's disease. *Alzheimers Dement.* 10, S12–S25. doi: 10.1016/J.JALZ.2013.12.007

Talbot, K., Wang, H.-Y., Kazi, H., Han, L.-Y., Bakshi, K. P., Stucky, A., et al. (2012). Demonstrated brain insulin resistance in Alzheimer's disease patients is associated with IGF-1 resistance, IRS-1 dysregulation, and cognitive decline. *J. Clin. Invest.* 122, 1316–1338. doi: 10.1172/JCI59903

Tchernof, A., Bélanger, C., Morisset, A. S., Richard, C., Mailloux, J., Laberge, P., et al. (2006). Regional differences in adipose tissue metabolism in women: minor effect of obesity and body fat distribution. *Diabetes* 55, 1353–1360. doi: 10.2337/db05-1439

Tchkonia, T., Lenburg, M., Thomou, T., Giorgadze, N., Frampton, G., Pirtskhalava, T., et al. (2007). Identification of depot-specific human fat cell progenitors through distinct expression profiles and developmental gene patterns. *Am. J. Physiol. Metab.* 292, E298–E307. doi: 10.1152/ajpendo.00202.2006

Tiemann Luecking, C., Yoshino, M., Klein, S., Samovski, D., Magkos, F., Okunade, A. L., et al. (2015). Metabolically normal obese people are protected from adverse effects following weight gain. *J. Clin. Invest.* 125, 787–795. doi: 10.1172/jci78425

Tilg, H., and Moschen, A. R. (2006). Adipocytokines: mediators linking adipose tissue, inflammation and immunity. *Nat. Rev. Immunol.* 6, 772–783. doi: 10. 1038/nri1937

Tiniakos, D. G., Vos, M. B., and Brunt, E. M. (2010). Nonalcoholic fatty liver disease: pathology and pathogenesis. *Annu. Rev. Pathol. Mech. Dis.* 5, 145–171. doi: 10.1146/annurev-pathol-121808-102132

Tobias, D. K., Chen, M., Manson, J. E., Ludwig, D. S., Willett, W., and Hu, F. B. (2015). Effect of low-fat diet interventions versus other diet interventions on long-term weight change in adults: a systematic review and meta-analysis. *Lancet Diabetes Endocrinol.* 3, 968–979. doi: 10.1016/S2213-8587(15)00367-8

Tomlinson, D. J., Erskine, R. M., Morse, C. I., Winwood, K., and Onambélé-Pearson, G. (2016). The impact of obesity on skeletal muscle strength and structure through adolescence to old age. *Biogerontology* 17, 467–483. doi: 10.1007/s10522-015-9626-4

Tong, Q., and Xu, Y. (2012). Central leptin regulation of obesity and fertility. *Curr. Obes. Rep.* 1, 236–244. doi: 10.1007/s13679-012-0025-8

Torres-Villalobos, G., Hamdan-Pérez, N., Díaz-Villaseñor, A., Tovar, A. R., Torre-Villalvazo, I., Ordaz-Nava, G., et al. (2016). Autologous subcutaneous adipose tissue transplants improve adipose tissue metabolism and reduce insulin resistance and fatty liver in diet-induced obesity rats. *Physiol. Rep.* 4:e12909. doi: 10.14814/phy2.12909

Townsend, K., and Tseng, Y.-H. (2012). Brown adipose tissue. *Adipocyte* 1, 13–24. doi: 10.4161/adip.18951

Tran, T. T., Yamamoto, Y., Gesta, S., and Kahn, C. R. (2008). Beneficial effects of subcutaneous fat transplantation on metabolism. *Cell Metab.* 7, 410–420. doi: 10.1016/j.cmet.2008.04.004

Trayhurn, P., Drevon, C. A., and Eckel, J. (2011). Secreted proteins from adipose tissue and skeletal muscle – adipokines, myokines and adipose/muscle cross-talk. *Arch. Physiol. Biochem.* 117, 47–56. doi: 10.3109/13813455.2010.535835

van Bloemendaal, L., Ijzerman, R. G., Ten Kulve, J. S., Barkhof, F., Diamant, M., Veltman, D. J., et al. (2016). Alterations in white matter volume and integrity in obesity and type 2 diabetes. *Metab. Brain Dis.* 31, 621–629. doi: 10.1007/s11011-016-9792-3

van den Berg, E., de Craen, A. J. M., Biessels, G. J., Gussekloo, J., and Westendorp, R. G. J. (2006). The impact of diabetes mellitus on cognitive decline in the oldest of the old: a prospective population-based study. *Diabetologia* 49, 2015–2023.

van den Berg, E., Reijmer, Y. D., de Bresser, J., Kessels, R. P. C., Kappelle, L. J., Biessels, G. J., et al. (2010). A 4 year follow-up study of cognitive functioning in patients with type 2 diabetes mellitus. *Diabetologia* 53, 58–65. doi: 10.1007/S00125-009-1571-9

Viljanen, A. P. M., Iozzo, P., Borra, R., Kankaanpää, M., Karmi, A., Lautamäki, R., et al. (2009). Effect of weight loss on liver free fatty acid uptake and hepatic insulin resistance. *J. Clin. Endocrinol. Metab.* 94, 50–55. doi: 10.1210/jc.2008-1689

Wadden, T. A., Volger, S., Sarwer, D. B., Vetter, M. L., Tsai, A. G., Berkowitz, R. I., et al. (2011). A two-year randomized trial of obesity treatment in primary care practice. *N. Engl. J. Med.* 365, 1969–1979. doi: 10.1056/NEJMoa1109220

Wajchenberg, B. L. (2000). Subcutaneous and visceral adipose tissue: their relation to the metabolic syndrome. *Endocr. Rev.* 21, 697–738. doi: 10.1210/edrv.21.6. 0415

Wallace, J. I., and Schwartz, R. S. (2002). Epidemiology of weight loss in humans with special reference to wasting in the elderly. *Int. J. Cardiol.* 85, 15–21.

Waragai, M., Ho, G., Takamatsu, Y., Sekiyama, K., Sugama, S., Takenouchi, T., et al. (2017). Importance of adiponectin activity in the pathogenesis of Alzheimer's disease. *Ann. Clin. Transl. Neurol.* 4, 591–600. doi: 10.1002/acn3.436

Waters, D. L., Ward, A. L., and Villareal, D. T. (2013). Weight loss in obese adults 65years and older: a review of the controversy. *Exp. Gerontol.* 48, 1054–1061. doi: 10.1016/j.exger.2013.02.005

Wayner, M., Armstrong, D., Phelix, C., and Oomura, Y. (2004). Orexin-A (Hypocretin-1) and leptin enhance LTP in the dentate gyrus of rats in vivo. *Peptides* 25, 991–996. doi: 10.1016/j.peptides.2004.03.018

Wen, J.-P., Liu, C., Hu, Y.-T., Chen, G., and Lin, L. (2010). Globular adiponectin regulates energy homeostasis through AMP-activated protein kinase–acetyl-CoA carboxylase (AMPK/ACC) pathway in the hypothalamus. *Mol. Cell. Biochem.* 344, 109–115. doi: 10.1007/s11010-010-0534-2

Wennberg, A. M. V., Gustafson, D., Hagen, C. E., Roberts, R. O., Knopman, D., Jack, C., et al. (2016). Serum adiponectin levels, neuroimaging, and cognition in the mayo clinic study of aging. *J. Alzheimers Dis.* 53, 573–581. doi: 10.3233/JAD-151201

West, R. K., Ravona-Springer, R., Schmeidler, J., Leroith, D., Koifman, K., Guerrero-Berroa, E., et al. (2014). The association of duration of type 2 diabetes with cognitive performance is modulated by long-term glycemic control. *Am. J. Geriatr. Psychiatry* 22, 1055–1059. doi: 10.1016/j.jagp.2014.01.010

Whitmer, R. A., Gustafson, D. R., Barrett-Connor, E., Haan, M. N., Gunderson, E. P., and Yaffe, K. (2008). Central obesity and increased risk of dementia more than three decades later. *Neurology* 71, 1057–1064. doi: 10.1212/01.wnl. 0000306313.89165.ef

Wiesner, G., Vaz, M., Collier, G., Seals, D., Kaye, D., Jennings, G., et al. (1999). Leptin is released from the human brain: influence of adiposity and gender 1. *J. Clin. Endocrinol. Metab.* 84, 2270–2274. doi: 10.1210/jcem.84.7.5854

Wilkinson, M., Brown, R., Imran, S. A., and Ur, E. (2007). Adipokine gene expression in brain and pituitary gland. *Neuroendocrinology* 86, 191–209. doi: 10.1159/000108635

Willner, I. R., Waters, B., Patil, S. R., Reuben, A., Morelli, J., and Riely, C. A. (2001). Ninety patients with nonalcoholic steatohepatitis: insulin resistance, familial tendency, and severity of disease. *Am. J. Gastroenterol.* 96, 2957–2961. doi: 10.1111/j.1572-0241.2001.04667.x

Wing, R. R., and Phelan, S. (2005). Long-term weight loss maintenance. *Am. J. Clin. Nutr.* 82, 222S–225S. doi: 10.1093/ajcn/82.1.222S

Wolf, P. A. (2012). Contributions of the framingham heart study to stroke and dementia epidemiologic research at 60 years. *Arch. Neurol.* 69, 567. doi: 10.1001/archneurol.2011.977

Wong, C., and Marwick, T. H. (2007). Obesity cardiomyopathy: diagnosis and therapeutic implications. *Nat. Clin. Pract. Cardiovasc. Med.* 4, 480–490. doi: 10.1038/ncpcardio0964

Wright, S. M., and Aronne, L. J. (2012). Causes of obesity. *Abdom. Imaging* 37, 730–732. doi: 10.1007/s00261-012-9862-x

Xiao, C., Dash, S., Morgantini, C., Hegele, R. A., and Lewis, G. F. (2016). Pharmacological targeting of the atherogenic dyslipidemia complex: the next frontier in CVD prevention beyond lowering LDL cholesterol. *Diabetes* 65, 1767–1778. doi: 10.2337/db16-0046

Xu, W. L., von Strauss, E., Qiu, C. X., Winblad, B., and Fratiglioni, L. (2009). Uncontrolled diabetes increases the risk of Alzheimer's disease: a population-based cohort study. *Diabetologia* 52, 1031–1039. doi: 10.1007/s00125-009-1323-x

Xu, Y., and Tong, Q. (2011). Expanding neurotransmitters in the hypothalamic neurocircuitry for energy balance regulation. *Protein Cell* 2, 800–813. doi: 10.1007/s13238-011-1112-4

Yaari, S., and Goldbourt, U. (1998). Voluntary and involuntary weight loss: associations with long term mortality in 9,228 middle-aged and elderly men. *Am. J. Epidemiol.* 148, 546–555.

Yaffe, K. (2007). Metabolic syndrome and cognitive decline. *Curr. Alzheimer Res.* 4, 123–126.

Yaffe, K., Falvey, C., Hamilton, N., Schwartz, A. V., Simonsick, E. M., Satterfield, S., et al. (2012). Diabetes, glucose control, and 9-year cognitive decline among older adults without dementia. *Arch. Neurol.* 69, 1170–1175. doi: 10.1001/archneurol.2012.1117

Yano, Y., Bakris, G. L., Inokuchi, T., Ohba, Y., Tamaki, N., Nagata, M., et al. (2014). Association of cognitive dysfunction with cardiovascular disease events in elderly hypertensive patients. *J. Hypertens.* 32, 423–431. doi: 10.1097/HJH.0000000000000025

Yates, K. F., Sweat, V., Yau, P. L., Turchiano, M. M., and Convit, A. (2012). Impact of metabolic syndrome on cognition and brain. *Arterioscler. Thromb. Vasc. Biol.* 32, 2060–2067. doi: 10.1161/ATVBAHA.112.252759

Yau, S. Y., Li, A., Hoo, R. L. C., Ching, Y. P., Christie, B. R., Lee, T. M. C., et al. (2014). Physical exercise-induced hippocampal neurogenesis and antidepressant effects are mediated by the adipocyte hormone adiponectin. *Proc. Natl. Acad. Sci. U.S.A.* 111, 15810–15815. doi: 10.1073/pnas.1415219111

Ye, J. (2013). Mechanisms of insulin resistance in obesity. *Front. Med.* 7, 14–24. doi: 10.1007/s11684-013-0262-6

Yoshiyama, Y., Higuchi, M., Zhang, B., Huang, S.-M., Iwata, N., Saido, T. C., et al. (2007). Synapse loss and microglial activation precede tangles in a p301s tauopathy mouse model. *Neuron* 53, 337–351. doi: 10.1016/j.neuron.2007.01.010

Young, S. E., Mainous, A. G., and Carnemolla, M. (2006). Hyperinsulinemia and cognitive decline in a middle-aged cohort. *Diabetes Care* 29, 2688–2693. doi: 10.2337/DC06-0915

Yu, Y.-H., and Ginsberg, H. N. (2005). Adipocyte signaling and lipid homeostasis. *Circ. Res.* 96, 1042–1052. doi: 10.1161/01.RES.0000165803.47776.38

Zhang, D., Guo, M., Zhang, W., and Lu, X.-Y. (2011). Adiponectin Stimulates Proliferation of Adult Hippocampal Neural Stem/Progenitor Cells through Activation of p38 Mitogen-activated Protein Kinase (p38MAPK)/Glycogen Synthase Kinase 3β (GSK-3β)/β-Catenin Signaling Cascade. *J. Biol. Chem.* 286, 44913–44920. doi: 10.1074/jbc.M111.310052

Zhang, D., Wang, X., and Lu, X.-Y. (2016). Adiponectin exerts neurotrophic effects on dendritic arborization, spinogenesis, and neurogenesis of the dentate gyrus of male mice. *Endocrinology* 157, 2853–2869. doi: 10.1210/en.2015-2078

Zhang, L., Hou, Y., and Po, S. S. (2015). Obstructive sleep apnoea and atrial fibrillation. *Arrhythmia Electrophysiol. Rev.* 4, 14–18. doi: 10.15420/aer.2015.4.1.14

Zhang, Y., Zitsman, J. L., Hou, J., Fennoy, I., Guo, K., Feinberg, J., et al. (2014). Fat cell size and adipokine expression in relation to gender, depot, and metabolic risk factors in morbidly obese adolescents. *Obesity* 22, 691–697. doi: 10.1002/oby.20528

Zhao, X., Han, Q., Lv, Y., Sun, L., Gang, X., and Wang, G. (2018). Biomarkers for cognitive decline in patients with diabetes mellitus: evidence from clinical studies. *Oncotarget* 9, 7710–7726. doi: 10.18632/oncotarget.23284

Zhao, Y.-F., Feng, D. D., and Chen, C. (2006). Contribution of adipocyte-derived factors to beta-cell dysfunction in diabetes. *Int. J. Biochem. Cell Biol.* 38, 804–819. doi: 10.1016/j.biocel.2005.11.008

Zlokovic, B. V. (2011). Neurovascular pathways to neurodegeneration in Alzheimer's disease and other disorders. *Nat. Rev. Neurosci.* 12, 723–738. doi: 10.1038/nrn3114

Zoico, E., Di Francesco, V., Guralnik, J. M., Mazzali, G., Bortolani, A., Guariento, S., et al. (2004). Physical disability and muscular strength in relation to obesity and different body composition indexes in a sample of healthy elderly women. *Int. J. Obes.* Relat. Metab. Disord. 28, 234–241. doi: 10.1038/sj.ijo.0802552

Permissions

All chapters in this book were first published by Frontiers; hereby published with permission under the Creative Commons Attribution License or equivalent. Every chapter published in this book has been scrutinized by our experts. Their significance has been extensively debated. The topics covered herein carry significant findings which will fuel the growth of the discipline. They may even be implemented as practical applications or may be referred to as a beginning point for another development.

The contributors of this book come from diverse backgrounds, making this book a truly international effort. This book will bring forth new frontiers with its revolutionizing research information and detailed analysis of the nascent developments around the world.

We would like to thank all the contributing authors for lending their expertise to make the book truly unique. They have played a crucial role in the development of this book. Without their invaluable contributions this book wouldn't have been possible. They have made vital efforts to compile up to date information on the varied aspects of this subject to make this book a valuable addition to the collection of many professionals and students.

This book was conceptualized with the vision of imparting up-to-date information and advanced data in this field. To ensure the same, a matchless editorial board was set up. Every individual on the board went through rigorous rounds of assessment to prove their worth. After which they invested a large part of their time researching and compiling the most relevant data for our readers.

The editorial board has been involved in producing this book since its inception. They have spent rigorous hours researching and exploring the diverse topics which have resulted in the successful publishing of this book. They have passed on their knowledge of decades through this book. To expedite this challenging task, the publisher supported the team at every step. A small team of assistant editors was also appointed to further simplify the editing procedure and attain best results for the readers.

Apart from the editorial board, the designing team has also invested a significant amount of their time in understanding the subject and creating the most relevant covers. They scrutinized every image to scout for the most suitable representation of the subject and create an appropriate cover for the book.

The publishing team has been an ardent support to the editorial, designing and production team. Their endless efforts to recruit the best for this project, has resulted in the accomplishment of this book. They are a veteran in the field of academics and their pool of knowledge is as vast as their experience in printing. Their expertise and guidance has proved useful at every step. Their uncompromising quality standards have made this book an exceptional effort. Their encouragement from time to time has been an inspiration for everyone.

The publisher and the editorial board hope that this book will prove to be a valuable piece of knowledge for researchers, students, practitioners and scholars across the globe.

List of Contributors

Paola Soto, Pablo S. Gaete, Christian Fuentes, Benjamin Lozano, Pamela A. Naulin, Xavier F. Figueroa and Nelson Patricio Barrera
Department of Physiology, Faculty of Biological Sciences, Pontificia Universidad Católica de Chile, Santiago, Chile

Lucas E. Cabrera Zapata and Mariana Bollo
Instituto de Investigación Médica Mercedes y Martín Ferreyra, INIMEC-CONICET, Universidad Nacional de Córdoba, Córdoba, Argentina

María Julia Cambiasso
Instituto de Investigación Médica Mercedes y Martín Ferreyra, INIMEC-CONICET, Universidad Nacional de Córdoba, Córdoba, Argentina
Cátedra de Biología Celular, Facultad de Odontología, Universidad Nacional de Córdoba, Córdoba, Argentina

Raquel Pascua-Maestro, Maria D. Ganfornina and Diego Sanchez
Instituto de Biología y Genética Molecular-Departamento de Bioquímica y Biología Molecular y Fisiología, Universidad de Valladolid-CSIC, Valladolid, Spain

Esperanza González
Exosomes Group, Metabolomics Unit and Platform, CIC bioGUNE, CIBERehd, Technology Park of Bizkaia, Derio, Spain

Concepción Lillo
Instituto de Neurociencias de Castilla y León, IBSAL, Universidad de Salamanca, Salamanca, Spain

Juan Manuel Falcón-Pérez
Exosomes Group, Metabolomics Unit and Platform, CIC bioGUNE, CIBERehd, Technology Park of Bizkaia, Derio, Spain
IKERBASQUE, Basque Foundation for Science, Bilbao, Spain

M. Victoria Simón, Facundo H. Prado Spalm, Marcela S. Vera and Nora P. Rotstein
Instituto de Investigaciones Bioquímicas de Bahía Blanca (INIBIBB), Departamento De Biología, Bioquímica y Farmacia, Universidad Nacional del Sur (UNS), Argentine National Research Council (CONICET), Bahía Blanca, Argentina

Lisandro Jorge Falomir-Lockhart and Gian Franco Cavazzutti
Instituto de Investigaciones Bioquímicas de La Plata (INIBIOLP), Centro Científico Tecnológico - La Plata, Consejo Nacional de Investigaciones Científicas y Técnicas (CONICET), La Plata, Argentina
Facultad de Ciencias Exactas, Universidad Nacional de La Plata (UNLP), La Plata, Argentina

Ezequiel Giménez and Andrés Martín Toscani
Instituto de Investigaciones Bioquímicas de La Plata (INIBIOLP), Centro Científico Tecnológico - La Plata, Consejo Nacional de Investigaciones Científicas y Técnicas (CONICET), La Plata, Argentina
Facultad de Ciencias Médicas, Universidad Nacional de La Plata (UNLP), La Plata, Argentina

Lin-Hui Zou
Department of Neurology, Xijing Hospital, Fourth Military Medical University, Xi'an, China
Frontier Medical Training Brigade, Army Medical University, Changji, China

Ya-Jun Shi, Xiao-Mu Wang, Fan Wu and Lei Ma
Department of Neurology, Xijing Hospital, Fourth Military Medical University, Xi'an, China

Hua He
Department of Specific Diagnosis, PLA 986 Hospital, Xi'an, China

Shi-Mei Jiang
Department of Acu-Moxibustion and Tuina, Henan University of Traditional Chinese Medicine, Zhengzhou, China

Fang-Fang Huo
Department of Medicine, Yulin Yuyang District Hospital of Traditional Chinese Medicine, Yulin, China

Lucia Rodríguez-Berdini and Beatriz L. Caputto
Centro de Investigaciones en Química Biológica de Córdoba (Consejo Nacional de Investigaciones Científicas y Técnicas), Departamento de Química Biológica "Ranwel Caputto", Facultad de Ciencias Químicas, Universidad Nacional de Córdoba, Córdoba, Argentina

Emeline Tanguy, Qili Wang and Nicolas Vitale
Institut des Neurosciences Cellulaires et Intégratives (INCI), UPR-3212 Centre National de la Recherche Scientifique & Université de Strasbourg, Strasbourg, France

Hervé Moine
Institut de Génétique et de Biologie Moléculaire et Cellulaire (IGBMC), CNRS UMR 7104, INSERM U964, Université de Strasbourg, Illkirch-Graffenstaden, France

Shuhu Liu, Zhihua Zhou, Ling Zhang, Siying Meng, Shuji Li and Xuemin Wang
Key Laboratory of Mental Health of the Ministry of Education, Guangdong Province Key Laboratory of Psychiatric Disorders, Department of Neurobiology, School of Basic Medical Sciences, Southern Medical University, Guangzhou, China

Viktoriya Morozova, Abdeslem El Idrissi, Alison Shur and Alejandra D. Alonso
Department of Biology and Center for Developmental Neuroscience, College of Staten Island, The City Universityof New York, Staten Island, NY, United States
Biology Program, The Graduate Center, The City University of New York, New York, United States

Leah S. Cohen and Ali El-Hadi Makki
Department of Biology and Center for Developmental Neuroscience, College of Staten Island, The City Universityof New York, Staten Island, NY, United States

Camila Fabiani and Silvia S. Antollini
Instituto de Investigaciones Bioquímicas de Bahía Blanca CONICET-UNS, Bahía Blanca, Argentina
Departamento de Biología, Bioquímica y Farmacia, Universidad Nacional del Sur, Bahía Blanca, Argentina
Instituto de Investigaciones Bioquímicas de Bahía Blanca (INIBIBB), Departamento de Biología, Bioquímica y Farmacia, Universidad Nacional del Sur-Consejo Nacional de Investigaciones Científicas y Técnicas (CONICET), Bahía Blanca, Argentina

Matías Lasala, Jeremías Corradi, Silvia Antollini and Cecilia Bouzat
Instituto de Investigaciones Bioquímicas de Bahía Blanca (INIBIBB), Departamento de Biología, Bioquímica y Farmacia, Universidad Nacional del Sur-Consejo Nacional de Investigaciones Científicas y Técnicas (CONICET), Bahía Blanca, Argentina

Melisa Malcolm, Lucía Saad, Laura Gabriela Penazzi and Eduardo Garbarino-Pico
Departamento de Química Biológica Ranwel Caputto, Facultad de Ciencias Químicas, Universidad Nacional de Córdoba (UNC), Córdoba, Argentina
CONICET-UNC, Centro de Investigaciones en Química Biológica de Córdoba (CIQUIBIC), Córdoba, Argentina

Maria Laura Bertoldi, Maria Ines Zalosnik, German A. Roth and Alicia L. Degano
Departamento de Química Biológica Ranwel Caputto, Facultad de Ciencias Químicas, Córdoba, Argentina
Centro de Investigaciones en Química Biológica de Córdoba (CIQUIBIC), CONICET, Universidad Nacional de Córdoba, Córdoba, Argentina

Maria Carolina Fabio
Instituto de Investigaciones Médicas Mercedes y Martin Ferreyra (INIMEC), CONICET, Córdoba, Argentina

Susan Aja
Center for Metabolism and Obesity Research, Johns Hopkins Medicine, Baltimore, MD, United States

Guillermo Pilar
Department of Neurosciences, Case Western Reserve University, Cleveland, OH, United States

Gabriele V. Ronnett
Center for Metabolism and Obesity Research, Johns Hopkins Medicine, Baltimore, MD, United States
Department of Neuroscience, The Johns Hopkins University, School of Medicine, Baltimore, MD, United States

Maximiliano N. Rios, Natalia A. Marchese and Mario E. Guido
Centro de Investigaciones en Química Biológica de Córdoba (CIQUIBIC), CONICET, Facultad de Ciencias Químicas, Universidad Nacional de Córdoba, Córdoba, Argentina
Departamento de Química Biológica "Ranwel Caputto," Facultad de Ciencias Químicas, Universidad Nacional de Córdoba, Córdoba, Argentina

Romina María Uranga
Instituto de Investigaciones Bioquímicas de Bahía Blanca, Universidad Nacional del Sur-Consejo Nacional de Investigaciones Científicas y Técnicas, Bahía Blanca, Argentina
Departamento de Biología, Bioquímica y Farmacia, Universidad Nacional del Sur, Bahía Blanca, Argentina

Jeffrey Neil Keller
Pennington Biomedical Research Center, Louisiana State University System, Baton Rouge, LA, United States

Index

www.ingramcontent.com/pod-product-compliance
Lightning Source LLC
LaVergne TN
LVHW082150200926
848484LV00008B/2136